SALIVARY GLAND PATHOLOGY
DIAGNOSIS AND MANAGEMENT

SALIVARY GLAND PATHOLOGY
DIAGNOSIS AND MANAGEMENT

Third Edition

Edited by

Eric R. Carlson
University of Tennessee Graduate School of Medicine,
University of Tennessee Cancer Institute,
Knoxville, TN, United States

Robert A. Ord
University of Maryland Medical Center,
Greenbaum Cancer Institute, Baltimore, MD,
United States

WILEY Blackwell

This edition first published 2022
© 2022 John Wiley & Sons, Inc.

Edition History
Wiley-Blackwell (1e, 2008); John Wiley & Sons, Inc. (2e, 2016)

All rights reserved. No part of this publication may be reproduced, stored in a retrieval system, or transmitted, in any form or by any means, electronic, mechanical, photocopying, recording or otherwise, except as permitted by law. Advice on how to obtain permission to reuse material from this title is available at http://www.wiley.com/go/permissions.

The right of Eric R. Carlson and Robert A. Ord to be identified as the authors of the editorial material in this work has been asserted in accordance with law.

Registered Office
John Wiley & Sons, Inc., 111 River Street, Hoboken, NJ 07030, USA

Editorial Office
111 River Street, Hoboken, NJ 07030, USA

For details of our global editorial offices, customer services, and more information about Wiley products visit us at www.wiley.com.

Wiley also publishes its books in a variety of electronic formats and by print-on-demand. Some content that appears in standard print versions of this book may not be available in other formats.

Limit of Liability/Disclaimer of Warranty
The contents of this work are intended to further general scientific research, understanding, and discussion only and are not intended and should not be relied upon as recommending or promoting scientific method, diagnosis, or treatment by physicians for any particular patient. In view of ongoing research, equipment modifications, changes in governmental regulations, and the constant flow of information relating to the use of medicines, equipment, and devices, the reader is urged to review and evaluate the information provided in the package insert or instructions for each medicine, equipment, or device for, among other things, any changes in the instructions or indication of usage and for added warnings and precautions. While the publisher and authors have used their best efforts in preparing this work, they make no representations or warranties with respect to the accuracy or completeness of the contents of this work and specifically disclaim all warranties, including without limitation any implied warranties of merchantability or fitness for a particular purpose. No warranty may be created or extended by sales representatives, written sales materials or promotional statements for this work. The fact that an organization, website, or product is referred to in this work as a citation and/or potential source of further information does not mean that the publisher and authors endorse the information or services the organization, website, or product may provide or recommendations it may make. This work is sold with the understanding that the publisher is not engaged in rendering professional services. The advice and strategies contained herein may not be suitable for your situation. You should consult with a specialist where appropriate. Further, readers should be aware that websites listed in this work may have changed or disappeared between when this work was written and when it is read. Neither the publisher nor authors shall be liable for any loss of profit or any other commercial damages, including but not limited to special, incidental, consequential, or other damages.

Library of Congress Cataloging-in-Publication Data applied for
[ISBN: 9781119730187]

Cover image:
Cover design by

Set in 10.5/12pt Slimbach by Straive, Pondicherry, India

Printed in Singapore

M110917_130721

Contents

Contributors		vii
Foreword to the First Edition		ix
Foreword to the Second Edition		xi
Foreword to the Third Edition		xiii
Preface to the First Edition		xv
Preface to the Second Edition		xvii
Preface to the Third Edition		xix
Acknowledgments		xxi
About the Companion Website		xxiii
Chapter 1	Surgical Anatomy, Embryology, and Physiology of the Salivary Glands *John D. Langdon*	1
Chapter 2	Diagnostic Imaging of Salivary Gland Pathology *J. Michael McCoy and Pradeep K. Jacob*	19
Chapter 3	Infections of the Salivary Glands	79
Chapter 4	Cysts and Cyst-Like Lesions of the Salivary Glands	117
Chapter 5	Sialolithiasis	145
Chapter 6	Systemic Diseases Affecting the Salivary Glands	175
Chapter 7	Salivary Gland Pathology in Children and Adolescents	201
Chapter 8	Classification, Grading, and Staging of Salivary Gland Tumors *J. Michael McCoy and John Sauk*	225
Chapter 9	The Molecular Biology of Benign and Malignant Salivary Gland Tumors *Randy Todd*	269
Chapter 10	Tumors of the Parotid Gland	301
Chapter 11	Tumors of the Submandibular and Sublingual Glands	345
Chapter 12	Tumors of the Minor Salivary Glands	373
Chapter 13	Radiation Therapy for Salivary Gland Malignancies *Joseph R. Kelley and Max Ofori*	435
Chapter 14	Systemic Therapy for Salivary Gland Cancer *Janakiraman Subramanian and Lara Kujtan*	455
Chapter 15	Non-salivary Tumors of the Salivary Glands	471

Chapter 16	Trauma and Injuries to the Salivary Glands	509
Chapter 17	Miscellaneous Pathologic Processes of the Salivary Glands	543
Chapter 18	Complications of Salivary Gland Surgery *Michael D. Turner*	569
Chapter 19	Innovations in Salivary Gland Surgery *Mark McGurk and Katherine George*	601
Index		625

Contributors

Eric R. Carlson, DMD, MD, EdM, FACS
Department of Oral and Maxillofacial Surgery, University of Tennessee Graduate School of Medicine, University of Tennessee Cancer Institute, Knoxville, TN, USA

Robert A. Ord, BDS, MB BCh (Hons), FRCS, FACS, MS, MBA
Department of Oral and Maxillofacial Surgery, University of Maryland Medical Center, Greenbaum Cancer Institute, Baltimore, MD, USA

Katherine George, BDS, BSc, MBBS, MFDS RCS (Eng), FRCS (OMFS)
Oral and Maxillofacial Surgeon, Kings College Hospital NHS Foundation Trust, Denmark Hill, London, UK

Pradeep Jacob, MD, MBA
Private Practice of Radiology, Chattanooga, TN, USA

Joseph Kelley, MD, PhD
Director of Clinical Research, GenesisCare USA of North Carolina

Lara Kujtan, MD, MSc
Department of Medicine, University of Missouri at Kansas City, Kansas City, MO, USA

John D. Langdon, FKC, MB BS, BDS, MDS, FDSRCS, FRCS, FMedSci
Department of Maxillofacial Surgery, King's College, London, England

J. Michael McCoy, DDS
Departments of Oral and Maxillofacial Surgery, Pathology, and Radiology, University of Tennessee Graduate School of Medicine, Knoxville, TN, USA

Mark McGurk, BDS, MD, FRCS, DLO, FDS, RCS
Head and Neck Academic Center, Department of Head and Neck Surgery, University College London Hospital, London, UK

Max Ofori, MD
Division of Radiation Oncology, University of Tennessee Medical Center, Knoxville, TN, USA

John J. Sauk, DDS, MS, FAAAS, FAHNS
School of Dentistry, University of Louisville, Louisville, KY, USA

Janikiraman Subramanian, MD
Department of Medicine, Thoracic Oncology and Center for Precision Oncology, Saint Luke's Cancer Institute, University of Missouri at Kansas City, Kansas City, MI, USA

Randy Todd, DMD, MD, DSc
Private Practice of Oral and Maxillofacial Surgery (retired), Peabody, MA, USA

Michael D. Turner, DDS, MD, FACS
Division of Oral and Maxillofacial Surgery, Mount Sinai Hospital, Icahn Mount Sinai School of Medicine, New York, NY, USA

Foreword First Edition

The mention of "head and neck cancer" immediately connotes the sobering realities and potentials of oral squamous cell carcinoma. Left to secondary recollection and awareness is the significance of salivary gland malignancy. The same can be said for the general perception of benign salivary neoplasia. In this brilliant new textbook, authors Carlson and Ord correct these notions, focusing proper emphasis on the group of diseases which, in their malignant form, represent some three percent of all North American head and neck tumors, affecting a minimum of 2500 victims per year.

One marvels at the dedication, energies, and resources – to say nothing of the expertise – mustered to produce a volume of this depth and expanse. While almost forty percent of the effort is directed toward the vitally significant elements of classification, diagnosis, and clinical care of neoplasia, there is more – much more – here, for both the training and practicing readerships. The whole array of salivary gland dysfunctions is marvelously displayed in meaningful clinical color, in easily grasped sketches and graphs, and in well-chosen descriptive imaging. From the mandatory fundaments for such an undertaking – John Langdon's discourse on macro- and microanatomy, Pradeep Jacob's presentation on imaging diagnostics (45 pages!), John Sauk's explanations of current classification and staging of tumors – to the surgical demonstrations of pathology, anatomy, and technique, the visual material is extraordinary.

What are the vagaries in defining the SMAS layer, can cell type be distinguished on the basis of imaging alone, what influence do genomics and biomarkers have in clinical classification, does contemporary understanding explain the etiology of mucous escape phenomena? Up-to-date propositions on such topics occupy these chapters. Clinical challenges, traditional and new, e.g., transection of ducts and nerves, intraductal micromanipulations, salivary diagnostics – they're all here, presented in clear, expansive, prose (28 pages of information on sialolithiasis alone!). The detriments of age and metabolic disorder on gland function, the genesis of non-salivary tumors inside the glands, and the lodging of metastatic disease within their confines receive emphasis in these pages. So do the presence of aberrant glands and the esoteric transplantation of salivary tissue in the management of xerophthalmia.

The *Textbook and Color Atlas of Salivary Gland Pathology* is authoritative. Its authors do not write anecdotally, but from the combined experience of decades which has elevated them both to international recognition in the field of head and neck neoplasia. Their clinical material here presented represents volumes in the operating room, and the comprehensive bibliographies in each of the text's chapters testify to the authors' awareness of their topic and their world-views. Eric Carlson displays the fruits of his earlier endeavors in Pittsburgh, Detroit, and Miami, and speaks now from his position as Professor and Chairman in the Department of Oral and Maxillofacial Surgery at the University of Tennessee Graduate School of Medicine in Knoxville. Robert Ord established his worthy reputation in Britain before resettling himself in Baltimore on the western shores of the Atlantic some 20 years ago, where he now serves as Professor and Chairman of the Department of Oral and Maxillofacial Surgery at the University of Maryland. Theirs is the first time in this domain engineered authoritatively by oral and maxillofacial surgeons, and does honor to their colleagues and forebears in the specialty who have toiled in the vineyards of salivary gland pathology. Neither in design nor execution, however, is their marvelous achievement directed to a parochial audience. Rather, surgeons or clinicians of whatever ilk will offer the authors a nod of appreciation in benefitting from this text.

Probably, one day, an expansion of this work will be written; and, undoubtedly, Carlson and Ord will write it.

R. Bruce MacIntosh, DDS
Detroit
June 2008

Foreword Second Edition

Casual students of surgery of pathology might be inclined to ask what can possibly have transpired over the past seven years to warrant a new edition of a text concerning salivary gland dysfunction only first published in 2008. The prevalence of salivary gland neoplasia in comparison to other oral tumors is very small, and to whole body cancer even smaller; significant trauma to the glands ranks low in incidence compared to the rest of maxillofacial injuries; no one dies from inflammatory or immune disease of the glands; don't these facts mitigate against the need for a new textbook on the salivary glands every few years?

Quite the contrary! Because the 2008 Carlson-Ord volume was one of the very few works – and certainly the most comprehensive – dedicated solely to their topic, it is almost mandatory that it be reviewed and up-dated on a regular basis to provide clinicians and educators an authoritative repository of new information in this specialized field of interest.

And, indeed, there is new information! The complexity, variety, and heterogeneity in the origins of salivary gland tumors (as discussed in the new Chapter 8) makes these lesions an ideal study group for the development of all malignant neoplasia; they give credence to the notion that all disease, particularly malignant, is ultimately individualized and not to be boxed into currently recognized classifications. Senior readers will well remember the teaching axiom that salivary gland malignancies are impervious to radiation therapy; this new edition's Chapter 12 effectively disassembles that contention. Concurrently with the burgeoning understanding of cellular pathology at the subcellular and molecular levels, the concept of systemic chemotherapy, even targeted therapy, for salivary gland cancers has demanded re-evaluation over the past decade; this is illuminated in the new Chapter 13. Further, the authors have combined their first-hand knowledge with a compilation of all pertinent literature to offer a unique assembly of pediatric salivary gland pathology in Chapter 15, another addition.

While new knowledge – most excitingly provided in Chapters 8, 12, and 13 – and updated bibliographies, sketches, highlighted algorithms, and investigational studies are features of the new text, the focus of these elements and the overall emphasis of the work remains the surgical treatment of patients. Illustrative surgeries from the first edition have been retained, and new cases added to demonstrate principles and additional techniques. Management of the more common salivary tumors, injuries, and infections is well exhibited, but room is provided for illustration of rarer entities (Primary desmoid melanoma of the parotid?! Central (osseous) mucoepidermoid carcinoma of the mandibular ramus?!). Mundane or rare, the range of these maladies, plus the scope and depth of their demonstrated knowledge, attest to the broad experiences of Carlson and Ord in the field of salivary gland abnormality, and deservedly position them in the upper echelons of American salivary gland surgeons.

One could anticipate in 2008 that Carlson-Ord would recognize the abiding need for pertinence and currency in their text; indeed, they have and have delivered again.

Robert Bruce MacIntosh, DDS
Department of Oral and Maxillofacial Surgery,
University of Detroit Mercy School of Dentistry,
Detroit, MI, USA

Foreword Third Edition

What defines dedication if not the willing contribution of countless hours, huge blocks of energy, and outpouring of intellect and meaningful experience to construct a landmark scientific text? Indeed, these were the elements that Eric Carlson and Robert Ord mobilized in 2008 in introducing to the surgical world their first – now landmark – textbook on salivary gland pathology and treatment. Their dedication to the topic was intense – they had elevated it to the level of subspecialty – and the volume's success prompted an updated second edition in 2016. Now, with Carlson-Ord-III, they have answered the continuing demand and – because of progress within the discipline – the need, for integration of previous writing with new information in the field.

To be a good scientific writer, an author must first be a good teacher, ready to anticipate uncertainties, confusion, or missed emphasis in the minds of his less-initiated readers, but also ready to anticipate the worthy critique of an experienced colleague. Both Carlson and Ord have easily answered this requirement, not only in their decades-long responsibilities in the resident education milieu but in countless lecture engagements, conferences, and surgical activities worldwide. Their word on the topic of salivary gland maladies is authority, and it is effectively transmitted both in the operating room and from the podium.

Some say today that a textbook is passé, that what is important in the literature can be much more efficiently harvested through one's fingertips on a computer. The good textbook is bifocal, however: It must be a lightning rod for all that is new and exciting at the time of printing, but also an entombed repository of everything pertinent that has been recorded up to that date. To honor the functions, the authors have labored diligently to review and update the bibliographies of the texted materials, including pertinent meta-analyses of earlier literature, and inserting more descriptive visuals of earlier material where appropriate. New features of this Third Edition include greater than 100 new full-color images, illustrated case presentations to demonstrate important clinical situations, and new chapters on minimally invasive surgery and the complications of surgery in the field. The roster of contributing faculty now numbers 14. With this detailed review and revision, the new edition provides an edited compilation of salivary gland pathology not readily recoverable through journal review, regardless how efficient.

From the perspective of 50 + years of navigation in the ablative and reconstructive precincts of oral and maxillofacial surgery, one can safely relate today's circumstances to those of "back when". In the earlier decades of the last half-century, imaging diagnosis of salivary gland disease depended chiefly on plain radiography and contrast sialography; microscopic diagnosis was dependent on the accommodation of a tumor to one of perhaps a dozen epithelial variants; chemotherapy protocols were essentially adaptions of those used for management of squamous cell carcinoma; salivary carcinoma was thought impervious to radiation therapy; surgical management of salivary malignancy fell almost exclusively to those few otolaryngologists, general surgeons, or, more infrequently, oral and maxillofacial surgeons, with special interests in treating these relatively uncommon lesions.

Immense progress in understanding the pathophysiology of salivary gland disease in later years has delivered incredibly complicated microscopic classifications and more precisely directed chemical treatment protocols, and over the past two decades, the earlier assumption that salivary gland disease was impervious to radiation therapy has been demolished. This improved understanding of salivary gland biology has brought in train the need for increasingly well-founded and sophisticated care within all interested surgical groups; Dr. Carlson in Knoxville, and Dr. Ord in Baltimore have answered this call with their surgical expertise and recognized educational efforts in oral and maxillofacial surgical training.

With this Third Edition, the authors have ensured their volume's position in the lexicon of surgical texts, a metric against which all future efforts will be scaled.

Robert Bruce MacIntosh, DDS
Department of Oral and Maxillofacial Surgery,
University of Detroit Mercy School of Dentistry,
Detroit, MI, USA

Preface First Edition

The concept of this book devoted to the diagnosis and management of salivary gland pathology arose from our longstanding friendship and professional relationship where we first collaborated in the early 1990s. This led to a trip to India with the Health Volunteers Overseas in 1996, where we operated numerous complex cancer cases, including many salivary gland malignancies. Dr. Carlson's interest in benign and malignant tumor surgery was fostered by the expert surgical tutelage of Dr. Robert E. Marx at the University of Miami Miller School of Medicine/Jackson Memorial Hospital in Miami, Florida. It was the training by Professor John Langdon who nurtured Dr. Ord's love of the parotidectomy. Over the years, following the publication of several papers and book chapters devoted to salivary gland surgery, we realized that a textbook and atlas related to this discipline should be produced. It was believed that a work written by two surgeons who shared similar surgical philosophies would be a unique addition to the current literature. This has been a project that we have approached with energy and enthusiasm which hopefully is evident to the reader.

The diagnosis and management of salivary gland pathology are an exciting and thought provoking discipline in medicine, dentistry, and surgery. It is incumbent on the clinician examining a patient with a suspected developmental, neoplastic, or non-neoplastic lesion of the major or minor salivary glands to obtain a comprehensive history and physical examination, after which time a differential diagnosis is established. A definitive diagnosis is provided with either an excisional or incisional biopsy depending on the gland involved and the differential diagnosis established preoperatively. A complete understanding of the anatomic barriers surrounding a salivary gland lesion is paramount when performing surgery for a salivary gland neoplasm.

It is the purpose of this Textbook and Color Atlas of Salivary Gland Pathology to provide both text and clinical images, thereby making this a singular work. The reader interested in the science and evidence based medicine associated with the management of salivary gland pathology will be attracted to our text. The reader interested in how to perform salivary gland surgery as a function of diagnosis and anatomic site will find the real-time images useful. To that end, artist sketches are limited in this book. Where appropriate, algorithms have been included as a guide for diagnosis and management. It is our hope that this text and atlas will find a home on the bookshelves of those surgeons who share our fascination with the diagnosis and management of salivary gland disease.

Eric R. Carlson, DMD, MD, FACS
Robert A. Ord, DDS, MD, FRCS, FACS, MS

Preface Second Edition

In 2008, we published our first work entitled Textbook and Color Atlas of Salivary Gland Pathology – Diagnosis and Management. In preparation for the development and publication of the second edition of this book, several issues became apparent that resulted in changes and additions to our first edition. The first change is the title. We selected Salivary Gland Pathology – Diagnosis and Management due to the inherent and obvious textbook nature of this work. In addition, our readership is aware that our teaching mission involves the use of high quality color images to illustrate the cases included in each chapter and to guide the reader through the workup and execution of the medical and surgical management of salivary gland pathology. The title was shortened accordingly. All chapters have been updated in terms of references and the addition of new cases to illustrate important points within each chapter. This includes Chapter 7, *Classification, Grading, and Staging of Salivary Gland Tumors*, where histomicrographs of most of the benign and malignant salivary gland neoplasms are now illustrated in the chapter. In keeping with our expanding knowledge base of the diagnosis and management of salivary gland pathology, we have included four new chapters in this second edition, including those devoted to the molecular biology of benign and malignant salivary gland tumors, radiation therapy for salivary gland tumors, systemic therapy for salivary gland cancer, and pediatric salivary gland pathology. Four new authors have been added including Drs. Joseph Kelley, J. Michael McCoy, Janakiraman Subramanian, and Randy Todd. Where appropriate, algorithms have been included in the chapters to assist in decision making processes associated with the management of salivary gland pathology.

As with the first edition of this textbook, it is our expressed purpose to make this second edition a singular work with extensive text and clinical images. It is our hope that this textbook will provide a useful update to our international colleagues who benefited from the first edition.

Eric R. Carlson, DMD, MD, FACS
Robert A. Ord, DDS, MD, FRCS, FACS, MS, MBA

Preface Third Edition

We enthusiastically present the third edition of Salivary Gland Pathology – Diagnosis and Management to practitioners and trainees, surgeons and pathologists, and clinicians and scientists alike. The World Health Organization's updated classification of head and neck tumors in 2017, including that of salivary gland tumors, is a reminder to the reader of the ephemeral nature of salivary gland pathology as well as the inherent need to frequently update our knowledge base. Therein, this third edition of our tome exploits the new information available regarding the taxonomy of salivary gland tumors as well as new neoplastic and non-neoplastic entities, image guided biopsies of salivary gland lesions, minimally invasive surgery to address these entities, and the complications encountered in traditional and nontraditional forms of salivary gland surgery. To this end, we introduce two new chapters and five new authors. Professor Mark McGurk of the United Kingdom requires no introduction as his contributions to oral and maxillofacial surgery, and especially salivary gland surgery, are extensive, innovative, highly meaningful, and transformational. Dr. Katherine George teamed up with Professor McGurk to review their experiences with innovative salivary gland surgery, including diagnostic and therapeutic sialendoscopy. Dr. Michael Turner of New York City is also an accomplished salivary gland surgeon and lends his expertise in the management of complications to our textbook. Dr. Laura Kujtan joins Dr. Subramanian in their update of chemotherapy and targeted therapy for salivary gland malignancies. Finally, Dr. Ofori collaborated with Dr. Joseph Kelley in their scholarly review of radiation therapy in the management of salivary gland tumors.

The practice of twenty-first century medicine and surgery exists within a data-driven world. To that end, all chapters are updated in terms of new references and many meta-analyses/systematic reviews are reviewed in the spirit of supporting evidence-based practice. New cases have been added to most chapters to illustrate important points. Algorithms continue to be offered to assist clinicians in decision-making processes associated with the management of salivary gland pathology. Most chapters also contain a new teaching element – case presentations that serve to illustrate and reinforce essential take-home messages either suggested or emphasized in their respective chapters. Finally, videos of salivary gland surgical procedures are included in the chapter devoted to innovative salivary gland surgery in this third edition.

As with the first and second editions of this textbook, it is our expressed purpose to brand this third edition a singular reference with extensive text and clinical images. It is our hope that this textbook will provide a useful update to our international colleagues and their patients who benefited from the prior editions.

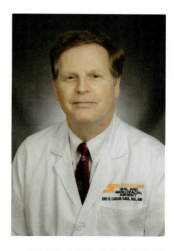

Eric R. Carlson, DMD, MD, EdM, FACS

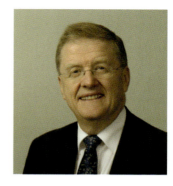

Robert A. Ord, BDS, MB BCh (Hons), FRCS, FACS, MS, MBA

Acknowledgments

I would like to thank my teachers, residents, fellows, and patients for their trust, encouragement, wisdom, and inspiration. I am grateful to all of you.

Eric R. Carlson

To my wife, Sue, my inspiration as always.

Robert A. Ord

About the Companion Website

Don't forget to visit the companion web site for this book:

www.wiley.com/go/carlson/salivary

There you will find valuable materials, including:

- Videos

Scan this QR code to visit the companion website:

Chapter 1
Surgical Anatomy, Embryology, and Physiology of the Salivary Glands

John D. Langdon, FKC, MB BS, BDS, MDS, FDSRCS, FRCS, FMedSci
Emeritus Professor of Maxillofacial Surgery King's College London, England

Outline

Introduction
Parotid Gland
  Embryology
  Anatomy
  Contents of the Parotid Gland
    Facial Nerve
    Auriculotemporal Nerve
    Retromandibular Vein
    External Carotid Artery
    Parotid Lymph Nodes
    Parotid Duct
    Nerve Supply to the Parotid
Submandibular Gland
  Embryology
  Anatomy
    Superficial Lobe
    Deep Lobe
    Submandibular Duct
    Blood Supply and Lymphatic Drainage
    Nerve Supply to the Submandibular Gland
      Parasympathetic innervation
      Sympathetic innervation
      Sensory innervation
Sublingual Gland
  Embryology
  Anatomy
    Sublingual Ducts
    Blood Supply, Innervations, and Lymphatic Drainage
Minor Salivary Glands
Tubarial Salivary Glands
Histology of the Salivary Glands
Control of Salivation
Summary
Case Presentation – *Wait, What?*
References

Introduction

There are three pairs of major salivary glands consisting of the parotid, submandibular, and sublingual glands. In addition, there are numerous minor glands distributed throughout the oral cavity within the mucosa and submucosa.

On average, about 1.5 l of saliva are produced each day but the rate varies throughout the day. At rest, about 0.3 ml/min is produced but this rises to 2.0 ml/min with stimulation. The contribution from each gland also varies. At rest, the parotid produces 20%, the submandibular gland 65%, and the sublingual and minor glands 15%. On stimulation, the parotid secretion rises to 50%. The nature of the secretion also varies from gland to gland. Parotid secretions are almost exclusively serous, the submandibular secretions are mixed, and the sublingual and minor gland secretions are predominantly mucinous.

Saliva is essential for mucosal lubrication, speech, and swallowing. It also performs an essential buffering role that influences demineralization of teeth as part of the carious process. When there is a marked deficiency in saliva production, xerostomia, rampant caries, and destructive periodontal disease ensues. Various digestive enzymes – salivary amylase – and antimicrobial agents – IgA, lysozyme, and lactoferrin – are also secreted with the saliva.

Salivary Gland Pathology: Diagnosis and Management, Third Edition. Edited by Eric R. Carlson and Robert A. Ord.
© 2022 John Wiley & Sons, Inc. Published 2022 by John Wiley & Sons, Inc.
Companion website: www.wiley.com/go/carlson/salivary

Parotid Gland

EMBRYOLOGY

The parotid glands develop as a thickening of the epithelium in the cheek of the oral cavity in the 15 mm Crown Rump length embryo (sixth week of intrauterine life) (Zhang et al. 2010; Berta et al. 2013; Chadi et al. 2017). This thickening extends backward toward the ear in a plane superficial to the developing facial nerve. The deep aspect of the developing parotid gland produces bud-like projections between the branches of the facial nerve in the third month of intrauterine life. These projections then merge to form the deep lobe of the parotid gland. By the sixth month of intrauterine life, the gland is completely canalized. Although not embryologically a bilobed structure, the parotid comes to form a larger (80%) superficial lobe and a smaller (20%) deep lobe joined by an isthmus between the two major divisions of the facial nerve. The branches of the nerve lie between these lobes invested in loose connective tissue. This observation is vital in the understanding of the anatomy of the facial nerve and surgery in this region (Berkovitz et al. 2003).

ANATOMY

The parotid is the largest of the major salivary glands. It is a compound, tubuloacinar, merocrine, exocrine gland. In the adult, the gland is composed entirely of serous acini.

The gland is situated in the space between the posterior border of the mandibular ramus and the mastoid process of the temporal bone. The external acoustic meatus and the glenoid fossa lie above together with the zygomatic process of the temporal bone (Figure 1.1). On its deep (medial) aspect lies the styloid process of the temporal bone. Inferiorly, the parotid frequently overlaps the angle of the mandible and its deep surface overlies the transverse process of the atlas vertebra.

The shape of the parotid gland is variable. Often it is triangular with the apex directed inferiorly. However, on occasion, it is essentially of even width and occasionally it is triangular with the apex superiorly. On average, the gland is 6 cm in length with a maximum of 3.3 cm in width. In 20% of subjects, a smaller accessory lobe arises from the upper border of the parotid duct approximately 6 mm in front of the main gland. This accessory lobe overlies the zygomatic arch.

The gland is surrounded by a fibrous capsule previously thought to be formed from the investing layer of deep cervical fascia. This fascia passes up from the neck and was thought to split to enclose the gland. The deep layer is attached to the mandible and the temporal bone at the tympanic plate and styloid and mastoid processes (McMinn et al. 1984; Berkovitz and Moxham 1988; Williams 1995; Ellis 1997). Recent investigations suggest that the superficial layer of the parotid capsule is not formed in this way, but is part of the superficial musculo-aponeurotic system (SMAS) (Mitz and Peyronie 1976; Jost and Levet 1983; Wassef 1987; Thaller et al. 1989; Zigiotti et al. 1991; Gosain et al. 1993; Flatau and Mills 1995). Anteriorly, the superficial layer of the parotid capsule is thick and fibrous but more posteriorly it becomes a thin translucent membrane. Within this fascia are scant muscle fibers running parallel with those of the platysma. This superficial

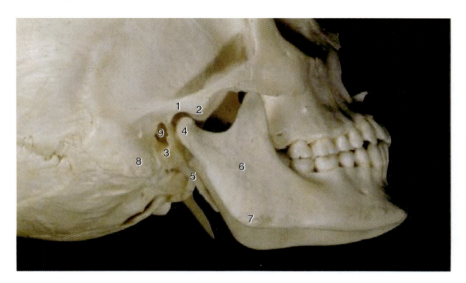

Figure 1.1. A lateral view of the skull showing some of the bony features related to the bed of the parotid gland. Source: Published with permission, Martin Dunitz, London, Langdon JD, Berkovitz BKB, Moxham BJ, editors, Surgical Anatomy of the Infratemporal Fossa. DOI: 10.1002/9781118949139.ch1.

layer of the parotid capsule appears to be continuous with the fascia overlying the platysma muscle. Anteriorly it forms a separate layer overlying the masseteric fascia which is itself an extension of the deep cervical fascia. The peripheral branches of the facial nerve and the parotid duct lie within a loose cellular layer between these two sheets of fascia. This observation is important in parotid surgery. When operating on the parotid gland, the skin flap can either be raised in the subcutaneous fat layer or deep to the SMAS layer. The SMAS layer itself can be mobilized as a separate flap and can be used to mask the cosmetic defect following parotidectomy by reattaching it firmly to the anterior border of the sternocleidomastoid muscle as an advancement flap (Meningaud et al. 2006).

The parotid capsule develops relatively late after the lymphoid tissue develops within the mesenchyme of the gland (Goldenberg et al. 2000). For this reason, the lymph nodes associated with the parotid gland are intraglandular as opposed to the extraglandular lymph nodes associated with the submandibular and sublingual salivary glands, in which the capsule forms earlier in their development.

Where the deep aspect of the superficial lobe overlies branches of the facial nerve, the capsule becomes very thin or even nonexistent, resulting in acinar tissue lying in direct contact with the nerve fibers.

The superior border of the parotid gland (usually the base of the triangle) is closely molded around the external acoustic meatus and the temporomandibular joint. An avascular plane exists between the gland capsule and the cartilaginous and bony acoustic meatus (Figure 1.2). The inferior border (usually the apex) is at the angle of the mandible and often extends beyond this to overlap the digastric triangle where it may lie very close to the posterior pole of the submandibular salivary

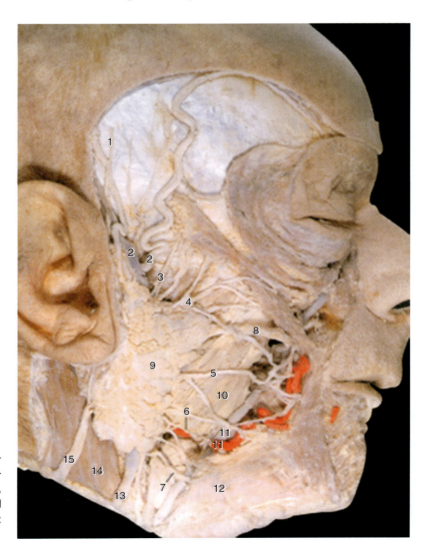

Figure 1.2. The parotid gland and associated structures. Source: Published with permission, Martin Dunitz, London, Langdon JD, Berkowitz BKB, Moxham BJ, editors, Surgical Anatomy of the Infratemporal Fossa. DOI: 10.1002/9781118949139.ch1.

gland. The anterior border just overlaps the posterior border of the masseter muscle and the posterior border overlaps the anterior border of the sternocleidomastoid muscle.

The superficial surface of the gland is covered by skin and platysma muscle. Some terminal branches of the great auricular nerve also lie superficial to the gland. At the superior border of the parotid, lie the superficial temporal vessels with the artery in front of the vein. The auriculotemporal branch of the mandibular nerve runs at a deeper level just behind the superficial temporal vessels.

The branches of the facial nerve emerge from the anterior border of the gland. The parotid duct also emerges to run horizontally across the masseter muscle before piercing the buccinator muscle anteriorly to end at the parotid papilla. The transverse facial artery (a branch of the superficial temporal artery) runs across the area parallel to and approximately 1 cm above the parotid duct. The anterior and posterior branches of the facial vein emerge from the inferior border.

The deep (medial) surface of the parotid gland lies on those structures forming the parotid bed. Anteriorly the gland lies over the masseter muscle and the posterior border of the mandibular ramus from the angle up to the condyle. As the gland wraps itself around the ramus, it is related to the medial pterygoid muscle at its insertion on to the deep aspect of the angle. More posteriorly, the parotid is molded around the styloid process and the styloglossus, stylohyoid, and stylopharyngeus muscles from below upwards. Behind this, the parotid lies on the posterior belly of the digastric muscle and the sternocleidomastoid muscle. The digastric and the styloid muscles separate the gland from the underlying internal jugular vein, the external and internal carotid arteries and the glossopharyngeal, vagus, accessory, and hypoglossal nerves and the sympathetic trunk.

The fascia that covers the muscles in the parotid bed thickens to form two named ligaments (Figure 1.3). The stylomandibular ligament passes from the styloid process to the angle of the mandible. The mandibulo-stylohyoid ligament (the angular tract) passes between the angle of the mandible and the stylohyoid ligament. Inferiorly, it usually extends down to the hyoid bone. These ligaments are all that separates the parotid gland anteriorly from the posterior pole of the superficial lobe of the submandibular gland.

CONTENTS OF THE PAROTID GLAND

Facial Nerve

From superficial to deep, the facial nerve, the auriculotemporal nerve, the retromandibular vein,

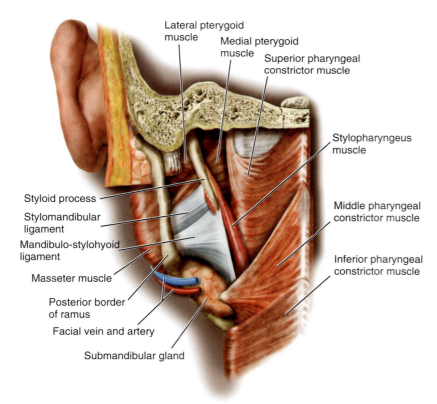

Figure 1.3. The mandibulo-stylohyoid ligament.

and the external carotid artery pass through the substance of the parotid gland.

The facial nerve exits the skull base at the stylomastoid foramen. The surgical landmarks are important (Figure 1.4). To expose the trunk of the facial nerve at the stylomastoid foramen, the dissection passes down the avascular plane between the parotid gland and the external acoustic canal until the junction of the cartilaginous and bony canals is palpated. A small triangular extension of the cartilage points toward the facial nerve as it exits the foramen (Langdon 1998b). This is the so-called tragal pointer. The main trunk of the nerve lies approximately 13.6mm from this landmark but there is considerable variation (Ji et al. 2018). The nerve lies about 9mm from the posterior belly of the digastric muscle where the digastric passes deep to the sternocleidomastoid muscle, and 11mm from the bony external meatus (Holt 1996). The facial nerve then passes downwards and forwards over the styloid process and associated muscles for about 1.3cm before entering the substance of the parotid gland (Hawthorn and Flatau 1990). The first part of the facial nerve gives off the posterior auricular nerve supplying the auricular muscles and also branches to the posterior belly of the digastric and stylohyoid muscles.

On entering the parotid gland, the facial nerve divides into two divisions, temporofacial and cervicofacial the former being the larger. The division of the facial nerve is sometimes called the pes anserinus due to its resemblance to the foot of a goose. From the temporofacial and cervicofacial divisions, the facial nerve gives rise to five named branches – temporal, zygomatic, buccal, mandibular, and cervical (Figure 1.5). The peripheral branches of the facial nerve form variable anastomotic arcades between adjacent branches to form the parotid plexus. These anastomoses are important during facial nerve dissection as accidental damage to a small branch often fails to result in any facial weakness due to dual innervation from adjacent branches. Davis et al. (1956) studied these patterns following the dissection of 350 facial nerves in cadavers. The anastomotic relationships between adjacent branches fell into six patterns (Figure 1.6). They showed that in only 6% of cases (type VI) is there any anastomosis between the mandibular branch and adjacent branches. This explains why, when transient facial weakness follows facial nerve dissection, it is usually the mandibular branch that is affected.

Auriculotemporal Nerve

The auriculotemporal nerve arises from the posterior division of the mandibular division of the trigeminal nerve in the infratemporal fossa. It runs backward beneath the lateral pterygoid muscle between the medial aspect of the condylar neck and the sphenomandibular ligament. It enters the anteromedial surface of the parotid gland passing upwards and outwards to emerge at the superior

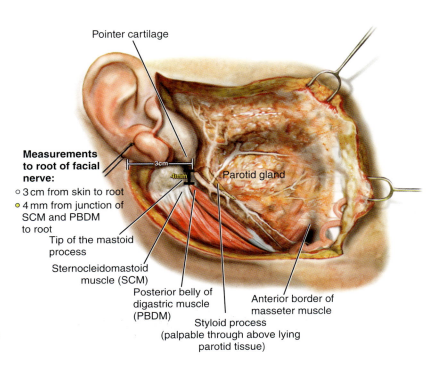

Figure 1.4. Anatomical landmarks of the extratemporal facial nerve.

border of the gland between the temporomandibular joint and the external acoustic meatus. This nerve communicates widely with the temporofacial division of the facial nerve and limits the mobility of the facial nerve during surgery (Flatau and Mills 1995). Further communications with the temporal and zygomatic branches loop around the transverse facial and superficial temporal vessels (Bernstein and Nelson 1984).

Retromandibular Vein

The vein is formed within the parotid gland by the union of the superficial temporal vein and the maxillary vein. The retromandibular vein passes downwards and close to the lower pole of the parotid where it often divides into two branches passing out of the gland. The posterior branch passes backward to unite with the posterior auricular vein on the surface of the sternocleidomastoid muscle to form the external jugular vein. The anterior branch passes forward to join the facial vein.

The retromandibular vein is an important landmark during parotid gland surgery. The division of the facial nerve into its temporofacial and cervicofacial divisions occurs just behind the retromandibular vein (Figure 1.7). The two divisions lie just superficial to the vein in contact with it. It is all too easy to tear the vein while exposing the division of the facial nerve!

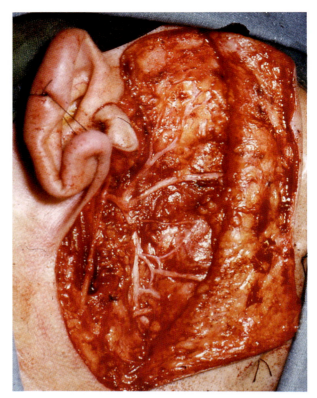

Figure 1.5. Clinical photograph of dissected facial nerve following superficial parotidectomy. Source: Published with permission, Martin Dunitz, London, Langdon JD, Berkowitz BKB, Moxham BJ, editors, Surgical Anatomy of the Infratemporal Fossa. DOI: 10.1002/9781118949139.ch1.

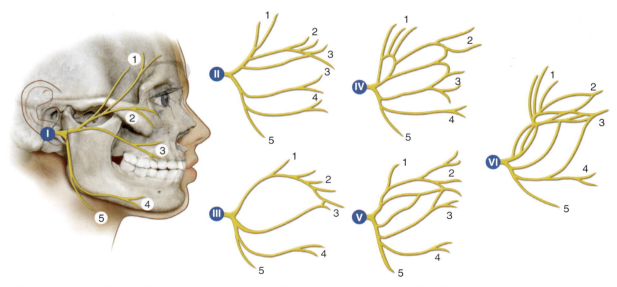

Figure 1.6. The branching patterns of the facial nerve. Source: Berkovitz et al. 2003/Taylor & Francis.
I Type I, 13%   **V** Type V, 9%   3 Buccal branch
II Type II, 20%   **VI** Type VI, 6%   4 Mandibular branch
III Type III, 28%   1 Temporal branch   5 Cervical branch
IV Type IV, 24%   2 Zygomatic branch

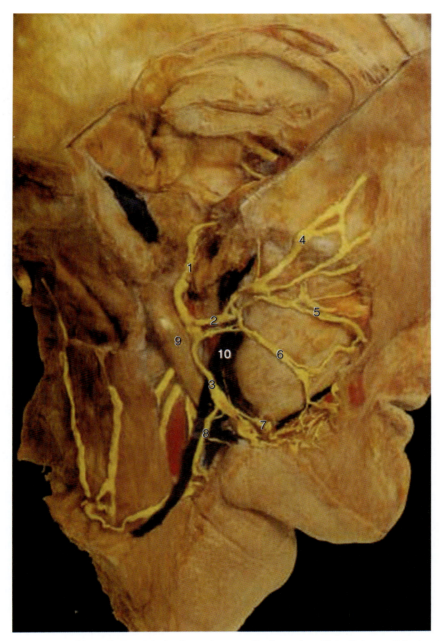

Figure 1.7. The facial nerve and its relationship to the retromandibular vein within the parotid gland. Source: Published with permission, Martin Dunitz, London, Langdon JD, Berkowitz BKB, Moxham BJ, editors, Surgical Anatomy of the Infratemporal Fossa. DOI: 10.1002/9781118949139.ch1.

1. Facial nerve at stylomastoid foramen
2. Temporofacial branch of facial nerve
3. Cervicofacial branch of facial nerve
4. Temporal branch of facial nerve
5. Zygomatic branch of facial nerve
6. Buccal branch of facial nerve
7. Mandibular branch of facial nerve
8. Cervical branch of facial nerve
9. Posterior belly of the digastric muscle
10. Retromandibular vein and external carotid artery

External Carotid Artery

The external carotid artery runs deeply within the parotid gland. It appears from behind the posterior belly of the digastric muscle and grooves the parotid before entering it. It gives off the posterior auricular artery before ascending and dividing into its terminal branches, the superficial temporal and maxillary arteries at the level of the condyle. The superficial temporal artery continues vertically to emerge at the superior border of the gland and crosses the zygomatic arch. Within the substance of the parotid, it gives off the transverse facial artery which emerges at the anterior border of the gland to run across the face above the parotid duct. The maxillary artery emerges from the deep aspect of the gland anteriorly to enter the infratemporal fossa. The maxillary artery gives off the deep auricular artery and the anterior tympanic artery within the substance of the parotid. All these branches from the external carotid also give off numerous small branches within the parotid to supply the gland itself.

Parotid Lymph Nodes

Lymph nodes are found within the subcutaneous tissues overlying the parotid to form the preauricular nodes and also within the substance of the gland (Goldenberg et al. 2000). There are typically 10 nodes within the substance of the gland, the majority being within the superficial lobe and therefore superficial to the plane of the facial nerve. Only one or two nodes lie within the deep lobe (Marks 1984; McKean et al. 1984; Garatea-Crelgo et al. 1993). All the parotid nodes drain into the upper deep cervical chain.

Parotid Duct

The parotid duct emerges from the anterior border of the parotid gland and passes horizontally across the masseter muscle. The surface markings of the duct are obtained by drawing a line from the midpoint of the tragal cartilage to the middle of a straight line from the ipsilateral ala to the commissure (Figure 1.8). This line is divided into three equal parts and the middle section corresponds to the position of the parotid duct. The duct lies approximately 1 cm below the transverse facial vessels. The accessory lobe of the parotid gland, when present, drains into its upper border via one or two tributaries (Kulkarni et al. 2011). Anastomosing branches between the buccal and

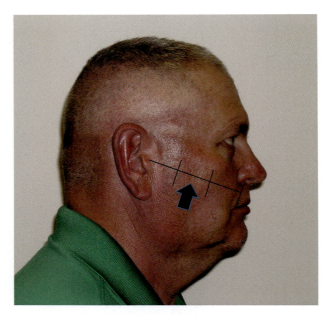

Figure 1.8. The surface markings for the location of the parotid duct.

zygomatic branches of the facial nerve cross the duct. At the anterior border of the masseter, the duct bends sharply to perforate the buccal pad of fat and the buccinator muscle at the level of the upper molar teeth. The duct then bends again to pass forward for a short distance before entering the oral cavity at the parotid papilla.

Nerve Supply to the Parotid

The parasympathetic secretomotor nerve supply comes from the inferior salivatory nucleus in the brain stem (Figure 1.9). From there, the fibers run in the tympanic branch of the glossopharyngeal nerve contributing to the tympanic plexus in the middle ear. The lesser petrosal nerve arises from the tympanic plexus leaving the middle ear and running in a groove on the petrous temporal bone in the middle cranial fossa. From here, it exits through the foramen ovale to the otic ganglion which lies on the medial aspect of the mandibular branch of the trigeminal nerve. Postsynaptic postganglionic fibers leave the ganglion to join the auriculotemporal nerve which distributes the parasympathetic secretomotor fibers throughout the parotid gland. Some authorities suggest that there are also some parasympathetic innervations to the parotid from the chorda tympani branch of the facial nerve.

The sympathetic nerve supply to the parotid arises from the superior cervical sympathetic ganglion. The sympathetic fibers reach the gland

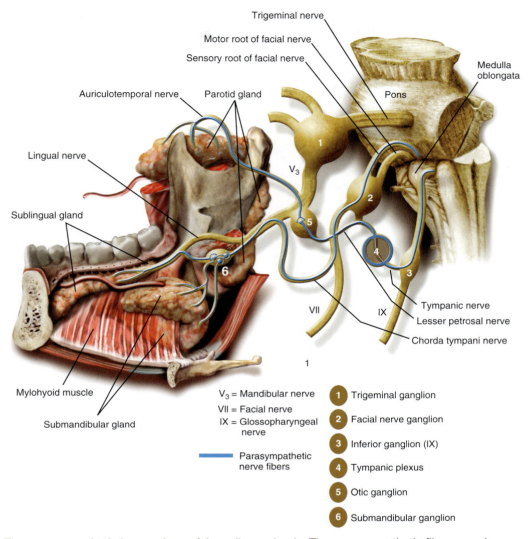

Figure 1.9. The parasympathetic innervations of the salivary glands. The parasympathetic fibers are shown as blue lines.

via the plexus around the middle meningeal artery. They then pass through the otic ganglion without synapsing and innervate the gland through the auriculotemporal nerve. There is also sympathetic innervation to the gland arising from the plexuses that accompany the blood vessels supplying the gland.

Sensory fibers arising from the connective tissue within the parotid gland merge into the auriculotemporal nerve and pass proximally through the otic ganglion without synapsing. From there, the fibers join the mandibular division of the trigeminal nerve. The sensory innervation of the parotid capsule is via the great auricular nerve.

Submandibular Gland

EMBRYOLOGY

The submandibular gland begins to form at the 13 mm stage in the seventh week of intrauterine life (Zhang et al. 2010; Berta et al. 2013; Chadi et al. 2017) as an epithelial outgrowth into the mesenchyme forming the floor of the mouth in the linguogingival groove. This proliferates rapidly giving off numerous branching processes which eventually develop lumina. Initially, the developing gland opens into the floor of the mouth posteriorly, lateral to the tongue. The walls of the groove into which it drains come together to form the submandibular duct. This process commences posteriorly and moves forwards so that ultimately the orifice of the duct comes to lie anteriorly below the tip of the tongue close to the midline.

ANATOMY

The submandibular gland consists of a larger superficial lobe lying within the digastric triangle in the neck and a smaller deep lobe lying within the floor of the mouth posteriorly (Figure 1.10).

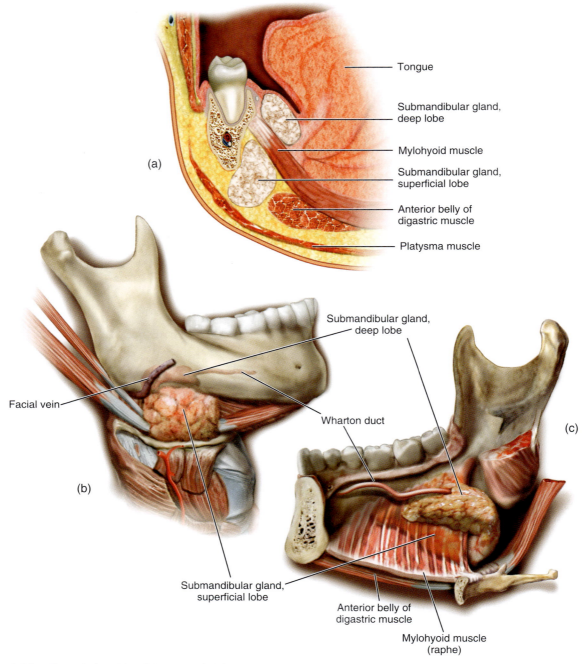

Figure 1.10. The relationship of the superficial and deep lobes of the submandibular gland. (a) cross-sectional anatomy. (b) The superficial lobe from outside. (c) The relationship of the deep and superficial lobes to the mylohyoid muscle.

The two lobes are continuous with each other around the posterior border of the mylohyoid muscle. As in the parotid gland, the two "lobes" are not true lobes embryologically as the gland arises as a single epithelial outgrowth (Langdon 1998a). However, surgically it consists of the two lobes as described above. It is a mixed seromucinous gland.

Superficial Lobe

The superficial lobe lies within the digastric triangle. Its anterior pole reaches the anterior belly of the digastric muscle and the posterior pole reaches the stylomandibular ligament. This structure is all that separates the superficial lobe of the submandibular gland from the parotid gland. It is important to realize just how close the lower pole of the parotid is to the posterior pole of the submandibular gland as confusion can arise if a mass in the region is incorrectly ascribed to the wrong anatomical structure (Figure 1.2). Superiorly, the superficial lobe lies medial to the body of the mandible. Inferiorly, it often overlaps the intermediate tendon of the digastric muscles and the insertion of the stylohyoid muscle. The lobe is partially enclosed between the two layers of the deep cervical fascia that arise from the greater cornu of the hyoid bone and is in intimate proximity of the facial vein and artery (Figure 1.11). The superficial layer of the fascia is attached to the lower border of the mandible and covers the inferior surface of the superficial lobe. The deep layer of fascia is attached to the mylohyoid line on the inner aspect of the mandible and therefore covers the medial surface of the lobe.

The inferior surface, which is covered by skin, subcutaneous fat, platysma, and the deep fascia, is crossed by the facial vein and the cervical branch of the facial nerve which loops down from the angle of the mandible and subsequently innervates the lower lip. The submandibular lymph nodes lie between the salivary gland and the mandible. Sometimes one or more lymph nodes may be embedded within the salivary gland.

The lateral surface of the superficial lobe is related to the submandibular fossa, a concavity on the medial surface of the mandible, and the attachment of the medial pterygoid muscle. The facial artery grooves its posterior part lying at first deep to the lobe and then emerging between its lateral surface and the mandibular attachment of the medial pterygoid muscle from which it reaches the lower border of the mandible.

The medial surface is related anteriorly to the mylohyoid from which it is separated by the mylohyoid nerve and submental vessels. Posteriorly, it is related to the styloglossus muscle, the stylohyoid ligament, and the glossopharyngeal nerve separating it from the pharynx. Between these, the medial aspect of the lobe is related to the hyoglossus muscle from which it is separated by the styloglossus muscle, the lingual nerve, the submandibular ganglion, the hypoglossal nerve, and the deep lingual vein. More inferiorly, the medial surface is related to the stylohyoid muscle and the posterior belly of digastric.

Deep Lobe

The deep lobe of the gland arises from the superficial lobe at the posterior free edge of the mylohyoid muscle and extends forward to the back of the sublingual gland (Figure 1.12). It lies between the mylohyoid inferolaterally, the hyoglossus, and the styloglossus muscles medially, the lingual nerve superiorly and the hypoglossal nerve and deep lingual vein inferiorly.

Submandibular Duct

The submandibular duct is about 62 mm long and 3 mm in diameter in the adult. The wall of the submandibular duct is thinner than that of the parotid duct. It arises from numerous tributaries in the

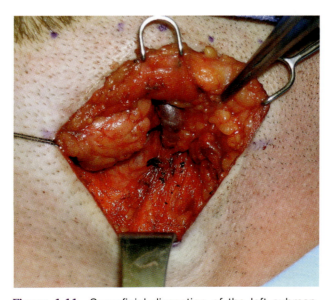

Figure 1.11 Superficial dissection of the left submandibular gland. The investing layer of the deep cervical fascia is elevated off the submandibular gland and the facial vein is identified.

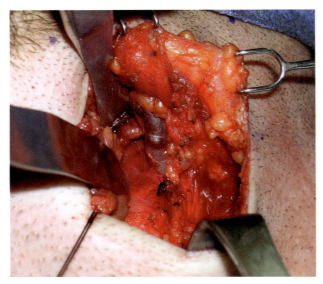

Figure 1.12. Deep dissection of the left submandibular gland. With the submandibular gland retracted, the facial artery is identified in proximity to the facial vein.

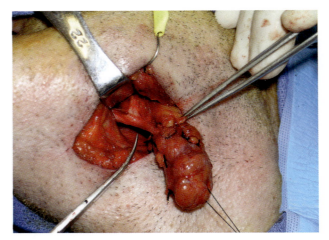

Figure 1.13. Clinical photograph showing the relationship of the lingual nerve to the submandibular gland.

superficial lobe and emerges from the medial surface of this lobe just behind the posterior border of the mylohyoid. It crosses the deep lobe, passing upwards, and slightly backward for 5 mm before running forwards between the mylohyoid and hyoglossus muscles. As it passes forward, it runs between the sublingual gland and genioglossus to open into the floor of the mouth on the summit of the sublingual papilla at the side of the lingual frenum just below the tip of the tongue. It lies between the lingual and hypoglossal nerves on the hyoglossus. At the anterior border of the hyoglossus muscle, it is crossed by the lingual nerve. As the duct traverses the deep lobe of the gland, it receives tributaries draining that lobe.

Blood Supply and Lymphatic Drainage

The arterial blood supply arises from multiple branches of the facial and lingual arteries. Venous blood drains predominantly into the deep lingual vein. The lymphatics drain into the deep cervical group of nodes, mostly into the jugulo-omohyoid node, via the submandibular nodes.

Nerve Supply to the Submandibular Gland

Parasympathetic innervation
The secretomotor supply to the submandibular gland arises from the submandibular (sublingual) ganglion. This is a small ganglion lying on the upper part of the hyoglossus muscle. There are additional ganglion cells at the hilum of the gland. The submandibular ganglion is suspended from the lingual nerve by anterior and posterior filaments (Figure 1.13).

The parasympathetic secretomotor fibers originate in the superior salivatory nucleus and the preganglionic fibers then travel via the facial nerve, chorda tympani, and lingual nerve to the ganglion via the posterior filaments connecting the ganglion to the lingual nerve. They synapse within the ganglion and the postganglionic fibers innervate the submandibular and sublingual glands (Figure 1.9). Some fibers are thought to reach the lower pole of the parotid gland.

Sympathetic innervation
The sympathetic root is derived from the plexus on the facial artery. The postganglionic fibers arise from the superior cervical ganglion and pass through the submandibular ganglion without synapsing. They are vasomotor to the vessels supplying the submandibular and sublingual glands. Five or six branches from the ganglion supply the submandibular gland and its duct. Others pass back into the lingual nerve via the anterior filament to innervate the sublingual and other minor salivary glands in the region.

Sensory innervation
Sensory fibers arising from the submandibular and sublingual glands pass through the ganglion without

synapsing and join the lingual nerve, itself a branch of the trigeminal nerve.

Sublingual Gland

EMBRYOLOGY

The sublingual gland arises in 20 mm embryos in the eighth week of intrauterine life as numerous small epithelial thickenings in the linguogingival groove and on the outer side of the groove. Each thickening forms its own canal and so many of the sublingual ducts open directly onto the summit of the sublingual fold. Those that arise within the linguogingival grove end up draining into the submandibular duct.

ANATOMY

The sublingual gland is the smallest of the major salivary glands. It is almond shaped and weighs approximately 4 g. It is predominantly a mucous gland. The gland lies on the mylohyoid and is covered by the mucosa of the floor of the mouth which is raised as it overlies the gland to form the sublingual fold. Posteriorly, the sublingual gland is in contact with the deep lobe of the submandibular gland. The sublingual fossa of the mandible is located laterally and the genioglossus muscle is located medially. The lingual nerve and the submandibular duct lie medial to the sublingual gland between it and the genioglossus.

Sublingual Ducts

The gland has a variable number of excretory ducts ranging from 8 to 20. The majority drain into the floor of the mouth at the crest of the sublingual fold. A few drain into the submandibular duct. Sometimes, a collection of draining ducts coalesce anteriorly to form a major duct (Bartholin's duct) which opens with the orifice of the submandibular duct at the sublingual papilla (Zhang et al. 2010).

Blood Supply, Innervation, and Lymphatic Drainage

The arterial supply is from the sublingual branch of the lingual artery and also the submental branch of the facial artery. Innervation is via the sublingual ganglion as described above. The lymphatics drain to the submental nodes.

Minor Salivary Glands

Minor salivary glands are distributed widely in the oral cavity and oropharynx. They are grouped as labial, buccal, palatoglossal, palatal, and lingual glands. The labial and buccal glands contain both mucous and serous acini whereas the palatoglossal glands are mucous secreting. The palatal glands which are also mucous secreting occur in both the hard and soft palates. The anterior and posterior lingual glands are mainly mucous secreting. The anterior glands are embedded within the muscle ventrally and they drain via four or five ducts near the lingual frenum. The posterior lingual glands are located at the root of the tongue. The deep posterior lingual glands are predominantly serous secreting. Additional serous glands (glands of von Ebner) occur around the circumvallate papillae on the dorsum of the tongue. Their watery secretion is thought to be important in spreading taste stimuli over the taste buds.

Tubarial Salivary Glands

In 2020, Valstar et al reported on the serendipitous presence of bilateral macroscopic salivary gland structures in the nasopharynx of humans. Their existence was visualized by positron emission tomography/computed tomography with prostate-specific membrane antigen ligands (PSMA PET/CT). The presence of the PSMA-positive nasopharyngeal regions was elucidated in a retrospective cohort of 100 consecutive patients with prostate or urethral gland cancer. The designated area of the posterior nasopharynx was also studied with hematoxylin and eosin (H&E) and PSMA and alpha-amylase) immunohistochemistry in two human cadavers. All 100 patients (99 males, one female; median age 69.5, range 53–84) demonstrated a well-demarcated bilateral PSMA-positive region on PSMA PET/CT. This 3.9 cm cranio-caudal structure (range 1.0–5.7 cm) extended from the skull base along the posterolateral pharyngeal wall on the pharyngeal aspect of the superior pharyngeal constrictor muscle with a PSMA-positive structure located predominantly over the torus tubarius. The tracer uptake in these structures was similar to the uptake of the sublingual glands. The dissected structures from the two human cadavers demonstrated a large aggregate of mucous salivary gland tissue with multiple visible draining duct openings in the dorsolateral pharyngeal wall. The authors concluded that the human body contains a pair of once overlooked and clinically significant salivary glands in the posterior nasopharynx, and the authors proposed the name tubarial glands. Their particular interest in these structures was in gland sparing radiation protocols for head and neck cancer in the best interests of maintaining salivary function and the quality of life of patients.

Histology of the Salivary Glands

The salivary glands are composed of large numbers of secretory acini that may be tubular or globular in shape. Each acinus drains into a duct. These microscopic ducts coalesce to form lobular ducts. Each lobule has its own duct and these then merge to form the main ducts. The individual lobes and lobules are separated by dense connective tissue that is continuous with the gland capsule. The ducts, blood vessels, lymphatics, and nerves run through and are supported by this connective tissue.

The acini are the primary secretory organs but the saliva is modified as it passes through the intercalated, striated, and excretory ducts before being discharged into the mouth and oropharynx (Figure 1.14). The lobules also contain significant amounts of adipose tissue particularly in the parotid gland. The proportion of adipose tissue relative to excretory acinar cells increases with age.

In the human parotid, the excretory acini are almost entirely serous. In the submandibular gland, again, the secretory units are mostly serous but there are additional mucous tubules and acini. In some areas, the mucinous acini have crescentic "caps" of serous cells called serous demilunes. In the sublingual gland, the acini are almost entirely mucinous although there are occasional serous acini or demilunes.

The serous cells contain numerous proteinaceous secretory (zymogen) granules. These granules contain high levels of amylase. In addition, the secretory cells produce kallikrein, lactoferrin, and lysozyme. In mucous cells, the cytoplasm is packed with large pale secretory droplets.

Initially the secretory acini drain into intercalated ducts. These ducts function mainly to conduct the saliva but they may also modify the electrolyte content and secrete immunoglobulin A. The intercalated ducts drain into striated ducts that coalesce into intralobular and extralobular collecting ducts. The intercalated duct cells are very active metabolically, and they transport potassium and bicarbonate into saliva. They reabsorb sodium and chloride ions so that the resulting saliva is hypotonic. They also secrete immunoglobulin A, lysozyme, and kallikrein. The immunoglobulin is produced by plasma cells adjacent to the striated duct cells, and it is then transported through the epithelial lining into the saliva. The main collecting ducts are simple conduits for saliva and do not modify the composition of the saliva.

Myoepithelial cells are contractile cells closely related to the secretory acini and much of the duct system. The myoepithelial cells lie between the basal lamina and the epithelial cells. Numerous cytoplasmic processes arise from them and surround the serous acini as basket cells. Those associated with the duct cells are more fusiform and are aligned along the length of the ducts. The cytoplasm of the myoepithelial cells contains actin myofilaments that contract as a result of both parasympathetic and sympathetic activity. Thus, the myoepithelial cells "squeeze" the saliva out of the secretory acini and ducts and add to the salivary secretory pressure.

Although the parotid capsule is a continuous structure covering the superficial and deep aspects of the gland, it becomes very attenuated where the gland envelopes the branches of the facial nerve. This is of some significance in parotid surgery as when peeling the gland off the branches of the nerve there may be none or a very thin capsule separating the gland from the nerve.

Control of Salivation

There is a continuous low background saliva production that is stimulated by drying of the oral and pharyngeal mucosa. A rapid increase in the resting levels occurs as a reflex in response to masticatory stimuli including the mechanoreceptors and taste fibers. Other sensory modalities such as smell are also involved. The afferent input is via the salivatory centers that are themselves influenced by the higher centers. The higher centers may be facilitory or inhibitory depending on the circumstances. The efferent secretory drive to the salivary glands passes via the parasympathetic and sympathetic pathways. There are no peripheral inhibitory mechanisms.

Cholinergic nerves (parasympathetic) often accompany ducts and branch freely around the

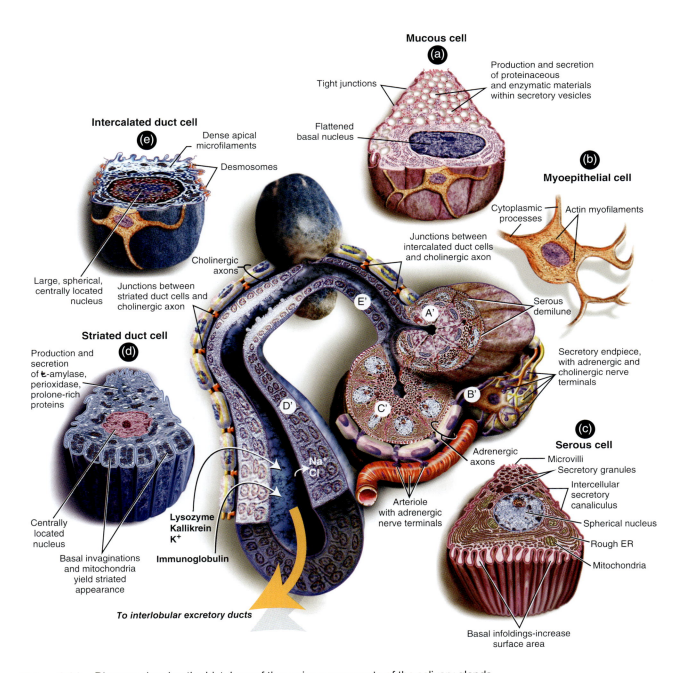

Figure 1.14. Diagram showing the histology of the major components of the salivary glands.

secretory endpieces (acini). Adrenergic nerves (sympathetic) usually enter the glands along the arteries and arterioles and ramify with them. Within the glands, the nerve fibers intermingle such that cholinergic and adrenergic axons frequently lie in adjacent invaginations of a single Schwann cell (Garrett and Kidd 1993). Secretion and vasoconstriction are mediated by separate sympathetic axons whereas a single parasympathetic axon may, through serial terminals, result in vasodilatation, secretion, and constriction of myoepithelial cells.

Secretory endpieces are the most densely innervated structures in the salivary glands. Individual acinar cells may have both cholinergic and adrenergic nerve endings. The secretion of water and electrolytes, which accounts for the volume of saliva produced, results from a complex set of stimuli which are largely parasympathetic. The active secretion of proteins into the saliva depends upon the relative levels of both sympathetic and parasympathetic stimulation.

Although the ducts are less densely innervated than secretory acini, they do influence the composition of the saliva. Adrenal aldosterone promotes resorption of sodium and secretion of potassium into the saliva by striated ductal cells. Myoepithelial cell contraction is stimulated predominantly by adrenergic fibers although there may be an additional role for cholinergic axons.

The cholinergic parasympathetic nerves release acetylcholine that binds to M3 and to a lesser extent M1 muscarinic receptors which result in the secretion of saliva by the acinar cells in the endpieces of the duct trees. The sympathetic nerves release noradrenaline that results in the release of stored protein from both the acinar cells and the ductal cells. There is also cross talk between the calcium and cyclic AMP intracellular pathways. Additionally, other non-adrenergic and non-cholinergic neuropeptides released from the autonomic nerves evoke saliva secretion and parasympathetically derived vasointestinal peptide acting through endothelial cell-derived nitric oxide. These neuropeptides play a role in the reflex vasodilatation that accompanies salivary secretion (as seen dramatically in Frey syndrome). Neuronal type, calcium activated, soluble nitric oxide within salivary cells seems to play a role in mediating salivary protein secretion in response to autonomimetics. The fluid secretion involves aquaporin 5 and the extent to which its expression on apical acinar cell membranes is upregulated by cholimimetics remains obscure (Proctor and Carpenter 2007).

Summary

- Although embryologically the parotid consists of a single lobe, anatomically the facial nerve lies in a distinct plane between the anatomical superficial and deep lobes.
- The parotid capsule is attenuated and incomplete where the gland lies in intimate contact with the branches of the facial nerve.
- There are fixed anatomical landmarks indicating the origin of the extracranial facial nerve as it leaves the stylomastoid foramen.
- The lower pole of the parotid gland is separated from the posterior pole of the submandibular gland by only thin fascia. This can lead to diagnostic confusion in determining the origin of a swelling in this area.
- The relationship of the submandibular salivary duct to the lingual nerve is critical to the safe removal of stones within the duct.
- Great care must be taken to identify the lingual nerve when excising the submandibular gland. The lingual nerve is attached to the gland by the parasympathetic fibers synapsing in the submandibular (sublingual) ganglion.
- The sublingual gland may drain into the submandibular duct or it may drain directly into the floor of the mouth via multiple secretory ducts.

Case Presentation – *Wait, What?*

A 67-year-old man presented to the emergency department with an abrupt onset of acute left visual loss. The patient had a known history of multiple cerebrovascular accidents and had chronic right visual loss and a chronic mild aphasia.

Past Medical History

The patient had a history of hypercoagulable state with methylenetetrahydrofolate reductase (MTHFR) mutation, hypertension, hyperlipidemia, peripheral vascular disease, and gastroesophageal reflux disease. He had undergone a left carotid endarterectomy in the past and a bypass surgery for peripheral vascular disease. He was taking a baby aspirin daily, atorvastatin, hydrochlorothiazide, metoprolol, niacin, ranitidine, and warfarin that was on hold for five days for a planned vascular surgery procedure.

Imaging

The patient underwent a CT of the head that demonstrated multiple remote infarcts with no acute findings. A CT angiogram of the brain and neck revealed occlusive disease of the left internal

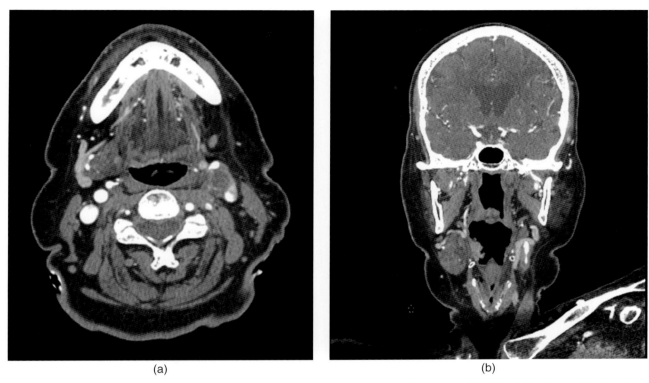

(a)   (b)

Figure 1.15. Axial (a) and coronal (b) CT angiogram of the neck demonstrating agenesis of the left submandibular gland. Hypertrophy of the right submandibular gland is noted.

carotid artery and absence of his left submandibular gland (Figure 1.15a and b).

Diagnosis

Congenital absence of the left submandibular gland. The patient's operative report for his left carotid endarterectomy made no mention of encountering or removing the left submandibular gland.

TAKE HOME POINTS

1. Unilateral or bilateral agenesis of the submandibular glands is extremely rare.
2. Unilateral submandibular gland agenesis is typically asymptomatic and discovered incidentally through imaging of the neck. Bilateral agenesis is more likely to produce symptoms in affected patients such as xerostomia, dysphagia, and dental problems.
3. Submandibular gland agenesis may be accompanied by genetic syndromes such as Treacher Collins syndrome, hemifacial microsomia, ectodermal dysplasia, and lacrimo-dento-digital syndrome.
4. Physical examination of the neck might not disclose unilateral or bilateral agenesis of the submandibular glands. It becomes necessary, therefore, to examine the oral cavity where the unilateral Wharton duct opening may not be present. CT or MR imaging of the neck will unequivocally establish the diagnosis of agenesis of the submandibular gland as this case demonstrated.

References

Berkovitz BKB, Moxham BJ. 1988. *A Textbook of Head and Neck Anatomy*. London, Wolfe.

Berkovitz BKB, Langdon JD, Moxham BJ. 2003. The Facial Nerve and the Parotid Gland. In: Langdon JD, Berkovitz BKB, Moxham BJ (eds.) *Surgical Anatomy of the Infratemporal Fossa*. London, Martin Dunitz, pp. 181–206.

Bernstein L, Nelson RH. 1984. Surgical anatomy of the extraparotid distribution of the facial nerve. *Arch Otolaryngol* 110:177–183.

Berta E, Bettega G, Jouk PS. 2013. Complete agenesis of major salivary glands. *Int J Pediatr Otorhinolaryngol* 77:1782–1785.

Chadi MJ, Saint Georges G, Albert F, Mainville G, Nguyen JM, Kauzman A. 2017. Major salivary gland aplasia and hypoplasia in Down syndrome: Review of the literature and report of a case. *Clin Case Rep* 5:939–944.

Davis RA, Anson BJ, Budinger JM, Kurth LE. 1956. Surgical anatomy of the facial nerve and parotid gland based on 350 cervicofacial halves. *Surg Gynecol Obstet* 102:385–412.

Ellis H. 1997. *Clinical Anatomy*, 9th edn. Oxford, Blackwell.

Flatau AT, Mills PR. 1995. Regional Aanatomy. In: de Norman JEB, McGurk M (eds.) *Color Atlas and Text of the Salivary Glands*. London, Mosby Wolfe, pp. 13–39.

Gareta-Crelgo J, Gay-Escoda C, Bermejo B, Buenechea-Imaz R. 1993. Morphological studies of the parotid lymph nodes. *J Cranio-Maxillo-Facial Surg* 21:207–209.

Garrett JR, Kidd A. 1993. The innervation of salivary glands is revealed by morphological studies. *Microsc Res Tech* 26:75–91.

Goldenberg D, Flax-Goldenberg R, Joachims HZ, Peled N. 2000. Misplaced parotid glands: Bilateral agenesis of parotid glands associated with bilateral accessory parotid tissue. *J Laryngol Otol* 114:883–885.

Gosain AK, Yousif NJ, Madiedo G et al. 1993. Surgical anatomy of the SMAS: A reinvestigation. *Plast Reconstr Surg* 92:1254–1263.

Hawthorn R, Flatau A. 1990. Temporomandibular Joint Anatomy. In: de Norman JEB, Bramley P (eds.) *A Textbook and Colour Atlas of the Temporomandibular Joint*. London, Mosby Wolfe, pp. 1–51.

Holt JJ. 1996. The stylomastoid area: Anatomic-histologic study and surgical approach. *Laryngoscope* 106:396–399.

Ji YD, Donoff RB, Peacock ZS, Carlson ER. 2018. Surgical landmarks to locating the main trunk of the facial nerve in parotid surgery: A systematic review. *J Oral Maxillofac Surg* 76:438–443.

Jost G, Levet Y. 1983. Parotid fascia and face lifting: A critical evaluation of the SMAS concept. *Plast Reconstr Surg* 74:42–51.

Kulkarni CD, Mittal SK, Katiyar V, Pathak O, Sood S. 2011. Accessory parotid gland with ectopic fistulous duct-diagnosis by ultrasound, digital fistulography, digital sialography and CT fistulography. A case report and review of current literature. *J Radiol Case Rep* 5:7–14.

Langdon JD. 1998a. Sublingual and Submandibular Gland Excision. In: Langdon JD, Patel MF (eds.) *Operative Maxillofacial Surgery*. London, Chapman & Hall, pp. 376–380.

Langdon JD. 1998b. Parotid Surgery. In: Langdon JD, Patel MF (eds.) *Operative Maxillofacial Surgery*. London, Chapman & Hall, pp. 386–388.

Marks NJ. 1984. The anatomy of the lymph nodes of the parotid gland. *Clin Otolaryngol* 9:271–275.

McKean ME, Lee K, McGregor IA. 1984. The distribution of lymph nodes in and around the parotid gland: An anatomical study. *Br J Plast Surg* 38:1–5.

McMinn RMH, Hutchings RT, Logan BM. 1984. *A Colour Atlas of Applied Anatomy*. London, Wolfe.

Meningaud J-P, Bertolus C, Bertrand J-C. 2006. Parotidectomy: Assessment of a surgical technique including facelift incision and SMAS advancement. *J Cranio-Maxillofacial Surg* 34:34–37.

Mitz V, Peyronie M. 1976. The superficial musculo-aponeurotic system (SMAS) in the parotid and cheek area. *Plast Reconstr Surg* 58:80–88.

Proctor GB, Carpenter GH. 2007. Regulation of salivary gland function by autonomic nerves. *Auton Neurosci* 133:3–18.

Thaller SR, Kim S Patterson H et al. 1989. The submuscular aponeurotic system (SMAS): A histologic and comparative anatomy evaluation. *Plast Reconstr Surg* 86:691–696.

Valstar MH, de Bakker BS, Steenbakkers RJHM et al. 2020. The tubarial salivary glands: A potential new organ at risk for radiotherapy. *Radiother Oncol*. https://doi.org/10.1016/j.radonc.2020.09.034.

Wassef M. 1987. Superficial fascia and muscular layers in the face and neck: A histological study. *Aesthetic Plast Surg* 11:171–176.

Williams PL (ed.). 1995. *Gray's Anatomy*, 38th edn. Oxford, Blackwell.

Zhang L, Xu H, Cai ZG, Mao C, Wang Y, Peng X. 2010. Clinical and anatomic study of the ducts of the submandibular and sublingual glands. *J Oral Maxillofac Surg* 68:606–610.

Zigiotti GL, Liverani MB, Ghibellini D. 1991. The relationship between parotid and superficial fasciae. *Surg Radiol Anat* 13:293–300.

Chapter 2
Diagnostic Imaging of Salivary Gland Pathology

J. Michael McCoy DDS, FACS[1] and Pradeep K. Jacob MD, MBA[2]
[1]Departments of Oral and Maxillofacial Surgery, Pathology, and Radiology, University of Tennessee Medical Center, Knoxville, TN, USA
[2]Private Practice of Radiology, Chattanooga, Tennessee

Outline

Introduction
Imaging Modalities
  Computed Tomography (CT)
    CT Technique
      Advanced computed tomography
  Magnetic Resonance Imaging (MRI)
    MRI Technique
      Spin-echo T1
      Spin-echo T2
      Proton density images (PD)
      Gradient recalled echo imaging (GRE)
      Short tau inversion recovery (STIR)
      Gadolinium (Gd) contrast
      Fluid attenuation inversion recovery (FLAIR)
      Diffusion weighted images (DWI)
      MR spectroscopy
      Dynamic contrast-enhanced magnetic resonance imaging
    Other Magnetic Resonance Imaging Techniques
  Ultrasonography (US)
    Ultrasound (US) Technique
  Sialography
  Image-Guided Biopsies of Salivary Gland Pathology
  Radionuclide Imaging (RNI)
  Positron Emission Tomography (PET)
  Positron Emission Tomography/Computed Tomography (PET/CT)
Diagnostic Imaging Anatomy
  Parotid Gland
  Submandibular Gland
  Sublingual Gland
  Minor Salivary Glands
Pathology of the Salivary Glands
  Vascular Lesions
    Lymphangioma (Cystic Hygroma)
    Hemangioma
  Acute Sialadenitis
  Chronic Sialadenitis
  HIV-Associated Lymphoepithelial Lesions
  Mucous Escape Phenomena
  Sialadenosis (Sialosis)
  Sialolithiasis
  Sjögren Syndrome
  Sarcoidosis
  Congenital Anomalies Salivary Glands
    First Branchial Cleft Cyst
  Neoplasms – Salivary, Epithelial
    Benign
      Pleomorphic adenoma
      Warthin tumor
      Oncocytoma
    Malignant Tumors
      Mucoepidermoid carcinoma
      Adenoid cystic carcinoma
  Neoplasms – Non-Salivary
    Benign
      Lipoma
      Neurogenic tumors
    Malignant
      Lymphoma
      Metastases
Summary
Case Presentation – *Duplicity*
References

Salivary Gland Pathology: Diagnosis and Management, Third Edition. Edited by Eric R. Carlson and Robert A. Ord.
© 2022 John Wiley & Sons, Inc. Published 2022 by John Wiley & Sons, Inc.
Companion website: www.wiley.com/go/carlson/salivary

Introduction

Anatomic and functional diagnostic imaging plays a central role in modern medicine. Virtually all specialties of medicine to varying degrees depend on diagnostic imaging for diagnosis, therapy, and follow-up of treatment. Because of the complexity of the anatomy, treatment of diseases of the head and neck, including those of the salivary glands, is particularly dependent on quality medical imaging and interpretation. Medical diagnostic imaging consists of two major categories, anatomic and functional. The *anatomic* imaging modalities include computed tomography (CT), magnetic resonance imaging (MRI) and ultrasonography (US). Although occasionally obtained, plain film radiography for the head and neck, including salivary gland disease, is mostly of historical interest. In a similar manner, the use of sialography is significantly reduced, although both plain films and sialography are of some use in imaging sialoliths. *Functional* diagnostic imaging techniques include planar scintigraphy, single photon emission computed tomography (SPECT), positron emission tomography (PET), and magnetic resonance spectroscopy (MRS), all of which are promising technologies. Recently, the use of a combined anatomic and functional modality in the form of PET/CT has proved invaluable in head and neck imaging. Previously widely employed procedures including gallium radionuclide imaging are less important today than in the past.

Imaging Modalities

COMPUTED TOMOGRAPHY (CT)

Computed tomography (CT) has become indispensable in the diagnosis, treatment, and follow-up of diseases of the head and neck. The latest generation of multiple-row detector CT (MDCT) provides excellent soft-tissue and osseous delineation. The rapid speed with which images are obtained, along with the high spatial resolution and tissue contrast, makes CT the imaging modality of choice in head and neck imaging. True volumetric data sets obtained from multi-detector row scanners allow for excellent coronal, sagittal, or oblique reformation of images as well as a variety of 3D renderings. This allows the radiologist and surgeon to characterize a lesion, assess involvement of adjacent structures or local spread from the orthogonal projections or three-dimensional rendering. The ability to manipulate images is critical when assessing pathology in complex anatomy, such as evaluation of parotid gland masses to determine deep lobe involvement, facial nerve involvement, or extension into the skull base. Images in the coronal plane are important in evaluating the submandibular gland in relation to the floor of mouth. Lymphadenopathy and its relationship to the carotid sheath and its contents and other structures are also well delineated. CT is also superior to MRI in demonstrating bone detail and calcifications. CT is also the fastest method of imaging head and neck anatomy. Other advantages of CT include widespread availability of scanners, high-resolution images, and speed of image acquisition that reduces motion artifacts. Exposure to ionizing radiation and the administration of IV contrast are the only significant disadvantages to CT scanning.

CT Technique

The CT scanner contains a gantry, which holds an X-ray tube and a set of detectors. The X-ray tube is positioned opposite the detectors and is physically coupled. A "fan beam" of X-rays are produced and pass through the patient to the detectors as the tube and detector rotate around the patient. In newer generation of scanners, the multiple rows of detectors are fixed around the gantry and only the tube rotates. A table carries the patient through the gantry. The detectors send signals, dependent on the degree of X-ray attenuation, to a computer that uses these data to construct an image using complex algorithms.

Intravenous contrast is administered for most CT studies, especially in the head and neck. IV contrast is a solution consisting of organic compounds bonded with iodine molecules. Iodine is a dense atom with an atomic weight of 127, which is good at absorbing X-rays, and is biocompatible. IV contrast readily attenuates the X-ray beam at concentrations optimal for vascular and soft tissue "enhancement," but short of causing attenuation-related artifacts. Streak artifacts, however, can occur if the concentration is too high, as seen occasionally at the thoracic inlet and supraclavicular region from dense opacification of the subclavian vein during rapid bolus injection of IV contrast.

CT of the neck should be performed with intravenous contrast whenever possible to optimize delineation of masses, inflammatory or infectious changes in the tissues, and enhance vascular structures. Imaging is obtained from the level of the orbits through the aortic arch in the axial plane with breath hold. The images are reconstructed using a computer algorithm to optimize soft tissue delineation, and displayed in soft tissue window and level settings (Figures 2.1 and 2.2). In a similar manner, images are reconstructed using a computer algorithm to optimize bone details as more sharp and defined (Figure 2.3). The lung apex is often imaged in a complete neck evaluation and displayed using lung window settings (Figure 2.4a). Dedicated CT scans of the chest are beneficial in the postoperative evaluation of patients with salivary gland malignancies as lung nodules can be observed, possibly indicative of metastatic disease (Figure 2.4b). Multiplanar reformatted images of the neck are obtained typically in the coronal and sagittal planes (Figures 2.5 and 2.6), although they may be obtained in virtually any plane desired or in a 3D rendering.

The Hounsfield unit (H) (named for Godfrey Hounsfield, inventor of the CT scanner) is the unit of density measurement for CT. These units are assigned based on the degree of attenuation of the X-ray beam by tissue in a given voxel (volume

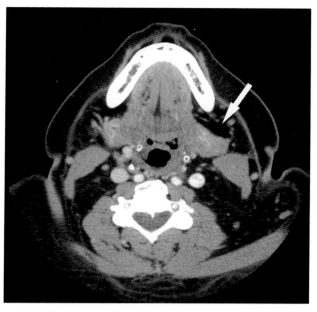

Figure 2.2. Axial CT of the neck in soft-tissue window with IV contrast demonstrates improved visualization of structures with enhancement of tissues and vasculature. Note the small lipoma (arrow) anterior to the left submandibular gland, which distorts the anterior aspect of the gland with slight posterior displacement.

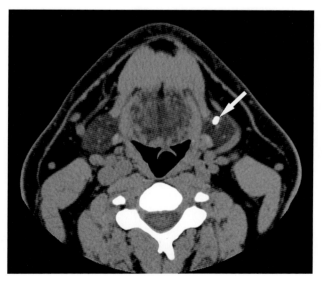

Figure 2.1. Axial CT of the neck in soft-tissue window without contrast demonstrating poor definition between soft-tissue structures. The blood vessels are unopacified and cannot be easily distinguished from lymph nodes. Note the sialolith (arrow) in the hilum of the left submandibular gland.

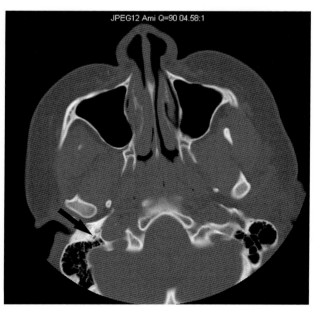

Figure 2.3. Axial CT of the skull base reconstructed in a sharp algorithm and in bone window and level display demonstrating sharp bone detail. Note the sharply defined normal right stylomastoid foramen (arrow).

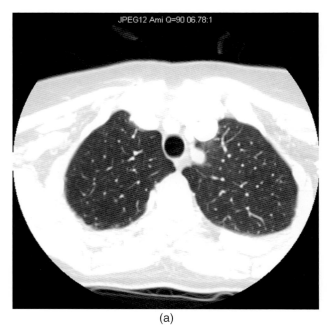

(a)

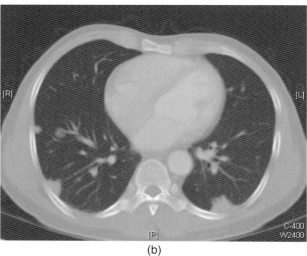

(b)

Figure 2.4. Axial CT of the neck at the thoracic inlet in lung windows demonstrating lung parenchyma (a). Axial image of dedicated CT of chest demonstrating cannon ball lesions in a patient previously treated for adenoid cystic carcinoma of the palate (b). These lesions are representative of diffuse metastatic disease of the lungs, but not pathognomonic of adenoid cystic carcinoma.

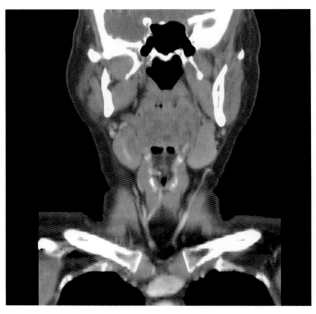

Figure 2.5. Coronal CT reformation of the neck in soft-tissue window at the level of the submandibular glands. Orthogonal images with MDCT offer very good soft-tissue detail in virtually any plane of interest to assess anatomic and pathologic relationships.

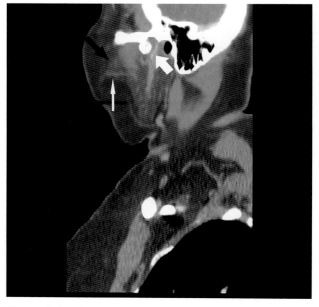

Figure 2.6. Sagittal CT reformation of the neck in soft-tissue window at the level of the parotid gland. Note the accessory parotid gland (black arrow) sitting atop the parotid (Stensen) duct (thin white arrow). Also, note the retromandibular vein (large white arrow) and external auditory canal.

element) and are assigned relative to water (0H) (Table 2.1). The scale ranges from −1024H for air, to +4000H for very dense bone. The images are created based on a gray scale from black (−1024H) to white (+4000H) and shades of gray. Despite the wide range of units, majority of tissues in the

Table 2.1. CT density in Hounsfield units (H).

Tissue or structure	Hounsfield unit (H)
Water or CSF	0
Fat	−30 to −100
Soft tissue, muscle[a]	50–60
Unclotted blood[b]	35–50
Clotted blood[b]	50–75
Parotid gland[c]	−10 to +30
Submandibular gland[c]	30–60
Sublingual gland[d]	60–90
Bone	1000
Lung	−850
Air	−1000
Calcification	150–200
Gray matter	35–40
White matter	25–35

[a] Depends on degree of fat deposition.
[b] Depends on the hemoglobin concentration and hematocrit.
[c] Depends on age and fat deposition.
[d] Very limited evaluation secondary to partial volume effect.
CSF = cerebrospinal fluid.

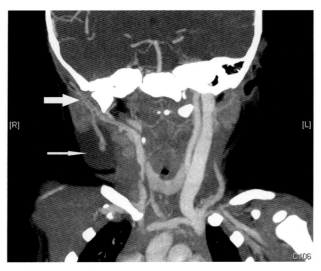

Figure 2.7. CT angiogram (CTA) of the neck at the level of the parotid gland demonstrating the retromandibular vein and adjacent external carotid artery (large white arrow). Note the right cervical lymphangioma (thin white arrow) associated with the tail of the right parotid gland.

human body are between −100 and +100 H. Soft tissues and parenchymal organs are in a range between 20 and 80 H, whereas fat is approximately −100 H. Simple fluid is 0 H, but proteinaceous fluid can be upward of 25 H. Unclotted and clotted blood varies depending on the hemoglobin concentration and hematocrit but average measurements are 50 and 80 H, respectively. CT images are displayed using a combination of "window widths" (WW, range of CT numbers from black to white), and "window levels" (WL, position of the window on the scale), which are based on the attenuation characteristics of tissues. Typically, head and neck images are interpreted using "soft-tissue windows" (WW 500 H, WL 30 H), "bone windows" (WW 2000, WL 500), or "lung windows" (WW 1500, WL 500). The "soft-tissue windows" demonstrate the slight density differences of soft tissues, whereas "bone windows" demonstrated cortical and medullary features of bones with sharp detail. "Lung windows" demonstrate the sharp interface of air and the fine soft-tissue components of lung parenchyma.

Although the density of the salivary glands is variable, the parotid glands tend to be slightly lower in density relative to muscle, secondary to a higher fat content and become progressively more fat replaced over time. The CT density of parotid glands varies from −10 to +30 H. The submandibular glands are denser than parotid glands and are equivalent in density to muscle. The submandibular glands vary in density from +30 to +60 H.

CT angiography (CTA) is a powerful method, which allows visualization of arterial vasculature, demonstrating the vascular anatomy of arteries and veins. CTA can be critical in preoperative evaluation to determine the degree of vascularity of lesions and plan an appropriate surgical approach to minimize blood loss or perform preoperative embolization. CTA is obtained with fast image acquisition over a defined region of interest while administering a rapid IV contrast bolus timed to arrive in the region of interest during image acquisition. CTA images may be rendered in 3D data sets and rotated in any plane (Figure 2.7). CTA is not only useful for preoperative planning, but it can also be quite useful in diagnosis of salivary gland vascular pathology such as aneurysms, or arteriovenous fistulas (AVFs) (Wong et al. 2004).

CT scanning, as with all imaging modalities, is prone to artifacts. Artifacts can be caused by motion, very dense or metallic implants (dental amalgam), and volume averaging. Motion artifact is common and may result from breathing, swallowing, coughing, or sneezing during the image acquisition or from an unaware or uncooperative patient. Metallic implants cause complete attenuation of X-rays in the beam and result in focal loss of data and bright and dark steaks in the image. Because the image is created from a three-dimensional section of tissue averaged to form a two-dimensional image, the partial volume or volume averaging artifact results from partial inclusion of structures in adjacent images. Finally, the beam hardening artifact is produced by attenuation of low-energy X-rays, by dense objects, from the energy spectrum of the X-ray beam, resulting in a residual average high-energy beam (or hard X-rays), which results in loss of data and dark lines on the image. This phenomenon is often seen in the posterior fossa of head CT scans caused by the very dense petrous bones. Multi-detector row CT scanner can help reduce metallic artifacts using advanced algorithms, and reduce motion artifacts secondary to faster scanning speeds.

Advanced computed tomography
Newer CT techniques including CT perfusion and dynamic contrast-enhanced multi-slice CT have been studied. Dynamic multi-slice contrast-enhanced CT is obtained while scanning over a region of interest and simultaneously administering IV contrast. The characteristics of tissues can then be studied as the contrast bolus arrives at the lesion and "washes in" to the tumor, reaches a peak presence within the mass, and then decreases over time, i.e. "washes out." This technique has demonstrated differences in various histologic types of tumors, for example, with early enhancement in Warthin's tumor with a time to peak at 30 seconds and subsequent fast washout. The malignant tumors show a time to peak at 90 seconds. The pleomorphic adenomas demonstrate a continued rise in enhancement in all four phases (Yerli et al. 2007).

CT perfusion attempts to study physiologic parameters of blood volume, blood flow, mean transit time, and capillary permeability surface product. Statistically significant differences between malignant and benign tumors have been demonstrated with the mean transit time measurement. A rapid mean transit time of less than 3.5 seconds is seen with most malignant tumors, but with benign tumors or normal tissue the mean transit time is significantly longer (Rumboldt et al. 2005).

MAGNETIC RESONANCE IMAGING (MRI)
Magnetic resonance imaging (MRI) represents imaging technology with great promise in characterizing salivary gland pathology. The higher tissue contrast of MRI, when compared to CT, enables subtle differences in soft tissues to be demonstrated. Gadolinium contrast-enhanced MRI further accentuates the soft-tissue contrast. Subtle pathologic states such as perineural spread of disease are better delineated when compared with CT. This along with excellent resolution and exquisite details make MRI a very powerful technique in head and neck imaging, particularly at the skull base. This notwithstanding, its susceptibility to motion artifacts and long imaging time as well as contraindication due to claustrophobia, pacemakers, aneurysm clips, deep brain and vagal nerve stimulators limit its usefulness in the general population as a *routine* initial diagnostic and follow-up imaging modality. Many of the safety considerations are well defined and detailed on the popular website, www.mrisafety.com.

MRI Technique
Although the physics and instrumentation of MRI are beyond the scope of this text, a fundamental understanding of the variety of different imaging sequences and techniques should be understood by clinicians to facilitate reciprocal communication of the clinical problem, and understanding of imaging reports.

In contrast to CT, which is based on the use of ionizing radiation, MRI utilizes a high magnetic field and pulsed radiofrequency waves to create an image or obtain spectroscopic data. MRI is based on the proton (hydrogen ion) distribution throughout the body. The basic concept is that protons are normally oriented in a random state. However, once placed in the imaging magnet, a high magnetic field, a large proportion of protons align with the magnetic field. The protons remain aligned and precess (spin) in the magnetic field until an external force acts upon them and forces them out of alignment. This force is an applied radiofrequency pulse, applied for a specified time and specified frequency by an antenna called a transmit coil. As the protons return to the aligned state, they give off energy in the form of their own radiofrequency pulse, determined by their local chemical state and tissue structure. The radiofrequency pulse given off is captured by an antenna, called a receive coil. The energy of the pulse and location are recorded and the process repeated multiple times and averaged, as the signal is weak. The recorded signal is used to form the image. Several different types of applied pulse sequences of radio waves result in different types of images.

The impact of MRI is in the soft-tissue contrast that can be obtained, noninvasively. The relaxation times of tissues can be manipulated to bring out soft-tissue detail. The routine sequences used in clinical scanning are spin-echo (SE), gradient echo (GRE), and echo-planar (EPI). Typical pulse sequences for head and neck and brain imaging include spin-echo T1, spin-echo T2, proton density (PD), fluid attenuation inversion recovery (FLAIR), diffusion weighted images (DWI), post-contrast T1 and STIR. A variant of the spin-echo, the fast spin-echo sequence (FSE) allows for a more rapid acquisition of spin-echo images. Any one of these can be obtained in the three standard orientations of axial, coronal, and sagittal planes. Oblique planes may be obtained in special circumstances.

Spin-echo T1

On T1 weighted images, a short repetition time (tr) and short echo time (te) are applied resulting in an image commonly used for anatomic depiction. Water signal is very low and is displayed as dark gray to black pixels on the gray scale. Fat is very bright, allowing tissue planes to be delineated. Fast flowing blood is devoid of signal and is therefore very black. Muscle tissue is an intermediate gray. Bone which has few free protons is also largely devoid of signal. Bone marrow, however, will vary depending on the relative percentage of red versus yellow marrow. Red marrow will have a signal slightly lower than muscle, whereas yellow marrow (fat replaced) will be bright. In the brain, cerebrospinal fluid (CSF) is dark, and flowing blood is black. Gray matter is dark relative to white matter (contains fatty myelin) but both are higher than cerebrospinal fluid (CSF) but less than fat. Cysts (simple) are dark in signal unless they are complicated by hemorrhage or infection or have elevated protein concentration, which results in an increased signal and slightly brighter display (Figure 2.8) (Table 2.2).

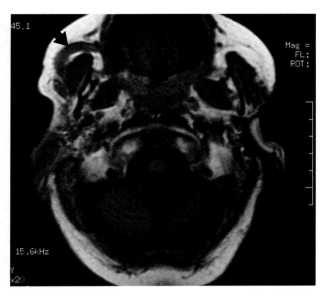

Figure 2.8. Axial MRI T1 weighted image at level of the skull base and brainstem without contrast demonstrating high signal in the subcutaneous fat, intermediate signal of the brain, and low signal of the CSF and mucosa. Note dilated right parotid duct (arrow).

Spin-echo T2

The T2 images are obtained with a long tr and te. The T2 image is sensitive to the presence of water in tissues and depicts edema as a very bright signal. Therefore, CSF or fluid containing structures such as cysts is very bright. Complicated cysts can vary in T2 images. If hemorrhagic, they can have heterogenous or even uniformly dark signal caused by a susceptibility artifact. These artifacts can be caused by metals, melanin, forms of calcium and the iron in hemoglobin. Increased tissue water from edema stands out as bright relative to the isointense soft tissue. The fast spin-echo T2 is a common sequence, which is many times faster than the conventional spin-echo T2 but does alter the image. Fat stays brighter on the fast spin-echo (FSE) sequence relative to the conventional (Figure 2.9) (Table 2.2).

Proton density images (PD)

Proton density images are obtained with a long tr but short te, resulting in an image with less tissue contrast but high signal-to-noise ratio. These are uncommonly used in the head and neck.

Table 2.2. Tissue characteristics on T1 and T2 MRI.[a]

	T1	T2
Increased signal	– Fat – Calcium[b] – Proteinaceous fluid (high)[c] – Slow flowing blood – Melanin – Hyperacute hemorrhage[d] (oxyhemoglobin) – Subacute hemorrhage (intracellular and extracellular methemoglobin) – Gadolinium contrast – Manganese – Cholesterol	– Water (CSF) or edema – Proteinaceous fluid – Hyperacute hemorrhage (oxyhemoglobin) – Subacute hemorrhage (extracellular methemoglobin) – Slow flowing blood – Fat (FSE T2 scans)
Intermediate signal	– Hyperacute hemorrhage (oxyhemoglobin) – Acute hemorrhage (deoxyhemoglobin) – Calcium[b] – Gray matter – White matter (brighter than gray matter) – Soft tissue (muscle) – Proteinaceous fluid[c]	– Grey matter (brighter than white matter) – White matter – Proteinaceous fluid[c] – Calcium[b]
Decreased signal	– Water (CSF) or edema – Fast flowing blood – Calcium[b] – Soft tissue – Acute hemorrhage (deoxyhemoglobin) – Chronic hemorrhage (hemosiderin) – Calcification – Air – Simple cyst (low protein)	– Calcium[b] – Melanin – Hemosiderin – Flowing blood – hemorrhagic cyst – Iron deposition – Acute hemorrhage (deoxyhemoglobin) – Early subacute hemorrhage (intracellular methemoglobin) – Chronic hemorrhage (hemosiderin) – Air – Fast flow – Fat (conventional or non-FSE T2 scan)

[a] MRI signal on T1 and T2 predominantly from intracranial exam at 1.5T (Tesla).
[b] Signal from calcium deposition is complex. Calcium concentrations of under 30% by weight have high T1 signal and intermediate T2 signal, but over 40% have decreasing signal on T1 and T2. The surface area of the calcium particle also has an effect, with large surface area resulting in increased T1 signal (Henkelman et al. 1991).
[c] Depends on the protein concentration (complex cysts, abscess).
[d] MRI signal of intracranial hemorrhage is quite complex and dependent on multiple factors with degrees of variability.
CSF = cerebrospinal fluid.

Gradient recalled echo imaging (GRE)

Gradient recalled echo imaging is the second most common type of imaging sequence after the spin-echo. This sequence is very susceptible (more than spin-echo T2) to magnetic field inhomogeneity and is commonly used in the brain to identify blood products, metal deposition such as iron, manganese, and nonmetals such as calcium. This sequence is very sensitive but not specific. The "flip angle" used in obtaining GRE can be altered, resulting in either T1 weighted (long flip angle) or T2 weighted (short flip angle) images (Figure 2.10).

Short tau inversion recovery (STIR)

Short tau inversion recovery (STIR) is commonly acquired because of its very high sensitivity to fluid and readily detects subtle edema in tissues.

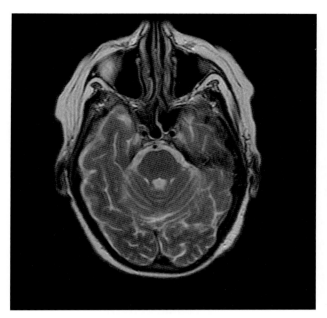

Figure 2.9. Axial MRI FSE T2 weighted image demonstrating the high signal of CSF and subcutaneous fat, intermediate signal of the brain and mucosa, and the low signal in the arteries.

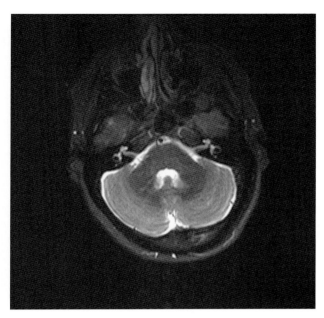

Figure 2.11. Axial MRI STIR image at the skull base demonstrating the high signal of CSF but suppression of subcutaneous fat signal.

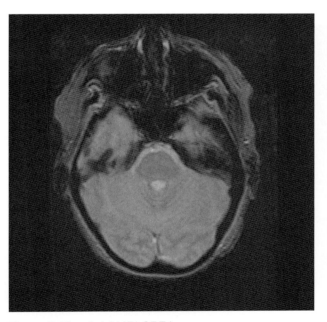

Figure 2.10. Axial MRI GRE image.

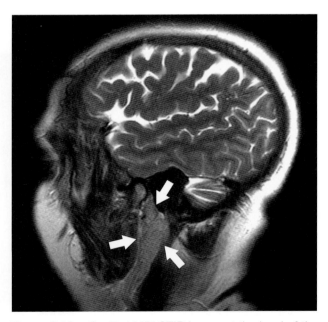

Figure 2.12. Sagittal MRI STIR image at the level of the parotid gland demonstrating the deep lobe seen through the stylomandibular tunnel (arrows). Note the parotid gland extending superiorly to the skull base.

When acquired in the conventional method, it also results in nulling the fat signal, thereby further increasing the signal of tissue fluid relative to background. This is the best sequence for edema, particularly when trying to determine bone invasion by tumors. It can also be useful in assessing skull base foramina (Figures 2.11 and 2.12).

Gadolinium (Gd) contrast

Intravenous contrast with gadolinium, a paramagnetic element, alters (shortens) T1 and T2 relaxation times, which results in a brighter signal. Its effect is greater on T1 than on T2 weighted images. Areas of tissue that accumulate Gd will have a higher or brighter signal and "enhance." In the head and neck, post-contrast T1 images should be produced with fat saturation to null the fat signal and therefore increase the signal of Gd accumulation (Figure 2.13).

Fluid attenuation inversion recovery (FLAIR)

Fluid attenuation inversion recovery (FLAIR) is not as commonly used in the neck but is a necessity in brain imaging. By nulling the CSF signal, brain tissue edema from a variety of causes stands out and is easily identified. It is however not specific. FLAIR can be useful for assessing skull base or foraminal invasion by tumors. However, artifacts can result from CSF pulsation or high FiO_2 administration and can mimic pathologic processes such as subarachnoid hemorrhage, or meningitis (bacterial, carcinomatous, viral, or aseptic) (Figure 2.14).

Diffusion weighted images (DWI)

Diffusion weighted images are not routinely clinically used in the neck or head but are indispensable in the brain. Typical intracranial application is for assessing acute stroke, but can be applied for the assessment of active multiple sclerosis (MS) plaques, and abscesses (Figure 2.15). The concept of DWI is based on the molecular motion of water and the sensitivity of certain MRI sequences to detect the diffusion or movement of water in tissues at the cellular level.

The use of DWI and specifically apparent diffusion coefficient (ADC) values and maps for salivary gland imaging are under investigation and show promise in differentiating benign from malignant tissues (Shah et al. 2003; Abdel-Razek et al. 2007; Eida et al. 2007; Habermann et al. 2007). The ADC values are affected by technical factors (b-value setting, image resolution, choice of region of interest, susceptibility artifacts, and adequate shimming) as well as physiologic factors (biochemical composition of tumors, hemorrhage, perfusion, and salivary flow) (Eida et al. 2007). The ADC values of salivary glands change with gustatory stimulation. Although mixed results

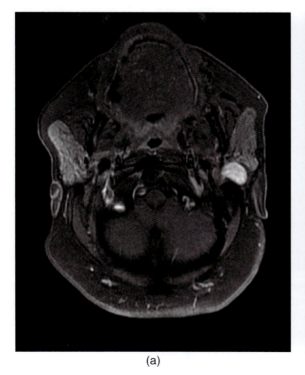
(a)

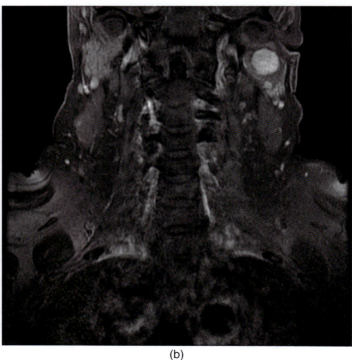
(b)

Figure 2.13. Axial (a) and coronal (b) MRI T1 post-contrast fat saturated image demonstrating a mass in the left parotid gland. Note the mild vascular enhancement and suppression of fat high signal on T1 weighted image.

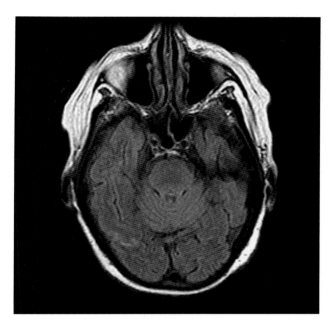

Figure 2.14. Axial MRI FLAIR image at the skull base demonstrating CSF flow-related artifactual increased signal in the right prepontine cistern.

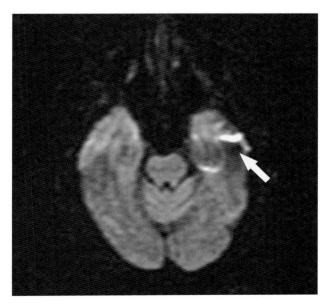

Figure 2.15. Axial MRI DWI image at the skull base demonstrating susceptibility artifact adjacent to the left temporal bone (arrow).

have been reported, there is generally an increase in the ADC value from pre-stimulation to post-stimulation measurements (Habermann et al. 2007). The normal parotid, submandibular, and sublingual glands have measured ADC values of $0.63 \pm 0.11 \times 10^{-3}$ mm²/s, $0.97 \pm 0.09 \times 10^{-3}$ mm²/s, and $0.87 \pm 0.05 \times 10^{-3}$ mm²/s, respectively (Eida et al. 2007). In pleomorphic adenomas, the ADC maps demonstrate areas of cellular proliferation to have intermediate ADC levels and areas of myxomatous changes to have high ADC values (Eida et al. 2007). Warthin's tumor showed lymphoid tissue to have a very low ADC, necrosis with intermediate ADC, and low ADC in cysts among the lymphoid tissue (Eida et al. 2007). Among the malignant lesions, mucoepidermoid carcinoma shows low ADC in a more homogenous pattern whereas the adenoid cystic carcinomas demonstrated a more speckled pattern with areas of low and high ADC likely from multiple areas of cystic or necrotic change (Eida et al. 2007). Lymphoma in salivary glands has been demonstrated to have a diffuse extremely low ADC likely from the diffuse uniform cellularity of lymphoma (Eida et al. 2007). In general, cystic, necrotic, or myxomatous changes tend to have higher ADC and regions of cellularity, low ADC. Malignant tumors tend to show very low to intermediate ADC whereas benign lesions have higher ADC, but with heterogenous pattern. Overlaps do occur for example with Warthin's tumor demonstrating very low ADC regions and adenoid cystic carcinoma with areas of high ADC (Eida et al. 2007).

Evaluating postoperative changes for residual or recurrent tumors is also an area where DWI and ADC may have a significant impact. In general, (with overlap of data) residual or recurrent lesions have been shown to have ADC values lower than post-treatment changes (Abdel-Razek et al. 2007). The lower ADC may be a result of smaller diffusion spaces for water in intracellular and extracellular tissues in hypercellular tumors. The benign post-treatment tissue with edema and inflammatory changes has fewer barriers to diffusion and increased extracellular space, resulting in a higher ADC (Abdel-Razek et al. 2007).

Evaluation of connective tissue disorders with DWI has demonstrated early changes with increase in ADC prior to changes on other MRI sequences. This may be a result of early edema and or early lymphocellular infiltration (Patel et al. 2004). Therefore, DWI and ADC may play an important role in early assessment of connective tissue disorders, preoperative evaluation of salivary tumors, as well as surveillance for recurrent disease.

MR spectroscopy

Magnetic resonance spectroscopy (MRS) falls under the category of functional MRI (fMRI), which contains a variety of different exams created to elucidate physiologic functions of the body. DWI, spectroscopy, perfusion weighted imaging (PWI), and activation studies are examples of fMRI. Of these, MRS of brain lesions is the most commonly performed functional study in clinical imaging. Spectroscopy is after all the basis for MRI. MRS attempts to elicit the chemical processes in tissues. Although a variety of nuclei may be interrogated, protons, demonstrating the highest concentration in tissues, are the most practical to evaluate. Most MRS studies are performed for the brain, but several recent studies have evaluated head and neck tumors. The need for a very homogenous magnetic field and patient cooperation (prevention of motion) are the keys to successful MRS. Susceptibility artifact and vascular pulsation artifact add to the challenge of MRS. With higher field strength magnets, MRS shows promise in determining the biochemical nature of tissues (King et al. 2005).

As in brain tumors, the most reliable markers for tumors are choline and creatine. Choline is thought to be an important constituent of cell membranes. Increased levels of choline are thought to be related to increased biosynthesis of cell membranes, which is seen in tumors, particularly those demonstrating rapid proliferation. The choline signal is comprised of signals from choline, phosphocholine, phosphatidylcholine, and glycerophosphocholine. Elevation of the choline peak in the MR spectra is associated with tumors relative to normal tissue. This unfortunately can be seen in malignant lesions, inflammatory processes, and hypercellular benign lesions (King et al. 2005). Another important constituent is creatine, a marker for energy metabolism. Its peak is comprised of creatine and phosphocreatine. The reduction of the creatine peak in neoplasms may represent the higher energy demands of neoplasms. The elevation of choline and, more importantly, the elevation of the ratio of choline to creatine have been associated with neoplasms relative to normal tissue. The elevation of choline is not tumor specific and may be seen with squamous cell carcinomas as well as a variety of salivary gland tumors, including benign tumors. It has been described in Warthin tumors, pleomorphic adenomas, glomus tumors, schwannomas, inflammatory polyps, and inverting papillomas (Shah et al. 2003). In fact, the Warthin tumor and pleomorphic adenoma demonstrate higher choline-to-creatine ratios than other tumors (King et al. 2005). King et al. also evaluated choline-to-water ratios and suggest that this may be an alternative method (King et al. 2005). Although the role of MRS in distinguishing between benign and malignant tumors may be limited, it nevertheless remains an important biomarker for neoplasms and plays a complementary role to other functional parameters and imaging characteristics (Shah et al. 2003). An area where MRS may play a more significant role is in a tumor's response to therapy and assessment of recurrence. Elevation of the choline-to-creatine ratio is seen in recurrent tumors whereas the ratio remains low in post-treatment changes. Progressive reduction of choline is seen with a positive response to therapy and persistent elevation is seen in failure of therapy (Shah et al. 2003). Use of artificial intelligence and neural network analysis of MR spectroscopy has demonstrated improved diagnostic accuracy of MRS using neural network analysis over linear discriminate analysis (Gerstle et al. 2000). Currently, MRS of salivary gland tumors is under study and not employed clinically.

Dynamic contrast-enhanced magnetic resonance imaging

Dynamic contrast-enhanced MRI has demonstrated improved diagnostic capability of tumor masses in the salivary glands and elsewhere in the body. Distinct enhancement curves can be generated based on the time points of acquisition, resulting in improved differentiation of tumors (Yabuuchi et al. 2003; Shah et al. 2003; Alibek et al. 2007). However, data demonstrate similar characteristics in Warthin's tumor and malignant tumors, with a rapid increase in the signal intensity post-contrast. Pleomorphic adenoma demonstrates a more gradual increase in intensity (Yabuuchi et al. 2003; Alibek et al. 2007). Primary salivary duct carcinomas have also demonstrated the rapid enhancement as well as low ADC values, as are seen with the more common primary malignancies of the salivary glands (Motoori et al. 2005).

Other magnetic resonance imaging techniques

Attempts have been made to develop MR sialography to replace the invasive technique of digital subtraction sialography. The techniques are based on acquiring heavily T2 weighted images to depict the ducts and branches. The lower spatial resolution and other technical factors have not allowed MR sialography to become a standard of care. This may change with newer single-shot MR sequences and higher field strength magnets (Kalinowski et al. 2002; Shah et al. 2003; Takagi et al. 2005b). Dynamic MR sialography has also been used to assess function of parotid and submandibular glands at rest and under stimulation (Tanaka et al. 2007).

An extension of this concept is MR virtual endoscopy. MR virtual endoscopy can provide high-resolution images of the lumen of salivary ducts comparable to sialendoscopy (Su et al. 2006). Although this initial experience was a preoperative assessment of the technology, it appears to be a promising method of noninvasive assessment of the ducts. In a similar manner, MR microscopy is a high-resolution imaging technique employing tiny coils enabling highly detailed images of the glands (Takagi et al. 2005a). This technique was used to demonstrate morphologic changes in Sjögren syndrome (SS).

Use of supraparamagnetic iron oxide particle MR contrast agents has been under investigation for several years. The particles used for evaluation of lymph nodes are 20 nm or smaller. These are intravenously injected and are taken up by the cells in the reticuloendothelial system (RES). Since normal lymph nodes have a RES that is intact, they readily take up the iron oxide agents. MR imaging using T2 and T2* weighted images demonstrates susceptibility to the iron oxide and results in signal loss at sites of iron accumulation. Therefore, normal lymph nodes lose signal whereas metastatic lymph nodes whose RES has been replaced by metastases do not take up the particles and do not lose signal (Shah et al. 2003). Although not a direct imaging technique for the salivary glands, it may prove to be useful in the evaluation of nodal metastases.

ULTRASONOGRAPHY (US)

Ultrasound is performed infrequently for head and neck imaging relative to CT and MRI. Although US can depict normal anatomy and pathology in the major salivary glands, it is limited in evaluation of the deep lobe of the parotid and submandibular gland (Figures 2.16 and 2.17). US is operator dependent and takes significantly longer to perform on bilateral individual salivary glands when compared to contrast-enhanced CT of the entire neck. US is quite effective at delineating cystic from solid masses, and determining degree of vascularity. US can be used to image calculi and observe the resulting ductal dilatation. Normal lymph nodes and lymphadenopathy can also be reliably distinguished. US can be used to initially stage disease. It is not, however, optimal for post-therapy follow-up, be it radiation or surgery. When compared with CT or MRI, US significantly lacks in soft-tissue resolution and contrast. Because of its real-time imaging capability and ease of hand-held imaging, US is quite good at image-guided fine needle aspiration and biopsy. The application of color Doppler or power Doppler US can distinguish arteries from veins, which are critical for

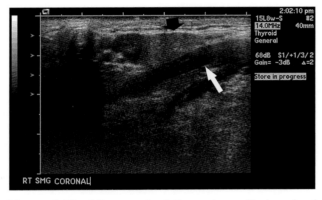

Figure 2.16. Ultrasound of the submandibular gland (black arrow) adjacent to the mylohyoid muscle (white arrow).

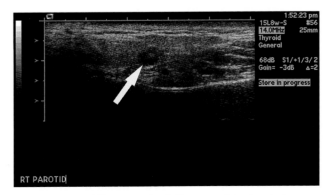

Figure 2.17. Ultrasound of the parotid gland demonstrating a normal intraparotid lymph node on a hyperechoic background. The lymph node is round and has a hypoechoic rim but demonstrates a fatty hyperechoic hilum (arrow).

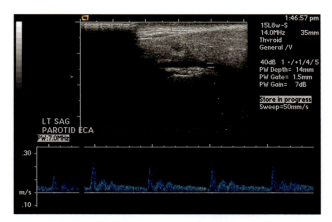

Figure 2.18. Ultrasound of the parotid gland in longitudinal orientation demonstrating the Doppler signal of the external carotid artery.

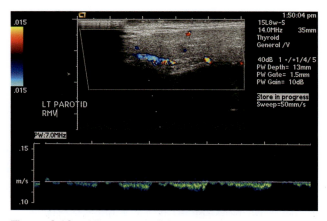

Figure 2.19. Ultrasound of the parotid gland in longitudinal orientation demonstrating the Doppler signal of the retromandibular vein.

image-guided biopsy (Figures 2.18 and 2.19). Eighteen-gauge core biopsies of the parotid may be safely performed under US guidance (Wan et al. 2004).

Ultrasound (US) Technique

High-frequency transducers such as 5, 7.5, or 10 MHz are typically applied to image superficial small parts. Real-time imaging and image acquisition are performed by a technologist or physician. Doppler US may be applied to observe the vascularity of the glands (increased in inflammatory conditions) or tumors within the glands. Doppler US can easily determine arterial from venous channels.

SIALOGRAPHY

Invasive salivary gland imaging was first introduced in 1904 when mercury was injected into surgical pathology and autopsy specimens. These injected tissue specimens were then visualized by X-rays. Sialography development continued, and in 1925 potassium iodide solution was injected into a human parotid gland, thereby initiating the radiographic technique of human sialography. Many modifications of sialography have been introduced since that time. These progressive changes brought sialography into the realm of practical salivary gland imaging. Since the advent of CT and MRI, sialography has to some extent been replaced as a diagnostic tool in salivary gland imaging. Only within the last few years has there be resurgence in its use, particularly in the diagnosis and treatment of obstructive and metabolic salivary gland disease (Mosier 2009). The specific choice of imaging depends predominately on the patient's clinical presentation as well as the patient's specific needs (Burke et al. 2011).

Most authorities believe the principal value of sialography is in the diagnosis of obstructive salivary gland disease. While most sialoliths are calcified and therefore opaque when visualized with X-ray, 20% of submandibular and 40% of parotid stones are either non-calcified or only partially calcified. Consequently, these stones are non-opaque when examined by way of plain X-ray and occasionally by CT imaging, as well (Sobrino-Guijarro et al. 2013) (Figure 2.20). Sialographic imaging was once essential in the delineation of benign and malignant masses, but imaging of such lesions has now been replaced by the more modern techniques of CT, US, and MRI. The major present-day indications of sialography are: (i) ductal anomalies such as sialoceles or salivary fistulas, (ii) obstructive and restrictive disease (Figure 2.21) including stones (Figure 2.22), mucous plugs, and intraductal neoplastic or inflammatory lesions, and (iii) chronic systemic parenchymal diseases of salivary gland such as those seen with Sjögren syndrome or sarcoidosis (Hasson 2010).

The only two paired salivary glands for which conventional sialography is suitable are the parotid and the submandibular glands. Even though the anatomy of every individual gland varies with the patient being studied, each separate gland has a single primary duct that excretes saliva. It is through this solitary duct that contrast can be introduced and the various anatomic and pathologic variances be imaged.

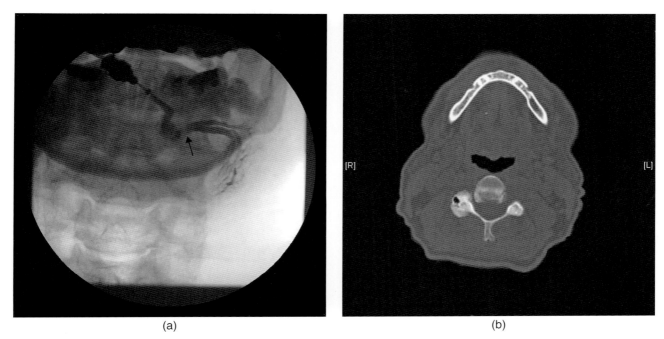

Figure 2.20. Submandibular sialogram (a). Note the continuity defect that represents a sialolith (arrow). The corresponding submandibular CT (b) demonstrates a partially calcified stone that is less impressive compared to the sialogram.

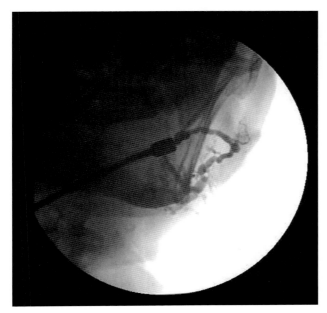

Figure 2.21. Parotid sialogram. Note the numerous areas of duct dilatation and stenosis. These features are diagnostic of obstructive disease.

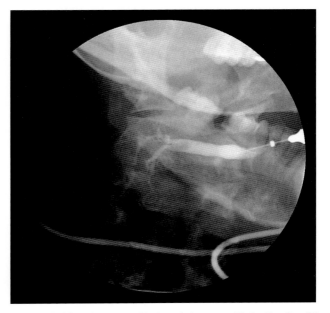

Figure 2.22. Submandibular sialogram: Note the "soft" noncalcified stone filling the duct.

Conventional sialography is a painless and minimally invasive technique that is generally quite successful. The mechanics of sialography are for the most part relatively simple. Initially, the patient is questioned regarding contrast allergies. In addition, it should be noted that the patient should not be imaged if there is evidence of an ongoing salivary gland infection, particularly acute inflammatory conditions or abscesses. Once the patient is placed supine on the examination table, they are given lemon juice to stimulate salivation. Using various sized lacrimal probes, the duct orifice is dilated for a length of 1–3 cm. Following dilation, a 23- to 25-gauge catheter is placed into the main duct and 1–3 cc of contrast is infused into the gland taking great care not to damage the duct. Even though non-water-soluble contrast usually delineates ductal walls more distinctly, water-soluble contrast also does quite well. In addition, the water-soluble contrast leaves no residual opacity with which to contend thereafter. Following contrast administration, images are acquired in various views (frontal, lateral, etc.). The patient is once again given lemon juice, allowing the residual contrast to be expelled. If the patient experiences pain during the procedure, a local anesthetic such as lidocaine can be infused into the ductal system in the same manner as the contrast agent. Occasionally, radiologists will also inject corticosteroids into the primary duct, which potentially can decrease the inflammatory component of the imaging study.

During sialography, there are two major phases of contrast filling: ductal and acinar. The initial or ductal phase will demonstrate the major or primary duct as well as the smaller secondary and tertiary ducts. The acinar phase is visualized as the contrast "blush" and demonstrates the parenchymal portion of the gland. Sialographic finding in obstructive disease will demonstrate the anatomy of the main, secondary, and occasionally tertiary ducts. Visualized will be strictures, obstructions, accessory glands, masses, and sialoliths. The observed obstructions include calcified and noncalcified sialoliths, mucous plugs, fibrin clots, other soft-tissue plugs, intraductal tumors, duct stenosis and strictures, and various anatomical kinking of the ducts.

The major parenchymal disorder of salivary gland that can be identified by sialography is the acinar change seen in Sjögren syndrome (Figure 2.23). This systemic autoimmune condition affects most of human exocrine glands but much more so the major and minor salivary glands (Golder and Stiller 2014). During the early phase of this syndrome, when imaged, these glands appear unremarkable but as Sjögren syndrome progresses, the salivary glands diffusely enlarge, mimicking chronic sialadenitis. Imaging of the salivary glands during this later time will demonstrate tiny discrete

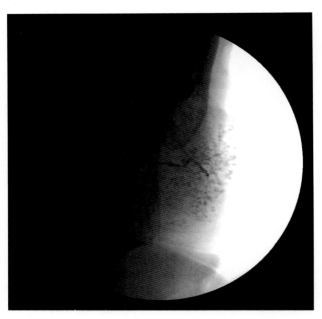

Figure 2.23. Parotid sialogram. Note the punctate filling areas without ductal involvement. These findings are seen predominately in Sjögren syndrome patients.

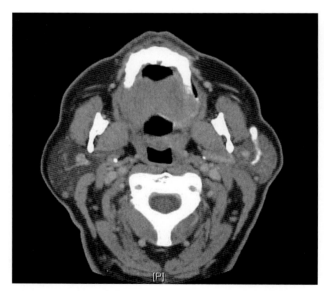

Figure 2.24. Parotid sialo-CT. Although the main duct is opacified, it is impossible to determine areas of stenosis and/or dilatation.

collections of contrast within the parenchyma of the salivary gland without interconnecting ducts. Advanced imaging techniques such as ultrasound, MRI, and CT have attempted to demonstrate these findings, but ultimately conventional sialography has proven to be the technique of choice for definitive imaging of patients afflicted with Sjögren syndrome.

In addition to conventional sialography, MR sialography, CT sialography (Figure 2.24), and digital subtraction sialography are also available. Each of these methods attempts to better identify the primary and secondary ductal systems and thus better define the exact nature of the clinical salivary malady.

Digital subtraction sialography utilizes the images obtained from conventional sialography and masks out the underlying osseous structures by means of computer revision to better visualize the duct system. This type of examination is more time consuming and can be quite difficult to interpret except by very experienced radiographers. In addition, this technique is considerably more expensive than conventional sialography and often without significant clinical benefit.

CT sialography allows better visualization of gland parenchyma and is widely available in many larger medical centers. In this method, contrast medium is injected into the primary duct followed by a CT exam. Contemporary multi-detector computed tomography allows reconstruction or reformatting of the original axial CT image into images representing many orthogonal planes. The major disadvantage of this method is one cannot visualize the dynamic duct filling and thus inadvertent overpressure may cause duct damage or rupture. In addition, it is very difficult to distinguish duct stenosis from anatomic variances of the normal duct system.

MR sialography (MRSIAL) appears to delineate the salivary ductal system as well as conventional sialography without the need of duct catheterization and subsequent contrast administration. Fluid-sensitive MR sequences now obviate this clinical need. MR can detect obstructions, stenosis, and strictures of the primary, secondary, and often tertiary ducts as well as conventional sialography. In addition, advances in 3D MRI will allow the production of virtual endoscopic views from available MR data. This noninvasive procedure does not depend on operator skill for definitive imaging. By using a heavily T2 weighted sequence, hyperintense saliva is visualized within the ductal system. This salivary flow functions much as does contrast during the conventional sialogram, thus allowing the detection of morphologic ductal alterations as well as parenchymal changes. Such studies have been shown to be helpful in not only obstructive salivary gland disease but also parenchymal diseases such as Sjögren syndrome (SS) (Andre' et al. 2021). It has been recently shown that MRSIAL is more sensitive in the detection of SS, than ultrasound (US). This technique also produces less false negatives than other imaging modalities. The major disadvantages of MRSIAL appear to be the much higher cost of both the equipment needed for the exam and the professional cost of the imaging exam itself.

IMAGE-GUIDED BIOPSIES OF SALIVARY GLAND PATHOLOGY

Salivary gland tumors are relatively rare, yet they encompass a wide range of benign and malignant diagnoses. Even though most of the primary tumors are epithelial in origin, the histology is often very diverse and complicated. Such diversity presents a diagnostic challenge to most contemporary pathologists.

To ensure proper surgical/medical intervention, a definitive diagnosis of parotid and other salivary gland masses is essential (Haldar et al. 2016). The primary techniques involved in such undertakings include (i) preoperative needle biopsy, both fine needle or core needle; (ii) intraoperative frozen section; and (iii) open biopsy or definitive excision. Clinicians have various imaging techniques that can be employed in conjunction with these invasive diagnostic procedures.

A surgical open biopsy has historically been used for obtaining biopsy tissue and providing a microscopic diagnosis of salivary gland neoplasia. In the early and mid-1980s, incisional biopsy of salivary gland tumors fell out of favor due to several factors including tumor seeding of the adjacent soft tissues, transient or permanent nerve damage of the facial nerve, and sialocele formation.

Needle biopsies of salivary gland, both fine needle (FNA) and core biopsies are utilized in most imaging facilities (Novoa et al. 2015). These procedures, particularly the FNA, are minimally invasive and most often will be completed with only local anesthesia. Imaging for such needle biopsies can now be accomplished with several imaging modalities including computerized tomography (CT), magnetic resonance (MR), and/or ultrasound (US). For very superficial lesions, hand-pressure localization without concurrent imaging will also accomplish the same objective in a short period. FNA biopsies were originally used in the late 1970s and proved a safe and accurate procedure in the hands of a well-trained cytopathology center. It has been demonstrated that such biopsies are often associated with inaccurate diagnoses outside such centers.

The most commonly performed salivary gland biopsy technique is the core needle biopsy, particularly when associated with US guidance (Figure 2.25). This method has gained great acceptance in the pathology, imaging, and surgical arenas. Ultrasound (US) has become the preferred imaging study of choice principally because it does not produce radiation to the patient as does CT, nor is US as time consuming and expensive as MRI (Kim and Kim 2018). Currently, US imaging when used with a core needle biopsy has been proven to produce accurate diagnoses with a high sensitivity and specificity. In their meta-analysis, Kim and Kim (2018) reviewed 10 observational studies and identified a sensitivity and specificity for the diagnosis of salivary gland pathology of 94 and 98%, respectively. Seven hematomas, one instance of temporary facial nerve paralysis thought to be caused by the local anesthesia, and no tumor seeding were reported from a total of 1315 procedures. Witt and Schmidt (2014) performed a systematic review and meta-analysis of ultrasound-guided core needle biopsy of salivary gland lesions. Five studies qualified for inclusion after an initial search of 7132 studies. The sensitivity and specificity of core needle biopsy were 96 and 100%, respectively in a total of 512 procedures, 88% of which were performed on the parotid gland and 12% were performed on the submandibular gland. The authors reported eight hematomas and one case of temporary facial nerve weakness secondary to local anesthesia. The authors concluded that the procedure is highly sensitive and specific and associated with a low risk of complications.

RADIONUCLIDE IMAGING (RNI)

Radionuclide imaging (RNI) has, throughout its history, been a functional imaging modality without the quality of anatomic depiction when compared with CT, MRI, or even US. Most radionuclide imaging has been performed with planar imaging systems, which produce single view images of functional processes. All RNI exams employ a radioactive tracer either bound to a ligand (radiopharmaceutical) or injected directly (radionuclide). As the radionuclide undergoes radioactive decay, it emits either a gamma ray (photon), and/or a particle such as an alpha particle (helium nucleus), beta particle (electron), or a positron (a positively charged electron). Gamma rays differ from X-rays in that, gamma rays (for medical imaging) are an inherent nuclear event and are emitted from the nucleus of an unstable atom to achieve stability. X-rays (in the conventional sense) are produced in the electron cloud surrounding the nucleus. In medical imaging, X-rays are artificially or intentionally produced on demand, whereas gamma rays (and other particles) are part of an ongoing nuclear decay, enabling unstable radioactive atoms to reach a stable state. The length of time it takes for one half of the unstable atoms to reach their stable state is called their half-life. Radionuclide imaging involves the emission of a photon that is imaged using a crystal or solid-state detector. The detector may be static and produces images of the event in a single plane or the detector may be rotated about the patient to gather three-dimensional data and reconstruct a tomographic image in the same manner as a CT scanner. This is the basis for single photon emission computed tomography (SPECT). Examples of planar images used in salivary gland diseases include gallium (^{67}Ga) for evaluation of inflammation, infection, and neoplasms (lymphoma). SPECT, which produces tomographic cross-sectional images, is less commonly used in oncologic imaging, although novel radionuclides and ligands are under investigation. The recent introduction of SPECT/CT, a combined functional and anatomic imaging machine may breathe new life into SPECT imaging.

POSITRON EMISSION TOMOGRAPHY (PET)

Positron emission tomography (PET) is a unique imaging modality that records a series of radioactive decay events. Positron emission is a form of radioactive decay in which a positron (positively charged electron) is emitted from the unstable atom to achieve a more stable state. The positron almost immediately collides with an electron (negatively charged) and undergoes

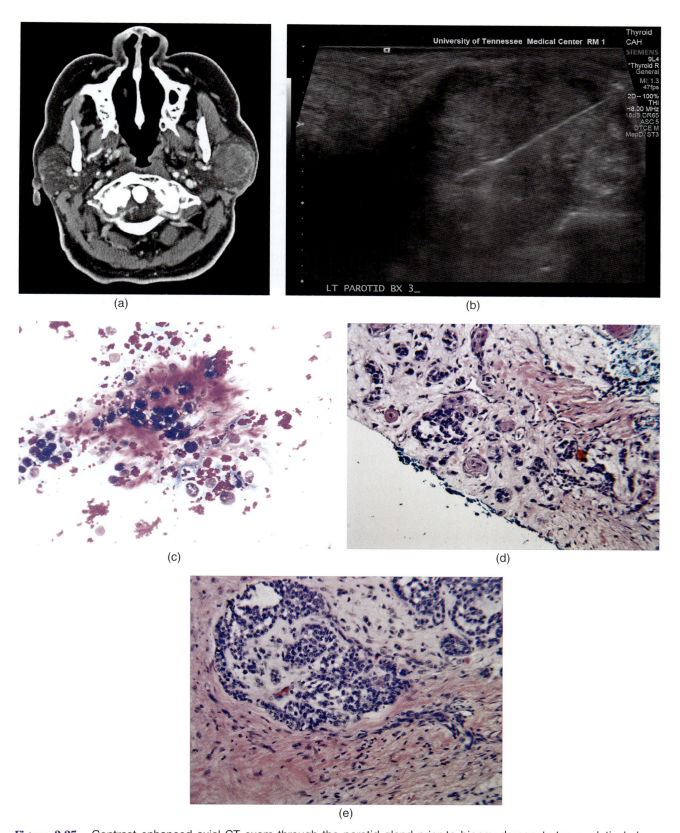

Figure 2.25. Contrast-enhanced axial CT exam through the parotid gland prior to biopsy demonstrates a relatively large heterogeneous mass with ill-defined borders (a). (b) Ultrasound-guided core needle biopsy. Note the biopsy needle passing into the hyperechoic mass within the parotid gland. (c) Fine needle aspiration biopsy: Note the darkly staining cells that appear atypical. A definitive diagnosis cannot be reached utilizing this cryptologic material. (d) Core needle biopsy. Note the darkly staining epithelial cells arranged in ductal groups. This biopsy was consistent with an atypical mixed tumor. (e) Surgical material from a parotidectomy. This lesion represents a carcinoma ex. mixed tumor. Note the similar cells seen in the core needle biopsy.

an annihilation event in which both particles are destroyed and converted into pure energy. The annihilation event produces two gamma rays, each with 511 Kev (kilo electron volt) of energy, and traveling in 180-degree opposition. By using sophisticated solid-state detectors, and coincidence circuitry, the PET system can record the source of the event, thereby localizing the event in three-dimensional space. Using a complex algorithm similar to SPECT and CT, a three-dimensional block of data is produced and can be "sliced" in any plane, but most commonly in axial, coronal, and sagittal planes, as well as a maximum intensity projection (MIP) rendering.

PET radionuclides are produced in a cyclotron and are relatively short lived. Typical radionuclides include ^{18}F, ^{11}C, ^{15}O, ^{82}Rb, and ^{13}N. A variety of ligands have been labeled and studied for the evaluation of perfusion, metabolism, and cell surface receptors. The most commonly available is ^{18}F-deoxyglucose (FDG), which is used to study glucose metabolism of cells. Most common uses of FDG include oncology, cardiac viability, and brain metabolism. PET has a higher spatial resolution than SPECT. Both systems are prone to multiple artifacts, especially motion. Acquisition times for both are quite long, limiting the exam to patients who can lie still for prolonged periods of time. Both systems, but PET in particular, are very costly to install and maintain. Radiopharmaceuticals are now widely available to most institutions through a network of nuclear pharmacies.

The oncologic principle behind FDG PET is that neoplastic tissues can have a much higher metabolism than normal tissues and utilize glucose at a higher rate (Warburg 1925). Glucose metabolism in the brain was extensively studied using autoradiography by Sokoloff and colleagues at The National Institutes of Health (NIH) (Sokoloff 1961). The deoxyglucose metabolism is unique in that it mimics glucose and is taken up by cells using the same transporter proteins. Both glucose and deoxyglucose undergo phosphorylation by hexokinase to form glucose-6-phosphate. This is where the similarities end. Glucose-6-phosphate continues to be metabolized, eventually to form CO_2 and H_2O. Deoxyglucose-6-phosphate cannot be further metabolized and becomes trapped in the cell as it cannot diffuse out through the cell membrane. Therefore, the accumulation of FDG reflects the relative metabolism of tissues (Sokoloff 1986). The characteristic increased rate of glucose metabolism by malignant tumors was initially described by Warburg and is the basis of FDG PET imaging of neoplasms (Warburg 1925).

FDG PET takes advantage of the higher utilization of glucose by neoplastic tissues to produce a map of glucose metabolism. Although the FDG PET system is sensitive, it is not specific. Several processes can elevate glucose metabolism, including neoplastic tissue, inflammatory or infected tissue, and normal tissue in a high metabolic state. An example of the latter includes uptake of FDG in skeletal muscle that was actively contracting during the uptake phase of the study (Figure 2.26). Another peculiar hypermetabolic phenomenon is brown adipose tissue (BAT) FDG uptake (Figure 2.27). BAT is distributed in multiple sites in the body including interscapular, paravertebral, around large blood vessels, deep cervical, axillary, mediastinal, and intercostal fat, but is concentrated in the supraclavicular regions (Cohade et al. 2003b; Tatsumi et al. 2004). BAT functions as a thermogenic organ producing heat in mammals and most commonly demonstrates uptake in the winter (Tatsumi et al. 2004). BAT is innervated by the sympathetic nervous system, has higher concentration of mitochondria, and is stimulated by cold temperatures (Cohade et al. 2003a; Tatsumi et al. 2004). Administration of ketamine anesthesia in rats markedly increased FDG uptake presumably from sympathetic stimulation (Tatsumi et al. 2004). Although typically described on FDG PET/CT exams, it can be demonstrated with ^{18}F-Fluorodopamine PET/CT, ^{99m}Tc-Tetrofosmin, and ^{123}I-MIBG SPECT as well as ^{201}TlCl, and ^{3}H-l-methionine (Baba et al. 2007; Hadi et al. 2007). Propranalol and reserpine administration appears to decrease the degree of FDG uptake whereas diazepam does not appear to have as significant an effect (Tatsumi et al. 2004). Exposure to nicotine and ephedrine also resulted in increased BAT uptake; therefore, avoiding these substances prior to PET scanning can prevent or reduce BAT uptake (Baba et al. 2007). Preventing BAT uptake of FDG can be accomplished by having the patient stay in a warm ambient temperature for 48 hours before the study and by keeping the patient warm during the uptake phase of FDG PET (Cohade et al. 2003a; Delbeke et al. 2006). Although somewhat controversial, diazepam or lorazepam and propranolol can reduce BAT uptake by blocking sympathetic activity, as well as reducing skeletal muscle uptake from

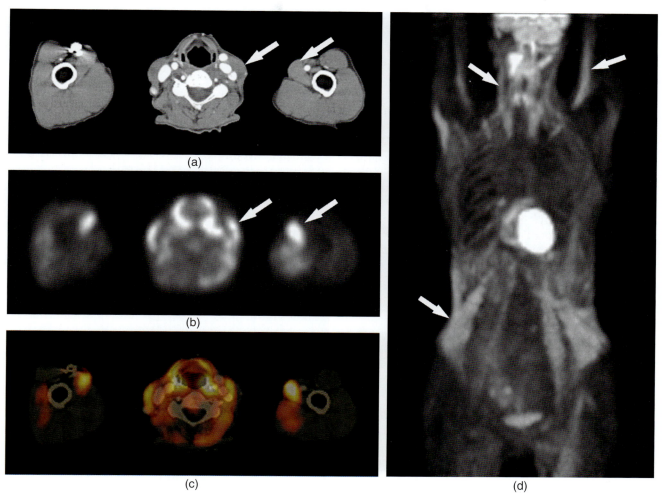

Figure 2.26. CT (a), PET (b), and fused PET/CT (c) images in axial plane and an anterior maximum intensity projection (MIP) image (d) demonstrating skeletal muscle uptake in the sternocleidomastoid muscle and biceps muscle (arrows). Note also the intense uptake in the abdominal, psoas, and intercostal muscles on the MIP image. The very high focal uptake in the middle of the image is myocardial activity.

reduced anxiety and improved relaxation (Delbeke et al. 2006). Understanding the distribution of BAT and the physiology that activates BAT, as well as recognizing the uptake of FDG in BAT in clinical studies, is critical in preventing false positive diagnosis of supraclavicular, paravertebral, and cervical masses or lymphadenopathy.

FDG uptake in all salivary glands in the normal state is usually mild and homogenous (Burrell and Van den Abbeele 2005; Wang et al. 2007) (Figures 2.28 and 2.29). After therapy, radiation or chemotherapy, the uptake can be very high (Burrell and Van den Abbeele 2005). Standardized uptake values (SUVs), a semiquantitative measurement of the degree of uptake of a radiotracer (FDG), may be calculated on PET scans. There are many factors that impact the measurement of SUVs, including the method of attenuation correction and reconstruction, size of lesion, size of region of interest, motion of lesion, recovery coefficient, plasma glucose concentration, body habitus and time from injection to imaging (Beaulier et al. 2003; Schoder et al. 2004; Wang et al. 2007).

A range of SUVs can be calculated in normal volunteers for each salivary gland. Wang et al. measured SUVs in normal tissues to determine the maximum SUV and mean SUV as well as assignment of an uptake grade ranging from none (mean SUV less than aortic blood pool) to mild (mean SUV greater than mean SUV of aortic blood pool

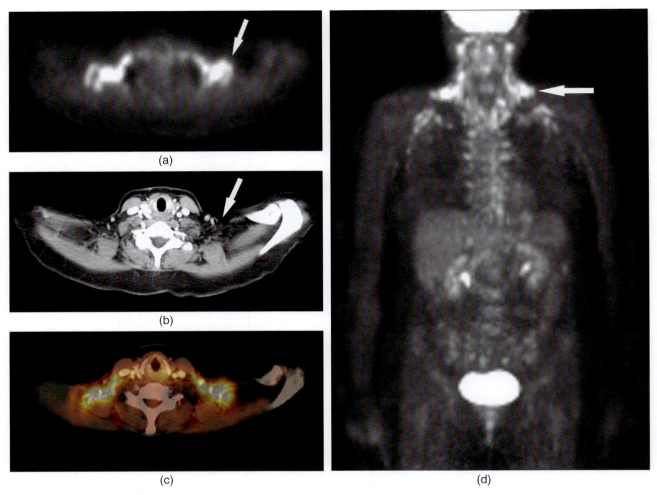

Figure 2.27. PET image (a), corresponding CT image (b) and a fused PET/CT image (c) in the axial plane demonstrating brown adipose tissue (BAT) uptake in the supraclavicular regions bilaterally, which could mimic lymphadenopathy (see arrows on a and b). Direct correlation enabled by the PET/CT prevents a false positive finding. Note the similar uptake on the MIP image (arrow) (d) including paraspinal BAT uptake.

but less than 2.5), moderate (mean SUV between 2.5 and 5.0), and intense (mean SUV greater than 5.0). SUV greater than 2.5 was considered significant (Wang et al. 2007). Parotid glands ($n = 97$) had a range of SUVmax of 0.78–20.45 and a SUVmean range of 1.75 ± 0.79. Fifty-three percent of the SUV measurements fell into the "none" category, 33% into the "mild" category, and 14% into the "moderate" category. No SUV measurement fell into the "intense" category. Submandibular glands ($n = 99$) had a SUVmax range of 0.56–5.14 and a SUVmean of 2.22 ± 0.77. The uptake grades consisted of the following: 25% were in the "none" category, 44% in the "mild," and 31% were in the "moderate." The sublingual gland ($n = 102$) had a SUVmax range of 0.93–5.91 and a SUVmean of 4.06 ± 1.76. Four percent of these fell into the "none" category, 19% in the "mild," 54% in the "moderate," and 23% in the "intense" group (Wang et al. 2007). Similar work by Nakamoto et al. demonstrated SUVmean of 1.9 ± 0.68 for the parotid gland, 2.11 ± 0.57 for the submandibular gland and 2.93 ± 1.39 for the sublingual gland (Nakamoto et al. 2005). This demonstrates the wide range of normal uptake values (Table 2.3).

Although, FDG does accumulate in the saliva, the concentration varies from 0.2–0.4 SUV but does not influence FDG imaging (Stahl et al. 2002).

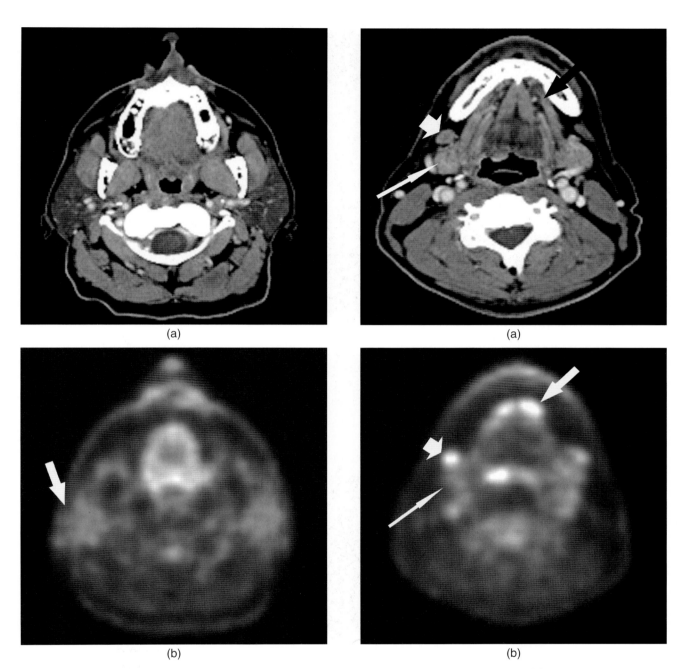

Figure 2.28. CT (a) and PET (b) images in axial plane demonstrating normal parotid gland activity (arrow).

Figure 2.29. CT (a) and PET (b) images in axial plane demonstrating normal submandibular (long thin arrow) and sublingual gland (medium arrow) activity. Note the abnormal uptake higher than and anterior to the submandibular glands (short fat arrow). Metastatic lymphadenopathy was diagnosed at the time of surgery.

SUV of greater than 2.5 has become a threshold for abnormal or neoplastic uptake (originally described by Patz et al.) (Patz et al. 1993; Wang et al. 2007). However, careful analysis must be undertaken when evaluating lesions based on SUVs as there is a significant overlap of SUVs for malignant and benign tumors and inflammatory conditions. One cannot depend on SUV measurements alone, and must take into consideration clinical data as well as radiologic imaging findings.

Table 2.3. Standard uptake value (SUV) of salivary glands.

Gland	SUV max (range)[a]	SUV mean ± SD[a]	SUV mean ± SD[b]
Parotid gland	0.78–20.45	1.75 ± 0.79	1.90 ± 0.68
Submandibular gland	0.56–5.14	2.22 ± 0.77	2.11 ± 0.57
Sublingual gland	0.93–5.91	4.06 ± 1.76	2.93 ± 1.39

[a] Wang (2007).
[b] Nakamoto (2005).
SD = standard deviation. Source: Data from Wang et al. (2007) and Nakamoto et al. (2005).

POSITRON EMISSION TOMOGRAPHY/ COMPUTED TOMOGRAPHY (PET/CT)

Head and neck imaging has greatly benefited from the use FDG PET imaging for the staging, restaging, and follow-up of neoplasms. The recent introduction of PET/CT has dramatically changed the imaging of diseases of the head and neck by directly combining anatomic and functional imaging.

The evaluation of the head and neck with FDG PET/CT has been significantly and positively affected with detection and demonstration of the extent of primary disease, lymphadenopathy, and scar versus recurrent or residual disease, pre-surgical staging, pre-radiosurgery planning and follow-up post-therapy.

The role of FDG PET or PET/CT and that of conventional CT and MRI on the diagnosis, staging, restaging, and follow-up post-therapy of salivary gland tumors has been studied (Keyes et al. 1994; Bui et al. 2003; Otsuka et al. 2005; Alexander de Ru et al. 2007; Roh et al. 2007). Although both CT and MRI are relatively equal in anatomic localization of disease and the effect of the tumors on local invasion and cervical nodal metastases, FDG PET/CT significantly improved sensitivity and specificity for salivary malignancies including nodal metastases (Otsuka et al. 2005; Uchida et al. 2005; Alexander de Ru et al. 2007; Jeong et al. 2007; Roh et al. 2007).

Early studies have demonstrated FDG PET's relative inability to distinguish benign from malignant salivary neoplasms (Keyes et al. 1994). The variable uptake of FDG by pleomorphic adenomas and the increased uptake and SUVs by Warthin tumors result in significant false positives (Jeong et al. 2007; Roh et al. 2007). In a similar manner, adenoid cystic carcinomas, which are relatively slower growing, may not accumulate significant concentrations of FDG and demonstrate low SUVs and therefore contribute to the false negatives (Jeong et al. 2007; Keyes et al. 1994). False negatives may also be caused by the relatively lower mean SUV of salivary tumors (SUV 3.8 ± 2.1) relative to squamous cell carcinoma (SUV 7.5 ± 3.4) (Roh et al. 2007). The low SUV of salivary neoplasms may also be obscured by the normal uptake of FDG by salivary glands (Roh et al. 2007). In general, FDG PET has demonstrated that lower grade malignancies tend to have lower SUV and vice versa for higher grade malignancies (Jeong et al. 2007; Roh et al. 2007). FDG PET has been shown to be more sensitive and specific compared to conventional CT or MRI (Otsuka et al. 2005; Cermik et al. 2007; Roh et al. 2007). Small tumor size can contribute to false negative results and inflammatory changes contribute to false positive results (Roh et al. 2007). The use of concurrent salivary scintigraphy with ^{99m}Tc-pertechnetate imaging can improve the false positive rate by identifying Warthin's tumors and oncocytomas, which tend to accumulate pertechnetate (and retain it after induced salivary gland washout) and have increased uptake of FDG (Uchida et al. 2005).

Diagnostic Imaging Anatomy

PAROTID GLAND

The average adult parotid gland measures 3.4 cm in AP, 3.7 cm in LR and 5.8 cm in SI dimensions and is the largest salivary gland. The parotid gland is positioned high in the suprahyoid neck directly inferior to the external auditory canal (EAC) and wedged between the posterior border of the mandible and anterior border of the styloid process, sternocleidomastoid muscle, and posterior belly of the digastric muscle (Figures 2.17 through 2.19; 2.30 through 2.36). This position, as well as the

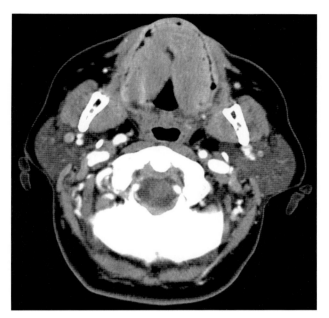

Figure 2.30. Axial CT of the neck demonstrates the intermediate to low density of the parotid gland.

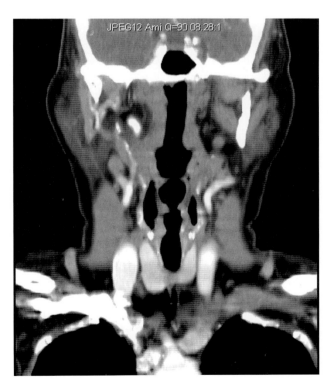

Figure 2.31. Reformatted coronal CT of the neck at the level of the parotid gland demonstrating its relationship to adjacent structures. Note the distinct soft-tissue anatomy below the skull base.

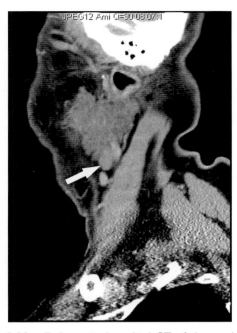

Figure 2.32. Reformatted sagittal CT of the neck at the level of the parotid gland demonstrating its relationship to adjacent structures including the external auditory canal. Note the slightly denser soft-tissue density in the parotid tail, the so-called "earring lesion" of the parotid gland. Cervical lymphadenopathy (arrow) was diagnosed at surgery.

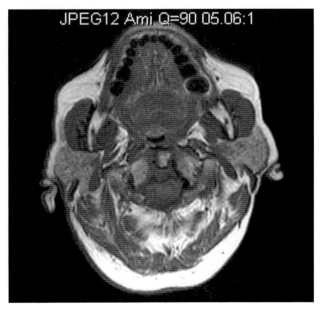

Figure 2.33. Axial T1 MRI image at the level of the parotid gland demonstrating the slightly higher signal as compared to skeletal muscle but less than subcutaneous fat.

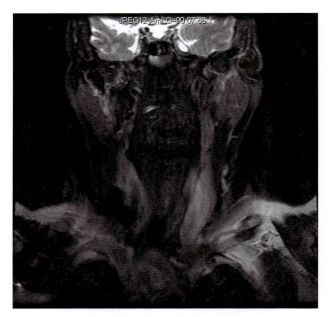

Figure 2.34. Coronal STIR MRI image at the level of the parotid gland demonstrating the nulling of the subcutaneous fat signal on STIR images and low signal from the partially fatty parotid gland.

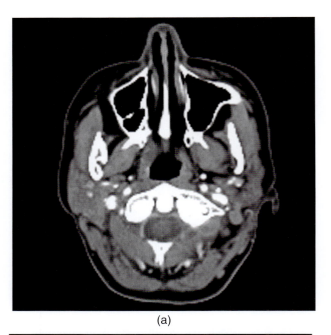

(a)

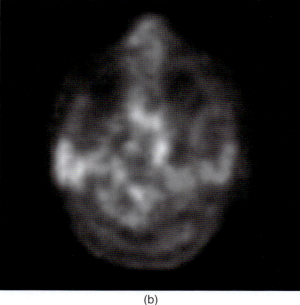

(b)

Figure 2.36. Axial CT scan (a) and corresponding PET scan (b) at the level of the parotid gland. Note the asymmetric slightly higher uptake on the right corresponding to partially resected parotid gland on the left, confirmed by CT.

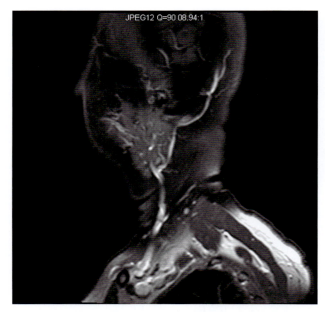

Figure 2.35. Sagittal fat suppressed T1 MRI image of the parotid gland demonstrating mild enhancement and lack of subcutaneous fat signal in the upper neck but incomplete fat suppression at the base of the neck.

seventh cranial nerve which traverses the gland, divides the gland functionally (not anatomically) into superficial and deep "lobes." Its inferior extent is to the level of the angle of the mandible where its "tail" is interposed between the platysma superficially and the sternocleidomastoid muscle (SCM) deep to the tail of the parotid. The parotid gland is surrounded by the superficial layer of the deep cervical fascia. The parotid space is bordered medially by the parapharyngeal space (PPS), the carotid space (CS), and the posterior belly of the digastric muscle. The anterior border is made up of the angle and ramus of the mandible along with the masticator space (MS). The posterior border is made up of the styloid and mastoid processes and the SCM. The gland traverses the stylomandibular tunnel that is formed by the posterior border of the mandibular ramus, the anterior border of the sternocleidomastoid muscle, the anterior border of the stylomandibular ligament, and the anterior border of the posterior belly of the digastric muscle and the skull base on its superior aspect (Som and Curtin 1996; Beale and Madani 2006). The external carotid artery (ECA) and retromandibular vein (RMV) traverse the gland in a craniocaudal direction, posterior to the posterior border of the mandibular ramus. The seventh cranial nerve (CN VII) traverses the gland in the slightly oblique anteroposterior direction from the stylomastoid foramen to the anterior border of the gland passing just lateral to the RMV. The seventh cranial nerve divides into five branches (temporal, zygomatic, buccal, mandibular, and cervical) within the substance of the gland. Prior to entering the substance of the parotid gland, the facial nerve gives off small branches, the posterior auricular, posterior digastric, and the stylohyoid nerves. The intraparotid facial nerve and duct can be demonstrated by MRI using surface coils and high-resolution acquisition (Takahashi et al. 2005). Because the parotid gland encapsulates later in development than other salivary gland, lymph nodes become incorporated into the substance of the gland. The parotid duct emanates from the superficial anterior part of the gland and is positioned along the superficial surface of the masseter muscle. Along the anterior aspect of the masseter muscle, the duct turns medially, posterior to the zygomaticus major and minor muscle to penetrate the buccinator muscle and terminates in the oral mucosa lateral to the maxillary second molar. Around 15–20% of the general population also has an accessory parotid gland which lies along the surface of the masseter muscle in the path of the parotid duct.

In the pediatric population, the parotid gland is isodense to skeletal muscle by CT and becomes progressively but variably fatty replaced with aging. The CT density will therefore progressively decrease over time (Drumond 1995). By MRI, the parotid gland is isointense to skeletal muscle on T1 and T2 weighted images, but with progressive fatty replacement demonstrates progressive increase in signal (brighter) similar to but remaining less than subcutaneous fat. Administration of iodinated contrast for CT results in slight enhancement (increase in density and therefore brightness). Administration of intravenous gadolinium (Gd) contrast results in an increase in signal (T1 shortening) and is therefore brighter on MRI scans. By US, the acoustic signature is isoechoic to muscle, but with fatty replacement becomes hyperechoic (more heterogenous gray). Therefore, masses tend to stand out as less echogenic foci. Normal uptake on FDG PET varies but is mild to moderate relative to muscle and decreases over age.

SUBMANDIBULAR GLAND

The submandibular gland (SMG) exists in the upper neck in the submandibular space (SMS) and the posterior oral cavity in the sublingual space (SLS). The SMG is more difficult to measure but the average adult superficial submandibular gland measures 3.5 cm in oblique AP, 1.4 cm in oblique LR, and 3.3 cm in SI dimensions. The gland "wraps" around the posterior border of the mylohyoid muscle and traverses the two spaces. The superficial portion is in the SMS adjacent to level one lymph nodes (level IB). The deep portion of the submandibular gland exists in the SLS. The SMS is bordered inferiorly by the hyoid bone and platysma and superiorly by the mylohyoid muscle. It is bordered laterally by the mandible and it is surrounded by the superficial layer of deep cervical fascia. Its medial border is a combination of the mylohyoid sling and anterior belly of the digastric muscle (Beale and Madani 2006) (Figures 2.37 through 2.43).

The submandibular duct emanates from the anterior-superior aspect of the gland and turns anteriorly and lies along the superior surface of the mylohyoid muscle between the genioglossus muscle medially and the sublingual gland laterally. The ducts open into the anterior medial (paramidline) floor of mouth at the sublingual papillae.

On CT scans the submandibular gland has a density that is isodense to slightly hyperdense relative to skeletal muscle. The gland does not become as fatty replaced as the parotid gland. The SMG demonstrates a signal characteristic like that of

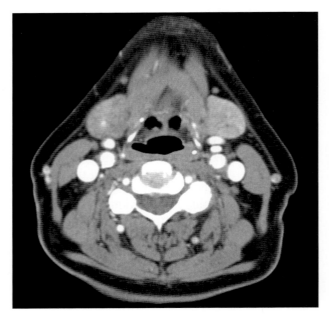

Figure 2.37. Axial CT at the level of the submandibular gland demonstrating density higher then skeletal muscle.

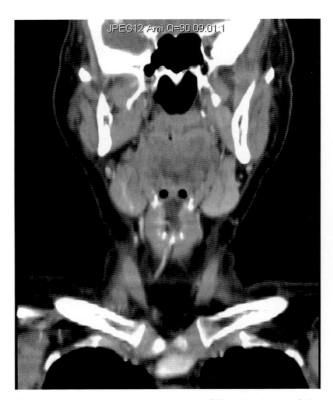

Figure 2.38. Reformatted coronal CT at the level of the submandibular gland demonstrating its relationship to the mylohyoid muscle and floor of mouth.

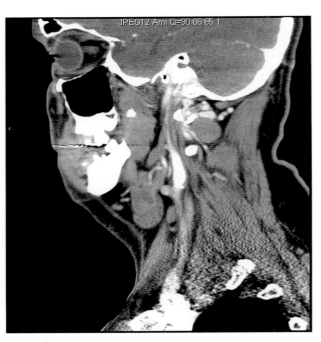

Figure 2.39. Reformatted sagittal CT at the level of the submandibular gland demonstrating its relationship to the floor of mouth. Note the slight notch at the hilum of the gland. Majority of the gland "hangs" below the mylohyoid muscle.

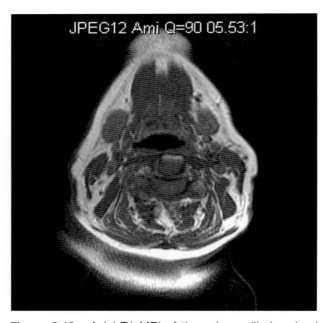

Figure 2.40. Axial T1 MRI of the submandibular gland demonstrating slight hyperintensity to muscle. Note the bright subcutaneous fat.

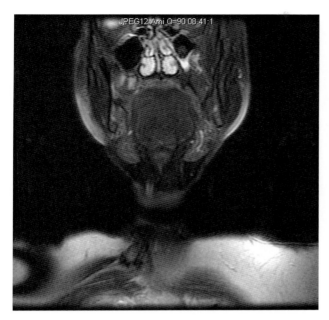

Figure 2.41. Coronal fat saturated T2 MRI of the submandibular gland. Note the slightly incomplete fat suppression and the engorged and edematous mucosa of the nasal cavity and turbinates.

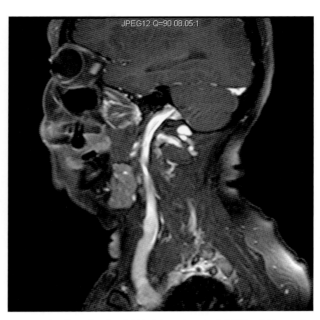

Figure 2.42. Sagittal T1 fat saturated MRI of the submandibular gland demonstrating the well-defined appearance on a fat suppressed background. Note the slight notch at the hilum. Note the entire internal jugular vein is visualized.

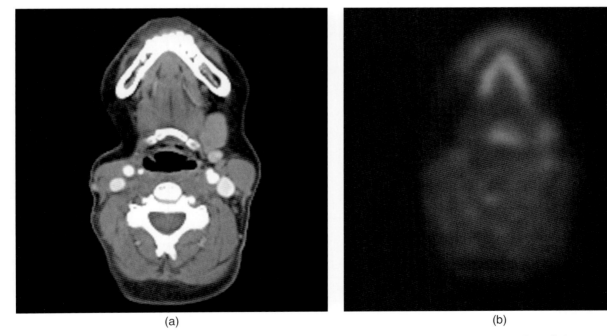

(a)   (b)

Figure 2.43. Axial CT (a) and corresponding PET (b) of the submandibular gland demonstrating slight normal uptake. Note the strong asymmetry of uptake on the PET corresponds to the absent submandibular gland on the right confirmed by the CT.

skeletal muscle on T1 and T2 weighted images and is less intense when compared to the parotid gland secondary to less fatty replacement. The FDG uptake is moderate but higher than that of the parotid gland. The SMG undergoes contrast enhancement by CT and MRI (Kaneda 1996).

SUBLINGUAL GLAND

The sublingual gland (SLG) is the smallest of the major salivary glands and is the least likely to be involved with pathology. The SLG measures an approximately 3.5 cm in oblique AP, 1.0 cm in oblique LR, and 1.5 cm in SI dimensions. Anatomically, the SLGs exist in the floor of mouth and lie on the superior surface of the mylohyoid muscle, bordered anteriorly and laterally by the mandible, and medially by the submandibular duct, genioglossus muscle, and geniohyoid muscle. The submandibular gland serves as its posterior border (Figures 2.44 through 2.46). The sublingual gland communicates with the oral cavity via multiple small ducts (ducts of Rivinus) opening into the floor of mouth adjacent to the sublingual papilla. These small ducts may be fused and form a larger single duct (duct of Bartholin) and empty into the submandibular duct (Beale and Madani 2006).

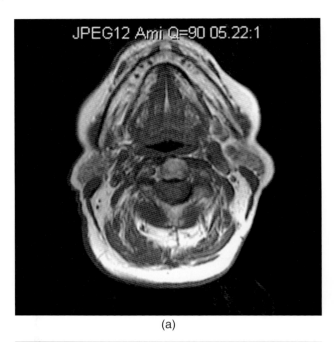

(a)

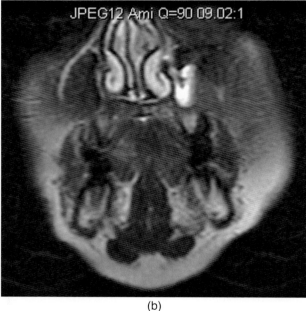

(b)

Figure 2.45. Axial contrast-enhanced T1 MRI of the sublingual gland demonstrating enhancement (a). Note the deep lobe of the submandibular glands seen at the posterior margin of the sublingual glands. Coronal T2 weighted image demonstrating the sublingual gland "cradled" between the mandible laterally, the genioglossus muscle medially, the geniohyoid muscle inferomedially, and the combined mylohyoid and digastric muscles inferiorly (b).

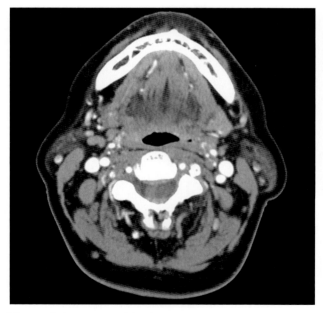

Figure 2.44. Axial CT of the neck at the level of the sublingual gland demonstrating mild normal enhancement along the lateral floor of mouth.

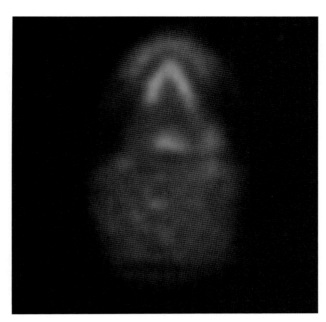

Figure 2.46. Axial PET of the sublingual gland demonstrating the intense uptake seen in the sublingual glands bilaterally medial to the mandible (photopenic linear regions).

The SLG can be seen by CT and MRI and is similar in appearance to the SMG, although smaller (Sumi et al. 1999a). FDG uptake is less well defined since it is small and closely approximated to adjacent skeletal muscle, but the uptake is moderate.

Occasionally, accessory salivary tissue is found in the SMS along the anterior aspect (anterior to the normal submandibular gland). This is caused by herniation of sublingual gland through defects in the mylohyoid muscle, called a mylohyoid boutonniere, which typically occurs between the anterior and posterior parts of the mylohyoid muscle. The accessory gland may be accompanied by sublingual branches of the facial artery and vein. Although the accessory tissue may mimic a tumor, this should be readily identified as normal since the accessory tissue has the same characteristics on CT and MRI as normal sublingual or submandibular gland (White et al. 2001; Hopp et al. 2004).

MINOR SALIVARY GLANDS

The minor salivary glands are unevenly distributed throughout the upper aerodigestive tract and are submucosal in location. They are more concentrated in the oral mucosa where they inhabit the mucosa of the hard and soft palate, buccal mucosa, floor of mouth, as well as the mucosa of the lips, gingiva, and tongue. They are also found in the pharynx (nasal and oral), sinonasal spaces, larynx, trachea, and bronchi. Functionally, they are either mucinous (predominantly in the palatal mucosa) or mixed seromucinous glands. The serous minor salivary glands are found only on the tongue at the circumvallate papilla. The minor salivary glands do not have large defined ducts but do contain multiple small excretory ducts. MRI of minor salivary glands has been achieved with high-resolution surface coils of the upper and lower lips. Patients with Sjogren disease had smaller gland area relative to normal, best demonstrated in the upper lip (Sumi et al. 2007).

Pathology of the Salivary Glands

Pathologic states of the salivary glands include tumors (epithelial and non-epithelial), infections and inflammation, autoimmune diseases, vascular lesion, and non-salivary tumors.

Of all salivary gland tumors, most (80%) are found in the parotid gland. The submandibular gland contains approximately 10% with the remainder in the sublingual and minor salivary glands. Of all parotid gland tumors, 80% are benign and 20% malignant. About 50% of submandibular gland tumors are benign and most of sublingual gland tumors are malignant. About 50% of minor salivary gland tumors are benign. The smaller the gland, the more likely that a mass within it is malignant. The pleomorphic adenoma and papillary cystadenoma lymphomatosum (Warthin tumor) account for most of benign salivary tumors, with the former being the more common at about 80% of benign and latter less common at about 15% of benign masses. Most of the malignant salivary gland tumors are represented by mucoepidermoid and adenoid cystic carcinomas.

Malignancies of the parotid gland may result in metastatic involvement of intraparotid and adjacent level II, and III jugular chain lymph nodes. The SMG drains primarily into adjacent level IB lymph nodes and then into the jugular chain and deep cervical nodes. The SLG drains into both level IA and IB nodes and then subsequently into the jugular chain and deep cervical nodes.

VASCULAR LESIONS

Lymphangioma (Cystic Hygroma)

The cystic hygroma is included in this discussion because of its transpatial location and that it might mimic other cystic masses. It is typically multilocular and has an epicenter in the posterior triangle, but may be found in the submandibular space and less commonly in the sublingual space. The imaging characteristics are those of cysts and follow fluid density on CT and signal intensity on MRI, although do typically demonstrate internal architecture from septation with varying thickness. CT typically demonstrates isodensity to simple fluid or slight hyperdensity if infected or contains products of hemorrhage (Koeller et al. 1999; Makariou et al. 2003) (Figure 2.47). US demonstrates anechoic spaces consistent with simple fluid with septa of variable thickness. Like cystic (and few solid lesions) lesions, there is increased thru transmission. Infection and hemorrhage cause variable degrees of echogenicity and thicker septations (Koeller et al. 1999; Makariou et al. 2003). MRI, however, can be variable on both T1 and T2 sequences based on the fluid characteristics. With simple fluid, T1 and T2 are isointense to simple fluid (CSF) but with infection, or hemorrhage products, the increased protein concentration as well as cellular debris and iron from hemoglobin can result in varying degrees of T1 hyperintensity and variable hypo- or hyperintensity on T2 (Figure 2.48). Any of these modalities may demonstrate fluid-fluid or fluid-debris layers. Both CT and MRI will demonstrate enhancement in the setting of infection (Macdonald et al. 2003). These lesions are more common in the pediatric age group, although small lesions may persist into adulthood. When found in the submandibular or sublingual space, they may be mistaken for a ranula (especially giant or plunging ranulae) and less likely hemangioma or thyroglossal duct cyst if midline (Kurabayashi et al. 2000; Macdonald et al. 2003). Although dermoids are in the differential diagnosis, they are usually identified by their imaging characteristics secondary to their contents of fat and dermal elements. Epidermoid cysts may be more difficult to differentiate from cystic hygromas and ranulae because of similar imaging characteristics (Koeller et al. 1999). Because the lymphangiomas have a vasculolymphatic origin, they may be associated with venous anomalies and rarely saccular venous aneurysms (Makariou et al. 2003).

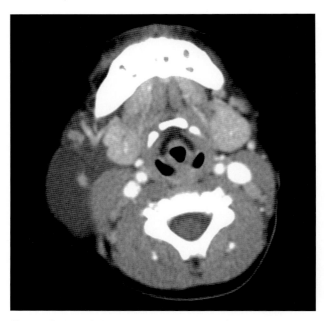

Figure 2.47. Axial contrast-enhanced CT of the neck at the level of the submandibular glands demonstrating a low-density structure on the right of approximately fluid density (compare to the CSF in the spinal canal), which is intermediate in density relative to the muscles and subcutaneous fat. A large lymphangioma associated with the right submandibular gland was diagnosed.

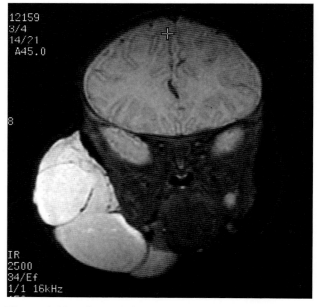

Figure 2.48. Coronal STIR MRI of the face of a different patient with a very large lymphangioma with large septations. Note the lymphangioma fluid is brighter than the CSF and there is fat suppression of the subcutaneous fat.

Vascular flow signals may be seen with Doppler US. The venous anomalies or aneurysms may be difficult to differentiate from other vascular malformations; however, their association with typical findings of lymphangiomas may assist in diagnosis.

Hemangioma

Hemangiomas are typically found in the pediatric age group. The majority are of the cavernous type and less likely the capillary type. They are best demonstrated by MRI and show marked enhancement. They are also very bright on T2 MRI. Foci of signal void may be vascular channels or phleboliths (Figures 2.49–2.51). They are typically slow flow lesions and may not be angiographically evident. US can vary from hypoechoic to heterogenous (Wong et al. 2004).

Other rare vascular lesions within salivary glands, most commonly the parotid gland, include aneurysms, pseudoaneurysms, and arteriovenous fistulae (AVFs). The aneurysms or pseudoaneurysms are most commonly associated with trauma or infection (mycotic). MRI in high flow lesions

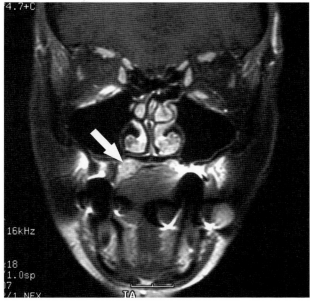

Figure 2.50. Coronal fat suppressed contrast-enhanced T1 MRI image corresponding to the same level as Figure 2.49, demonstrating a sharply marginated homogenously enhancing mass (arrow).

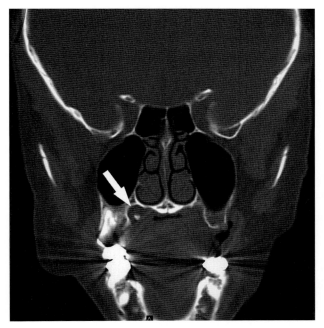

Figure 2.49. Direct coronal CT displayed in bone window demonstrating smooth erosion of the hard palate on the right lateral aspect, along with a dense calcification consistent with a phlebolith (arrow). A hemangioma is presumed based on this CT scan.

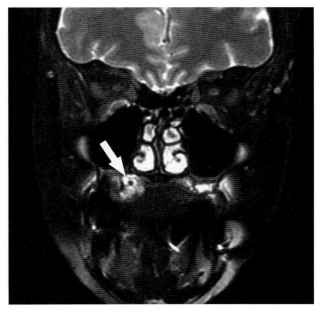

Figure 2.51. Coronal fat saturated T2 MRI image demonstrating a well-demarcated hyperintense mass with a focal signal void centrally. A hemangioma containing a phlebolith (arrow) was presumed based on this MRI.

demonstrates "flow voids" or an absence of signal but slow flow lesions or turbulent flow can demonstrate heterogenous signal mimicking a mass. Contrast enhancement and MRA can help delineate vascular lesions from masses. CT without contrast however demonstrates a mass or masses isodense to skeletal muscle or normal blood vessels. With contrast, large vascular channels become more obvious, although smaller lesions may still mimic a mass. US (especially Doppler US) can reveal characteristic flow patterns of arterial waveforms in the venous channels for AVFs. US can also delineate aneurysms with their turbulent flow patterns. Angiography is typically reserved for endovascular treatment. CTA or MRA is useful for noninvasive assessment of arterial feeders and venous anatomy in AVFs and in defining aneurysms (Wong et al. 2004).

ACUTE SIALADENITIS

Acute sialadenitis may be bacterial or viral in nature and may be a result of obstruction from a calculus, stricture or mass (see Chapters 3 and 5). Viral parotitis or mumps may be caused by a variety of viruses but most commonly the paromyxovirus is the culprit. The patient presents with an enlarged, tender, and painful gland. Acute suppurative parotitis (sialadenitis) presents in a similar manner as viral parotitis with the additional sign of purulent exudate. Oral bacterial pathogens are the causative agents, with staphylococcal and streptococcal species being the most common. CT scan demonstrates an enlarged gland with ill-defined margins and infiltration of the surrounding fat by edema fluid. The gland, especially the parotid, is increased in density because of the edema fluid, which is of higher density than fat. CT contrast demonstrates heterogenous enhancement and may show an abscess. On T1 MRI scan, the overall gland signal may be decreased slightly from the edema but does enhance heterogeneously with contrast. T2 MRI scan shows increased signal secondary to edema. Both CT and MRI may demonstrate enhancement and enlargement of the parotid (or sublingual) duct. US shows slight decrease in echogenicity relative to normal. These patterns are not unique to bacterial or viral infection or inflammation and may be seen with autoimmune diseases such as Sjögren syndrome or a diffusely

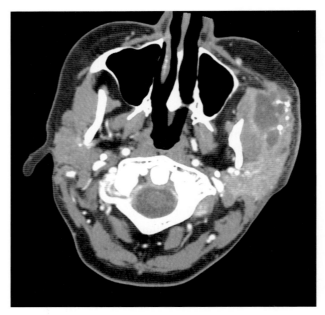

Figure 2.52. Axial CT with contrast at the level of the masseter muscles demonstrating a left accessory parotid gland abscess.

infiltrating mass. The surrounding subcutaneous fat also demonstrates heterogenous increased density from edema, resulting in a "dirty fat" appearance. There is also thickening of fascia and the platysma muscle (Shah 2002; Bialek et al. 2006; Madani and Beale 2006a).

With acute submandibular sialadenitis, the gland becomes enlarged and may be associated with a dilated duct if a sialolith is present. By CT, the calculus may be readily identified but not as easily seen by MRI. There may be varying degrees of cellulitis or frank abscess formation. The inflamed gland undergoes greater contrast enhancement. MRI demonstrates an enlarged heterogenous gland with dilated fluid-filled duct and gland which on T2 images is of high signal. On ultrasound, the acutely inflamed gland demonstrates enlargement with focal hypoechoic foci (Shah 2002; Bialek et al. 2006; Madani and Beale 2006a), (Figures 2.52 through 2.54).

CHRONIC SIALADENITIS

The etiology of chronic inflammatory states of the salivary glands varies by the specific gland in question. Chronic inflammatory changes in the

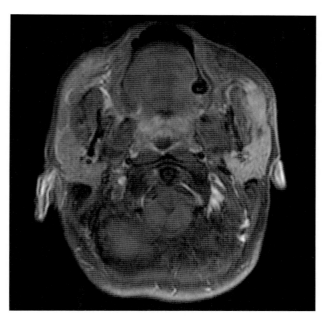

Figure 2.53. Axial contrast-enhanced fat saturated T1 MRI demonstrating heterogenous enhancement consistent with abscess of the left accessory parotid gland.

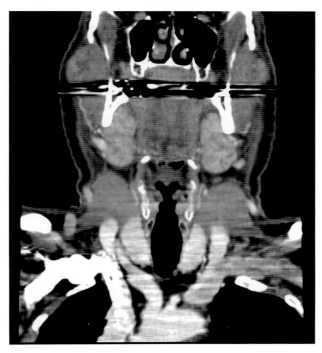

Figure 2.54. Reformatted coronal CT demonstrating enlargement and enhancement of the submandibular glands consistent with viral sialadenitis.

parotid gland tend to be related to autoimmune disease (Sjögren syndrome), recurrent suppurative parotitis, or radiation injury. Other etiologies include granulomatous infections such as tuberculosis or sarcoidosis. Chronic inflammation of the submandibular gland and, to a lesser degree, the sublingual gland is more commonly due to obstructive disease, particularly sialolithiasis. In the chronically inflamed state, the glands are enlarged but over longer periods of time progressively reduced in size, and heterogenous density may be seen on CT with extensive fibrosis and small focal (punctate) calcification. The density on CT is often increased due to cellular infiltration and edema during acute phases of exacerbation. The surrounding subcutaneous fat may not show signs of edema as is seen with acute sialadenitis. MRI demonstrates similar changes with heterogenous signal on both T1 and T2. The duct or ducts may be dilated, strictured, or both. Both may be visible by contrast CT and MRI (Sumi et al. 1999b; Shah 2002; Bialek et al. 2006; Madani and Beale 2006a). Chronic sclerosing sialadenitis (aka Kuttner tumor, or IgG4-related disease [see Chapter 6]) can mimic a mass of the salivary (most commonly submandibular) glands (Huang et al. 2002). It presents with a firm, enlarged gland mimicking a tumor. The most common etiology is sialolithiasis (50–83%) but other etiologies include chronic inflammation from autoimmune disease (Sjögren syndrome), congenital ductal dilatation and stasis, disorders of secretion (Huang et al. 2002). It is best diagnosed by gland removal and pathologic examination as fine needle aspiration biopsy may be misleading (Huang et al. 2002). Chronic sialadenitis can also be caused by chronic radiation injury. US studies have demonstrated a difference in imaging characteristics between submandibular sialadenitis caused by acalculus versus calculus disease. The acalculus sialadenitis submandibular gland US demonstrates multiple hypoechoic lesions, mimicking cysts, with diffuse distribution throughout a heterogenous hypoechoic gland. They did not, however, demonstrate increased thru transmission, which is typically seen with cysts and some soft-tissue tumors. Sialadenitis caused by calculus disease demonstrates hyperechoic glands relative to the adjacent digastric muscle, but some are iso- or hypoechoic relative to the contralateral gland (Ching et al. 2001).

HIV-ASSOCIATED LYMPHOEPITHELIAL LESIONS

These lesions are comprised of mixed cystic and solid masses within the parotid (much less in the SMG and SLG). CT shows multiple cystic and solid masses with associated parotid enlargement. IV contrast shows mild peripheral enhancement in the cysts and more heterogenous enhancement in the solid lesions (Figure 2.55). MRI images of the cysts are typical with low signal on T1 and high on T2. The more solid lesions are of heterogenous soft-tissue signal on T1 and increase on T2. Contrast MRI images follow the same pattern as CT (Holliday 1998). The US images show heterogenous cystic lesions with internal architecture of septation and vascularity and slightly hypoechoic signal of the solid masses. Mural nodules may be seen in predominantly cystic lesion. Associated cervical lymphadenopathy is commonly seen as well as hypertrophy of tonsillar tissues. Differential diagnosis of these findings includes Sjögren syndrome, lymphoma, sarcoidosis, other granulomatous diseases, metastases, and Warthin tumor (Kirshenbaum et al. 1991; Som et al. 1995; Martinoli et al. 1995; Shah 2002; Madani and Beale 2006a).

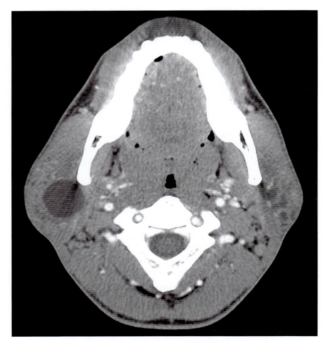

Figure 2.55. Axial CT demonstrating a large cystic lesion in the right parotid gland and multiple small lesions in the left parotid diagnosed as lymphoepithelial cysts.

MUCOUS ESCAPE PHENOMENA

The mucous escape phenomenon most commonly results from obstruction in the sublingual gland, resulting in a backup of salivary secretions (see Chapter 4). Ductal obstruction may be caused by calculi, stricture from prior infection or trauma. The chronic dilatation of the duct and accumulation of fluid produces a cystic mass by CT, MRI, and US. The simple ranula remains in the sublingual space and typically presents with a unilocular, well-demarcated and homogenous structure unless complicated by hemorrhage or infection. The walls may enhance slightly if a ranula remains contained above the mylohyoid muscle. It may rupture into the surrounding tissues and extravasate along a path of least resistance and extend inferiorly into the submandibular space or posteriorly into the parapharyngeal space under which circumstances it is termed a plunging ranula (see Chapter 4). The non-plunging ranula has a dilated ovoid configuration on axial images, but when it herniates into the submandibular space the dilated space shrinks into a tail-like configuration in the sublingual space. The tail sign is pathognomonic for ranulae and may be seen in both simple and plunging types. The ranula can usually be differentiated from a hemangioma and lymphangioma by its lack of internal architecture (unless complicated). The ranulas are typically homogenous internally with well-defined margins, unless infected or hemorrhagic, follow fluid density on CT (isodense to simple fluid) and intensity on MRI (low on T1 and high on T2). Both simple and plunging ranulae have these characteristics. The plunging component may be in the parapharyngeal space if the lesion plunges posterior to the mylohyoid muscle or in the anterior submandibular space if it plunges through the anterior and posterior portions of the mylohyoid muscle or through a defect in the muscle. Involvement of the parapharyngeal space and the submandibular space results in a large cystic mass termed "giant ranula" and may mimic a cystic hygroma (Cholankeril and Scioscia 1993; Kurabayashi et al. 2000; Macdonald et al. 2003; Makariou et al. 2003).

SIALADENOSIS (SIALOSIS)

Sialadenosis, also known as sialosis, is a painless bilateral enlargement of the parotid glands and less commonly the submandibular and sublingual glands (see Chapter 6). It is typically bilateral and without inflammatory changes. No underlying mass is present. It has been associated with malnutrition, alcoholism, medications, and a variety of endocrine abnormalities, the most common of which is diabetes mellitus. In the early stages, there is gland enlargement but may progress to fatty replacement and reduction in size by late stages. By CT, there is slight increase in density of the entire gland in the early setting but the density decreases in the late stage when the gland is predominantly fatty. On T1 weighted MRI images in the early stage, the gland demonstrates a slight decrease in signal corresponding to the lower fat content and increased cellular component. T2 images show a slight increase in signal (Som and Curtin 1996; Bialek et al. 2006; Madani and Beale 2006a).

SIALOLITHIASIS

Approximately 80–90% of salivary calculi form in the submandibular gland due to the chemistry of the secretions as well as the orientation and size of the duct in the floor of mouth. Eighty percent of submandibular calculi are radio-opaque while approximately 40% of parotid sialoliths are radio-opaque (see Chapter 5). CT without contrast is the imaging modality of choice as it easily depicts the dense calculi (Figures 2.56 through 2.58). MRI is less sensitive and may miss calculi. Vascular flow voids can be false positives on MRI. MR sialography as previously discussed may become more important in the assessment of calculi not readily visible by CT or for evaluation of strictures and is more important as part of therapeutic maneuvers. US can demonstrate stones over two millimeters with distal shadowing (Shah 2002; Bialek et al. 2006; Madani and Beale 2006a).

SJÖGREN SYNDROME

This autoimmune disease affects the salivary glands and lacrimal glands and is designated primary Sjogren if no systemic connective tissue disease is present but designated secondary Sjogren if the salivary disease is associated with systemic connective tissue disease (Madani and Beale 2006a). The presentations vary radiographically according to stage. Typically, early in the disease the gland may appear normal on CT and MRI. Early during

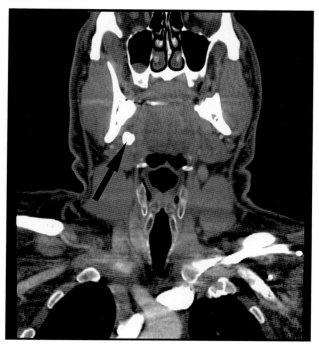

Figure 2.56. Reformatted coronal contrast-enhanced CT of the submandibular gland demonstrating a sialolith in the hilum of the right submandibular gland.

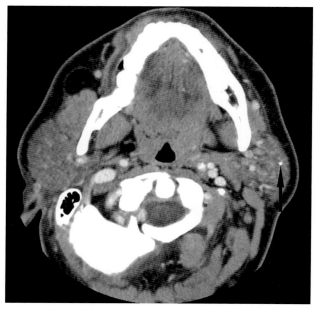

Figure 2.57. Axial contrast-enhanced CT of the parotid gland demonstrating a small left parotid sialolith (arrow).

the disease, there may be premature fat deposition, which may be demonstrated radiographically and may be correlated with abnormal salivary flow

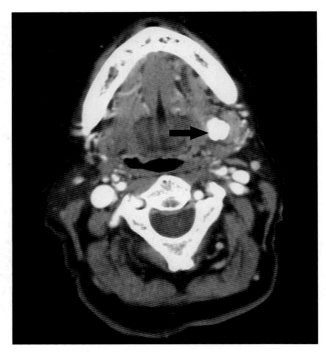

Figure 2.58. Axial contrast-enhanced CT at the level of the submandibular glands with a very large left hilum sialolith (arrow).

(Izumi et al. 1997). Also, in the early course of disease, tiny cysts may form consistent with dilated acinar ducts and either enlarge or coalesce as the disease progresses. These can give a mixed density appearance of the gland with focal areas of increased and decreased density by CT and areas of increased and decreased signal on T1 and T2 MRI, giving a "salt and pepper" appearance (Takashima et al. 1991, 1992). There may be either diffuse glandular swelling from the inflammatory reaction or this may present as a focal area of swelling. The diffuse swelling may mimic viral or bacterial sialadenitis. The focal swelling may mimic a tumor, benign or malignant, including lymphoma. Pseudotumors may be cystic lesions from coalescence or formation of cysts or dilatation of ducts, or they may be solid from lymphocytic infiltrates (Takashima et al. 1991, 1992). As glandular enlargement and cellular infiltration replaces the fatty elements, the gland appears denser on CT and lower in signal on T1 and T2 MRI. But when chronic inflammatory changes have progressed, tiny or course calcifications may develop. The cysts are variable in size, and the larger cysts may represent confluent small cysts or abscesses.

The CT and MRI appearance can be like that of lymphoepithelial lesions seen with HIV but does include calcifications. Typically, there is no diffuse cervical lymphadenopathy. The development of cervical adenopathy may indicate development of lymphoma (Takashima et al. 1992). Solid nodules or masses can also represent underlying lymphoma (non-Hodgkin type) to which these patients are prone (Sugai 2002). The latter stages of the disease produce a smaller and more fibrotic gland (Shah 2002; Bialek et al. 2006; Madani and Beale 2006a).

SARCOIDOSIS

Sarcoidosis is a granulomatous disease of unknown etiology (see Chapter 6). It typically presents with bilateral parotid enlargement. It may be an asymptomatic enlargement or may mimic a neoplasm with facial nerve palsy. The parotid gland usually demonstrates multiple masses bilaterally, which is a nonspecific finding and can also be seen with lymphoma, tuberculosis (TB) or other granulomatous infections, including cat-scratch disease. There is usually associated cervical lymphadenopathy. The CT characteristics of the masses are slightly hypodense to muscle but hyperdense to the more fatty parotid gland. MRI also demonstrates nonspecific findings. Doppler US demonstrates hypervascularity, which may be seen with any inflammatory process. The classically described "panda sign" seen with uptake of ^{67}Ga-citrate in sarcoidosis is also not pathognomonic for this disease and may be seen with Sjögren syndrome, mycobacterial diseases, and lymphoma.

CONGENITAL ANOMALIES OF THE SALIVARY GLANDS

First Branchial Cleft Cyst

This congenital lesion is in the differential diagnosis of cystic masses in and around the parotid gland along with lymphoepithelial lesions, abscesses, infected or necrotic lymph nodes, cystic hygromas, and Sjögren syndrome. Pathologically, the first branchial cleft cyst is a remnant of the first branchial apparatus. Radiographically, it has typical characteristics of a benign cyst if uncomplicated by infection or hemorrhage, with water density by CT and signal intensity by MRI. It may demonstrate slightly increased signal on T1 and T2 images if the protein concentration is elevated and may be heterogenous if infected or hemorrhagic. Contrast enhancement by either modality is seen if infection is present. Ultrasound demonstrates hypoechoic or anechoic signal if uncomplicated and hyperechoic if infected or hemorrhagic. There is no increase in FDG uptake unless complicated. Anatomically, it may be intimately associated with the facial nerve or branches. They are classified as type I (Figure 2.59) (less common of the two types) if found in the external auditory canal and type II if found in the parotid gland or adjacent to the angle of the mandible (Figure 2.60) and may extend into the parapharyngeal space. It may have a fistulous connection to the external auditory canal or the skin surface. Infected or previously infected cysts may mimic a malignant tumor. Although not typically associated with either the parotid or submandibular glands, the second branchial cleft cyst, which is found associated with the sternocleidomastoid muscle and carotid sheath, may extend superiorly to the tail of the parotid or anteroinferiorly to the posterior border of the submandibular gland. It has imaging characteristics like the first branchial cleft cyst. Therefore, the second branchial cleft cyst must be differentiated from cervical chain lymphadenopathy or exophytic salivary masses. The third and fourth branchial cleft cysts are rare and are not associated with the salivary glands and are found in the posterior triangle and adjacent to the thyroid gland, respectively (Koeller et al. 1999).

NEOPLASMS – SALIVARY, EPITHELIAL

Benign

Pleomorphic adenoma

Pleomorphic adenoma (PA) is the most common tumor of the salivary glands and is comprised of epithelial, myoepithelial, and stromal components. It is also the most common benign tumor of the minor salivary glands (Jansisyanant et al. 2002). Most commonly unilateral, lobulated and most commonly sharply marginated, the PA can vary in size and be up to 8 cm long and involve superficial and deep parotid lobes. The lobulated regions are sometimes referred to as a "cluster of grapes" (Shah 2002). The majority (80%) exist in the superficial lobe of the parotid gland. Small lesions are better circumscribed, have homogenous enhancement, and are of uniform soft tissue density (skeletal muscle). There can be mild to moderate enhancement and the lesion is relatively

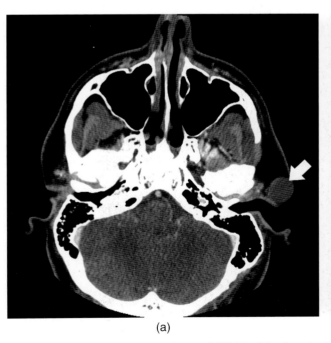
(a)

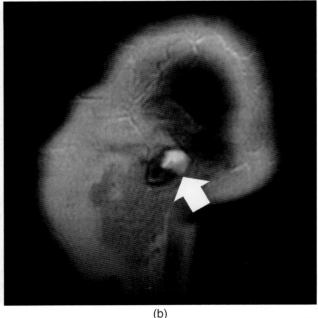
(b)

Figure 2.59. Axial contrast-enhanced CT (a) of the head with a cystic mass at the level of the left external auditory canal and sagittal T2 MRI of a different patient (b) consistent with a type 1 branchial cleft cyst.

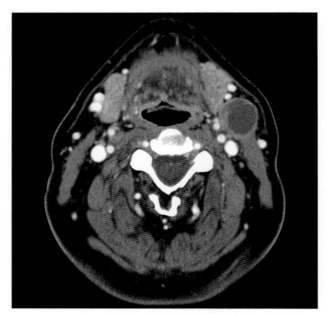

Figure 2.60. Axial contrast-enhanced CT of the maxillofacial soft tissues with a cystic mass interposed between the left submandibular gland and sternocleidomastoid muscle, consistent with a type 2 branchial cleft cyst.

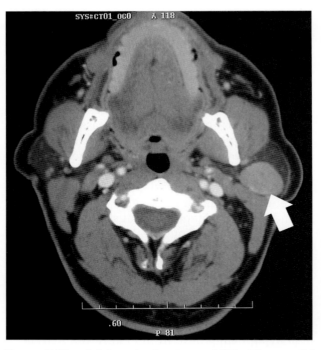

Figure 2.61. Axial contrast-enhanced CT of the parotid gland with a heterogenous mass with cystic changes. A pleomorphic adenoma (arrow) was diagnosed at surgery.

homogenous. The larger lesions have heterogenous density, enhancement pattern, and low attenuation foci from necrosis and cyst formation as well as calcification. The T1 signal can be as variable as the density on CT but tends to follow muscle or soft tissue signal against a background of fat of the normal parotid gland (Figure 2.61). The masses may be hypointense when small, and then become heterogenous with the cystic and calcific changes, and can be hyperintense secondary to areas of hemorrhage and calcifications. The T2 imaging characteristic is that of high signal intensity, with a thin low signal rim, except when hemorrhage may cause the signal to be heterogenous. The cystic or necrotic regions will tend to be low to intermediate signals on T1 and high on T2. There is mild homogenous enhancement when small and heterogenous when large. US usually demonstrates a homogenous hypoechoic mass but may also have heterogenous hypoechoic features with slight increase in thru transmission (Madani and Beale 2006b). These features may be shared with other benign and malignant lesions but only tumors that have both lobulation of the contour and a well-defined pseudocapsule are benign (Ikeda et al. 1996). The tumor components, cellular or myxoid, determine the MRI signal. The hypercellular regions have lower signal on T2 and STIR sequences as well as reduced ADC values on DWI and earlier TIC (time versus signal intensity curves) peak on dynamic MRI (Motoori et al. 2004). The high cellular components may be seen with other tumor types including malignant types. The myxoid components, which are more diagnostic of PAs, result in high T2 and STIR signal, high ADC values on DWI, and progressive enhancement on dynamic MRI (Motoori et al. 2004). In fact, of the three types of PAs, myxoid, cellular, and classic, the myxoid is the most common the most likely to recur (Moonis et al. 2007). MRI with T2 and STIR sequences has been shown to be quite sensitive in detecting recurrent PA of the myxoid type by demonstrating the focal, diffuse, or multifocal high signal of the myxoid material (Kinoshita and Okitsu 2004; Moonis et al. 2007). While most PAs demonstrate the benign and nonaggressive features of smooth margins and homogenous enhancement, the more aggressive and invasive features may be seen with carcinoma ex-pleomorphic adenoma, which is seen in areas of previously or concurrently benign PAs. Carcinoma ex-pleomorphic adenomas can result in distance metastatic foci, including the

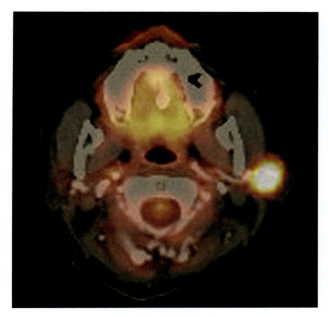

Figure 2.62. Axial PET/CT fused image demonstrating intense FDG uptake in a parotid mass. Pleomorphic adenoma was diagnosed at surgery.

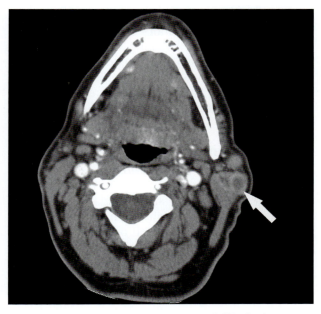

Figure 2.63. Axial contrast-enhanced CT of a heterogenous parotid mass at the tail of the gland, with multiplicity and cystic or necrotic changes, diagnosed as a Warthin tumor (arrow).

brain (Sheedy et al. 2006). Heterogeneous signal within PAs can indicate a concurrent high-grade malignancy, which can be low on T1 and T2 (Kinoshita and Okitsu 2004). FDG PET can be variable but tends to have increased uptake (Figure 2.62). Benignancy cannot be determined by imaging and therefore the differential includes primary parotid malignancy, metastases, and lymphoma as well as benign Warthin tumors (Shah 2002; Madani and Beale 2006b; Thoeny 2007).

Warthin tumor

Papillary cystadenoma lymphomatosum, or Warthin tumor, is the second most common benign lesion of the salivary glands. These tumors are typically well marginated but inhomogenous and found in the parotid tail of the superficial lobe and 15% present as bilateral or multicentric disease (Madani and Beale 2006b). There is by CT a heterogenous density and very mild enhancement (Figure 2.63). They typically have small cysts but do not demonstrate calcifications. The differential diagnosis therefore includes lymphoepithelial cysts, primary neoplasms, metastatic disease, and lymphoma. MRI signal on T1 is generally low but may be heterogenous, and T2 is either high signal based on its more cystic features or heterogenous. If the tumor is primarily solid, the imaging characteristics may mimic a PA with relatively homogenous hypoechoic architecture. Contrast with Gd follows CT characteristics. FDG uptake can be high on PET imaging. Warthin tumors contain oncocytes and are thought to be the mechanism by which they tend to accumulate ^{99}mTc-pertechnetate. The ^{99}mTc-pertechnetate uptake and retention after lemon juice-stimulated washout by the normal tissue is a good indicator of the diagnosis of Warthin tumor (Miyaki et al. 2001). This pattern is much less commonly seen by other lesions such as lymphoepithelial cysts, PAs, and oncocytomas. This technique allows visualization of Warthin tumors as small as 9 mm (Miyaki et al. 2001). By its peripheral location and cystic components, it can be mistaken for a necrotic lymph node or second branchial cleft cyst (Ikeda et al. 2004). The tail of the parotid region can be difficult to differentiate from adjacent cervical lymphadenopathy. However, coronal images can aid in determining the site of origin. If the lesion is medial to the parotid tail, it is more likely cervical jugular chain lymphadenopathy and if it is more laterally located, it is more likely an exophytic tumor from the parotid gland (Hamilton et al. 2003).

Oncocytoma

These relatively rare tumors exist primarily in the parotid gland. Their imaging characteristics are that of PAs except that they do accumulate ^{99m}Tc-pertechnetate. They are also reported to have high 18F-FDG uptake. They are considered benign but may have some invasive features.

Malignant Tumors
Mucoepidermoid carcinoma

Mucoepidermoid carcinoma is the most common malignant lesion of the salivary glands. They are also the most common salivary malignancy in the pediatric population. One half occur in the parotid gland and the other half in minor salivary glands (Jansisyanant et al. 2002; Shah 2002). The imaging characteristics of mucoepidermoid carcinoma are based on histologic grade. The low-grade lesions are sharply marginated and inhomogenous, mimicking PA and Warthin tumor. These well-differentiated lesions can have increased signal on T2 weighted sequences. The low-grade lesions are more commonly cystic (Madani and Beale 2006b). The high-grade, invasive lesions mimic adenoid cystic carcinoma and lymphoma or large heterogeneous PAs or carcinoma ex-pleomorphic adenoma. They tend to have a lower signal of T2. Contrast-enhanced studies demonstrate enhancement in the more solid components (Sigal et al. 1992; Lowe et al. 2001; Bialek et al. 2006; Madani and Beale 2006b) (Figures 2.64 through 2.66). Therefore, standard imaging cannot exclude a malignant neoplasm. Defining the tumor's extent is critical. Contrast MRI, especially in the coronal or sagittal plane, is essential to identify perineural invasion into the skull base.

Adenoid cystic carcinoma

Adenoid cystic carcinoma has similar characteristics as mucoepidermoid carcinoma in that their imaging findings are based on histologic grade. Adenoid cystic carcinoma is the most common malignant neoplasm of the submandibular and sublingual glands as well as the minor salivary glands in the palate. These tumors have a high rate of local recurrence, higher rate of distance metastases as opposed to nodal disease, and may recur after a long latency period (Madani and Beale 2006b). MRI is the imaging method of choice, demonstrating high signal due to increased water

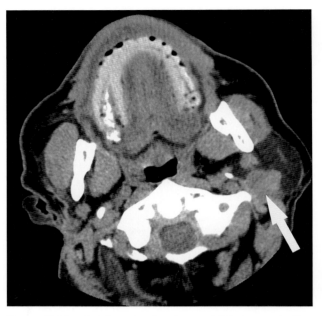

Figure 2.64. Axial contrast-enhanced CT demonstrating an ill-defined mass diagnosed as a mucoepidermoid carcinoma (arrow).

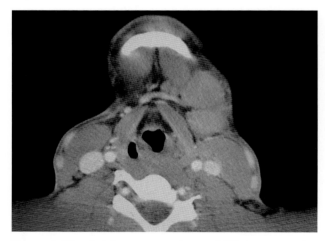

Figure 2.65. Axial contrast-enhanced CT demonstrating large bulky cervical lymphadenopathy with ill-defined borders, diagnosed as a mucoepidermoid carcinoma.

content. Contrast-enhanced fat saturated images are critical to evaluate for perineural spread, which is demonstrated by nerve thickening and enhancement (Madani and Beale 2006b; Shah 2002). CT can be helpful to evaluate bone destruction or foraminal widening. It is important to define the tumors' extent and identify perineural invasion into the skull base (Figures 2.67 through 2.71).

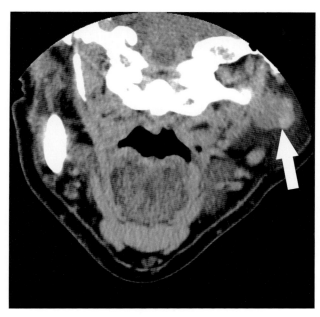

Figure 2.66. Reformatted coronal contrast-enhanced CT demonstrating an ill-defined heterogeneous density mass diagnosed as a mucoepidermoid carcinoma (arrow).

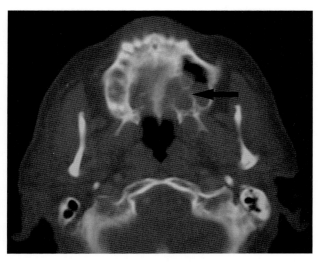

Figure 2.68. Axial CT in bone window demonstrating a mass eroding through the left side of the hard palate and extending into the maxillary sinus (arrow) diagnosed as adenoid cystic carcinoma.

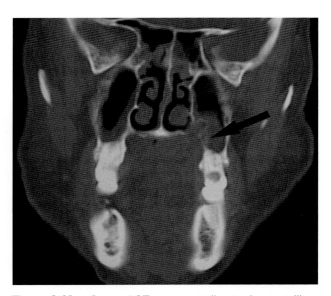

Figure 2.69. Coronal CT corresponding to the case illustrated in Figure 2.68 with a mass eroding the hard palate and extending into the left maxillary sinus (arrow).

NEOPLASMS – NON-SALIVARY

Benign
Lipoma
In the cervical soft tissues, lipomas are slightly more commonly seen within the parotid gland rather than periparotid. Lipomas of the salivary glands are uncommon (Shah 2002). The CT and

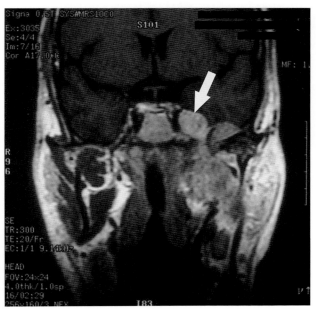

Figure 2.67. Coronal contrast-enhanced MRI of the skull base demonstrating a mass extending through the skull base via the left foramen ovale (arrow), diagnosed as an adenoid cystic carcinoma originating from a minor salivary gland of the pharyngeal mucosa.

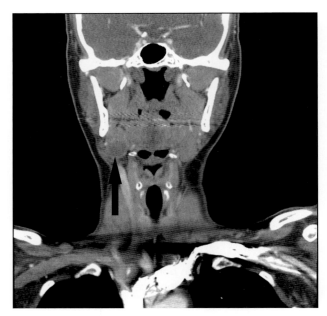

Figure 2.70. Reformatted contrast-enhanced coronal CT with a mass in the right submandibular gland (arrow) diagnosed as an adenoid cystic carcinoma.

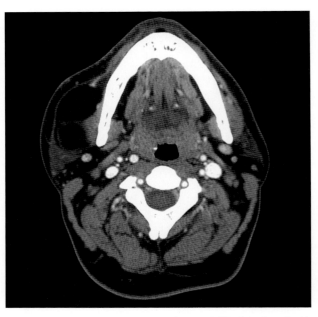

Figure 2.72. Axial contrasted-enhanced CT of the head with a fat density mass at the level of the parotid gland and extending to the submandibular gland, diagnosed as a lipoma.

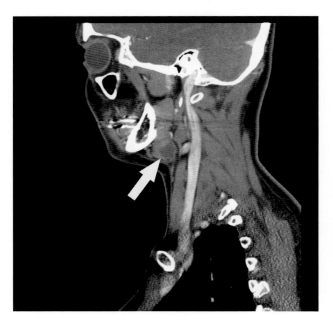

Figure 2.71. Reformatted sagittal contrast-enhanced CT corresponding to the case illustrated in Figure 2.65.

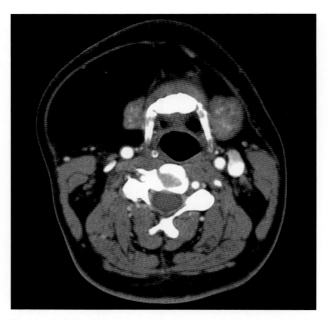

Figure 2.73. Axial contrast-enhanced CT through the submandibular gland with fat density mass partially surrounding the gland. A lipoma was diagnosed.

MRI characteristics are those of subcutaneous fat with CT density very low (approximately 100 H) and hyperintense on both T1 and T2. Lipomas tend to be echogenic on US. They may be uniform on imaging but may have areas of fibrosis. The heterogenous density from fibrosis, or hemorrhage, carries the additional differential diagnosis of liposarcoma or other neoplasms (Som et al. 1995), (Figures 2.72 and 2.73).

Neurogenic tumors

Neurogenic tumors are uncommon in the salivary glands but when encountered are most commonly found in the parotid gland. Most facial nerve schwannomas are on the intratemporal facial nerve with only 9% extra-temporal and in the parotid gland (Shimizu et al. 2005), (Figures 2.74 through 2.76). These are difficult to preoperatively diagnose as they do not typically present with facial nerve dysfunction. As seen in other parts of the body, they tend to be sharply marginated and have an ovoid shape along the axis of the involved nerve, such as the facial nerve. The CT density is that of soft tissue but post-contrast, both enhance (schwannoma slightly greater than neurofibroma). Both are noted as low signal on T1 and high on T2. MRI enhancement pattern follows that of CT. They may demonstrate a target sign appearance with peripheral hyperintensity relative to a central hypointensity (Martin et al. 1992; Suh et al. 1992; Shimizu et al. 2005). However, this sign is not pathognomonic and may be seen in schwannomas or neurofibromas. Increased uptake is seen on FDG PET in both diseases. The neurofibroma may be associated with Von Recklinghausen's disease. Although, most schwannomas and neurofibromas are benign, they are reported as demonstrating increased uptake (hypermetabolism of glucose) of 18F-FDG on PET imaging (Hsu et al. 2003). Although the calculated standard uptake value (SUV) can be helpful in differentiating benign from malignant lesions, there is a significant overlap (Ioannidis and Lau 2003). There is difficulty in

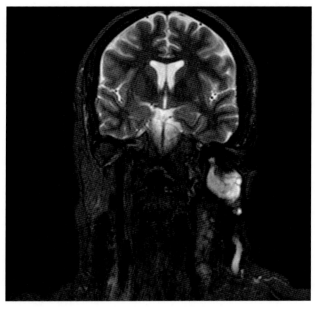

Figure 2.75. Coronal T2 MRI corresponding to the case illustrated in Figure 2.74.

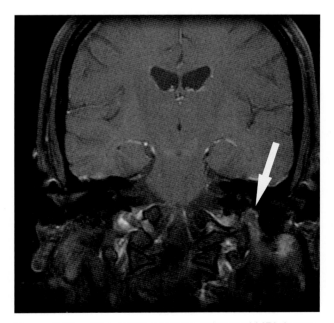

Figure 2.74. Coronal T1 contrast-enhanced MRI demonstrating a mass in the left parotid gland with smooth margins. The mass extends superiorly into the skull base at the stylomastoid foramen (arrow). A benign schwannoma was diagnosed.

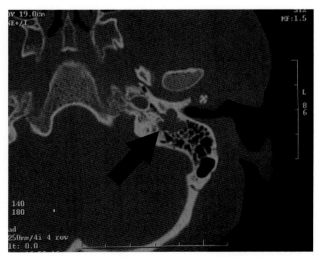

Figure 2.76. Axial CT at the skull base displayed in bone window showing dilatation of the stylomastoid foramen with soft tissue mass (arrow). A benign schwannoma was diagnosed.

separating low-grade malignant lesions from benign lesions (Ioannidis and Lau 2003), (Figures 2.77 and 2.78). Plexiform neurofibromas are also slow-growing and rare. They present with multiple cord-like masses and are far more common in the parotid gland relative to other salivary glands. By CT and MRI, they are sometimes described as a "branching" pattern or "bag of worms" secondary to the multiple lesions growing along nerve branches. They have CT and MRI signal characteristics like neurofibromas and schwannomas including the "target sign" (Lin and Martel 2001; Aribandi et al. 2006). The target sign may also be seen by US as a hypoechoic periphery surrounding a subtle and slightly hyperechoic center. There may also be slight increase through-transmission (Lin and Martel 2001).

Malignant
Lymphoma

Both primary and secondary lymphomas of the salivary glands are rare. Primary lymphoma of the salivary glands is the mucosa-associated lymphoid tissue subtype (MALT). MALT lymphomas constitute about 5% of non-Hodgkin lymphomas (Jhanvar and Straus 2006). These lymphomas are seen in the gastrointestinal tract and are associated with chronic inflammatory or autoimmune diseases. The salivary glands do not typically contain MALT but may in the setting of chronic inflammation (Ando et al. 2005). The MALT lymphomas found in the gastrointestinal tract are not typically associated with Sjögren syndrome. The MALT lymphoma, a low-grade B-cell type, tends to be a slow-growing neoplasm. Metastases tend to occur at other mucosal sites, a demonstration of tissue tropism. The MALT lymphomas are amenable to radiotherapy but can relapse in the contralateral gland, demonstrating tropism for the glandular tissue (MacManus et al. 2007). In Sjögren syndrome, there is an approximately 40-fold increased incidence of developing lymphoma compared to age-controlled populations. Of the various subtypes of lymphoma that are seen associated with Sjögren syndrome (follicular, diffuse large B-cell, large cell, and immunoblastic), the MALT subtype is the most common, at around 50% (Tonami et al. 2002). The parotid gland is the most commonly affected (80%). Less commonly, the submandibular and rarely the sublingual gland may be involved. Clinically, it may present with a focal mass or diffuse unilateral or bilateral glandular swelling.

[67]Ga-citrate scintigraphy had been the standard imaging modality used to assess staging and post-therapy follow-up for lymphomas (Hodgkin

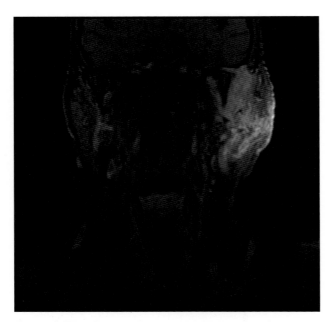

Figure 2.77. Coronal T1 contrast image showing a very ill-defined mass with heterogenous enhancement in the parotid gland with skull base extension via the stylomastoid foramen. A malignant schwannoma was diagnosed.

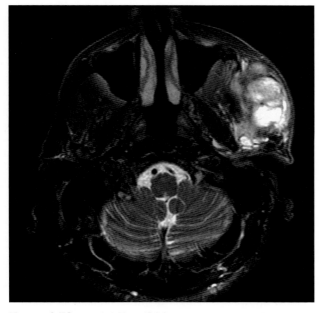

Figure 2.78. Axial T2 MRI image corresponding to the case illustrated in Figure 2.77.

and non-Hodgkin) for many decades. PET/CT with FDG is quickly becoming the standard for staging and follow-up for many lymphoma subtypes (Jhanvar and Straus 2006).

The imaging findings in salivary lymphomas, however, are not specific. CT may demonstrate focal or diffuse low- to intermediate-density mass with cystic areas and calcifications. MRI shows the soft-tissue areas to be isointense to skeletal muscle on T1 images and hypointense relative to fat on T2 images along with diffuse enhancement post-contrast (Tonami et al. 2002). Although, there may be cystic changes demonstrated by CT, MRI, or US, they are thought to be dilated ducts resulting from compression of terminal ducts (Ando et al. 2005). The US characteristics of MALT lymphoma may demonstrate multifocal hypoechoic intraparotid nodules and cysts (which may be dilated ducts) and calcification as well. Large B-cell intraparotid lymphoma has been described as hypoechoic, homogenous, well-marginated mass exhibiting increased thru transmission (a characteristic of cysts) and hypervascularity (Eichhorn et al. 2002). Although there are reports of hypermetabolism in MALT lymphomas, PET imaging findings are also not conclusive (MacManus et al. 2007). Uptake in the tumor and a background of chronic inflammatory changes of chronic sialadenitis may result in variably elevated uptake of FDG.

Secondary lymphomas (Hodgkin and non-Hodgkin) are also quite rare, with the histology most commonly encountered being of the large cell type. There is typically extra-glandular lymphadenopathy associated. The imaging features are also non-specific, although there is usually no associated chronic sialadenitis (Figures 2.79 through 2.81).

Metastases

Intraglandular lymph nodes are found in the parotid gland due to its early encapsulation during development. The sublingual gland and submandibular gland do not contain lymph nodes. The parotid and periparotid lymph nodes are the first order nodal site for lesions that affect the scalp, skin of the upper face, and external ear (Ollila et al. 1999). The most common malignancy to metastasize to the parotid nodes is squamous cell carcinoma followed by melanoma and, less commonly, Merkel cell carcinoma (Bron et al. 2003) (Figures 2.82 through 2.84).

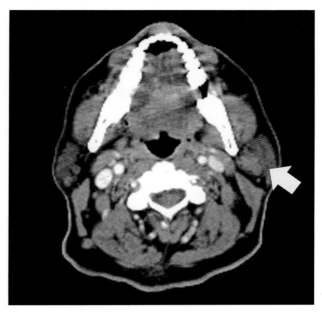

Figure 2.79. Axial CT scan with contrast at the level of the parotid tail demonstrating an ill-defined heterogeneously enhancing mass adjacent to or exophytic from the parotid tail medially (arrow). Lymphoma in cervical lymphadenopathy was diagnosed at surgery.

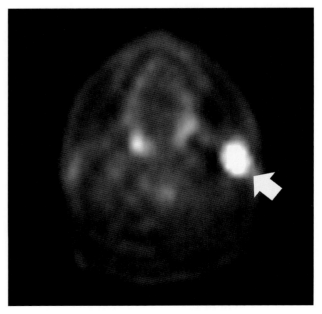

Figure 2.80. Axial PET scan image corresponding to the case in Figure 2.79. A large mass of the left parotid gland (arrow) is noted.

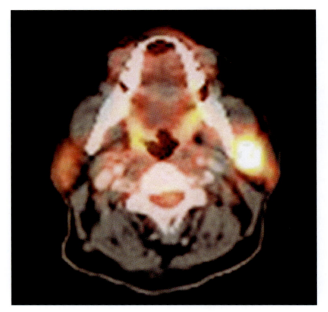

Figure 2.81. Fused axial PET/CT image corresponding to the case illustrated in Figure 2.79.

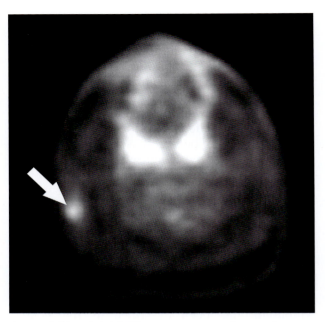

Figure 2.83. Axial PET scan corresponding to the case illustrated in Figure 2.82. The mass in the right parotid gland (arrow) is hypermetabolic. Note two foci of intense uptake corresponding to inflammatory changes in the tonsils.

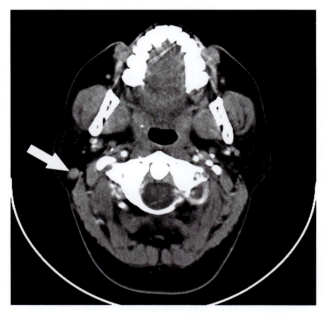

Figure 2.82. Axial CT of a mass in the right parotid gland with homogenous enhancement. The patient had a history of right facial melanoma. Metastatic melanoma was diagnosed at surgery.

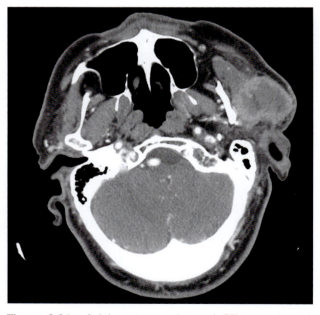

Figure 2.84. Axial contrast-enhanced CT scan through the parotid glands demonstrating a large mass of heterogenous density and enhancement partially exophytic from the gland. Metastatic squamous cell carcinoma from the scalp was diagnosed.

The imaging findings are not specific. CT in early stages demonstrates the nodes to have sharp margins, round or ovoid architecture but without a fatty hilum. Late in the disease, mass can mimic infected or inflammatory nodes with heterogenous borders, enhancement, and necrosis. Late in the disease with extranodal spread, the margins blur and are ill-defined. Contrast enhancement is heterogenous. Similar findings are seen on MRI with T1 showing low to intermediate signal pre-contrast and homogenous to heterogenous signal post-contrast depending on intranodal versus extranodal disease. PET with FDG is abnormal in infectious, inflammatory, and neoplastic etiology and is not typically helpful within the parotid, but can aid in localizing the site of the primary lesion as well as other sites of metastases. This can be significant since the incidence of clinically occult neck disease is high in skin cancer metastatic to the parotid gland (Bron et al. 2003). Local failure was highest with metastatic squamous cell carcinoma and distant metastases were higher in melanoma (Bron et al. 2003).

With either squamous cell carcinoma or melanoma, there is also a concern for perineural invasion and spread. Tumors commonly known to have perineural spread in addition to the above include adenoid cystic carcinoma, lymphoma, and schwannoma. The desmoplastic subtype of melanoma has a predilection for neurotropism (Chang et al. 2004). The perineural spread along the facial nerve in the parotid gland and into the skull base at the stylomastoid foramen must be carefully assessed. MRI with contrast is the best means of evaluating the skull base foramina for perineural invasion. Gadolinium contrast-enhanced T1 MRI in the coronal plane provides optimal view of the skull base (Chang et al. 2004). There may also be symptomatic facial nerve involvement with lymphadenopathy from severe infectious adenopathy, or inflammatory diseases such as sarcoidosis.

Summary

- Among the choices for imaging of the salivary glands, CT with IV contrast is the most commonly performed procedure. Coronal and sagittal reformatted images provide excellent evaluation soft tissues in orthogonal planes. The latest generation MDCT scanners provide rapid image acquisition, reducing motion artifact and produce exquisite multiplanar reformatted images.
- US has the inherent limitation of being operator dependent, poor at assessing deep lobe of the parotid gland, and surveying the neck for lymphadenopathy, as well as time consuming relative to the latest generation MDCT scanners.
- MRI should not be used as a primary imaging modality but reserved for special situations, such as assessment of the skull base for perineural spread of tumors. Although MRI provides similar information to CT, it is more susceptible to motion and has longer image acquisition time but has better soft-tissue delineation.
- PET/CT can also be utilized for initial diagnosis and staging but excels in localizing recurrent disease in postsurgical or radiation fields. Its limitations are specificity, as inflammatory diseases and some benign lesions can mimic malignant neoplasms, and malignant lesions such as adenoid cystic carcinoma may not demonstrate significantly increased uptake of FDG. A major benefit is its ability to perform combined anatomic and functional evaluation of the head and neck as well as upper and lower torso in the same setting. The serial acquisitions are fused to provide a direct anatomic correlate to a focus of radiotracer uptake.
- Newer MRI techniques such as dynamic contrast enhancement, MR sialography, diffusion weighted imaging, MR spectroscopy, and MR microscopy are challenging PET/CT in functional evaluation of salivary gland disease and delineation of benign versus malignant tumors. However, PET/CT with novel tracers may repel this challenge.
- Conventional radionuclide scintigraphic imaging has largely been displaced. However, conventional scintigraphy with ^{99m}Tc-pertechnetate can be useful for the evaluation of masses suspected to be Warthin tumors or oncocytomas, which accumulate the tracer and retain it after washout of the normal gland with acid stimulants. The advent of SPECT/CT in a similar manner to PET/CT may breathe new life into older scintigraphic exams.
- Radiology continues to provide a very significant contribution to clinicians and surgeons in the diagnosis, staging, and post-therapy

follow-up of disease. Because of the complex anatomy of the head and neck, imaging is even more important in evaluation of diseases affecting this region. The anatomic and functional imaging, as well as the direct fusion of data from these methods, has had a beneficial effect on disease treatment and outcome. A close working relationship is important between radiologists, pathologists, and surgeons to achieve these goals.

Case Presentation – *Duplicity*

A 58-year-old patient (Figure 2.85a–c) was referred regarding swelling of the left face. The patient's history of present illness included six weeks of a painless left facial swelling, and no associated fever or weight loss.

Past Medical History
Hypertension treated with metoprolol and quinapril
    Hypercholesterolemia treated with simvastatin
    Type 2 diabetes treated with Metformin

Social History
The patient is a smoker and has accumulated a 40-pack year history of cigarette smoking

Examination
The patient demonstrated an obvious mass of the left parotid region. There was no tenderness to palpation of the mass. There was no palpable mass of the right parotid gland. Cranial nerve VII was intact. Saliva was present at the left Stensen duct. There were no oral mucosal lesions and no oropharyngeal mucosal lesions.

Imaging
The patient had undergone a CT scan of the maxillofacial region prior to referral that identified multicentric enhancing masses of the left parotid gland (Figure 2.85d–f) and a smaller mass of the right parotid gland (Figure 2.85g). The patient underwent fine needle aspiration biopsy of his largest left parotid mass that demonstrated an oncocytic proliferation.

Diagnosis
With a preoperative clinical diagnosis of synchronous, multicentric bilateral Warthin tumors, the patient underwent staged superficial parotidectomies beginning with the larger tumors in the left parotid gland. With a modified Blair incision (Figure 2.85h), the patient underwent left superficial parotidectomy that began with the identification of the parotid capsule (Figure 2.85i). The main trunk of the facial nerve was identified and preserved with superficial elevation of the specimen (Figure 2.85j). The specimen was delivered (Figure 2.85k and l). Two Warthin tumors were later diagnosed in the specimen on permanent sections (Figure 2.85m). The resultant tissue bed and facial nerve dissection is appreciated (Figure 2.85n). At five months following left superficial parotidectomy, the patient was prepared for right superficial parotidectomy (Figure 2.85o–q). His facial nerve was intact bilaterally. He underwent repeat CT scanning (Figure 2.85g) that demonstrated one tumor in the superficial lobe of the right parotid gland (Figure 2.85r–t) that was larger than that noted on the initial CT scan obtained five months earlier. He underwent right superficial parotidectomy with identification and preservation of the facial nerve (Figure 2.85u–x). Final pathology confirmed the presence of one Warthin tumor (Figure 2.85y). The patient's postoperative course was unremarkable and he sustained no morbidity with either surgical procedure.

TAKE-HOME POINTS

1. Warthin tumors should be suspected when patients present with multicentric unilateral and/or bilateral tumors of the parotid glands.
2. Staging the performance of the bilateral superficial parotidectomies is prudent to avoid the possibility of bilateral facial nerve palsies if bilateral surgery was performed synchronously and postoperative facial nerve weaknesses were noted bilaterally.
3. Repeat CT scanning in staged parotid surgeries permits the assessment of interval growth of masses prior to the second parotid surgery. The increased growth of the mass in this case increased the pretest probability of a neoplastic process, and specifically a Warthin tumor.

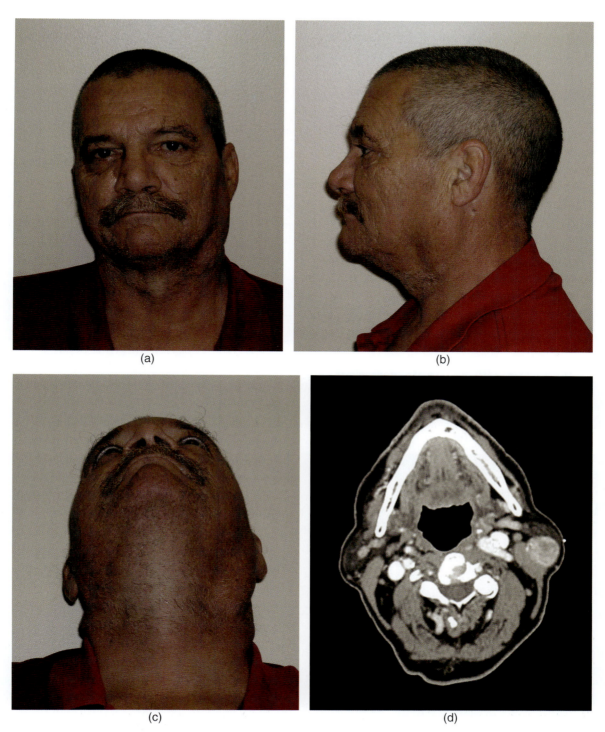

Figure 2.85. The patient demonstrates obvious left facial swelling in the region of the parotid gland (a–c). Axial (d), coronal (e), and sagittal (f) views demonstrate two tumors in the superficial lobe of the left parotid gland. Additionally, an enhancing but smaller tumor is noted in the right parotid gland (g). Synchronous, bilateral Warthin tumors are the suspected diagnoses. The patient underwent left superficial parotidectomy via a modified Blair incision (h). The skin flap is elevated anteriorly, superficial to the parotid capsule (i). The main trunk of the facial nerve and its peripheral branches are identified as the specimen is elevated (j). The specimen is delivered and inspected on its lateral (k) and medial surfaces (l). Final pathology identifies Warthin tumors of the left parotid gland (m). The resultant tissue bed and dissected facial nerve are noted (n). The patient is noted at five months postoperatively (o–q). A repeat CT scan is obtained and axial (r), coronal (s), and sagittal (t) images identify a larger tumor of the right parotid gland than was noted at the time of the patient's original presentation. He underwent a right superficial parotidectomy via a modified Blair incision (u). The specimen is elevated off the identified and preserved facial nerve (v). The specimen is delivered (w) and the resultant tissue bed is noted (x). Final pathology confirmed the clinical suspicion of Warthin tumor of the right parotid gland (y). (m = Hematoxylin and eosin, original magnification × 100; y = Hematoxylin and eosin, original magnification × 100).

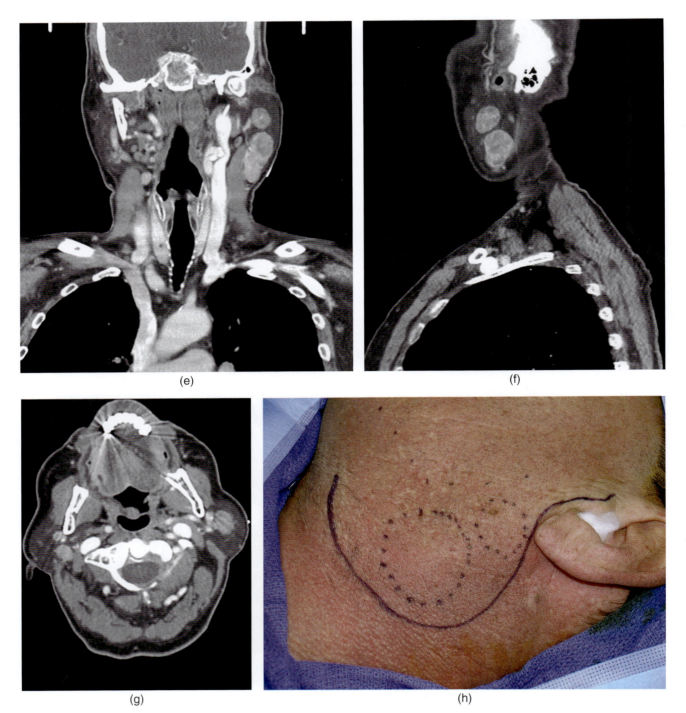

Figure 2.85. (Continued).

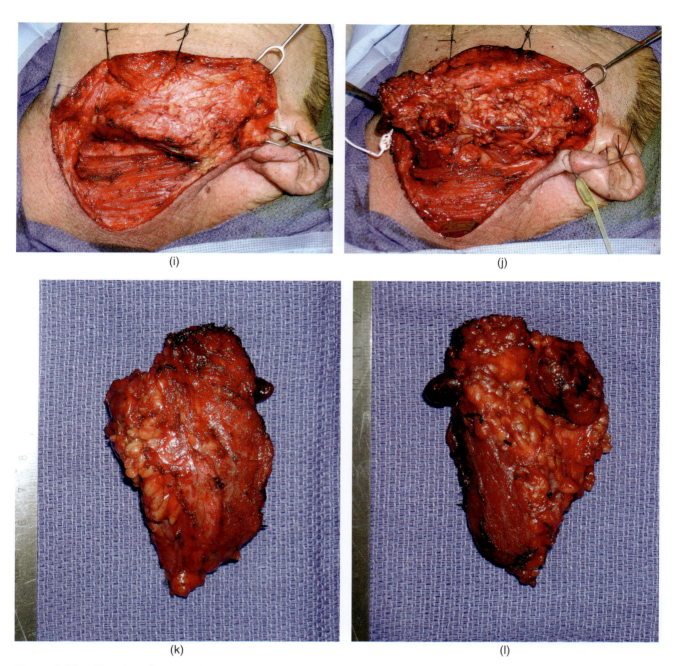

Figure 2.85. (*Continued*).

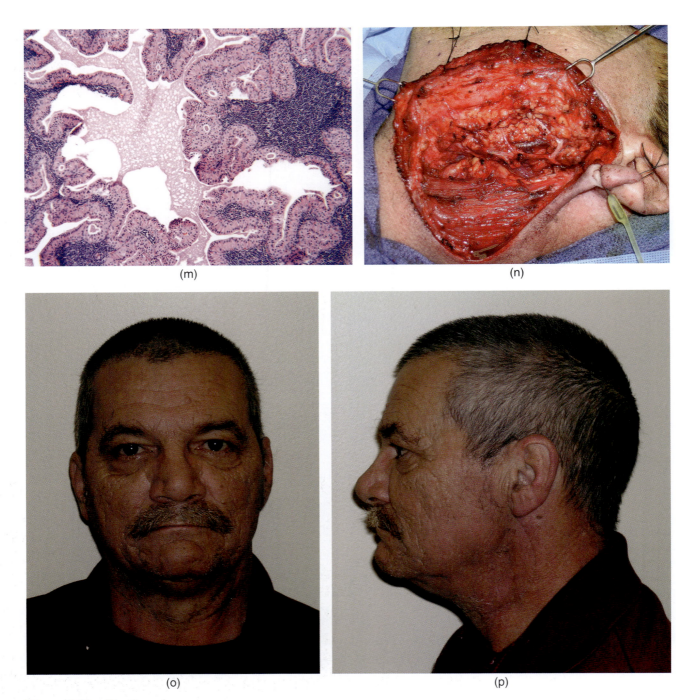

Figure 2.85. (Continued).

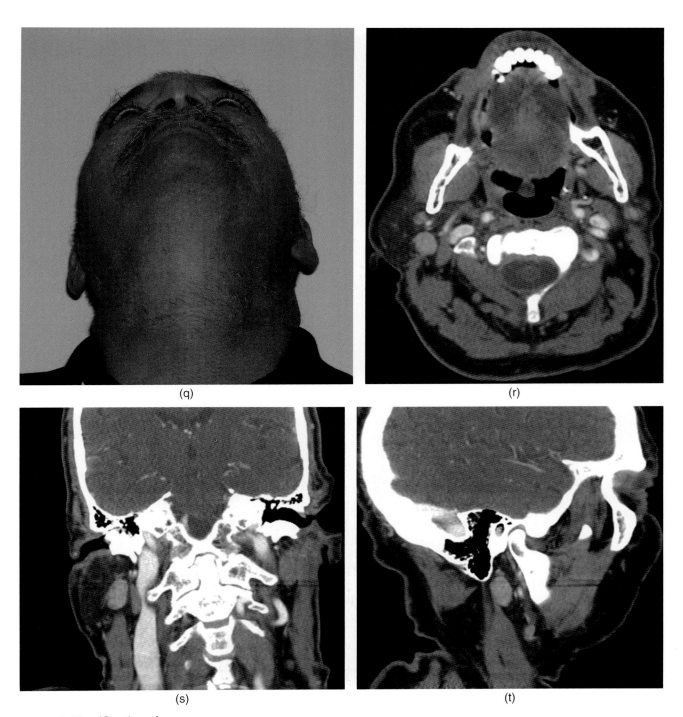

Figure 2.85. (*Continued*).

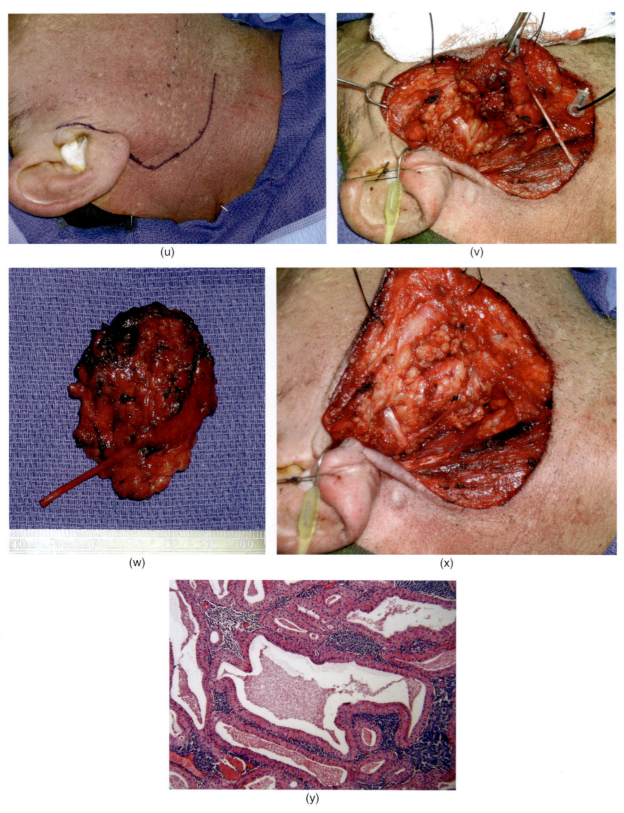

Figure 2.85. (Continued).

References

Abdel-Razek A, Kandeel A, Soliman N et al. 2007. Role of diffusion-weighted echo-planar MR imaging in differentiation of residual or recurrent head and neck tumors and post-treatment changes. *Am J Neuroradiol* 28:1146–1152.

Alexander de Ru J, Van Leeuwen M, Van Benthem P et al. 2007. Do magnetic resonance imaging and ultrasound add anything to the workup of parotid gland tumors? *J Oral Maxillofac Surg* 65:945–952.

Alibek S, Zenk J, Bozzato A et al. 2007. The value of dynamic MRI studies in parotid tumors. *Acad Radiol* 14:701–710.

Ando M, Matsuzaki M, Murofushi T. 2005. Mucosa-associated lymphoid tissue lymphoma presents as diffuse swelling of the parotid gland. *Am J Otolaryngol* 26:285–288.

Andre' R, Becker M, Lombardi T, Buchholzer S, Marchal F, Seebach JD. 2021. Comparison of clinical characteristics and magnetic resonance imaging of salivary glands with magnetic resonance sialography in Sjogren's syndrome. *Laryngoscope* 131 (1):E83–E89.

Aribandi M, Wood W, Elston D, Weiss D. 2006. CT features of plexiform neurofibroma of the submandibular gland. *Am J Neuroradiol* 27:126–128.

Baba S, Engles J, Huso D et al. 2007. Comparison of uptake of multiple clinical radiotracers into brown adipose tissue under cold-stimulated and nonstimulated conditions. *J Nucl Med* 48:1715–1723.

Beale T, Madani G. 2006. Anatomy of the salivary glands. *Semin Ultrasound CT MRI* 27:436–439.

Beaulier S, Kinaha P, Tseng J et al. 2003. SUV varies with time after injection in 18F-FDG PET of breast cancer: Characterization and method to adjust for time differences. *J Nucl Med* 44:1044–1050.

Bialek E, Jakubowski W, Zajkowski P et al. 2006. US of the major salivary glands: Anatomy and spatial relationships, pathologic conditions and pitfalls. *Radiographics* 26:745–763.

Bron L, Traynor S, McNeil E et al. 2003. Primary and metastatic cancer of the parotid: Comparison of clinical behavior in 232 cases. *Laryngoscope* 113(6):1070–1075.

Bui C, Ching A, Carlos R et al. 2003. Diagnostic accuracy of 2-[fluorine-18]-fluro-2-deoxy-D-Glucose Positron Emission Tomography imaging in non-squamous tumors of the head and neck. *Invest Radiol* 38:593–601.

Burke CJ, Thomas RH, Howlett D. 2011. Imaging the major salivary glands. *Br J Oral Maxillofac Surg* 49:261–269.

Burrell S, Van den Abbeele A. 2005. 2-Deoxy-2-(F-18)-Fluoro-D-glucose--Positron Emission tomography of the head and neck: An atlas of normal uptake and variants. *Mol Imaging Biol* 7:244–256.

Cermik T, Mavi A, Acikgoz G et al. 2007. FDG PET in detecting primary and recurrent malignant salivary gland tumors. *Clin Nucl Med* 32(4):286–291.

Chang P, Fischbein N, McCalmont T et al. 2004. Perineural spread of malignant melanoma of the head and neck: Clinical and imaging features. *Am J Neuroradiol* 25:5–11.

Ching A, Ahuja A, King A et al. 2001. Comparison of the sonographic features of acalculous and calculous submandibular sialadenitis. *J Clin Ultrasound* 29(6):332–338.

Cholankeril J, Scioscia P. 1993. Post-traumatic sialoceles and mucoceles of the salivary glands. *Clin Imaging* 17(1):41–45.

Cohade C, Mourtzikos K, Wahl R. 2003a. USA-fat: Prevalence is related to ambient outdoor temperature-evaluation with 18F-FDG PET/CT *J Nucl Med* 44:1267–1270.

Cohade C, Osman M, Pannu H, Wahl R. 2003b. Uptake in supraclavicular area fat (USA-Fat): Description on 18F-FDG PET/CT *J Nucl Med* 44:170–176.

Delbeke D, Coleman R, Guiberteau M et al. 2006. Procedure guidelines for tumor imaging with 18F-FDG PET/CT *J Nucl Med* 47:887–895.

Drumond J. 1995. Tomographic measurements of age changes in the human parotid gland. *Gerodontology* 12(1):26–30.

Eichhorn K, Iakovos A, Ridder G. 2002. Malignant non-Hodgkin's lymphoma mimicking a benign parotid tumor: Sonographic findings. *J Clin Ultrasound* 30(1):42–44.

Eida S, Sumi M, Sakihama N et al. 2007. Apparent diffusion coefficient mapping of salivary gland tumors: Prediction of the benignancy and malignancy. *Am J Neuroradiol* 28:116–121.

Gerstle R, Aylward S, Kromhout-Schiro S et al. 2000. The role of neural networks in improving the accuracy of MR spectroscopy for the diagnosis of head and neck squamous cell carcinoma. *Am J Neuroradiol* 21:1133–1138.

Golder W, Stiller M. 2014. Distribution pattern of Sjogren's syndrome: A sialographical study. *Z Rheumatol* 10:1–6.

Habermann C, Gossrau P, Kooijman H et al. 2007. Monitoring of gustatory stimulation of salivary glands by diffusion weighted MR imaging: Comparison of 1.5T and 3T. *Am J Neuroradiol* 28:1547–1551.

Hadi M, Chen C, Millie W et al. 2007. PET/CT, and 123I-MIBG SPECT: A study of patients being evaluated for pheochromocytoma. *J Nucl Med* 48:1077–1083.

Haldar S, Sinnott JD, Tekeli KM, Turner SS, Howlett DC. 2016. Biopsy of parotid masses: Review of current techniques. *World J Radiol* 8(5):501–505.

Hamilton B, Salzman K, Wiggins R, Harnsberger H. 2003. Earring lesions of the parotid tail. *Am J Neuroradiol* 24:1757–1764.

Hasson O. 2010. Modern sialography for screening of salivary gland obstruction. *J Oral Maxillofac Surg* 68:276–280.

Henkelman R, Watts J, Kucharczyk W. 1991. High signal intensity in MR images in calcified brain tissue. *Radiology* 179:199–206.

Holliday R. 1998. Benign lymphoepithelial parotid cysts and hyperplastic cervical adenopathy in AIDS-risk patients: A new CT appearance. *Radiology* 168:439–441.

Hopp E, Mortensen B, Kolbenstvedt A. 2004. Mylohyoid herniation of the sublingual gland diagnosed by magnetic resonance imaging. *Dentom Radiol* 33:351–353.

Hsu C, Lee C, Wang F, Fang C. 2003. Neurofibroma with increased uptake of F-18-fluoro-2-deoxy-D-glucose interpreted as a metastatic lesion. *Ann Nucl Med* 17:609–611.

Huang C, Damrose E, Bhuta S, Abemayor E. 2002. Kuttner tumor (chronic sclerosing sialadenitis). *Am J Otolaryngol* 23(6):394–397.

Ikeda K, Tsutomu K, Ha-Kawa S et al. 1996. The usefulness of MR in establishing the diagnosis of parotid pleomorphic adenoma. *Am J Neuroradiol* 17:555–559.

Ikeda M, Motoori K, Hanazawa T et al. 2004. Warthin tumor of the parotid gland: Diagnostic value of MR imaging with histopathologic correlation. *Am J Neuroradiol* 25:1256–1262.

Ioannidis J, Lau J. 2003. 18F-FDG PET for the diagnosis and grading of soft-tissue sarcoma: A meta-analysis. *J Nucl Med* 44:717–724.

Izumi M, Eguchi K, Hideki N et al. 1997. Premature fat deposition in the salivary glands associated with Sjogren's syndrome: MR and CT evidence. *Am J Neuroradiol* 18(5):951–958.

Jansisyanant P, Blanchaert R, Ord R. 2002. Intraoral minor salivary gland neoplasm: A single institution experience of 80 cases. *Int J Oral Maxillofac Surg* 31(3):257–261.

Jeong H, Chung M, Son Y et al. 2007. Role of 18-F-FDG PET/CT in management of high-grade salivary gland malignancies. *J Nucl Med* 48:1237–1244.

Jhanvar Y, Straus D. 2006. The role of PET in lymphoma. *J Nucl Med* 47:1326–1334.

Kalinowski M, Heverhagen J, Rehberg E et al. 2002. Comparative study of MR sialography and digital subtraction sialography for benign salivary gland disorders. *Am J Neuroradiol* 23:1485–1492.

Kaneda T. 1996. MR of the submandibular gland: Normal and pathologic states. *AJR* 17:1575–1581.

Keyes J, Harkness B, Greven K et al. 1994. Salivary gland tumors: Pretherapy evaluation with PET. *Radiology* 192:99–102.

Kim HJ, Kim JS. 2018. Ultrasound-guided Core needle biopsy in salivary glands: A meta-analysis. *Laryngoscope* 128:118–125.

King A, Yeung D, Ahuja A et al. 2005. Salivary gland tumors at in-vivo proton MR spectroscopy. *Radiology* 237:563–569.

Kinoshita T, Okitsu T. 2004. MR imaging findings of parotid tumors with pathologic diagnostic clues: A pictorial essay. *Clin Imaging* 28:93–101.

Kirshenbaum K, Nadimpalli S, Rehberg E et al. 1991. Benign lymphoepithelial parotid tumors in AIDS patients: CT and MR findings in nine cases. *Am J Neuroradiol* 12:271–274.

Koeller K, Alamo L, Adair C, Smirniotopoulos J. 1999. Congenital cystic masses of the neck: Radiologic-pathologic characteristics. *Radiographics* 19:121–146.

Kurabayashi T, Ida M, Yasumoto M et al. 2000. MRI of ranulas. *Neuroradiology* 42(12):917–922.

Lin J, Martel W. 2001. Cross-sectional imaging of peripheral nerve sheath tumors: Characteristics signs on CT, MR imaging and sonography. *AJR* 176:75–82.

Lowe L, Stokes L, Johnson J et al. 2001. Swelling at the angle of the mandible: Imaging of the pediatric parotid gland and periparotid region. *Radiographics* 21:1211–1227.

Macdonald A, Salzman K, Hansberger H. 2003. Giant ranula of the neck: Differentiation from cystic hygroma. *Am J Neuroradiol* 24:757–761.

MacManus M, Ryan G, Lau E, Wirth A, Hicks R. 2007. Positron emission tomography of stage IV mucosa-associated lymphoid tissue lymphoma confined to the four major salivary glands. *Aust Radiol* 51:68–70.

Madani G, Beale T. 2006a. Inflammatory conditions of the salivary glands. *Semin Ultrasound CT MRI* 27:440–451.

Madani G, Beale T. 2006b. Tumors of the salivary glands. *Semin Ultrasound CT MRI* 27:452–464.

Makariou E, Pikis A, Harley E. 2003. Cystic hygroma of the neck: Associated with a growing venous aneurysm. *Am J Neuroradiol* 24:2102–2104.

Martin N, Serkers O, Mompoint D, Nahum H. 1992. Facial nerve neuromas: MR imaging-report of four cases. *Neuroradiology* 34:62–67.

Martinoli C, Pretolesi F, Del Bono V et al. 1995. Benign lymphoepithelial parotid lesion in HIV-positive patients: Spectrum of findings at gray-scale and Doppler sonography. *AJR* 165:975–979.

Miyaki H, Matsumoto A, Hori Y et al. 2001. Warthin's tumor of parotid gland on Tc-99m pertechnetate scintigraphy with lemon juice stimulation: Tc99m uptake, size, and pathologic correlation. *Eur Radiol* 11(12):2472–2478.

Moonis G, Patel P, Koshkareva Y et al. 2007. Imaging characteristics of recurrent pleomorphic adenoma of the parotid gland. *Am J Neuroradiol* 28:1532–1536.

Mosier KM. 2009. Diagnostic radiographic imaging for salivary endoscopy. *Otolaryngol Clin North Am* 42:949–972.

Motoori K, Yamamoto S, Ueda T et al. 2004. Inter- and intratumoral variability in magnetic resonance imaging of pleomorphic adenoma. *J Comput Assist Tomogr* 28:233–246.

Motoori K, Iida Y, Nagai Y et al. 2005. MR imaging of salivary duct carcinoma. *Am J Neuroradiol* 26:1201–1206.

Nakamoto Y, Tatsumi M, Hammoud D et al. 2005. Normal FDG distribution patterns in the head and neck: PET/CT evaluation. *Radiology* 234:879–885.

Novoa E, Gurrier N, Arnoux A, Kraft M. 2015. Diagnostic value of core needle biopsy and fine-needle aspiration in salivary gland lesions. *Head Neck* 38:E346–E352.

Ollila DW, Foshag LJ, Essner R et al. 1999. Parotid region lymphatic mapping and sentinel lymphadenopathy for cutaneous melanoma. *Ann Surg Oncol* 6(2):150–154.

Otsuka H, Graham M, Kogame M, Nishitani H. 2005. The impact of FDG-PET in the management of patients with salivary gland malignancy. *Ann Nucl Med* 19(8):691–694.

Patel R, Carlos R, Midia M, Mukherji S. 2004. Apparent diffusion coefficient mapping of the normal parotid gland and parotid involvement in patients with systemic connective tissue disorders. *Am J Neuroradiol* 25:16–20.

Patz E, Lowe V, Hoffman J et al. 1993. Focal pulmonary abnormalities: Evaluation with F-18 fluorodeoxyglucose PET scanning. *Radiology* 188:487–490.

Roh J, Ryu C, Choi S et al. 2007. Clinical utility of 18F-FDG PET for patients with salivary gland malignancies. *J Nucl Med* 48:240–246.

Rumboldt Z, Al-Okkaili R, Deveikis J. 2005. perfusion CT for head and neck tumors: A pilot study. *Am J Neuroradiol* 26:1178–1185.

Schoder H, Yusuf E, Chao K et al. 2004. Clinical implications of different image reconstruction parameters for interpretation of whole-body PET studies in cancer patients. *J Nucl Med* 45:559–566.

Shah G. 2002. MR imaging of salivary glands. *Mag Reson Clin N Am* 10:631–662.

Shah G, Fischbein N, Patel R, Mukherji S. 2003. Newer MR imaging techniques for head and neck. *Magn Reson Clin N Am* 11:449–469.

Sheedy S, Welker K, Delone D, Gilbertson J. 2006. CNS metastases of carcinoma ex pleomorphic adenoma of the parotid gland. *Am J Neuroradiol* 27:1483–1485.

Shimizu K, Iwai H, Ikeda K et al. 2005. Intraparotid facial nerve schwannoma: A report of five cases and an analysis of MR imaging results. *Am J Neuroradiol* 26:1328–1330.

Sigal R, Monnet O, De Baere T et al. 1992. Adenoid cystic carcinoma of the head and neck: Evaluation with MR imaging and clinical-pathologic correlation in 27 patients. *Radiology* 184:95–101.

Sobrino-Guijarro B, Cascarini L, Lingam RK. 2013. Advances in imaging of obstructed salivary gland can improve diagnostic outcomes. *Oral Maxillofac Surg* 17:11–19.

Sokoloff L. 1961. Local Cerebral Circulation at Rest and During Altered Cerebral Activity Induced by Anesthesia or Visual Stimulation. In: S.S. Kety, J. Elkes (eds.) *The Regional Chemistry, Physiology and Pharmacology of the Nervous System.* Oxford, Pergamon Press, pp. 107–117.

Sokoloff L. 1986. Cerebral circulation, energy metabolism, and protein synthesis: General characteristics and principles of measurement. In: M. Phelps, J. Mazziotta, H. Schelbert (eds.) *Positron Emission Tomography and Autoradiography: Principles and Applications for the Brain and Heart.* Raven Press, pp. 1–71.

Som P, Curtin H (eds.). 1996. *Head and Neck Imaging*, 3rd edn. Mosby-Year Book Inc, pp. 823–914.

Som P, Brandwein M, Silver A. 1995. Nodal inclusion cysts of the parotid gland and parapharyngeal space: A discussion of lymphoepithelial, AIDS-related parotid and branchial cysts, cystic Warthin's tumors, and cysts in Sjogren's syndrome. *Laryngoscope* 105(10):1122–1128.

Stahl A, Dzewas B, Schwaige W, Weber W. 2002. Excretion of FDG into saliva and its significance for PET imaging. *Nuklearmedizin* 41:214–216.

Su Y, Liao G, Kang Z, Zou Y. 2006. Application of magnetic resonance virtual endoscopy as a presurgical procedure before sialoendoscopy. *Laryngoscope* 116:1899–1906.

Sugai S. 2002. Mucosa-associated lymphoid tissue lymphoma in Sjogren's syndrome. *AJR* 179:485–489.

Suh J, Abenoza P, Galloway H et al. 1992. Peripheral (extracranial) nerve tumors: Correlation of MR imaging and histologic findings. *Radiology* 183:341–346.

Sumi M, Izumi M, Yonetsu K, Nakamura T. 1999a. Sublingual gland: MR features of normal and diseased states. *AJR* 172(3):717–722.

Sumi M, Izumi M, Yonetsu K, Nakamura T. 1999b. The MR imaging assessment of submandibular gland sialoadenitis secondary to sialolithiasis: Correlation with CT and histopathologic findings. *Am J Neuroradiol* 20:1737–1743.

Sumi M, Yamada T, Takagi Y, Nakamura T. 2007. MR imaging of labial glands. *Am J Neuroradiol* 28:1552–1556.

Takagi Y, Sumi M, Sumi T et al. 2005a. MR microscopy of the parotid glands in patients with Sjogren's syndrome: Quantitative MR diagnostic criteria. *Am J Neuroradiol* 26:1207–1214.

Takagi Y, Sumi M, Van Cauteren M, Nakamura T. 2005b. Fast and high resolution MR sialography using a small surface coil. *J Magn Reson Imaging* 22:29–37.

Takahashi N, Okamoto K, Ohkubo M, Kawana M. 2005. High-resolution magnetic resonance of the extracranial facial nerve and parotid duct: Demonstration of the branches of the intraparotid facial nerve and its relation to parotid tumours by MRI with a surface coil. *Clin Radiol* 60:349–354.

Takashima S, Takeuchi N, Morimoto S et al. 1991. MR imaging of Sjogren's syndrome: Correlation with sialography and pathology. *J Comput Assist Tomogr* 15(3):393–400.

Takashima S, Tomofumi N, Noguchi Y et al. 1992. CT and MR appearances of parotid pseudotumors in Sjogren's syndrome. *J Comput Assist Tomogr* 16(3):376–383.

Tanaka T, Ono K, Habu M et al. 2007. functional evaluation of the parotid and submandibular glands using dynamic magnetic resonance sialography. *Dentom Radiol* 36:218–223.

Tatsumi M, Engles J, Ishimori T et al. 2004. Intense 18F-FDG uptake in Brown fat can be reduced pharmacologically. *J Nucl Med* 45:1189–1193.

Thoeny H. 2007. Imaging of Salivary gland tumors. *Cancer Imaging* 7:52–62.

Tonami H, Munetaka M, Yokata H et al. 2002. Mucosa-associated lymphoid tissue lymphoma in Sjogren's syndrome: Initial and follow-up imaging features. *AJR* 179:485–489.

Uchida Y, Minoshima S, Kawata T et al. 2005. Diagnostic value of FDG PET and salivary gland scintigraphy for parotid tumors. *Clin Nucl Med* 30:170–176.

Wan Y, Chan S, Chen Y. 2004. Ultrasonography-guided core-needle biopsy of parotid gland masses. *Am J Neuroradiol* 25:1608–1612.

Wang Y, Chiu E, Rosenberg J, Gambhir S. 2007. Standardized uptake value atlas: Characterization of physiological 2-deoxy-2-[18F]fluoro-D-glucose uptake in normal tissues. *Mol Imaging Biol* 9(2):83–90.

Warburg O. 1925. Uber den Stoffwechsel der Carcinom-Zelle. *Klin Wochenschr* 4:534–536.

White D, Davidson H, Harnsberger H et al. 2001. Accessory salivary tissue in the mylohyoid boutonnière: A clinical and radiologic pseudolesion of the oral cavity. *Am J Neuroradiol* 22:406–412.

Witt BL, Schmidt RL. 2014. Ultrasound-guided core needle biopsy of salivary gland lesions: A systematic review and meta-analysis. *Laryngoscope* 124:695–700.

Wong K, Ahuja A, King A et al. 2004. Vascular lesion in the parotid gland in adult patients: Diagnosis with high-resolution ultrasound and MRI. *British J Radiol* 77:600–606.

Yabuuchi H, Fukuya T, Tajima T et al. 2003. Salivary gland tumors: Diagnostic value of gadolinium enhanced dynamic MR imaging with histopathologic correlation. *Radiology* 226:345–354.

Yerli H, Aydin E, Coskum M et al. 2007. Dynamic multislice CT of parotid gland. *J Comput Assist Tomogr* 31(2):309–316.

Chapter 3
Infections of the Salivary Glands

Outline

Introduction
General Considerations
Bacterial Salivary Gland Infections
  Acute Bacterial Parotitis
    Variants of ABP and Their Etiology
    Diagnosis of Acute Bacterial Parotitis
    Treatment of Acute Bacterial Parotitis
  Chronic (Recurrent or Refractory) Bacterial Parotitis
    Treatment of Chronic Bacterial Parotitis
  Chronic Recurrent Juvenile Parotitis
    Treatment of Chronic Recurrent Juvenile Parotitis
  Acute Bacterial Submandibular Sialadenitis
    Treatment of Acute Bacterial Submandibular Sialadenitis
  Chronic Recurrent Submandibular Sialadenitis
  Bartonella Henselae (Cat-Scratch Disease)
  Tuberculous Mycobacterial Disease
  Nontuberculous Mycobacterial Disease
Viral Salivary Gland Infections
  Mumps
  Human Immunodeficiency Virus
  Influenza A
Bacterial Sialadenitis in Pregnancy
Autoimmune Sialadenitis and IgG4-Related Disease
Summary
Case Presentation – *Gadzooks*
References

Introduction

Most non-neoplastic swellings of the major salivary glands represent acute or chronic infections of these glands. Sialadenitis, a generic term used to describe infection of the salivary glands, has a diverse range of signs and symptoms and predisposing factors. Although any of the major and minor salivary glands can become infected, these conditions most commonly occur in the parotid (Figure 3.1) and submandibular glands (Figure 3.2), with minor salivary gland and sublingual gland infections being very rare. From an etiologic standpoint, these infections may be related to underlying bacterial, viral, fungal, mycobacterial, parasitic, or immunologically mediated inflammation/infections (Miloro and Goldberg 2002). The most common of these diagnoses include acute bacterial parotitis and acute submandibular sialadenitis (see Table 3.1). Numerous risk factors may predispose patients to sialadenitis. The classic risk factor is the hospitalized patient who recently underwent surgery with general anesthesia. Additionally, dehydration (insufficient intake) may contribute to sialadenitis, as may chronic nausea/vomiting (excessive output) in hospitalized patients. Both conditions decrease intravascular volume, thereby decreasing perfusion of salivary gland tissue with resultant decreased salivary flow. In general terms, stasis and decreased salivary flow predispose patients to sialadenitis, although, medications and comorbid diagnoses may also contribute to this diagnosis (see Table 3.2).

Salivary Gland Pathology: Diagnosis and Management, Third Edition. Edited by Eric R. Carlson and Robert A. Ord.
© 2022 John Wiley & Sons, Inc. Published 2022 by John Wiley & Sons, Inc.
Companion website: www.wiley.com/go/carlson/salivary

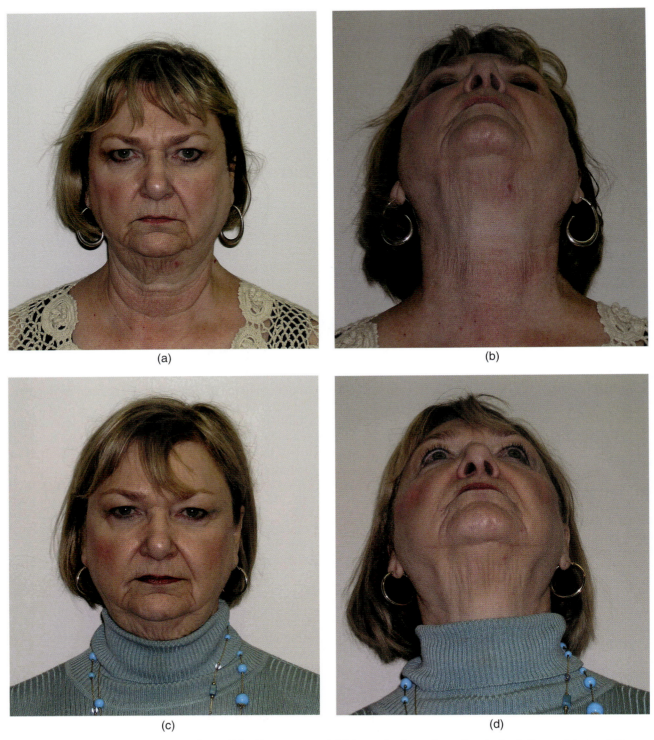

Figure 3.1. A 55-year-old woman (a and b) with a one-week history of pain and swelling in the left parotid gland. No pus was present at Stensen duct. The diagnosis was community acquired acute bacterial parotitis. Conservative measures were instituted including the use of oral antibiotics, warm compresses to the left face, sialogogues, and digital massage. Two weeks later, she was asymptomatic, and physical examination revealed resolution of her swelling (c and d).

Infections of the Salivary Glands 81

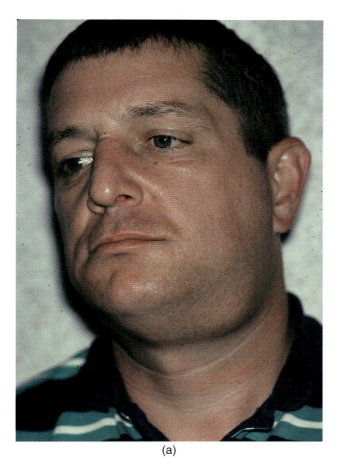

(a)

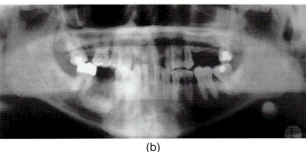

(b)

Figure 3.2. A 45-year-old man (a) with a six-month history of left submandibular pain and swelling. A clinical diagnosis of chronic submandibular sialadenitis was made. A screening panoramic radiograph was obtained that revealed the presence of a large sialolith in the gland (b). As such, the obstruction of salivary outflow by the sialolith was responsible for the chronic sialadenitis. This case underscores the importance of obtaining a screening panoramic radiograph in all patients with a clinical diagnosis of sialadenitis, as it permitted expedient diagnosis of sialolithiasis in this case.

Table 3.1. Classification of salivary gland inflammation/infection.

Bacterial infections
   Acute bacterial parotitis
   Chronic bacterial parotitis
   Chronic recurrent juvenile parotitis
   Acute suppurative submandibular sialadenitis
   Chronic recurrent submandibular sialadenitis
   Acute allergic sialadenitis
Viral infections
   Mumps
   HIV/AIDS
   Cytomegalovirus
Fungal infections
Mycobacterial infections
   Tuberculosis
   Atypical mycobacteria
Parasitic infections
Autoimmune-related inflammation
   Systemic lupus erythematosus
   Sarcoidosis
   Sjögren syndrome

Table 3.2. Risk factors associated with salivary gland inflammation/infection.

Modifiable risk factors
   Decreased intravascular volume
      Decreased input (dehydration/prerenal azotemia)
      Increased output (chronic vomiting/diarrhea)
   Recent surgery and anesthesia
   Malnutrition
   Medications
      Antihistamines
      Diuretics
        Tricyclic antidepressants
      Phenothiazines
      Antihypertensives
      Barbiturates
      Anti-sialogogues
      Anticholinergics
      Chemotherapeutic agents
   Sialolithiasis
   Oral infection
Non-modifiable risk factors
   Advanced age

(*Continued*)

Table 3.2. (Continued)

Relatively non-modifiable risk factors
  Radiation therapy where cytoprotective agents were not administered
  Renal failure
  Hepatic failure
  Congestive heart failure
  HIV/AIDS
  Diabetes mellitus
  Anorexia nervosa/bulimia
  Cystic fibrosis
  Cushing disease

General Considerations

Evaluation and treatment of the patient with sialadenitis begins with a thorough history and physical examination. The setting in which the evaluation occurs, for example a hospital ward vs. an office, may provide information as to the underlying cause of the infection. Many cases of acute bacterial parotitis (ABP) occur in elderly debilitated patients, some of whom are admitted to the hospital, who demonstrate inadequate intravenous fluid resuscitation (insufficient intake) or excessive volume loss (excessive output) (Figure 3.3) or third-spacing of fluid resulting in hypovolemia. This notwithstanding, many cases of acute bacterial parotitis and submandibular sialadenitis are evaluated initially in an outpatient setting.

The formal history taking process begins by obtaining the patient's chief complaint. Sialadenitis commonly begins as swelling of the salivary gland with pain due to stretching of that gland's sensory innervated capsule. Patients may or may not describe the perception of pus associated with salivary secretions, and the presence or absence of pus may be confirmed on physical examination.

History taking is important to disclose the acute or chronic nature of the problem that will significantly impact on how the sialadenitis is ultimately managed. Regarding the prognosis and the anticipation for the possible need for future surgical intervention, an acute sialadenitis is somewhat arbitrarily classified as one where symptoms are less than one month in duration, while a chronic sialadenitis is defined as having been present for longer than one month. In addition, the history will permit the clinician to assess the risk factors associated with the condition. In so doing, the realization of modifiable versus relatively non-modifiable versus non-modifiable risk factors can be determined. For example, dehydration, recent surgery, oral infection, and some medications represent modifiable risk factors predisposing patients to sialadenitis. On the other hand, advanced age is a non-modifiable risk factor, and chronic medical illnesses and radiation therapy constitute relatively non-modifiable risk factors associated with these infections. The distinction between modifiable and relatively non-modifiable risk factors is not intuitive. For example, dehydration is obviously modifiable. The sialadenitis associated with diabetes mellitus may abate clinically as evidenced by decreased swelling and pain; however, the underlying medical condition is not reversible. The same is true for HIV/AIDS. While much medical comorbidity can be controlled and palliated, these conditions often are not curable such that patients may be fraught with recurrent sialadenitis at unpredictable time frames following the initial event. As such, these and many other risk factors are considered relatively non-modifiable.

Other features of the history, such as the presence or absence of prandial pain, may direct the physical and radiographic examinations to the existence of an obstructive phenomenon. The presence of medical conditions and the use of medications to manage these conditions are very important elements of the history taking of a patient with a chief complaint suggestive of sialadenitis. They may be determined to be of etiologic significance when the physical examination confirms the diagnosis of sialadenitis. Musicians playing wind instruments who present for evaluation of bilateral parotid swelling and pain after a concert may have acute air insufflation of the parotid glands as part of the "trumpet blower's syndrome" (Miloro and Goldberg 2002). Recent dental work, specifically the application of orthodontic brackets, may result in traumatic introduction of bacteria into the ductal system with resultant retrograde sialadenitis. Deep facial lacerations proximal to an imaginary line connecting the lateral canthus of the eye to the oral commissure, and along an imaginary line connecting the tragus to the mid-philtrum of the lip may violate the integrity of Stensen duct. While a thorough exploration of these wounds with cannulation and repair of Stensen duct is meticulously performed, it is possible for foreign bodies to result in obstruction of salivary flow with resultant parotid swelling. Numerous autoimmune diseases

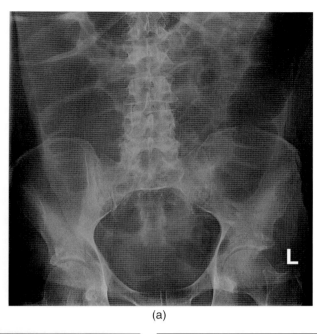
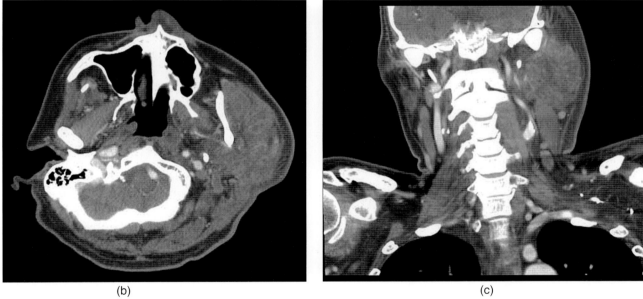

Figure 3.3. A 35-year-old man with a toxic megacolon (a) associated with *Clostridium difficile* diarrhea. He developed a left parotitis (b and c) due to a severe depletion of his intravascular volume.

with immune complex formation can also be responsible for sialadenitis, and confirmation of their diagnosis should be sought during the history and physical examination.

After the patient's history has been obtained, the physical examination should be performed. In the patient with suspected sialadenitis, the examination is focused on the head and neck and begins with the extraoral examination followed by the intraoral examination. Specifically, the salivary glands should be assessed in a bimanual fashion for asymmetries, erythema, tenderness to palpation, swellings, induration, and warmth. In so doing, one of the most important aspects of this examination is to rule out the presence of a tumor (Carlson 2013). A neoplastic process of the parotid gland presents as a *discrete* mass within the gland, with or without symptoms of pain. An infectious process presents as a *diffuse* enlargement of the parotid gland that is commonly symptomatic. It is possible for an indurated inflammatory lymph node within the parotid gland to simulate neoplastic disease. The distinction in the character of the parotid gland is important to not waste time treating a patient for an infectious process when they have a tumor in the parotid gland, particularly in the event of a malignancy. Evidence of facial trauma, including healing facial lacerations or ecchymoses, should be ascertained. The intraoral examination focuses on the observation of the quality and quantity of spontaneous and stimulated salivary flow. It is important to understand, however, that the anxiety and sympathomimetic response associated with the examination is likely to decrease the patient's salivary flow. Nonetheless, an advanced case of sialadenitis will often allow the clinician to appreciate the flow of pus from the salivary ducts (Figures 3.4 and 3.5). If pus is not observed, mucous plugs, small stones, or "salivary sludge" may be noted. As part of the examination, it may be appropriate to perform cannulation of the salivary duct with a series of lacrimal probes (Figure 3.6). This maneuver may dislodge obstructive material or diagnose an obstruction. The decision to perform this instrumentation, however, must not be made indiscriminately. This procedure may introduce bacteria into the salivary duct that normally colonize around

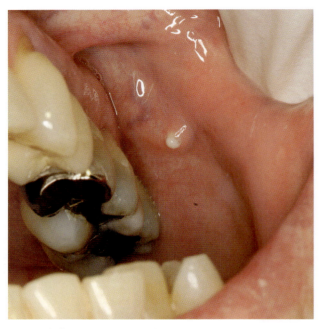

Figure 3.5. A mild case of community acquired parotitis is noted by the expression of pus at the left Stensen duct.

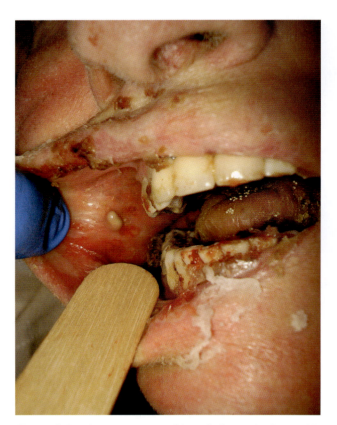

Figure 3.4. A severe case of hospital acquired parotitis related to insufficient rehydration of this patient.

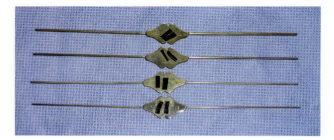

Figure 3.6. Lacrimal probes are utilized to probe the salivary ducts. The four shown in this figure incrementally increase in size. Cannulation of salivary ducts begins with the smallest probe and proceeds sequentially to the largest to properly dilate the duct. It is recommended that patients initiate a course of antibiotics prior to probing salivary ducts to not exacerbate the sialadenitis by introducing oral bacteria proximally into the gland.

the ductal orifice, thereby permitting retrograde contamination of the gland. Prepping the Wharton duct or Stensen duct with a Betadine solution prior to lacrimal probe cannulation is therefore advised. This procedure is probably contraindicated in patients with acute bacterial parotitis and acute bacterial submandibular sialadenitis. The head and neck examination concludes by palpating the regional lymph nodes, including those in the preauricular and cervical regions.

Radiographs of the salivary glands may be obtained after performing the history and physical examination. Since radiographic analysis of the salivary glands is the subject of Chapter 2, this discipline will not be discussed in detail in this chapter. Nonetheless, plain films and specialized imaging studies may be of value in evaluating patients with a clinical diagnosis of sialadenitis. Obtaining screening plain radiographs such as a panoramic radiograph and/or an occlusal radiograph is important data to obtain when a history exists that suggests an obstructive phenomenon. The presence of a sialolith on plain films, for example, represents very important diagnostic information to direct therapy. It permits the clinician to identify the etiology of the sialadenitis and to remove the stone at an expedient time frame. Such expedience may permit the avoidance of chronicity such that gland function can be maintained.

Bacterial Salivary Gland Infections

ACUTE BACTERIAL PAROTITIS

World history indicates that acute bacterial parotitis (ABP) played a significant role in its chronicles, particularly in the United States. We are told that the first case of acute bacterial parotitis occurred in Paris in 1829 in a 71-year-old man where the parotitis progressed to gangrene (McQuone 1999; Miloro and Goldberg 2002). As mumps plays a role in the differential diagnosis of infectious parotitis, Brodie's distinction between acute bacterial parotitis and viral mumps in 1834 represents a major inroad into the understanding of this pathologic process (Brodie 1834; Goldberg and Bevilacqua 1995). Prior to the modern surgical era, ABP was not uncommonly observed, and indeed represented a dreaded complication of major surgery, with a mortality rate as high as 50% (Goldberg and Bevilacqua 1995). Ineffective postoperative intravascular volume repletion with resultant diminished salivary flow and dry mouth were the norm rather than the exception. President Garfield sustained a gunshot wound to the abdomen in July 1881 and developed chronic peritonitis and ultimately died several weeks later. The terminal event was described as suppurative parotitis that led to sepsis (Goldberg and Bevilacqua 1995; Carlson 2009).

It has been pointed out that upper and lower aerodigestive tract surgeries require patients to be without oral nutritional intake or with limited oral intake postoperatively (McQuone 1999). The reduction of salivary stimulation predisposes these patients to acute bacterial parotitis, with an estimated incidence of 1 in 1000 postoperative patients (Andrews et al. 1989). Other statistics showed 3.68 cases per 10,000 operations in the preantibiotic era compared with 0.173 in 10,000 operations in the antibiotic era (Robinson 1955). The prophylactic use of antibiotics has probably contributed to the reduction of cases of acute bacterial parotitis. In addition, intraoperative and postoperative intravenous hydration became well accepted in the 1930s, particularly during World War II, therefore also contributing to the reduction in the incidence of ABP. In 1958, Petersdorf reported seven cases of staphylococcal parotitis and the 1960s ushered in several reports of ABP as a disease making a comeback (Petersdorf et al. 1958; Goldberg and Bevilacqua 1995). Of Petersdorf's seven cases, five of the patients had undergone surgery, and two of the patients died in the hospital. Oral and maxillofacial surgeons began to report cases of ABP in the literature in the 1960s (Goldberg and Harrigan 1965; Guralnick et al. 1968). These cases were most likely due to the emergence of penicillin-resistant bacteria (Lewis 1995), like contemporary reports of methicillin-resistant Staphylococcus aureus parotitis (Nicolasora 2009).

The parotid gland's relative propensity for infection results from physiologic and anatomic factors. Parotid saliva differs from that of the submandibular and sublingual glands. Parotid saliva is predominantly serous compared to the mucinous saliva from the submandibular and sublingual glands. Mucoid saliva contains lysosomes and IgA antibodies, which protect against bacterial infection. Mucins also contain sialic acid, which agglutinates bacteria, thereby preventing its adherence to host tissues. Glycoproteins found in mucins bind epithelial cells, thereby inhibiting bacterial attachment to the epithelial cells of the salivary duct.

Variants of ABP and Their Etiology

Over the past several decades, changes have occurred in the bacterial flora of the oral cavity that directly reflect the identification of organisms in ABP. In part, this change is evident due to the increased incidence of nosocomial and opportunistic infections in patients who are immunocompromised as well as those critically ill patients in hospital intensive care units whose mouths became colonized with microorganisms that were previously only rarely found in the oral cavity (Figure 3.4). Moreover, improved culturing techniques have permitted the identification of anaerobes that were previously difficult to recover in the microbiology laboratory. Finally, the occasionally indiscriminate use of antibiotics has allowed for the occupation of other organisms in the oral cavity such as Gram negative enteric organisms. Bacterial Darwinism has also occurred such that iatrogenically and genetically altered staphylococcal organisms have developed penicillin resistance.

Acute bacterial parotitis has two well-defined presentations, *hospital acquired* (Figure 3.4) and *community acquired* (Figure 3.5) variants. Numerous factors predispose the parotid gland to sialadenitis. Retrograde infection is recognized as the major cause of ABP. Resulting from acute illness, sepsis, trauma, or surgery, depleted intravascular volume may result in diminished salivary flow that in turn diminishes the normal flushing action of saliva as it passes through Stensen duct. Patients with salivary secretions of modest flow rates show bacteria at the duct papillae and in cannulated ducts, while patients with salivary secretions of high rates show bacteria at the duct papillae but not within the duct (Katz et al. 1990). In a healthy state, fibronectin exists in high concentrations within parotid saliva, which promotes the adherence of *Streptococcus* species and *Staphylococcus aureus* around the ductal orifice of the Stensen duct (Katz et al. 1990). Low levels of fibronectin such as those occuring in the unhealthy host are known to promote the adherence of *Pseudomonas* and *Escherichia coli*. This observation explains the clinical situation whereby colonization resulting from dehydration leads to a Gram positive sialadenitis in ABP compared to the development of Gram negative sialadenitis of the parotid gland in immunocompromised patients (Miloro and Goldberg 2002). Depending on the health of the host, therefore, specific colonized bacteria can infect the parotid gland in a retrograde fashion. Hospital acquired ABP still shows cultures of *Staphylococcus aureus* in over 50% of cases (Goldberg and Bevilacqua 1995). Methicillin-resistant *Staphylococcus aureus* should be ruled out in this population of inpatients. Critically ill and immunocompromised inpatients may also show *Pseudomonas, Klebsiella, Escherichia coli, Proteus, Eikenella corrodens, Haemophilus influenzae, Prevotella* and *Fusobacterium* species. Postoperative parotitis has been reported from 1 to 15 weeks following surgery, but most commonly occurs within 2 weeks after surgery (McQuone 1999). The peak incidence of this disease seems to be between postoperative days 5 and 7.

Community acquired ABP is diagnosed five times more commonly than hospital acquired ABP and is diagnosed in emergency departments, offices, and outpatient clinics. This variant of ABP is most commonly associated with staphylococcal and streptococcal species. As community acquired methicillin-resistant *Staphylococcus aureus* becomes more common in society, this organism will become more prevalent in community acquired ABP. Etiologic factors in community acquired ABP include medications that decrease salivary flow, trauma to Stensen duct, cheek biting, toothbrush trauma, trumpet blower's syndrome and medical conditions such as diabetes, malnutrition, and dehydration from acute or chronic gastrointestinal disorders with loss of intravascular volume. Sialoliths present in Stensen duct with retrograde infection are less common than in Wharton duct, but this possibility should also be considered in the patient with community acquired ABP.

Diagnosis of Acute Bacterial Parotitis

Diagnosis of ABP requires a thorough history and physical examination followed by laboratory and radiographic corroboration of the clinical diagnosis. Whether occurring in outpatient or inpatient arenas, a history of use of anti-sialogogue medications, dehydration, malnutrition, diabetes mellitus, immunosuppression, surgery, or systemic disease supports this diagnosis. A predilection for males exists for ABP, and the average age at presentation is 60 years (Miloro and Goldberg 2002). A systemic disorder will result in both glands being affected, but when one gland is affected, the right gland seems to be involved more commonly than the left gland (Miloro and Goldberg 2002). The declaration of acute requires that the parotitis has been present for one month or shorter.

The classic symptoms include an abrupt history of painful swelling of the parotid region, typically when eating. The physical findings are commonly dramatic, with parotid enlargement, often displacing the ear lobe, and tenderness to palpation. If the Stensen duct is patent, milking the gland may produce pus (Figures 3.4 and 3.5). A comparison of salivary flow should be performed by also examining the contralateral parotid gland as well as the bilateral submandibular glands. The identification of pus should alert the clinician to the need to obtain a sterile culture and sensitivity. Constitutional symptoms may be present, including fever and chills, and temperature elevation may exist provided the gland is infected. If glandular obstruction is present without infection, temperature elevation may not be present. Laboratory values will show a leukocytosis with a bandemia in the presence of true bacterial infection, with elevated hematocrit, blood urea nitrogen, and urine specific gravity if the patient is dehydrated. Electrolyte determinations should be performed in this patient population, particularly in inpatients and outpatients who are malnourished. Probing of Stensen duct is considered contraindicated in ABP. The concern is for pushing purulent material proximally in the gland, although an argument exists that probing may relieve duct strictures and mucous plugging.

The radiographic assessment of ABP is discussed in detail in Chapter 2. Briefly, plain films are of importance to rule out sialoliths, and special imaging studies may be indicated to further image the parotid gland depending on the magnitude of the swelling and the patient's signs and symptoms (Figure 3.7). The presence of an intraparotid abscess on special imaging studies, for example, may direct the clinician to the need for expedient incision and drainage.

Treatment of Acute Bacterial Parotitis

The treatment of ABP is a function of the setting in which ABP is diagnosed, as well as the severity of the disease within the parotid gland and the presence of medical comorbidities (Figure 3.8). In the outpatient setting, the presence or absence of pus will assist in directing specific therapy. The presence of pus should result in culture and sensitivity. Early species-specific antibiotic therapy is the sine qua non of treatment of ABP. Empiric antibiotic

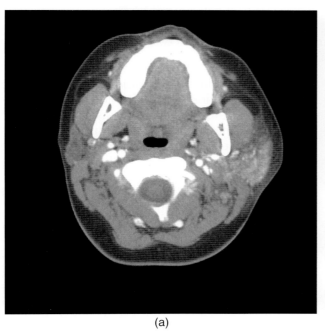
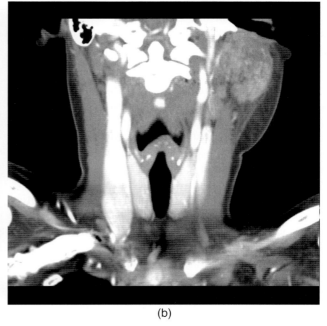

(a)   (b)

Figure 3.7. Axial (a) and coronal (b) CT scans of a patient with a hospital acquired parotitis. The degree of swelling led to the acquisition of these scans to rule out intraparotid abscess. No abscess was identified, thereby not requiring incision and drainage in this patient.

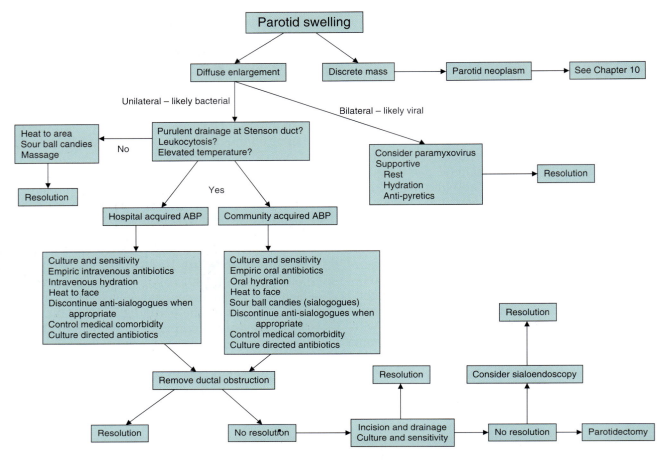

Figure 3.8. The algorithm for diagnosis and treatment of a unilateral or bilateral parotid swelling.

therapy should be based on a Gram stain of ductal exudates. In general terms, an anti-staphylococcal penicillin or a first-generation cephalosporin is a proper choice. Antibiotics should be changed if cultures and sensitivities show methicillin-resistant staphylococcal species, in which case clindamycin is indicated in community acquired ABP. In the absence of pus, empiric antibiotic therapy should be instituted as described above. Antibiotic compliance is often difficult for patients such that once or twice daily antibiotics are always preferable. In all patients with community acquired ABP, other general measures should be followed including the stimulation of salivary flow with digital massage, the use of dry heat, and the use of sour ball candies. Sugarless sour ball candies should be recommended for diabetics or those with impaired glucose tolerance. Some elderly and debilitated outpatients may require admission to the hospital in which case intravenous antibiotic therapy will be instituted and incision and drainage may be required. Alteration of anti-sialogogue medications should be accomplished as soon as possible. In the outpatient setting, these commonly include urinary incontinence medications, loop diuretics, beta blockers, and antihistamines. Glycemic control in diabetics is beneficial in the control of ABP. Finally, effective control of viral load in HIV-infected patients is of utmost importance.

Imaging of outpatients with community acquired ABP is based on the severity of the clinical disease, its chronicity, and the clinician's suspicion for intraparotid abscess. Obtaining routine plain films, such as a panoramic radiograph, is certainly indicated to investigate for the presence of a sialolith. It may be acceptable, however, to defer special imaging studies in these patients until refractory infection develops. Patients with severe symptoms, fever, and concern for abscess formation within the parotid gland should be imaged with CT scans in an expedient fashion (Figures 3.7 and 3.9). Except in the presence of severe immunosuppression or other medical comorbidity, refractory infections are uncommonly seen in ABP.

The general principles of the management of hospital acquired ABP are identical to those of the community acquired ABP. As previously described, however, the risk factors differ. In these inpatients, rehydration should be performed with caution to avoid cardiac overload. Empiric intravenous antibiotics should be instituted in these patients, and confirmed as to their efficacy with culture and sensitivity of purulent parotid exudates whenever possible. The use of heat to the affected gland is appropriate in this setting, as well. The inpatient should be monitored closely for clinical improvement. Despite the institution of conservative measures, if the patient's course deteriorates within 48–72 hours as evident by increased swelling and pain, or an increase in white blood cell count, an incision and drainage procedure is indicated (Figure 3.9). Such a procedure must be guided by CT scans to explore all loculations of pus. A needle aspiration of a parotid abscess is unlikely to represent a definitive drainage procedure, although it will permit the procurement of a sample of pus prior to instituting antibiotic therapy in preparation for incision and drainage.

CHRONIC (RECURRENT OR REFRACTORY) BACTERIAL PAROTITIS

Chronic bacterial parotitis occurs in at least three clinical settings. The first is in which the patient defers evaluation such that the condition has persisted for at least one month. The second includes the setting in which acute bacterial parotitis was managed conservatively, but without resolution (refractory sialadenitis). Finally, it is possible for a successfully treated parotitis to become recurrent such that periods of remission separate recurrent episodes of ABP. The parotid gland may demonstrate evidence of latent infection despite clinical resolution of the disease. The result is scarring in the gland such that function is impaired. Histology will show dilation of glandular ducts, abscess formation, and atrophy (Patey 1965). Pus is rarely observed in chronic bacterial parotitis (Baurmash 2004). Rather, there is a marked reduction of salivary flow, and the parotid secretions are viscous and milky in appearance. The microbiologic etiology of chronic bacterial parotitis is most commonly streptococci and staphylococci, but other organisms may be found as a function of the patient's immune status, the setting in which the parotitis originally occurred, and medical comorbidity. It has been suggested that the accumulation of a semisolid material that obstructs the parotid duct is the culprit in chronic bacterial parotitis (Baurmash 2004). The clinical course of the disease shows pain and swelling waxing and waning. As with acute bacterial parotitis, a screening panoramic radiograph or CT scans should be obtained to rule out the presence of a sialolith (Carlson 2009).

Treatment of Chronic Bacterial Parotitis

Treatment of chronic bacterial parotitis centers on palliative therapy with parotidectomy reserved as a last resort (Figure 3.10). Effective treatment is centered on the gland inflammation as well as the precipitated intraductal material. Patients should be treated with culture-specific systemic antibiotics, ductal antibiotic irrigations during periods of remission, analgesics, and avoidance of dehydration and anti-sialogogue medications (Goldberg and Bevilacqua 1995). The identification of a sialolith should result in expedient removal. Sialendoscopy represents a technique that may obviate the need for aggressive surgical intervention (Nahlieli et al. 2006; Hasson 2007). Sialendoscopy is a minimally invasive procedure with a low rate of complications. A Danish study published in 2016 demonstrated a 26% reduction in the number of salivary gland excisions for benign processes after the introduction of sialendoscopy in 2004 compared to the five years prior (Rasmussen et al. 2016). Sialendoscopic findings of patients with chronic obstructive parotitis include ductal stricture, mucous plugs, and desquamative epithelial cells and inflammatory cells (Qi et al. 2005). A sialendoscopic procedure may address any or all of these problems, thereby sparing the gland (Figure 3.11). If pain and swelling become intolerable for the patient, or if special imaging studies reveal abscess formation in the parotid gland, then nerve sparing parotidectomy is the treatment of choice (Figure 3.12)

van der Lans et al. (2019) retrospectively reviewed 46 parotidectomies performed on 37 patients with chronic bacterial parotitis. Total parotidectomy was performed in 41 cases (89%) and superficial parotidectomy was performed in 5 cases (11%). No information was included in this report regarding the chronicity of symptoms, nor the type of symptoms in their cohort. Temporary paresis of the facial nerve was noted in 12 operations (26%) with a mean duration of 7.7 weeks, with no incidence of permanent paresis. Frey syndrome was noted after 20 parotidectomies. Recurrence of the parotitis was noted in six cases (15%) and was successfully treated with conservative measures in four patients. The authors concluded that parotidectomy is a safe and effective means to resolve chronic recurrent parotitis. These authors did not find differences in resolution of disease between superficial parotidectomy and total parotidectomy. Therein, they indicated that successful treatment is

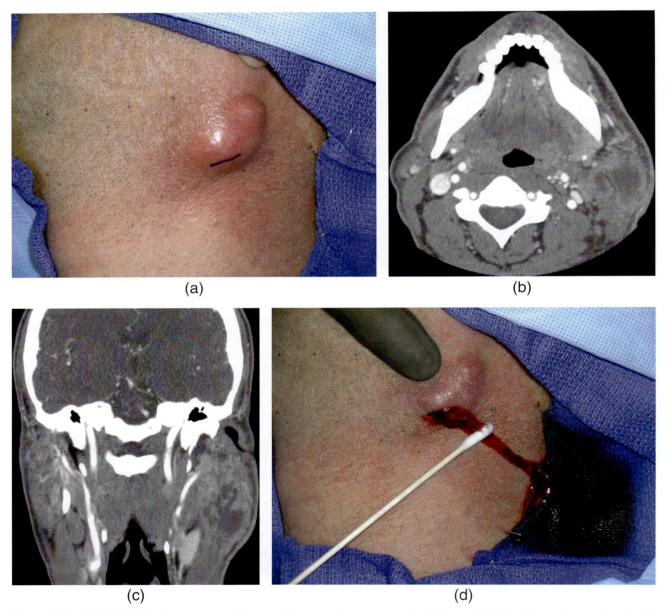

Figure 3.9. A left facial abscess in a 45-year-old man with a two-week history of left facial swelling and pain (a). Computerized tomograms (b and c) demonstrate an abscess within the tail of the left parotid gland. The patient underwent incision and drainage (d) in the operating room for a diagnosis of community acquired acute bacterial parotitis with abscess formation. Methicillin-resistant *Staphylococcus aureus* species were cultured. He showed resolution of his disease at two months postoperatively (e and f).

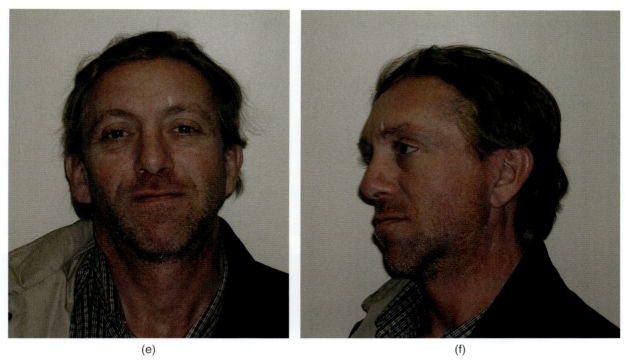

Figure 3.9. (*Continued*).

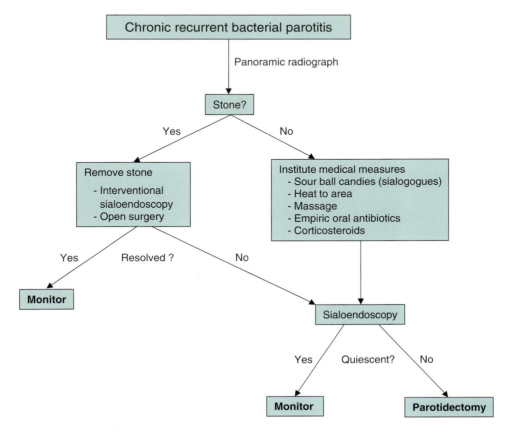

Figure 3.10. Algorithm for the management of chronic recurrent bacterial parotitis.

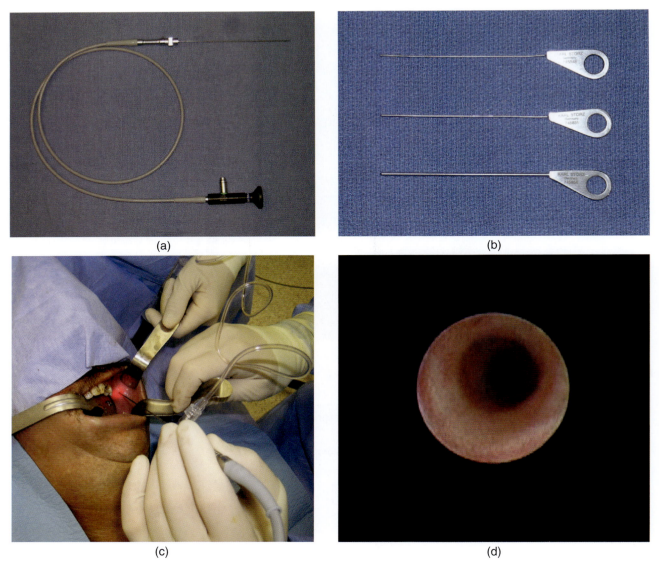

Figure 3.11. The miniature endoscope for diagnostic and interventional sialendoscopic procedures (a – Karl Storz Endoscopy, Germany). The instrumentation seen here is utilized for diagnostic procedures only. The endoscope may be connected to an operating sheath for interventional procedures (see Chapter 5). A series of duct dilators (b) are inserted in Stensen duct prior to placing the sialendoscope (c). A representative image is noted in (d) that demonstrates normal findings in a patient with chronic parotid pain. The sialendoscopy procedure, including dilatation and irrigation of the duct, resulted in resolution of symptoms. A 76-year-old man with a chronic history of right parotid swelling that waxed and waned (e–g) and he was noted to have the forced expression of pus from right Stensen duct (h). He underwent imaging studies (i and j) due to the chronicity of his diagnosis of chronic parotitis. A sialendoscopy was performed (k) that identified thick mucus in his main Stensen duct (l) and strictures in his distal ductwork within the gland (m).

Infections of the Salivary Glands 93

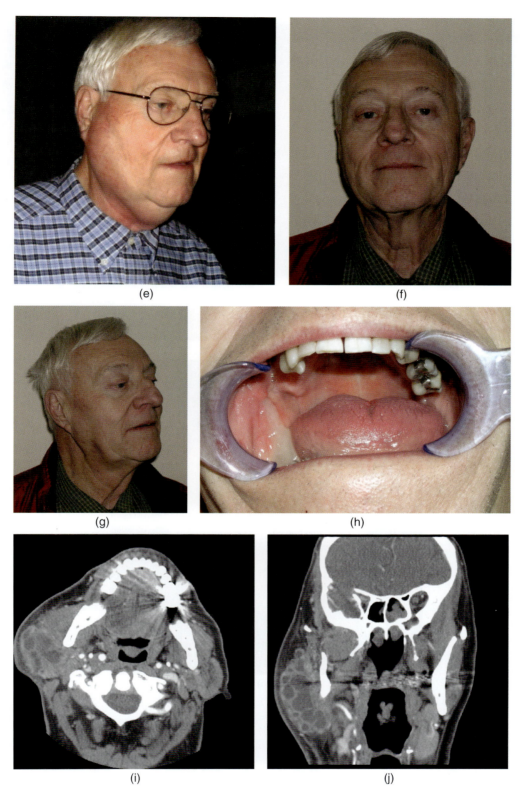

Figure 3.11. (*Continued*).

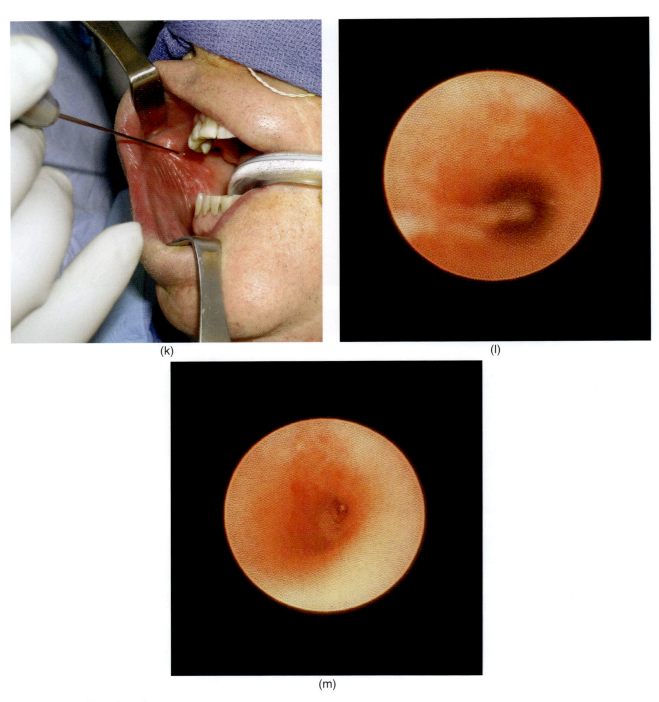

Figure 3.11. (*Continued*).

Infections of the Salivary Glands

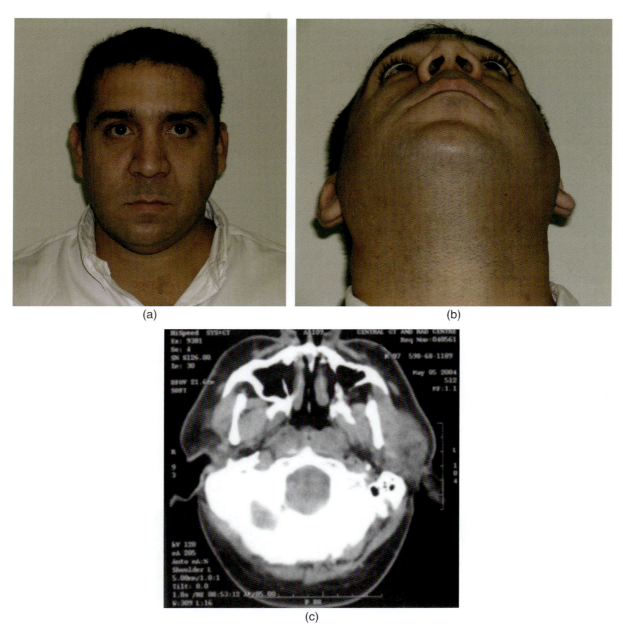

Figure 3.12. A 35-year-old man with a two-year history of left parotid pain and swelling (a and b). Computerized tomograms (c) showed sclerosis of the parotid parenchyma as well as a suspected abscess. The patient underwent left superficial parotidectomy with a clinical and radiographic diagnosis of chronic bacterial parotitis with abscess formation. The superficial parotidectomy was accessed with a standard incision (d). A nerve sparing approach was followed (e) that allowed for delivery of the specimen (f). Histopathology showed chronic sialadenitis with abscess formation (g). The patient displayed resolution of his disease at three years postoperatively (h and i) he displays resolution of his disease.

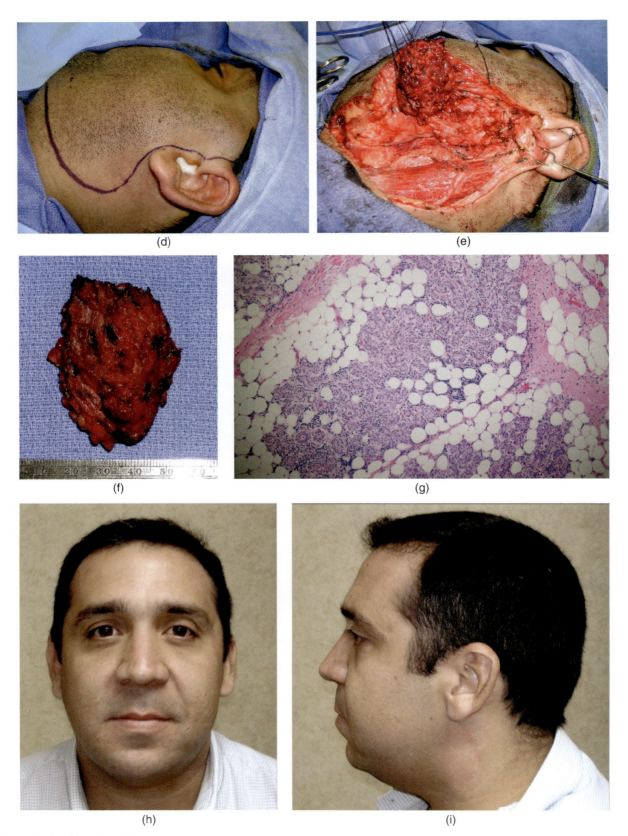

Figure 3.12. (*Continued*).

realized in removal of as much affected glandular tissue as possible while identifying and preserving the facial nerve.

CHRONIC RECURRENT JUVENILE PAROTITIS

Chronic recurrent juvenile parotitis is the second most common inflammatory disease of the salivary glands in children after mumps (Erkul and Gillespie 2016; Xie et al. 2016). In terms of its frequency, chronic recurrent parotitis in adults is 10 times more common than chronic recurrent parotitis in children (Baurmash 2004). It is characterized by recurrent inflammation of one or both parotid glands, with 73% of cases occurring bilaterally (Shacham et al. 2009). Pain may be present or absent, and the lack of pus is one of the main clinical features associated with this disease. Episodes typically occur every three to four months and each episode lasts four to seven days. Recurrent juvenile parotitis is commonly noted prior to puberty with the peak incidence of chronic recurrent juvenile parotitis being between the ages of three and six years (Shacham et al. 2009). This disease is thought to be self-limiting with many cases resolving by puberty, although some cases persist in adulthood. It is more common in boys than girls. The disease is made on a clinical basis and is confirmed by ultrasonography or sialography that demonstrates the pathognomonic sialectasis.

Several theories exist regarding the etiology and pathophysiology of chronic recurrent juvenile parotitis. Microbiologic analysis of these cases has identified *Streptococcus pneumoniae* and *Haemophilus influenza* in high concentrations in these cases, thereby suggesting that microorganisms are of etiologic significance. An autosomal dominant pattern of inheritance has also been suggested to be involved in some cases. It has also been suggested that congenital abnormalities or strictures of Stensen duct, trauma, foreign bodies with the duct, or a history of viral mumps are etiologic. Regardless of the exact etiology, the pathophysiology of the disease is decreased salivary production with inadequate outflow through the duct that encourages ascending salivary gland infections via the oral cavity (Tucci et al. 2019).

Treatment of Chronic Recurrent Juvenile Parotitis

Treatment recommendations range from conservative measures including antibiotics, massage, and sialagogues and surgical procedures with sialendoscopy. Gland preservation should be the goal of treatment since cases typically resolve (Erkul and Gillespie 2016). Shacham et al. (2009) reported on 70 children with chronic recurrent juvenile parotitis who were treated with sialendoscopy and lavage of the gland with 60ml of normal saline bilaterally. Dilatation of Stensen ducts was performed in four patients and 100mg of hydrocortisone was injected into each gland. In 93% of patients treated in this fashion, a single treatment was sufficient to resolve the parotitis and prevent its recurrence. Although encouraging studies demonstrate the benefit of sialendoscopy for chronic recurrent juvenile parotitis, there is a lack of prospective, randomized controlled studies comparing this modality to conservative measures alone. It has been recommended to adopt a watchful waiting approach with conservative measures followed by the performance of sialendoscopy if three episodes occur within a six-month period or four episodes within one year (Erkul and Gillespie 2016). This approach seems valid since spontaneous regeneration of salivary function has been reported (Galili and Marmary 1985).

Tucci et al. (2019) performed a retrospective study of 110 patients with a diagnosis of chronic recurrent juvenile parotitis who underwent sialography without local anesthesia or sedation. The outcome of the sialography was measured by comparing the number and magnitude of episodes of parotid swelling before and after the procedure. Marked improvement was defined by an outcome that saw no episode of parotid swelling or a reduction of more than 80% of episodes in the first year after the procedure. A nonresponder was defined by no improvement in swelling events or by a reduction of less than 30% events. Partial improvement was defined as decreased but not complete resolution of swelling or with a reduction of episodes from 30 to 80% of episodes in the year after sialography. After performing the sialography, a statistically significant overall recovery of pathology was noted in 98 (89%) of patients with a mean 67.4% reduction in the number of acute episodes of parotid swelling in the year after the procedure. Seventy-five patients demonstrated a marked improvement in symptoms with a mean reduction of 80.6% of acute attacks. Partial improvement was noted in 23 patients with a mean reduction of the number of episodes of 36.5% in the year after sialography. No remission of swelling was noted in 12 patients. The authors concluded that sialography is an effective therapeutic method for chronic recurrent juvenile parotitis and is associated with low cost and with a low rate of complications.

ACUTE BACTERIAL SUBMANDIBULAR SIALADENITIS

Acute bacterial submandibular sialadenitis (ABSS) is usually associated with physical obstruction of the Wharton duct and therefore presents as swelling associated with the submandibular gland. That said, physical examination of the patient with submandibular swelling may not immediately disclose whether the swelling is related to sialadenitis of the submandibular gland, to neoplastic disease of the submandibular gland, or due to a process extrinsic to the submandibular gland. As such, CT scans become required when the distinction cannot be made entirely on physical findings alone (Figure 3.13a). This notwithstanding, sialolithiasis, the likely cause of obstruction of the duct with resultant submandibular gland swelling, is discussed in Chapter 5, it is only briefly mentioned here. Suffice it to say that the submandibular ductal system is prone to stone formation. The common features of ABSS are swelling in the submandibular region associated with prandial pain. ABSS is a community acquired disease that less frequently is associated with dehydration and hospitalization as compared to ABP. Purulence may be expressed from the opening of the Wharton duct, but in many cases, complete obstruction to pus and saliva occurs. As in the case of acute bacterial parotitis, imaging studies are also obtained in patients with clinically unequivocal acute bacterial submandibular sialadenitis when signs and symptoms are of a magnitude to justify acquiring CT scans (Figure 3.13b).

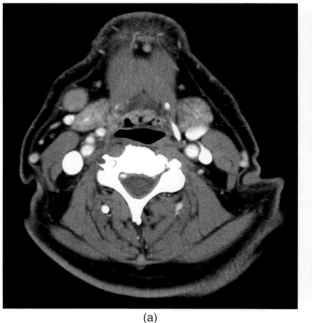
(a)

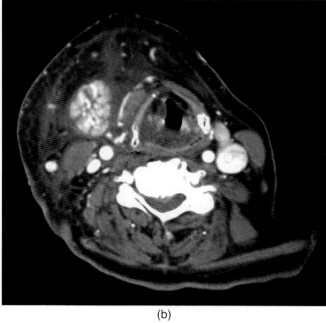
(b)

Figure 3.13. The CT scan (a) of a 73-year-old man with a one-year history of right submandibular swelling. Physical examination of the neck identified a mass with a differential diagnosis of submandibular gland mass vs. enlarged lymph node in the submandibular region. This CT scan was obtained due to the equivocal nature of the finding on physical examination. Fine needle aspiration biopsy of this mass led to a diagnosis of low-grade lymphoma. By distinction, a 24-year-old woman with right submandibular swelling and pain who underwent a CT scan that identified intense uptake of intravenous contrast of the right submandibular gland indicative of acute bacterial submandibular sialadenitis (b). Fat stranding in the left neck indicative of inflammation is also noted.

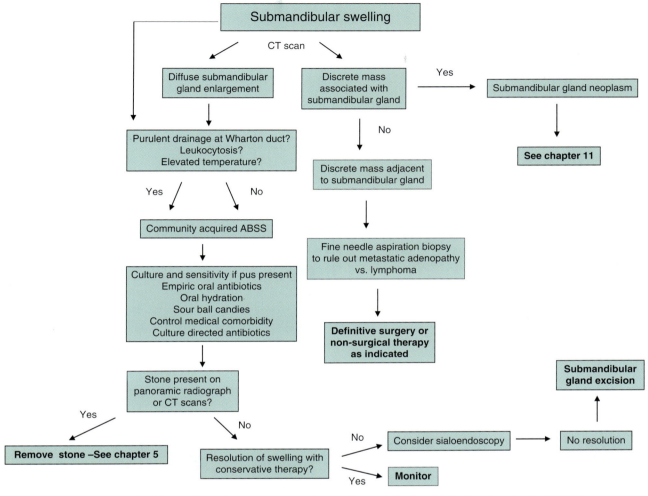

Figure 3.14. Algorithm for diagnosis and management of acute bacterial submandibular sialadenitis (ABSS).

Treatment of Acute Bacterial Submandibular Sialadenitis

Treatment of ABSS consists of antibiotic therapy, hydration, avoidance of anti-sialogogues, and removal of a sialolith, if one is identified (Figure 3.14). Empiric antibiotics used to treat ABSS are similar to those antibiotics used in ABP, including an extended spectrum penicillin, a first-generation cephalosporin, clindamycin, or a macrolide. Patients are also encouraged to use sialogogues, such as sour ball candies.

CHRONIC RECURRENT SUBMANDIBULAR SIALADENITIS

Chronic recurrent submandibular sialadenitis usually follows ABSS and is associated with untreated sialolithiasis. Chronic recurrent submandibular sialadenitis occurs more commonly than chronic recurrent bacterial parotitis. Initial treatment for chronic recurrent submandibular sialadenitis begins with antibiotic therapy, sialogogues, and hydration. Sialolithotomy is required if diagnosed. Sialendoscopic intervention may also be of benefit in the treatment of chronic recurrent submandibular sialadenitis prior to subjecting the patient to submandibular gland removal. Ultimately, removal of the submandibular gland is often necessary (Figure 3.15).

BARTONELLA HENSELAE (CAT-SCRATCH DISEASE)

Cat-scratch disease (CSD) is a granulomatous lymphadenitis that most commonly results from cutaneous inoculation caused by a scratch from a

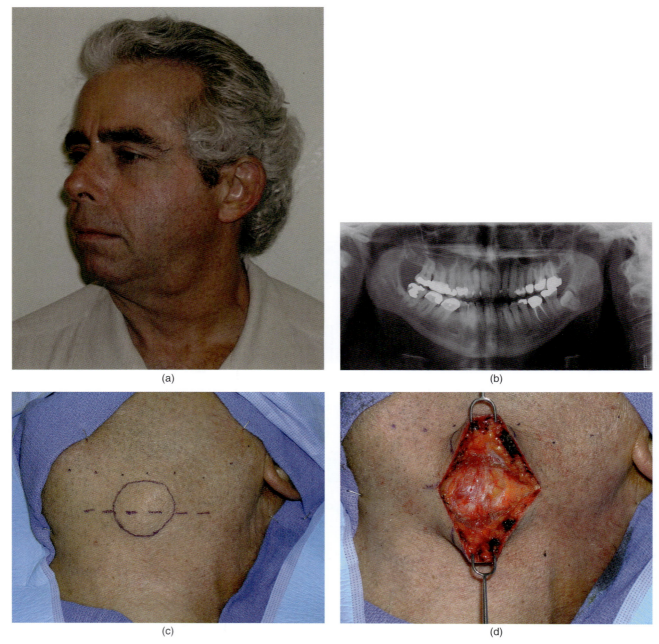

Figure 3.15. A 52-year-old man (a) with a one-year history of vague discomfort in the left upper neck. Screening panoramic radiograph (b) showed no evidence of a sialolith. His diagnosis was chronic submandibular sialadenitis and he was prepared for left submandibular gland excision (c). The surgery was carried through anatomic planes, including the investing layer of the deep cervical fascia (d). The dissection is carried deep to this layer since a cancer surgery is not being performed that would require a dissection superficial to the investing fascia. Exposure of the gland demonstrates a small submandibular gland due to scar contracture (e). Inferior retraction of the gland allows for identification and preservation of the lingual nerve (f). The specimen (g) is bivalved (h), which allows for the appreciation of scar within the gland. The resultant tissue bed (i) shows the hypoglossal nerve, which is routinely preserved in excision of the submandibular gland. Histopathology shows a sclerosing sialadenitis (j). The patient's symptoms were eliminated postoperatively, and he healed uneventfully, as noted at one year following the surgery (k).

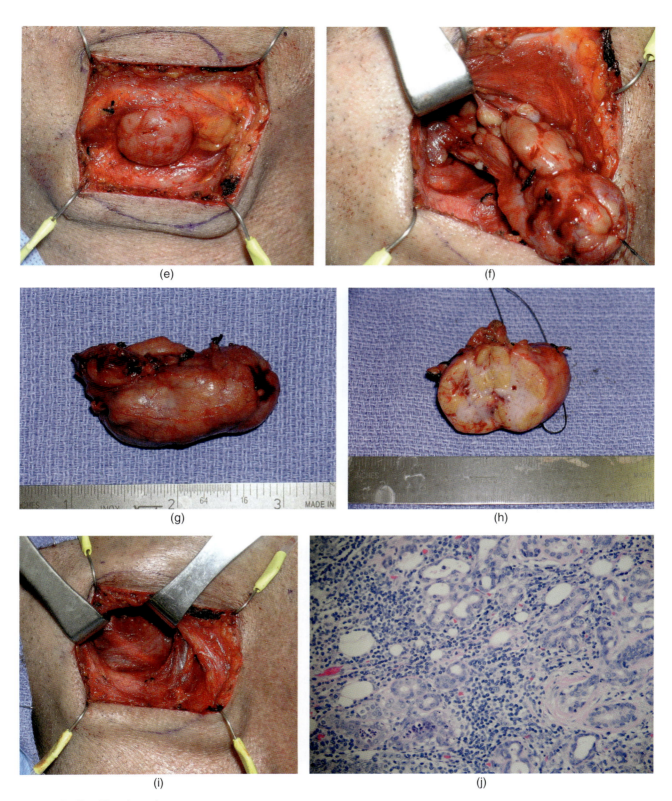

Figure 3.15. (Continued).

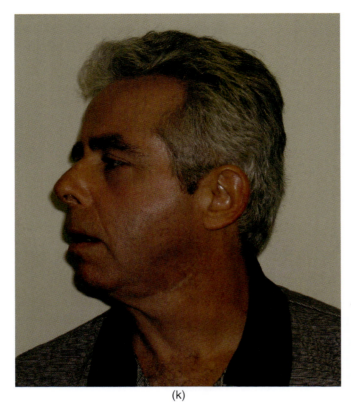

(k)

Figure 3.15. (Continued).

domestic cat. The causative microorganism is *Bartonella henselae*, a Gram negative bacillus. Approximately 90% of patients who have cat-scratch disease have a history of exposure to cats, and 75% of these patients report a cat scratch or bite (Arrieta and McCaffrey 2005). Dogs have been implicated in 5% in these cases. This disease process begins in the preauricular and cervical lymph nodes as a chronic lymphadenitis and may ultimately involve the salivary glands, most commonly the parotid gland by contiguous spread (English et al. 1988).

The diagnosis of CSD has changed with advances in serologic and molecular biologic techniques. These methods have replaced the need for the Rose Hanger skin test previously used to establish the diagnosis of CSD. Testing for the presence of antibodies to *B. henselae* is now the most commonly used test to confirm the diagnosis. The two methods used for antibody detection are the indirect fluorescent antibody (IFA) and the enzyme immunoassay (EIA). When tissue is removed for diagnosis, histologic examination might demonstrate bacilli with the use of Warthin–Starry staining or a Steiner stain. Lymph node involvement shows reticular cell hyperplasia, granuloma formation, and occasionally a stellate abscess.

In most cases, no active therapy is required. The patient should be reassured that the lymphadenopathy is self-limited and will spontaneously resolve in two to four months. Antibiotic therapy is indicated when patients are symptomatic. Antibiotics reported to be most effective include rifampin, erythromycin, gentamycin, azithromycin, and ciprofloxacin. Surgery becomes necessary when the diagnosis is equivocal, or when incision and drainage is indicated (Figure 3.16).

TUBERCULOUS MYCOBACTERIAL DISEASE

Tuberculosis is a chronic infectious disease with worldwide distribution, although more commonly seen in developing countries. While primarily noted in the lungs and characterized by caseous necrosis, extrapulmonary forms of the disease account for approximately 20% of active tuberculosis and can affect any organ in the body (Maurya et al. 2019). The most common head and neck manifestation of mycobacterium tuberculosis is infection of the cervical lymph nodes. Tuberculous infection of the salivary glands is very rare and generally seen in older children and adults. Parotid tuberculous constitutes 2.5–10% of salivary gland tuberculosis (Maurya et al. 2019). Salivary glands are thought to resist the growth of mycobacterium tuberculosis due to the continuous flow of saliva that prevents colonization of the bacteria. The infection is believed to originate in the tonsils or gingiva and most commonly ascends to the parotid gland via its duct (Arrieta and McCaffrey 2005). Secondary infection of the salivary glands occurs by way of the lymphatic or hematogenous spread from the lungs. Clinically, tuberculous salivary gland infection presents in two different forms. The first is an acute inflammatory lesion with diffuse glandular edema that may be confused with an acute sialadenitis or abscess. The chronic lesion occurs as a slow-growing painless mass with or without cervical adenopathy that mimics a tumor. Patients with tuberculous parotitis have been further classified into three groups: group 1 – patients with asymptomatic unilateral preauricular swelling; group 2 – patients with recurrent swelling with fistula; and group

McCaffrey 2005). The disease primarily affects children younger than five years of age. The specific organisms are *M. Kansasii, Mycobacterium avium-intracellulare*, and *M. scrofulaceum*. The typical clinical presentation is that of a rapidly enlarging and persistent parotid and/or neck mass that has failed to resolve with antibiotic therapy (Mitchell and Ord 1988) (Figure 3.17). A characteristic violaceous discoloration to the skin develops. The treatment of choice is surgical removal of the involved salivary gland and associated lymph nodes.

Viral Salivary Gland Infections

MUMPS

Viral mumps is an acute, nonsuppurative communicable disease that often occurs in epidemics during the spring and winter months. The term mumps is derived from the Danish "mompen," which refers to mumbling, thereby describing the difficulty with speech because of inflammation and trismus (McQuone 1999; Arrieta and McCafrey 2005). The nearly routine administration of the measles–mumps–rubella (MMR) vaccination has decreased the incidence of mumps in industrialized nations. Since the introduction of the live attenuated vaccine in the United States in 1967 and its administration as part of the MMR vaccine, the yearly incidence of mumps cases has declined from 76 to two cases per 100,000 (Murray et al. 1994). Mumps characteristically occurs in the parotid glands. Although the disease is typically seen in children between six and eight years of age, it may occur in adults who have avoided childhood infection, as well, and displays an equal sex predilection. The disease is caused most commonly by a paramyxovirus, a ribonucleic acid virus related to the influenza and parainfluenza virus groups. Several other non-paramyxoviruses may cause mumps, including coxsackie A and B viruses, Epstein-Barr virus, influenza and parainfluenza viruses, enteric cytopathic human orphan (ECHO) virus, and human immunodeficiency virus (HIV). Mumps is transmitted by infected saliva and urine. The incubation period between exposure and the development of signs and symptoms is 15–18 days. A prodromal period occurs that lasts 24–48 hours and involves fever, chills, headache, and preauricular tenderness. Following the prodromal period, rapid and painful unilateral or bilateral swelling of the parotid glands occurs. Features that distinguish sialadenitis due to mumps versus bacteria include a lack of purulent discharge, positive serum titers for mumps, and a relative lymphocytosis in mumps. In addition, the clinical presentation of mumps is mild; not infrequently, patients may be asymptomatic (Schreiber and Hershman 2009). The diagnosis is made by demonstrating complement-fixing soluble (S) antibodies to the nucleoprotein core of the virus, which are the earliest antibodies to appear. These antibodies peak at 10 days to 2 weeks and disappear within eight to nine months. The S antibodies are therefore associated with active infection. The complement-fixing viral (V) antibodies are against outer surface hemagglutinin and appear later than S antibodies but persist at low levels for years. The diagnosis may also be made by isolating the virus from urine, which is possible up to 6 days prior and 13 days after the salivary gland symptoms occur (Rice 1998. Serum amylase levels may be elevated regardless of an associated pancreatitis. Abdominal pain is often indicative of mumps pancreatitis. Mumps orchitis occurs in 20% of adult males who have mumps parotitis (Goldberg and Bevilacqua 1995). Approximately half of these males will experience secondary testicular atrophy that may result in sterility if the testicular atrophy occurs bilaterally. Other rare complications of mumps include mumps hepatitis, mumps myocarditis, and mumps thyroiditis.

Treatment of mumps is supportive as spontaneous resolution of the disease occurs within 5–10 days. Such supportive care includes bed rest, proper hydration, and dietary modifications to minimize glandular activity. Persistent or recurrent parotid swelling may indicate the presence of sialadenitis. In the presence of such symptoms, a CT scan may be ordered that will frequently identify generalized sialadenitis to all salivary glands (Figure 3.18).

HUMAN IMMUNODEFICIENCY VIRUS

HIV infection is associated with numerous pathologic processes involving the salivary glands, with the parotid gland being the most common. Parotid gland enlargement is estimated to occur in 1–10% of HIV-infected patients (Shanti and Aziz 2009). HIV-associated salivary gland disease (HIV-SGD) is a term used to describe the diffuse enlargement of the salivary glands. HIV-SGD may affect patients throughout all stages of the infection, and may be

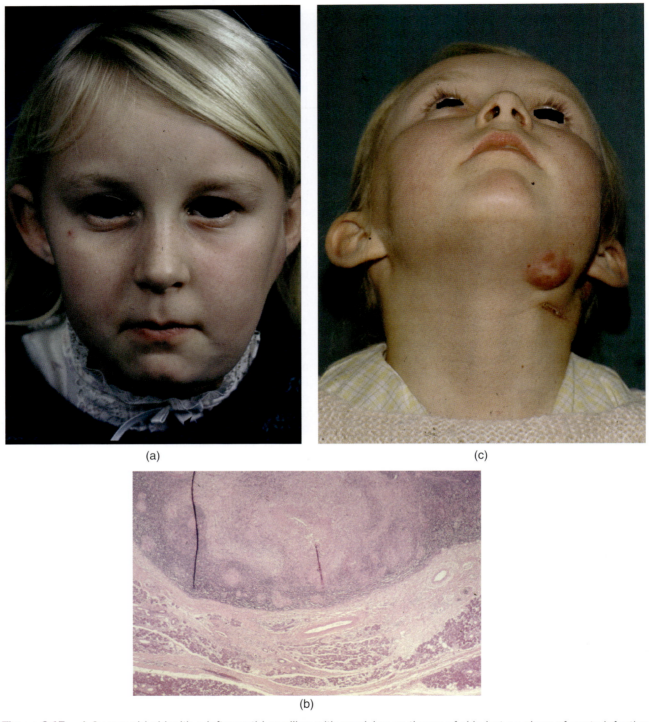

Figure 3.17. A 9-year-old girl with a left parotid swelling with overlying erythema of skin but no signs of acute infection (a). The patient underwent left superficial parotidectomy and excision of a submandibular lymph node. Histopathology showed noncaseating granulomas (b), and cultures showed mycobacterium avium-intracellulare. Two months following the parotidectomy, a left submandibular lymph node became enlarged (c) and was treated with medical therapy.

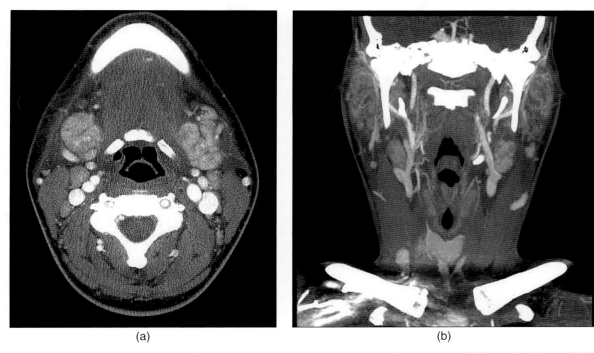

Figure 3.18. Axial (a) and coronal (b) CT images demonstrating contrast enhancement of bilateral submandibular and parotid glands in a patient with a clinical viral prodrome.

the initial manifestation of HIV infection (Schiodt et al. 1992).

Patients with HIV-SGD present with a history of nontender swelling of one or more of the salivary glands (Figure 3.19). These swellings may fluctuate, but are generally persistent. Imaging studies are generally beneficial to diagnose lymphoepithelial cysts in this patient population that may clinically resemble the nontender swellings of the parotid glands in this patient population. Decreased salivary gland function results in xerostomia and sicca symptoms. This sicca symptom complex mimics Sjögren syndrome and has resulted in the classification of another HIV-related salivary gland process known as the diffuse infiltrative lymphocytosis syndrome (DILS). This pathologic process is characterized by the presence of persistent circulating CD8 lymphocytes and infiltration of organs by CD8 lymphocytes that occur predominantly in the salivary glands and lungs. While DILS appears clinically like Sjögren syndrome, it can be differentiated by the presence of extraglandular involvement of the lungs, kidneys, and gastrointestinal tract. In addition, Sjogren's autoantibodies will be absent in patients with DILS.

Medical management of HIV-SGD involves the use of antiretrovirals, observing meticulous oral hygiene, and the use of sialogogues. Corticosteroids may also be of use.

INFLUENZA A

Annual influenza outbreaks result in seasonal flu epidemics of acute viral respiratory disease related to influenza A or B infection. These outbreaks typically cause fever, headache, malaise, and myalgia with symptoms of upper respiratory infection including cough, rhinorrhea, and sore throat. During one month in 2018, Stafford et al. (2018) diagnosed and managed four patients with sialadenitis related to influenza A. Two cases involved the bilateral submandibular glands, one case involved bilateral parotid glands and one submandibular gland, and one case involved one parotid gland. These authors indicated that the Centers for Disease Control and Prevention reported hundreds of confirmed influenza cases with associated parotitis during the 2014–2015 influenza season, primarily related to influenza A (H3N2) infection. The cause of the association of influenza A and sialadenitis is not clear. Dehydration related to

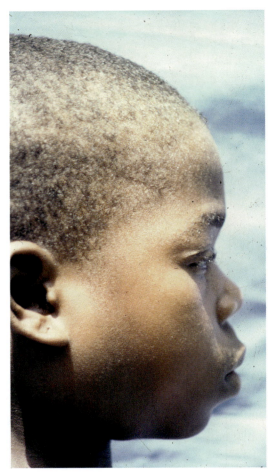

Figure 3.19. A 6-year-old African female with AIDS showing involvement of the right parotid gland by diffuse infiltrative lymphocytosis syndrome (DILS).

respiratory influenza infection might make patients prone to salivary stasis, or it is possible that the virus may directly involve salivary tissue with resultant sialadenitis.

Bacterial Sialadenitis in Pregnancy

The female patient with inflammation of any major salivary gland and a superimposed gravid uterus represents a routine clinical diagnostic challenge but a radiographic and treatment dilemma (Figure 3.20). Under such circumstances, the clinician must exert proper judgment in terms of the utility and timing of contrast-enhanced CT or MRI as well as the administration of oral and intravenous antibiotics. Although evidence-based guidelines report the safety to the fetus in using iodinated contrast during pregnancy, intravenous gadolinium is contraindicated due to its teratogenicity (Chen et al. 2008). These authors also indicate that the first two weeks of embryogenesis are associated with a risk of blastocyst implant failure when the radiation dose exceeds 0.1 Gy (10 cGy). Further, between the second and twentieth week of embryonic age, the fetus is most susceptible to radiation and its teratogenic sequelae including microcephaly, growth restriction, behavioral defects, cataracts, and others. The precise threshold dose of radiation to the fetus when teratogenicity occurs is estimated to range from 5 to 15 cGy (Chen et al. 2008). Most maxillofacial CT scans that would be ordered to image submandibular and parotid sialadenitis are likely to not exceed this threshold, but individual practitioners are encouraged to confirm such in consultation with their radiology departments. In terms of contrast media for use in CT, iodine has the potential to induce neonatal hypothyroidism, although iodinated contrast media are generally not believed to be teratogenic. Given that it is standard practice to screen all neonates for hypothyroidism, this test is particularly important in neonates of women who underwent iodine contrast CT during pregnancy. In the final analysis, guidelines of the American College of Radiology state that it is not possible to establish definitive conclusions regarding the risks of iodinated contrast use in pregnant women and therefore recommend that such contrast should only be administered if absolutely essential and only after informed consent has been obtained from the patient.

The potential use of MRI in pregnant women with sialadenitis conjures two concerns, including teratogenicity and acoustic damage, although most studies evaluating MRI in pregnant women show no ill effects (Chen et al. 2008). Potential mechanisms for damage of the developing fetus include the heating effect of magnetic resonance gradient changes and direct nonthermal interaction of the electromagnetic field with biological structures. In terms of acoustic damage, loud noises generated by the MRI scanner coils, particularly with echo planar imaging, the noisiest sequence in clinical use, could be deleterious to the developing fetus. Finally, intravenous gadolinium is teratogenic in animal studies, although at high and repeated doses. It is classified as a category C drug by the Food and Drug Administration. Gadolinium crosses the placenta where it is likely excreted by the fetal kidneys into the amniotic fluid. In terms of

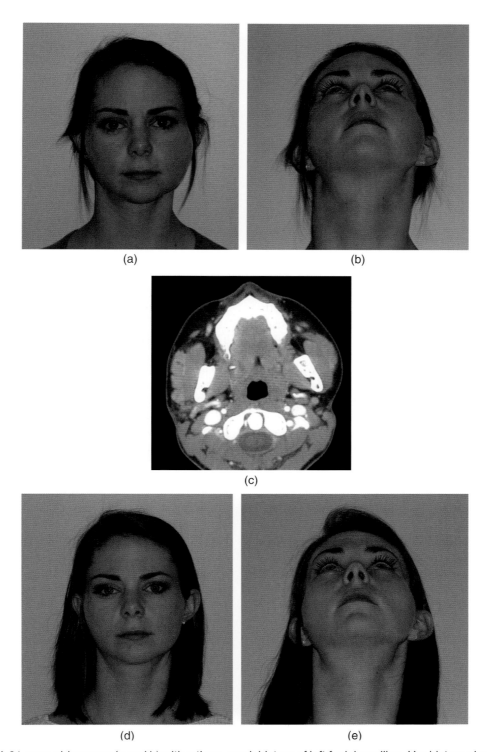

Figure 3.20. A 21-year-old woman (a and b) with a three-week history of left facial swelling. Her history also divulged a first trimester pregnancy. Conservative measures were accomplished including heat, the use of sour ball candies, massage, and an anti-staphylococcal antibiotic × one week. She responded incompletely to these conservative measures and a CT scan (c) was obtained during her second trimester of pregnancy. No stone was identified and no surgical intervention was required. The patient ultimately resolved her chronic parotitis (d and e) and she did not experience a recurrent episode.

gadolinium-induced nephrogenic systemic fibrosis, this raises the theoretical issue of toxicity due to disassociation and persistence of free gadolinium (Chen et al. 2008). As such, gadolinium should be avoided during pregnancy and CT with intravenous contrast should be substituted under proper considerations and judgment.

Antibiotics account for approximately 80% of all medications prescribed during pregnancy and approximately 20–55% of women will receive an antibiotic during pregnancy (Bookstaver et al. 2015). Although the use of an oral or intravenous antibiotic during pregnancy is a risk–benefit decision-making exercise, any untreated infection is associated with significant fetal risk including spontaneous abortion, low birth rate, and prematurity. That said, antibiotic exposure during pregnancy may result in short-term and long-term effects on infant weight, specifically lower birth weight; childhood obesity; neurologic disease, including cerebral palsy and epilepsy; and childhood asthma (Bookstaver et al. 2015).

In addition to fetal safety related to antibiotic use during pregnancy, there are physiologic changes in pregnancy that may lead to pharmacokinetic changes and impact pregnancy. For example, increases in total body water, blood volume (40–50%), and plasma volume (40–50%) contribute to increases in volume of distribution of various antibiotics. Renal blood flow increases by 50%, serum creatinine decrease, and glomerular filtration rate increases elimination of renally excreted antibiotics. Changes in gastrointestinal motility may alter absorption, oral bioavailability, and delayed onset of action of certain antibiotics. The beta-lactam antibiotics, vancomycin, metronidazole, and clindamycin are generally considered safe in pregnancy, while fluoroquinolones and tetracyclines are generally avoided in pregnancy (Bookstaver et al. 2015). In the final analysis, consultation with the pregnant women's obstetrician is recommended when antibiotics are required for the treatment of sialadenitis.

Autoimmune Sialadenitis and IgG4-Related Disease

Collectively, the collagen vascular diseases, including polymyositis, dermatomyositis, scleroderma, and systemic lupus erythematosus, may all affect the salivary glands, although Sjogren disease and sarcoidosis are most commonly responsible (Kessler and Bhatt 2018). Sjogren disease-related sialadenitis is predominantly seen in females and most commonly in postmenopausal women (50–70 years of age). A juvenile subtype is seen in men younger than 20 years of age that typically resolves at puberty. Sjogren disease-related sialadenitis is classified into two types. Sjogren type 1 disease (Mikulicz disease or sicca syndrome without a connective disorder) refers to autoimmune sialadenitis without a systemic collagen vascular disorder. These patients demonstrate xerostomia and are incorporated into the IgG4 spectrum of disease. Sjogren type 2 disease refers to autoimmune inflammation of the salivary glands with a systemic autoimmune diagnosis (rheumatoid arthritis > systemic lupus erythematosus > scleroderma).

Systemic lupus erythematosus is most frequently seen in fourth and fifth-decade women. Any of the salivary glands may become involved, and a slowly enlarging gland is the presentation. The diagnosis is made by identification of the underlying systemic disorder, and salivary chemistry levels will reveal sodium and chloride ion levels that are elevated to two three times normal levels (Miloro and Goldberg 2002).

Sarcoid-related sialadenitis is seen in 10–30% of patients with sarcoidosis and patients typically present with painless bilateral parotid swelling. The treatment of autoimmune sialadenitis involves treatment of the responsible systemic disease. The reader is referred to Chapter 6 in which autoimmune sialadenitis is more granularly reviewed and illustrated.

Immunoglobulin G4-related disease (IgG4-RD) is a condition characterized by an immune-mediated fibroinflammatory pathologic process with a tendency to form tumefactive lesions in organs, the most common of which are the pancreas and salivary glands (Lang et al. 2016)(see Chapter 6). Clinical and serologic findings include swollen organs and elevated serum IgG4. Common histologic findings in tissues include fibrosis with a storiform pattern, a diffuse lymphoplasmacytic infiltrate, obliterative phlebitis, abundance of IgG4 plasma cells, and mild to moderate tissue eosinophilia (Puxeddu et al. 2018). The increase of IgG4 seems to be a reactive phenomenon rather than the primary etiology of the disease. Involvement of the salivary glands is seen in 27–53% of patients with IgG4-related disease (Puxeddu et al. 2018). Unlike classic autoimmune diseases such as systemic lupus erythematosus and Sjögren syndrome that affect mainly females, IgG4-related disease occurs in a subacute form in most patients without the rapid onset of general symptoms such as fever. Mikulicz disease affecting the lacrimal and parotid glands and Kuttner tumor affecting the submandibular glands are two examples of IgG4-related disease of the salivary gland.

Summary

- Sialadenitis is an infection of salivary glands that has numerous etiologies including microorganisms, and autoimmune diseases.
- Staphylococcal and streptococcal species are involved in community acquired acute bacterial parotitis, and *Pseudomonas, Klebsiella, Prevotella, Fusobacterium, Haemophilus,* and *Proteus* species are cultured from hospital acquired cases of acute bacterial parotitis. Methicillin-resistant *Staphylococcus aureus* may be cultured from cases of community acquired and hospital acquired acute bacterial parotitis.
- The clinician must rule out a neoplastic process in a prompt fashion while diagnosing and treating the sialadenitis.
- The presence of a sialolith must be considered in the initial workup of patients with a clinical diagnosis of sialadenitis. A screening panoramic radiograph or occlusal radiograph should be obtained. If identified, the expedient removal of a sialolith may permit functional recovery of the salivary gland.
- The parotid and submandibular glands are the most commonly affected salivary glands by sialadenitis.
- The purpose of initial treatment for sialadenitis is to provide medical therapy for the disorder, with surgical therapy being introduced if the disorder becomes refractory to medical treatment.
- Minimally invasive strategies have a role to play in the surgical treatment of sialadenitis, as well as surgical removal of the salivary gland.
- Sialadenitis in pregnant women is a clinical diagnosis worthy of expert consultation in terms of acquiring special imaging studies and initiating antibiotic therapy.

Case Presentation – *Gadzooks*

A 71-year-old man was transferred from an outside hospital with a large left facial abscess (Figure 3.21a). Prior to urgent intubation due to concern for airway patency, the patient reported a history of recent trauma to the left face related to a trip and fall. He was a resident in a nursing home at the time of his admission.

Past Medical History
A review of the patient's medical record and the patient's report revealed a history of coronary heart disease, hypertension, hyperlipidemia, severe left ventricular systolic dysfunction (ejection fraction 15%), and a cardiomyopathy. He was medicated with lisinopril, carvedilol, donepezil, furosemide, and famotidine. The patient reported no known drug allergies. He reported no tobacco history.

Physical Examination
The patient was orally intubated at the time of comprehensive examination. There was significant left facial swelling and substantial pus expressed from the left Stensen duct during left parotid massage (Figure 3.21b). The left parotid gland was indurated. There were no oral mucosal or oropharyngeal lesions.

Imaging
CT scans were obtained at the outlying hospital that revealed left parotid, masseteric, buccal, submandibular, lateral pharyngeal, and pterygomandibular abscesses (Figure 3.21c and d). The CT scans also demonstrated airway deviation, thereby resulting in urgent intubation in the emergency department.

Diagnosis
A clinical diagnosis of left suppurative parotitis was established. He was subjected to urgent incision and drainage of the left parotid abscess and multiple fascial space abscesses in the operating room (Figure 3.21e) and three Penrose drains were placed (Figure 3.21f). Final culture and sensitivity identified methicillin-resistant *Staphylococcus aureus* sensitive to vancomycin. The patient received one week of intravenous vancomycin postoperatively with monitoring of his peaks and troughs and his renal function. He recovered well and was discharged from the hospital following a one-week admission. He is noted at six months following the incision and drainage procedure (Figure 3.21g). The left parotid gland swelling resolved and his gland recovered from the suppurative parotitis as noted by the production of saliva.

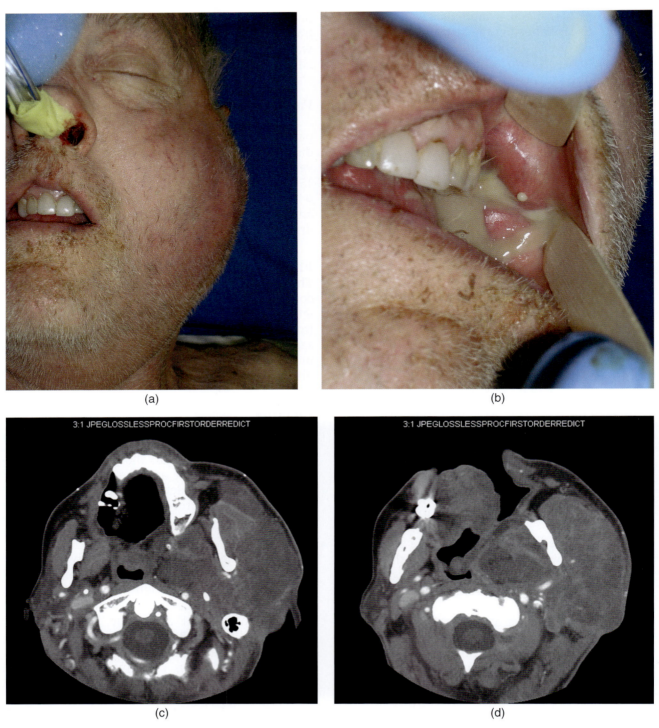

Figure 3.21. A 71-year-old man (a) demonstrated significant left facial swelling related to his acute left parotitis. Examination of the oral cavity identified thick pus at the left Stensen duct (b) and the ability to express significant pus at this site by massage of the left parotid gland. (c and d) CT imaging identified obvious abscess of the left parotid gland and involvement of numerous fascial spaces. (e) The patient underwent urgent incision and drainage that liberated substantial pus from the left parotid gland. Three Penrose drains were placed (f). Culture and sensitivity identified methicillin-resistant *Staphylococcus aureus*, sensitive to vancomycin. (g) The patient improved in the hospital and resolved his parotitis as noted at six months postoperatively.

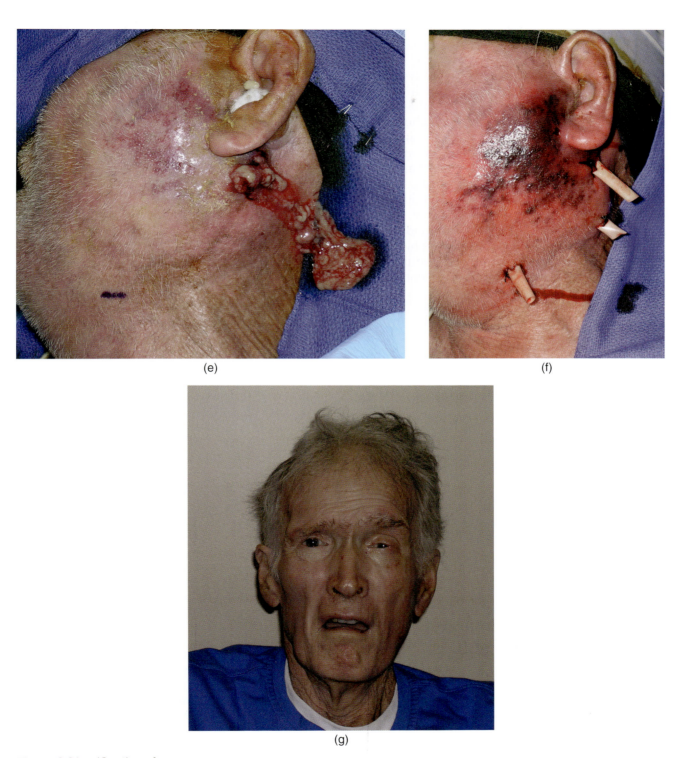

Figure 3.21. (Continued).

TAKE-HOME POINTS

1. Incision and drainage of parotitis is uncommonly required as patients typically resolve their parotitis with antibiotics while investigating for the possible presence of a sialolith.
2. Incision and drainage is warranted when physical examination demonstrates a significant magnitude of suppurative infection and when CT scans demonstrate the presence of an intraparotid abscess. Under these circumstances, culture-directed antibiotic therapy is required.
3. A suppurative parotitis is typically of intrinsic origin, e.g. sialolithiasis or retrograde infections. This case demonstrates a possible extrinsic etiology of the suppurative parotitis due to his recent facial trauma, or possibly both intrinsic and extrinsic etiologies.

References

Andrews JC, Abemayor E, Alessi DM et al. 1989. Parotitis and facial nerve dysfunction. *Arch Otolaryngol Head Neck Surg* 115:240-242.

Arrieta AJ, McCaffrey TV. 2005. Inflammatory Disorders of the Salivary Glands. In: Cummings CW (ed.) *Cummings Otolaryngology Head and Neck Surgery*, 4th edn. Philadelphia, Elsevier Mosby, pp. 1323-1338.

Baurmash HD. 2004. Chronic recurrent parotitis: A closer look at its origin, diagnosis, and management. *J Oral Maxillofac Surg* 62:1010-1018.

Bookstaver PB, Bland CM, Griffin B et al. 2015. A review of antibiotic use in pregnancy. *Pharmacotherapy* 35:1052-1062.

Brodie BC. 1834. Inflammation of the parotid gland and salivary fistulae. *Lancet* 1:450-452.

Carlson ER. 2009. Diagnosis and management of salivary gland infections. *Oral Maxillofac Surg Clin N Am* 21:293-312.

Carlson ER. 2013. The diagnosis and management of parotid disease. *Oral Maxillofac Surg Clin N Am* 25:31-48.

Chen MM, Coakley FV, Kaimal A, Laros RK, Jr. 2008. Guidelines for computed tomography and magnetic resonance imaging use during pregnancy and lactation. *Obstet Gynecol* 112:333-340.

English CK, Wear DJ, Margileth AM et al. 1988. Cat-scratch disease. *JAMA* 259:1347-1352.

Erkul E, Gillespie B. 2016. Sialendoscopy for non-stone disorders: The current evidence. *Laryngoscope Investig Otolaryngol* 1:140-145.

Galili D, Marmary Y. 1985. Spontaneous regeneration of the parotid salivary gland following juvenile recurrent parotitis. *Oral Surg* 60:605-606.

Goldberg MH, Bevilacqua RG. 1995. Infections of the Salivary Glands. In: Carlson ER (ed.) *The Comprehensive Management of Salivary Gland Pathology*. Philadelphia, W.B. Saunders Company, pp. 423-430.

Goldberg M, Harrigan W. 1965. Acute suppurative parotitis. *Oral Surg* 20:281-286.

Guralnick W, Donoff R, Galdabini J. 1968. Parotid swelling in a dehydrated patient. *J Oral Surg* 26:669-675.

Hasson O. 2007. Sialoendoscopy and sialography: Strategies for assessment and treatment of salivary gland obstructions. *J Oral Maxillofac Surg* 65:300-304.

Katz J, Fisher D, Levine S. 1990. Bacterial colonization of the parotid duct in xerostomia. *Int J Oral Maxillofac Surg* 19:7-9.

Kessler AT, Bhatt AA. 2018. Review of the major and minor salivary glands, part 1: Anatomy, infectious, and inflammatory processes. *J Clin Imaging Sci* 8:47.

Lang D, Zwerina J, Pieringer H. 2016. IgG4-related disease: Current challenges and future prospects. *Ther Clin Risk Manag* 12:189-199.

van der Lans RJL, Lohuis PJFM, van Gorp JMHH, Quak JJ. 2019). Surgical treatment of chronic parotitis. *Int Arch Otorhinolaryngol* 23:83-87.

Lewis MA, Parkhurst CL, Douglas CW et al. 1995. Prevalence of penicillin resistant bacteria in acute suppurative oral infection. *J Antimicrob Chemother* 35:785-791.

Maurya MK, Kumar S, Singh HP, Verma A. 2019. Tuberculous parotitis: A series of eight cases and review of literature. *Natl J Maxillofac Surg* 10:118-122.

McQuone SJ. 1999. Acute viral and bacterial infections of the salivary glands. *Otolaryngol Clin North Am* 32:793-811.

Miloro M, Goldberg MH. 2002. Salivary Gland Infections. In: Topazian RG, Goldberg MH, Hupp JR (eds.) *Oral and Maxillofacial Infections*, 4th edn. Philadelphia, W.B. Saunders Company, pp. 279-293.

Mitchell DA, Ord RA. 1988. Atypical mycobacterial infection presenting as a parotid mass in a child. *J Cranio-Max-Fac Surg* 16:221-223.

Murray PR, Kobayashi GS, Pfaller KS. 1994. Paramyxoviruses. In: *Medical Microbiology*, 2nd edn. St. Louis, Mosby, pp. 629-640.

Nahlieli O, Nakar LH, Nazarian Y, Turner MD. 2006. Sialoendoscopy: A new approach to salivary gland obstructive pathology *JADA* 137:1394-1400.

Nicolasora NP, Zacharek MA, Malani AN. 2009. Community-acquired Methicillin-resistant staphylococcus aureus: An emerging cause of acute bacterial parotitis. *South Med J* 102:208-210.

Patey DH. 1965. Inflammation of the salivary glands with particular reference to chronic and recurrent parotitis. *Ann R Coll Surg Engl* 36:26-44.

Petersdorf R, Forsyth B, Bernanke D. 1958. Staphylococcal parotitis. *N Engl J Med* 259:1250-1254.

Puxeddu I, Capecchi R, Carta F, Tavoni AG, Migliorini P, Puxeddu R. 2018. Salivary gland pathology in

IgG4-related disease: A comprehensive review. *J Immunol Res* 6936727.

Qi S, Xiaoyong L, Wang S. 2005. Sialoendoscopic and irrigation findings in chronic obstructive parotitis. *Laryngoscope* 115:541-545.

Rasmussen ER, Lykke E, Wagner N, Nielsen T, Waersted S, Arndal H. 2016. The introduction of sialendoscopy has significantly contributed to a decreased number of excised salivary glands in Denmark. *Eur Arch Otorhinolaryngol* 273:2223-2230.

Rice DH. 1998. Diseases of the Salivary Glands – Nonneoplastic. In: Bailey BJ (ed.) *Head and Neck Surgery – Otolaryngology*, 2nd edn. Philadelphia, Lippincott Raven Publishers, pp. 561-570.

Robinson JR. 1955. Surgical parotitis, vanishing disease. *Surgery* 38:703-707. *Oral Maxillofac Surg Clin N Am* 21:339–343.

Schiodt M, Dodd C, Greenspan D et al. 1992. Natural history of HIV-associated salivary gland disease. *Oral Surg Oral Med Oral Pathol* 74:326-331.

Schreiber A, Hershman G. 2009. Non-HIV viral infections of the salivary glands. *Oral Maxillofac Surg Clin N Am* 21:331-338.

Shacham R, Droma EB, London D, Bar T, Nahlieli O. 2009. Long-term experience with endoscopic diagnosis and treatment of juvenile recurrent parotitis. *J Oral Maxillofac Surg* 67:162-167.

Shanti RM, Aziz SR. 2009. HIV-associated salivary gland disease. *Oral Maxillofac Surg Clin N Am* 21:339-343.

Stafford JA, Moore CA, Mark JR. 2018. Acute sialadenitis associated with 2017-2018 influenza A infection: A case series. *Laryngoscope* 128:2500-2502.

Tucci RM, Roma R, Bioanchi A, De Voncentiis GC, Bianchi PM. 2019. Juvenile recurrent parotitis: Diagnostic and therapeutic effectiveness of sialography. Retrospective study on 110 children. *Int J Pediatr Otolorhinolaryngol* 124:179-184.

Xie L, Pu Y, Zheng L, Yu C, Wang Z, Shi H. 2016. Function of the parotid gland in juvenile recurrent parotitis: A case series. *Br J Oral Maxillofac Surg* 54:270-274.

Chapter 4
Cysts and Cyst-Like Lesions of the Salivary Glands

Outline

Introduction
Mucous Escape Reaction
  Clinical Features and Treatment of the Mucus Escape Reaction
  Mucocele
  Ranula and Plunging Ranula
  Submandibular Gland Mucocele
  Cyst of Blandin and Nuhn's Gland
Mucous Retention Cyst
Parotid Cysts Associated with Human Immunodeficiency Virus Infection
Branchial Cleft Cysts
Parotid Neoplasms Masquerading as Cysts
Summary
Case Presentation – *Down Yonder*
References

Introduction

Cysts of the salivary glands may originate as benign non-neoplastic entities, or in association with benign and malignant tumors of the salivary glands. Cystic development as part of specific neoplasms of the salivary glands is well recognized, including those that occur in the pleomorphic adenoma, Warthin tumor, mucoepidermoid carcinoma, acinic cell carcinoma, and the adenoid cystic carcinoma. The histologic features of these neoplasms are sufficiently distinctive; however, non-neoplastic salivary gland cysts do require differentiation from cystadenoma, mucoepidermoid carcinoma, and acinic carcinoma (Dardick 1996). This notwithstanding, clinically and radiographic appearing cysts of the salivary glands, particularly in the parotid gland, should entertain a differential diagnosis that includes malignant diagnoses.

Many cysts of the salivary glands may be generically attributed to an obstructive process. They can occur because of traumatic severance of salivary gland ducts, partial or complete blockage of the excretory ducts, or stasis of salivary flow in ducts. Salivary cysts are categorized in many ways in this chapter, including those that originate directly from the salivary gland and those entities that are associated with the salivary glands. In addition, there are those salivary cysts that exhibit a true cystic epithelium and those that are lined with a non-epithelial lining, i.e. pseudocysts. Finally, it is possible to categorize these lesions as acquired (obstructive due to stricture, neoplasms, sialoliths, or trauma) and developmental (dermoid, branchial cleft, branchial pouch and ductal). It is the purpose of this chapter to discuss those salivary gland cysts and cyst-like lesions that are developmental and acquired in a non-neoplastic nature (see Table 4.1). The reader is reminded to not dismiss cystic lesions of the salivary glands as benign entities without executing a strategy for definitive microscopic diagnosis.

Mucous Escape Reaction

The mucous escape reaction can be defined as a pooling of salivary mucus within a connective tissue lining. This concept is defined by several names including mucocele, ranula, mucous retention phenomenon, and mucus retention cyst. Of these, mucocele and ranula are the two best known entities to clinicians diagnosing and managing pathology in the head and neck region. It was once believed that the lesion developed from obstruction of a salivary gland's excretory duct with the subsequent formation of an epithelially lined cyst (Thoma 1950). Early studies investigated the result of ligation of the excretory ducts of the submandibular and sublingual glands

---

Salivary Gland Pathology: Diagnosis and Management, Third Edition. Edited by Eric R. Carlson and Robert A. Ord.
© 2022 John Wiley & Sons, Inc. Published 2022 by John Wiley & Sons, Inc.
Companion website: www.wiley.com/go/carlson/salivary

Table 4.1. Cysts and cyst-like lesions of the salivary glands – nomenclature and classification.

Nomenclature
   Mucous escape reaction
      Mucocele
      Ranula
   Mucous retention cysts
   Lymphoepithelial cysts
      HIV-associated lymphoepithelial cysts
   Developmental cysts
      Branchial cleft cysts
      Dermoid cysts
      Polycystic (dysgenetic) disease

Classification
   I Etiology
      a *Origination from* salivary gland tissue
         i Mucous escape reaction
         ii Mucous retention cyst
      b *Association with* salivary gland tissue
   II Lining
      a True cystic lining
         i Mucous retention cyst
      b Non-epithelial lining (pseudocyst)
         i Mucous escape reaction
            1 Mucocele
            2 Ranula
   III Occurrence
      a Acquired
         i Mucous escape reaction
         ii Mucous retention cyst
      b Developmental

(Bhaskar et al. 1956b). A mucous escape reaction did not result, thereby leading to further investigation. The complete obstruction of a salivary duct by the presence of a sialolith without the development of a mucous escape reaction substantiates the lack of a cause and effect relationship. Subsequent studies determined that severance of the excretory duct was required to produce extravasation of salivary mucin into the surrounding tissues with the development of a lesion histologically identical to the mucus escape reaction observed in humans (Bhaskar et al. 1956a). It is now accepted that severance of a salivary duct with resultant pooling of mucus into surrounding tissues is the pathophysiology of the mucus escape reaction. The fibrous connective tissue encasing the pooled saliva is presumably due to the foreign body nature of the saliva. The occasional report of an epithelial-like lining can be explained as a misinterpretation of compressed macrophages resembling a layer of cuboid-shaped cells (van den Akker et al. 1978). When these lesions occur in the floor of mouth, a designation of ranula is given, while a similar lesion in the lower lip carries a designation of mucocele.

CLINICAL FEATURES AND TREATMENT OF THE MUCUS ESCAPE REACTION

The mucus escape reaction may develop from a major or minor salivary gland, but seems to be more commonly observed in the minor glands. Armed Forces Institute of Pathology data of 2339 cases indicate that the minor glands are the site of predilection of this lesion, with 2273 (97.2%) of the 2339 lesions occurring in these glands. The lip accounted for 1502 of these lesions (64.2%) with the lower lip being the most common site (98.8% when the site was specified). This figure is consistent with other series that indicate a predilection of lower lip lesions (Cataldo and Mosadomi 1970). The major glands showed a nearly equal distribution of occurrence in the parotid, submandibular, and sublingual glands, and collectively accounted for only 2.9% of the 2339 cases.

Most investigators consider these lesions to be most common in children and young adults, with a mean age of 25 years. No significant sex predilection has been offered. The clinical appearance of these lesions differs depending on their depth within surrounding soft tissues. Superficial lesions present as blue, raised, soft tissue swellings with a fluctuant character on palpation (Figure 4.1). The blue hue is generally reflective of the color of pooled saliva at the mucosal surface. Lesions that are located more deeply in the soft tissues take on the color of the surrounding soft tissues; however, they may retain their fluctuant character. The most common clinical course of mucous escape reactions is that of a painless mucosal swelling that develops during a period of between a few days to one week and ruptures with apparent resolution with subsequent recurrence occurring within one month. Mild symptoms of pain may accompany mucus escape reactions if secondary trauma or inflammation occurs. Pain may also occur in the rare event that the mucus escape reaction impedes the flow of saliva due to obstruction (Figure 4.2).

Cysts and Cyst-Like Lesions of the Salivary Glands 119

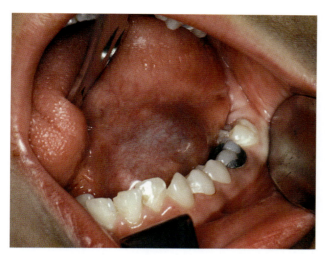

Figure 4.1. The typical appearance of a ranula of the floor of mouth. The characteristically raised nature of the lesion, as well as its blue hue are appreciated.

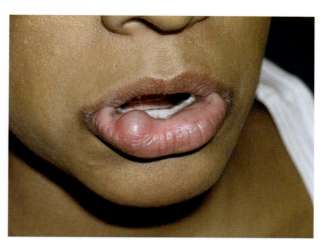

Figure 4.3. The classic appearance of a mucocele of the lower lip. Similar to a ranula of the floor of mouth, it shows an elevated blue lesion.

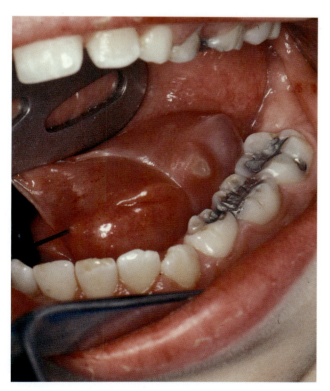

Figure 4.2. This ranula has resulted in significant pain experienced by the patient. The size of the ranula has resulted in obstruction of the sublingual gland.

Mucocele

Mucoceles are common lesions of the oral mucosa, and perhaps the most common benign salivary gland lesion in the oral cavity. The incidence of mucoceles is understandable due to the prevalence of minor salivary gland tissue in the oral cavity and the frequent occurrence of trauma to these tissues, which results in their formation. These lesions are painless, freely movable, smooth, and fluctuant. Their appearance is so characteristic that the clinical diagnosis is most frequently confirmed by subsequent histopathologic diagnosis following removal (Figure 4.3). As such, an incisional biopsy is not required for proper surgical treatment of the mucocele. Clearly, the most common location for these lesions is the lip, and specifically the lower lip. This notwithstanding, mucoceles occur on the buccal mucosa, tongue, and palate. Patients often give a history of the lesions spontaneously bursting with predictable recurrence. Mucoceles occur most commonly in children and young adults, probably due to the relatively high incidence of oral trauma in younger patients. Treatment with surgical excision of the mucocele and its associated minor salivary gland tissue is highly curable.

Ranula and Plunging Ranula

The ranula represents the prototypical mucus escape reaction occurring in the floor of mouth. Specifically, the ranula originates in the body of the sublingual gland in the ducts of Rivinus of this gland and infrequently from the minor salivary glands at this location (Kokong et al. 2017). Its nomenclature stems from its derivation from the Latin diminutive "rana," or frog that refers to its resemblance to the belly of a frog (Figure 4.4). The ranula was first described in the sixteenth century and its curative treatment was

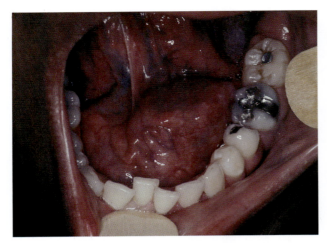

Figure 4.4. A ranula of the left floor of mouth. While the lesion is clearly elevated, only subtle signs exist of its blue color.

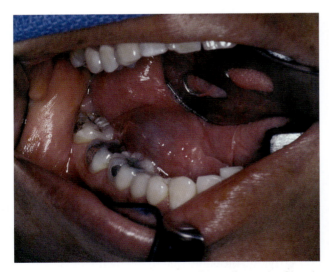

Figure 4.5. A ranula of the right floor of mouth. Classic signs of elevation and the blue discoloration are present.

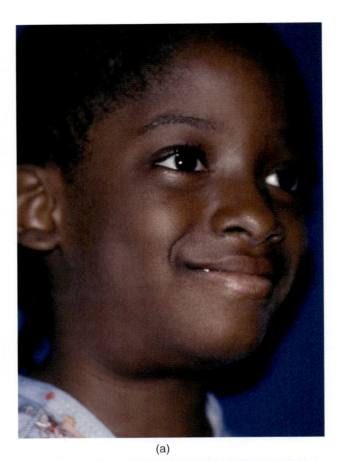

(a)

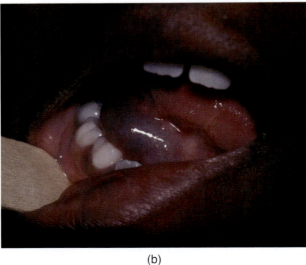

(b)

Figure 4.6. An 8-year-old girl with obvious right submandibular swelling (a) as well as simultaneous clinical evidence of a ranula in the right floor of mouth (b).

described in the seventeenth century (Carlson 2015). The precise tissue of origin was elucidated in the nineteenth century and its pathophysiologic mechanism was elaborately described in 1956 (Carlson 2015). The lesion has a characteristic appearance and history, commonly exhibiting a blue color and displaying periods of bursting of the lesion with liberation of saliva, only to relapse some time thereafter (Figure 4.5).

The development of a cervical component of the ranula has been a subject of fascination for centuries (Catone 1995). The oral and cervical mucus escape reactions may exist simultaneously (Figure 4.6), or they may occur independently of one another. As such, it was once considered possible that they had different etiologies, with the oral lesion being derived from the sublingual gland and the cervical lesion being derived from the submandibular gland. Some observed that the neck mass was often preceded by repeated spontaneous evacuations or surgical drainages of the oral lesion. This was perhaps the first explanation that scar tissue formation in the mucosa of the floor of mouth was responsible for the development of the cervical mass as it descended through the cleft of the posterior extent of the mylohyoid muscle as a path of least resistance (Figure 4.7) (Braun and Sotereanos 1982). The anatomy of the mylohyoid muscle and its hiatus, or cleft, and herniations within the mylohyoid muscle have been studied to explain the development of a plunging ranula. In their study of 23 adult cadavers, Harrison et al. identified a bilateral mylohyoid hiatus to exist in 10 of their 23 specimens (43%), with the hiatus being unilateral in 6 (26%) and bilateral in 4 (17%) cadavers (Harrison et al. 2013). The median anteroposterior dimension of the hiatus was 7 mm with a range of 2–11 mm, and the median mediolateral dimension was 14 mm with a range of 7–20 mm. The authors identified

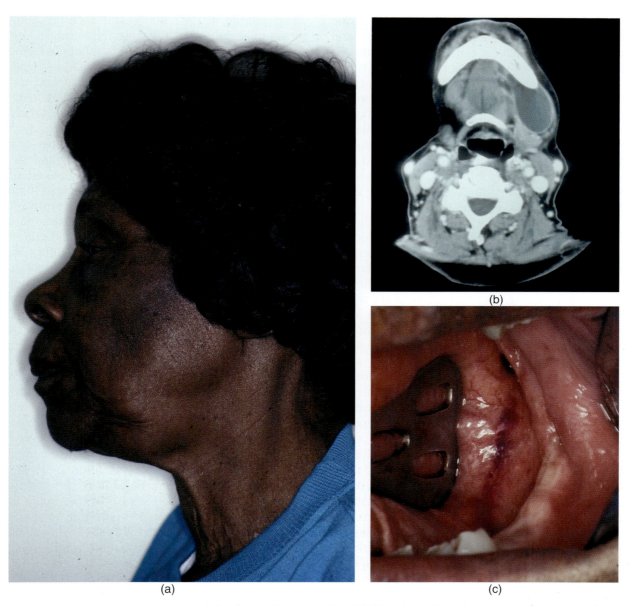

Figure 4.7. This elderly woman shows left submandibular swelling (a). Her history includes numerous aspirations of fluid within a ranula of the left floor of mouth. Computerized tomograms of the neck show a fluid-filled lesion of the submandibular region (b). A diagnosis of plunging ranula was made and the patient underwent left sublingual gland excision (c). Examination of the left floor of mouth did not show signs of ranula in this region. Scar tissue formation from her previous aspirations resulted in the development of a plunging ranula.

sublingual gland tissue in nine hernias and fat in six hernias. Other authors have demonstrated that approximately one-third of the population has discontinuities of the mylohyoid muscle such that direct invasion of the pseudocyst through these defects of the muscle permits extension into the neck (McClatchey et al. 1984). Morton et al. (2010) reported on 80 consecutive plunging ranulas in 77 patients. The clinical findings of their patients and supporting data from the international literature, when considered based on information relating to the known anatomical defect of dehiscence in the mylohyoid muscle and ectopic sublingual gland lying below the mylohyoid muscle, seem to support a genetic basis for the plunging ranula.

While the pathophysiology of the plunging ranula is now well understood from an anatomic perspective, the literature continues to identify controversy regarding the most appropriate means to treat the ranula and plunging ranula including aspiration, isolated excision of the ranula, and excision of the ranula and sublingual gland combined (Patel et al. 2009; Harrison 2010; Lesperance 2013; Sigismund et al. 2013; Kokong et al. 2017).

If anything has been learned by reading the scientific literature on the topic of cyst-like lesions of the salivary glands, it is the common pathogenesis of three clinical entities: the mucocele, the oral ranula, and the plunging ranula. Specifically, it is their lack of an epithelial lining, and their association with a salivary gland, whether major or minor, that these entities share in common. If the offending sublingual salivary gland is not removed, the lesion has a statistical likelihood of recurrence (Catone et al. 1969; Suresh and Vora 2012). Kokong et al. (2017) reviewed 12 cases of ranula. They identified 100% recurrence of the ranula following aspiration while excision of the ranula alone was associated with recurrence of 50%. There were no recurrences of ranulas when managed with excision of the ranula and sublingual gland combined. In their clinical review of 580 ranulas, Zhao et al. (2004) indicated that excision of the sublingual gland is necessary in the management of the ranula and reported recurrence rates for marsupialization, excision of the ranula, and excision of the sublingual gland or gland combined with the ranula as 66.7, 57.7, and 1.2%, respectively.

This notwithstanding, while the diagnosis of the conventional, non-plunging ranula remains straightforward, its management has historically been variable and controversial, ranging from incision and marsupialization to sublingual gland excision. Interestingly, most mucoceles are located in the lower lip and are treated with an excision of the mucocele and associated etiologic minor salivary gland tissue of the lower lip. Ironically, although the ranula of the floor of mouth is the second most common type of mucocele, removal of the ranula and the associated salivary gland, in this case, the sublingual gland, has not been uniformly accepted as standard treatment of the ranula as it is for the lower lip mucocele. To this end, there are several published papers adamantly recommending that more conservative procedures be performed as first-line therapy (Baurmash 1992, 2007). One such procedure is marsupialization with packing (Baurmash 1992). The author contends that routine sublingual removal is inappropriate therapy for several reasons. The first is that the term "ranula" is loosely applied to any cyst-like structure of the floor of mouth. He believes that some of these lesions are unrelated to the sublingual gland, such that its removal is not indicated. Specifically, he cites the existence of mucoceles arising from the mucus-secreting incisal gland in the anterior floor of mouth, single or multiple retention cysts involving the openings of the ducts of Rivinus, and retention cysts at the Wharton duct orifice that can resemble the sublingual gland-associated ranula, but that would possibly not be cured with sublingual gland removal. Moreover, the author states that sublingual gland excision is potentially associated with significant morbidity such as injury to the Wharton duct with resultant salivary obstruction or salivary leakage, and lingual nerve injury (Baurmash 1992). Zhao and his group presented an objective assessment of complications associated with surgical management of ranulas treated with a variety of procedures (Zhao et al. 2005). These included 9 marsupializations, 28 excisions of the ranula only, 356 sublingual gland excisions, and 213 excisions of both the sublingual gland and ranula. A total of 569 sublingual gland excisions were performed in 571 patients undergoing 606 operations. Injury to the Wharton duct occurred in 11 of 569 patients who underwent excision of the sublingual gland with or without excision of the ranula compared to zero of 37 patients who did not undergo sublingual gland excision. Injury to the lingual nerve occurred in 21 of patients who underwent sublingual gland excision compared to zero patients who did not undergo sublingual gland excision. Of particular note is that recurrence of the ranula occurred in 1.2% of patients who underwent excision of their sublingual glands compared to 60% of patients who underwent marsupialization or excision of the ranula only. Baurmash laments that simple marsupialization has fallen into disfavor because of the excessive number of failures associated with this procedure (Baurmash 1992). The recurrence patterns have been confirmed by other authors as well (Yoshimura et al. 1995). As such, he recommends packing the cystic cavity with gauze for 7–10 days. In so doing, he reports that the recurrence rate is reduced to 10–12% (Baurmash 2007). McGurk points out that the disadvantage of this procedure is that the results are unpredictable and that the packing is uncomfortable for the patient (McGurk 2007). He concluded by stating that reliable eradication of the ranula comes from removal of the sublingual gland. Further work by this author has led to a recommendation for conservative treatment of the oral ranula by partial excision of the sublingual gland (McGurk et al. 2008). It is true that the sublingual gland excision requires an anatomically precise approach such that some surgeons may wish to defer the sublingual gland excision for recurrences. Unfortunately, the development of scar tissue in the floor of mouth is such that the anatomy may be more obscured related to a recurrence after a marsupialization and packing procedure. With this issue in mind, a sublingual gland excision should probably be performed from the outset (Figure 4.8). While the anatomy of the floor of

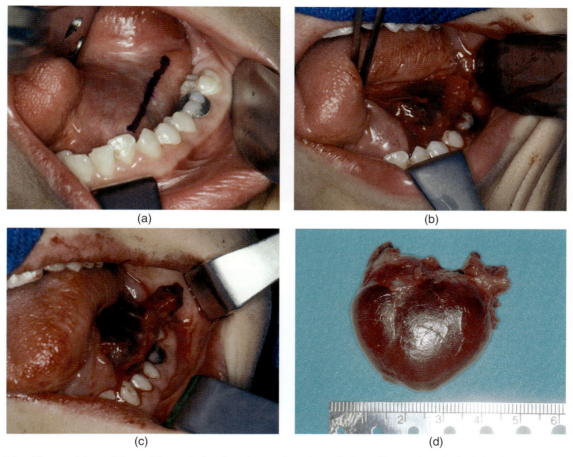

Figure 4.8. The excision of the sublingual gland and associated ranula from Figure 4.1. An incision is designed over the prominence of the sublingual gland and ranula, and lateral to Wharton duct (a). Careful dissection allows for separation of the mucosa from the underlying pseudocystic membrane (b). The dissection continues to separate the sublingual gland from surrounding tissues, including the underlying Wharton duct and the lingual nerve beneath Wharton's duct (c). The specimen and ranula are delivered en bloc (d). If the pseudocyst bursts intraoperatively, no compromise in cure exists provided the sublingual gland is completely excised. The histopathology shows the non-epithelial lining (e) and the intimate association of the sublingual gland and mucus escape reaction (f). The remaining tissue bed shows the anatomic relationship of the preserved superficial Wharton duct and underlying lingual nerve (g). The Wharton duct originates posteriorly in a medial position to the lingual nerve and terminates in a position lateral to the nerve. The sublingual vein can be visualized in the tissue bed lateral to the anterior aspect of Wharton duct (g). Healing is uneventful as noted in the one month postoperative image (h).

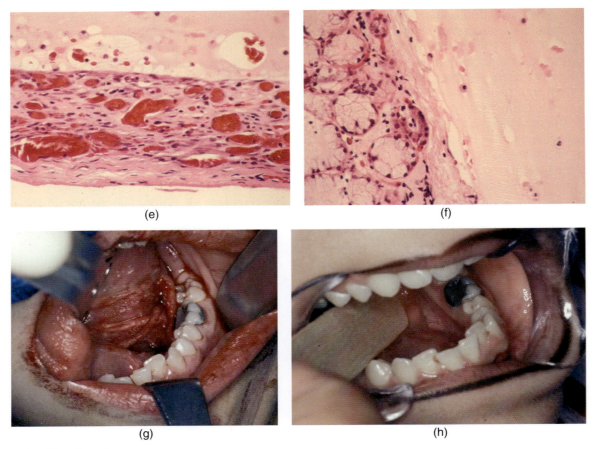

Figure 4.8. (*Continued*).

mouth might be considered foreign and intimidating to some surgeons, preservation of the lingual nerve and Wharton's duct is not a difficult task, and treatment of this pathologic process with sublingual excision should be a curative procedure. One pathologic and clinical similarity of the ranula and mucocele is their derivation from salivary gland tissue. As stated previously, there does not seem to be a dispute among clinicians as to the best surgical therapy for the mucocele, with complete surgical excision of the etiologic minor salivary tissue along with the mucus escape reaction being highly accepted (Figure 4.9). As such, it is advisable to apply the same approach to the ranula that only differs from the mucocele in the anatomic region in which it occurs. Regarding the ranula and plunging ranula, even the most extensive lesions are predictably treated for cure with excision of the offending sublingual gland. While it is not essential to remove the non-epithelial lined pseudocyst with the sublingual gland, it is common for the tightly adherent pseudocyst to be delivered

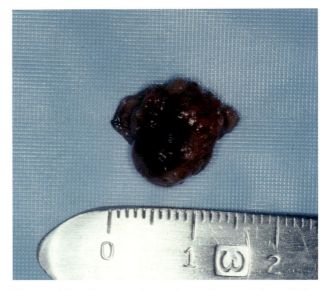

Figure 4.9. The specimen from the excision of the mucocele seen in Figure 4.3. The minor salivary gland tissue remains attached to the mucus escape reaction.

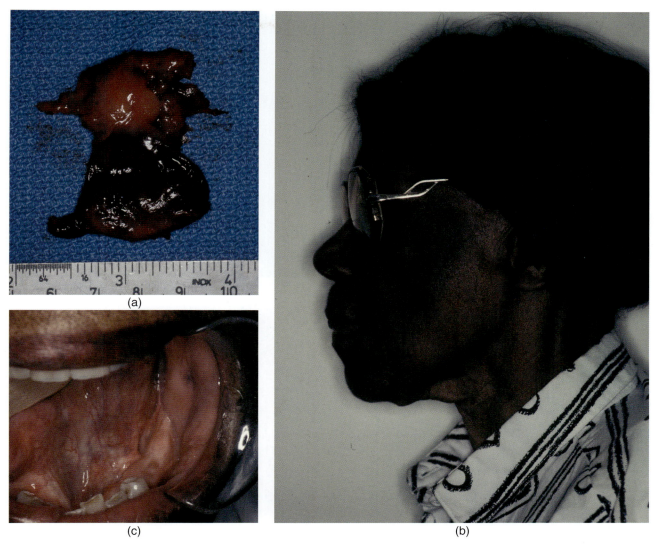

Figure 4.10. The patient seen in Figure 4.7 underwent excision of her left sublingual gland for her plunging ranula. The specimen (a) includes the sublingual gland and associated mucus escape reaction. Her two-year postoperative examination shows no mass in the submandibular region (b) and a normal oral examination without recurrence of the ranula (c).

with the sublingual gland specimen (Figure 4.10). As such, documentation of a plunging component to the ranula serves a matter of medical completeness rather than representing an implication for surgical treatment.

Submandibular Gland Mucocele

Clinical experience demonstrates that patients occasionally present with a neck examination consistent with a diagnosis of plunging ranula, yet without signs of ranula on oral examination. Moreover, many of these patients will demonstrate CT evidence of a fluid-filled lesion originating from the submandibular gland rather than from the sublingual gland. These rare cases are typically diagnosed as submandibular gland mucoceles (Ozturk et al. 2005; Hze-Khoong et al. 2012) on clinical grounds and should be treated with excision of the offending submandibular gland and associated mucocele (Figure 4.11). A thorough analysis of the CT scans is thought to be able to distinguish the sublingual gland ranula from the submandibular mucocele by identifying the tail-like extension of the ranula to the sublingual gland that is absent in the submandibular gland mucocele (Anastassov et al. 2000). This notwithstanding, the

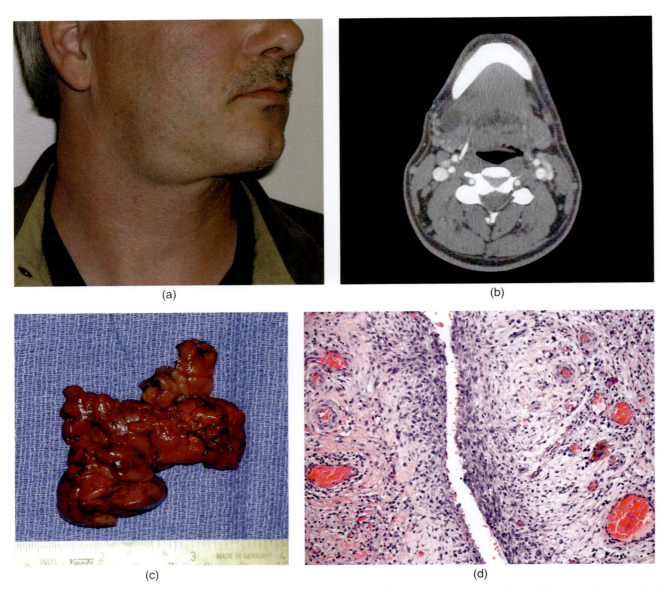

Figure 4.11. A 48-year-old man with a swelling of the right submandibular region (a). Palpation of this swelling revealed a ballotable mass. A CT scan revealed a fluid-filled lesion intimately associated with the right submandibular gland (b). A clinical diagnosis of submandibular gland mucocele was made and the patient underwent excision of his right sublingual gland and submandibular gland/mucocele (c). The presence of a submandibular gland mucocele was confirmed by histopathology (d). Hematoxylin and eosin, original magnification ×100.

management of the submandibular gland mucocele requires removal of the submandibular gland and its associated mucocele. Excision of the sublingual gland en bloc with the submandibular gland and mucocele may be performed when the mucocele appears to be intimately associated the sublingual gland (Ozturk et al. 2005). The surgeon's intraoperative discretion dictates whether the sublingual gland is indicated for removal when providing surgical treatment for the submandibular gland mucocele. As with the mucocele and the ranula, appropriate surgical management of the submandibular mucocele represents a curative procedure for this diagnosis.

Cyst of Blandin and Nuhn's Gland

On rare occasions, the mucosa of the ventral surface of the tongue may become a source for the development of a mucous escape reaction. This process is referred to as a cyst of Blandin and Nuhn's gland (Figure 4.12). This designation is a misnomer, as this process represents a mucous escape reaction, rather than a true cyst. In this sense, then, it represents a ranula of the tongue. Simple excision of the "cyst" and the associated gland of Blandin and Nuhn is the treatment of choice with recurrence being uncommon.

Mucous Retention Cyst

The mucus retention cyst is less common than the mucus escape reaction. This entity is a true cyst that is lined by epithelium. The exact classification of this lesion seems to be in question. Some prefer to simply include it with the more common mucus escape reaction, whereas others describe it as a separate entity (Koudelka 1991). The pathogenesis seems to be related to partial obstruction of a duct, as opposed to complete severance of the salivary duct that is seen in the mucus escape reaction. The increased pressure in the salivary duct causes dilatation without rupture such that proliferation of the ductal epithelium occurs. The Armed Forces Institute of Pathology reviewed 178 cases of mucus retention cysts, accounting for 0.9% of all salivary gland pathology cases in their files (Koudelka 1991). One hundred seventy-one cases (96%) occurred in the major salivary glands with 156 (87.6%) occurring in the parotid gland (Figure 4.13), 14 cases (7.8%) occurring in the submandibular gland, and only 1 case occurring in the sublingual gland. Only one case was specifically documented as occurring in the minor salivary glands. The mean age of patients is late 40s, with a nearly equal gender predilection. The clinical presentation of the mucus retention cyst is that of a slowly enlarging, painless, fluctuant, soft tissue swelling that may persist from months to years. These cysts vary in their size, and the color of the overlying tissues depends on their depth within the soft tissue. Superficial lesions are blue in color, whereas deep lesions take on the same color of the overlying tissue. Some pathologists have split the mucus retention cysts into separate categories. Eversole has categorized these lesions as mucus retention cysts, reactive oncocytoid cysts, and mucopapillary cysts (Eversole 1987). In his series of 121 mucus retention cysts, he found 70 mucus retention cysts, 41 reactive oncocytoid cysts, and 10 mucopapillary cysts. From a pathologic and surgical standpoint, perhaps the most striking piece of information in this report was the need to distinguish the mucopapillary cyst from the low-grade mucoepidermoid carcinoma.

Treatment of mucus retention cysts is most commonly surgical excision (Figure 4.13). Cysts within or closely associated with a salivary gland should include that salivary gland with the excision. Some mucus retention cysts, however, may be removed without the inclusion of the salivary gland, a distinct departure from the recommendations associated with mucus escape reactions.

Parotid Cysts Associated with Human Immunodeficiency Virus Infection

Infection with the human immunodeficiency virus has been shown to manifest in variety of ways. Symptoms related to the head and neck have historically been encountered in this disease. It has been reported that 41% of patients with acquired immunodeficiency syndrome (AIDS) initially presented with signs or symptoms of head and neck disease (Marcussen and Sooy 1985). Salivary gland diseases include the enlargement of major salivary glands with or without hypofunction and xerostomia

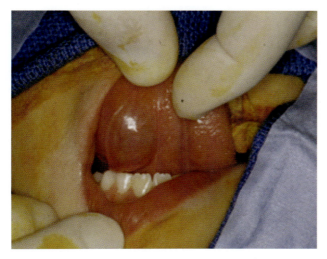

Figure 4.12. A cyst of Blandin and Nuhn of the ventral surface of the tongue. Simple excision of the cyst and associated minor salivary gland tissue is curative for this mucus escape phenomenon.

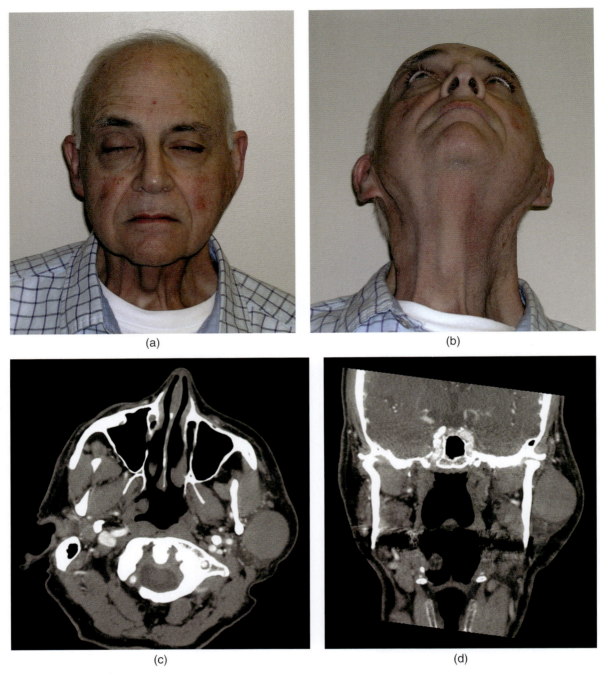

Figure 4.13. A 71-year-old man was referred with a six-month history of a progressively enlarging left parotid mass (a and b). A needle biopsy had been performed on two occasions yet without definitive results. CT scans were obtained that identified a 3.8 cm low attenuating homogenous and well-defined lesion within the superficial lobe of the left parotid gland (c and d). The patient underwent a left superficial parotidectomy through a modified Blair incision (e). The main trunk of the facial nerve was identified (f) and a complete dissection of the facial nerve branches was performed, thereby permitting delivery of the specimen (g and h). A salivary duct cyst, oncocytic variant, was diagnosed microscopically (i). The resultant defect is noted (j).

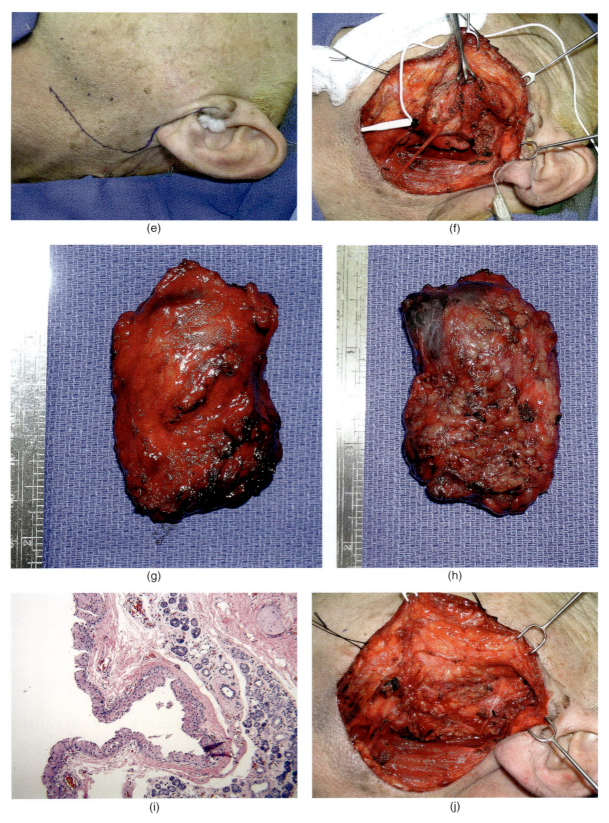

Figure 4.13. (*Continued*).

(Owotade et al. 2005). In early lesions, the submandibular and sublingual glands are often initially affected and enlarged. As the disease progresses, however, parotid gland swelling is more commonly noted. Approximately 1–10% of patients with HIV-1 infection have been reported to have parotid swelling (Sekikawa and Hongo 2017) with the incidence increasing to approximately 20% in AIDS patients (Owotade et al. 2005). Ryan and his group were the first to describe salivary gland involvement in HIV disease as intrasalivary gland lymphadenopathy (Ryan et al. 1985). Shortly thereafter, parotid gland cysts were reported, and were noted to resemble the benign lymphoepithelial lesion (BLL) histologically (Colebunders et al. 1988). The BLL is a benign sialadenopathy associated with Sjögren syndrome with pathognomonic epimyoepithelial islands. It is felt to represent an autoimmune reaction in Sjögren syndrome, but the BLL is felt to be of unknown pathogenesis in HIV (Sperling et al. 1990). It remains unclear whether lymphoepithelial cysts within parotid glands in HIV/AIDS patients develop from pre-existing salivary gland inclusions in intraparotid lymph nodes or from a lymphoepithelial lesion of the parenchyma of the salivary gland. HIV-1 p24 antigen immunostaining may be a useful study in distinguishing a suspected lymphoepithelial cyst in an HIV-positive patient from lymphoma as the follicular dendritic cells and interfollicular macrophages in lymphoepithelial cysts are positive for HIV-1 p24 antigen (Sekikawa and Hongo 2017).

Treatment of lymphoepithelial cysts of the parotid gland in HIV/AIDS patients is a function of the size of the cysts, the patient's concern for cosmetics, and compliance with medical therapy. Following their original description, these cysts were managed in a variety of ways including periodic aspirations, simple excision of the cysts, and nerve sparing superficial parotidectomy (Figure 4.14). Shaha and his group reported an early experience with 50 patients with lymphoepithelial cysts of the bilateral parotid glands (Shaha et al. 1993). Their initial approach involved superficial parotidectomy with identification and preservation of the facial nerve. They subsequently performed excision of the cyst only. Ferraro and his group recommended against superficial parotidectomy due to possible subsequent recurrence in the deep lobe (Ferraro et al. 1993). They indicated that aspiration is usually ineffective as a long-term solution because of the high rates of recurrence, in addition to the inability to obtain a tissue diagnosis of the cyst wall. Their solution to recurrence of the cyst was a second enucleation procedure.

Improved and evolving pharmacologic therapy of HIV/AIDS has changed the observation and management of these cysts. Highly active antiretroviral therapy (HAART) uses combinations of drugs to maximize viral suppression and minimize selection of drug-resistant strains. Most commonly, HAART consists of a backbone of two nucleoside analog reverse transcriptase inhibitors in combination with either a protease inhibitor or a nonnucleoside reverse transcriptase inhibitor. Gland enlargement has been shown to be significantly and positively associated with viral load in a linear fashion (Mulligan et al. 2000). Compliance with HAART, therefore, has led to the observation that this therapy will result in these cysts subsiding without the need for surgery (Figure 4.15).

Branchial Cleft Cysts

Patients with first branchial anomalies usually present with a unilateral painless swelling of the parotid gland. Bilateral swelling is rare. Work has classified these cysts as types I and II (Work 1977). Type I branchial defects are duplication anomalies of the membranous external auditory canal. These defects are composed of ectoderm only. They are located within the preauricular soft tissues and parotid gland and present as sinus tracts or areas of localized swelling near the anterior tragus. Complete surgical removal is curative. Type II branchial anomalies are less common than type I anomalies. This defect is a duplication anomaly consisting of an anomalous membranous and cartilaginous external auditory canal. Unlike type I cysts, type II cysts are composed of ectoderm and mesoderm. They commonly present in the upper neck and are located posterior or inferior to the angle of the mandible and can extend into the external auditory canal or middle ear cavity. Sinus tracts are common and abscess formation may also occur. Complete surgical excision during an asymptomatic period is the treatment of choice. The reader is directed to Chapter 17 for a more detailed discussion and illustration of these pathologic processes.

Parotid Neoplasms Masquerading as Cysts

Most masses of the parotid gland are classified as solid lesions but 3–9% of parotid lesions have been described as cysts (Boursiquot et al. 2020). Numerous neoplasms can be described as cystic

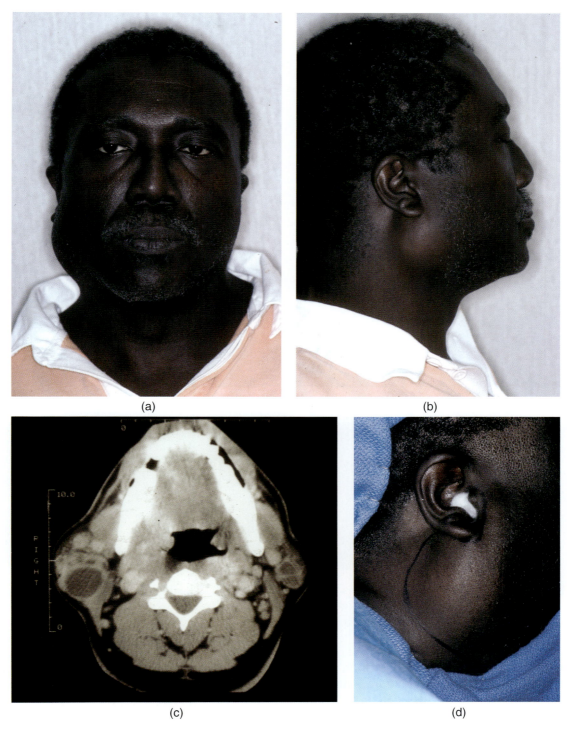

Figure 4.14. A 50-year-old HIV positive male presented in 1994 with obvious right parotid swelling (a and b). This time period predated the development of HAART. Examination of the bilateral parotid gland regions revealed a large mass of the right parotid gland, and a smaller mass of the left parotid gland. Computerized tomograms (c) confirmed the findings of the physical examination. A clinical diagnosis of bilateral lymphoepithelial cysts was made. The patient requested removal of these cysts. A standard incision was made (d). This permitted unroofing of the large cyst in the right parotid gland (e) and the smaller cysts in the left parotid gland (f). The specimen from the right parotid gland (g) and the left parotid gland (h) showed typical gross signs of lymphoepithelial cysts. The resultant right parotid tissue bed is noted (i). Six months postoperatively, the patient showed well-healed surgical sites without signs of recurrent lymphoepithelial cysts (j–m).

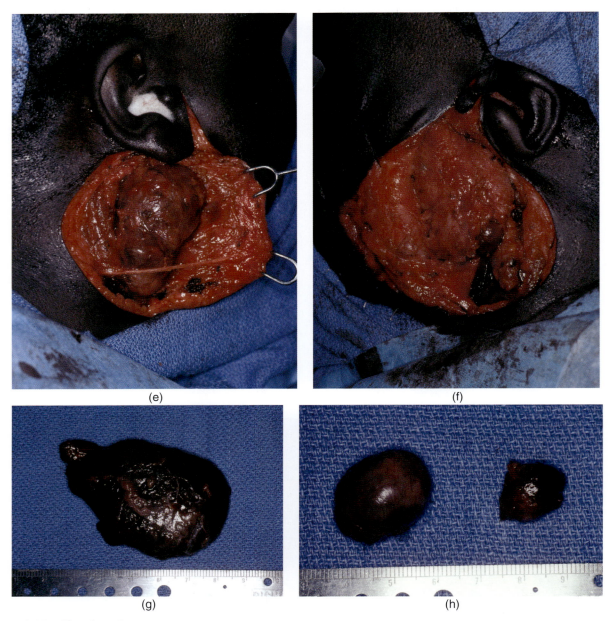

Figure 4.14. (*Continued*).

microscopically, including Warthin tumor, sebaceous adenoma, pleomorphic adenoma, mucoepidermoid carcinoma, acinic cell carcinoma, and secretory carcinoma (Ata and Unverdi 2000; Pantanowitz et al. 2018). Non-neoplastic lesions such as second branchial cleft cyst and cystic hygroma can also be described as cystic salivary gland lesions. As many as 20% of parotid lesions are believed to be cystic, based on preoperative examination that includes physical examination and imaging studies. Takita et al. (2017) have discussed cystic lesions of the parotid gland and provided a pathoradiologic correlation of these cysts according to the 2017 World Health Organization Classification of Head and Neck Tumors. These authors emphasize that the etiologies of parotid cysts are quite diverse and can be classified as non-neoplastic cysts, benign tumors with macrocystic changes, and malignant tumors with macrocystic changes (Table 4.2).

Cysts and Cyst-Like Lesions of the Salivary Glands **133**

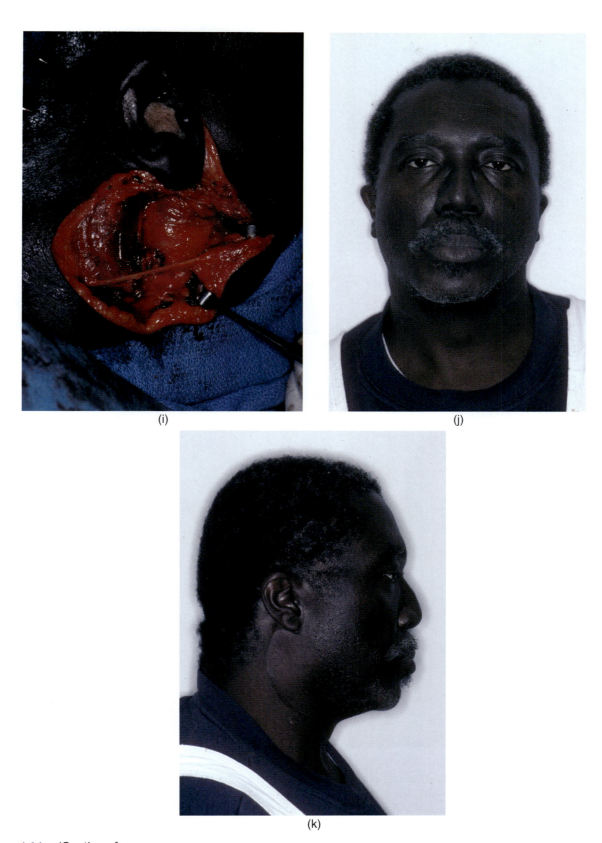

Figure 4.14. (Continued).

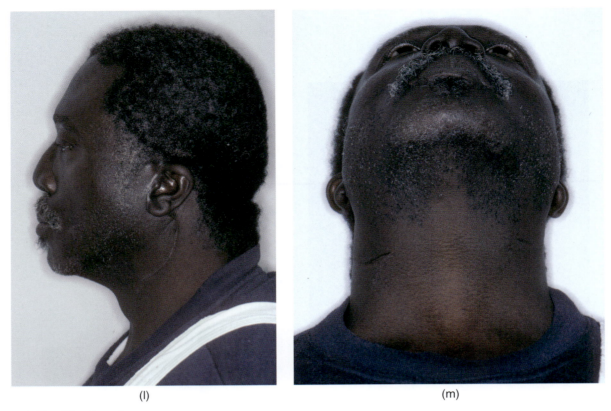

(l)　　　　　　　　　　　　　　　　　　(m)

Figure 4.14. *(Continued).*

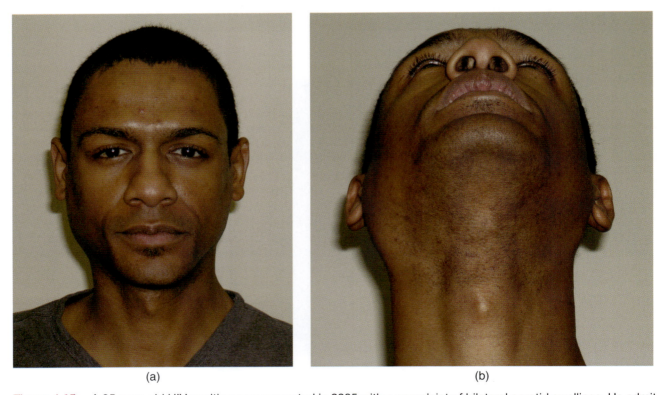

(a)　　　　　　　　　　　　　　　　　　(b)

Figure 4.15. A 35-year-old HIV positive man presented in 2005 with a complaint of bilateral parotid swellings. He admitted to noncompliance with his HAART. His CD4/CD8 was 0.69 at the time of initial consultation. Physical examination revealed an obvious right parotid swelling and a subtle mass of the left parotid gland (a and b). Computerized tomograms (c and d) confirmed these findings. A fine needle aspiration biopsy was performed that yielded thick white fluid. A diagnosis of lymphoepithelial cysts was made. The patient resumed his HAART and the cysts regressed as noted on an examination four months later (e and f). His CD4/CD8 was 1.12 at that time.

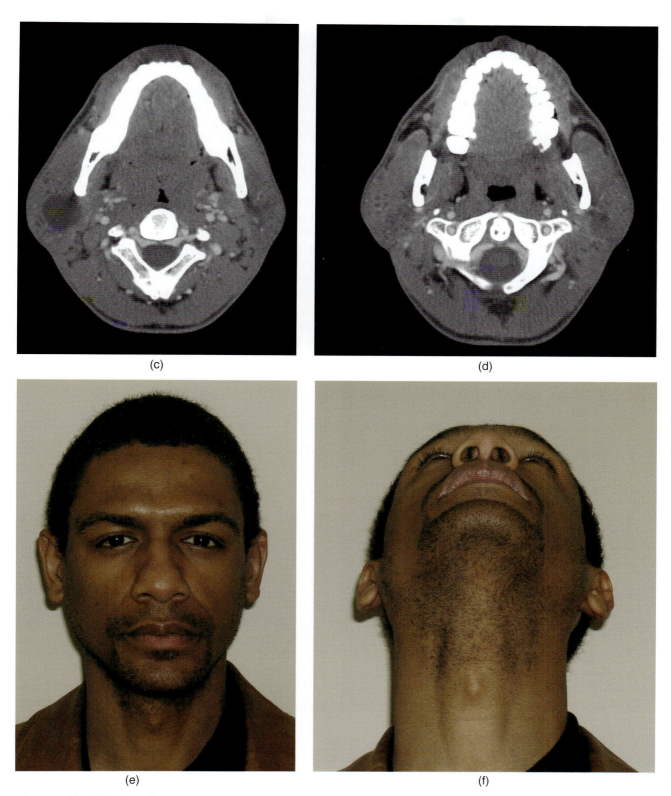

Figure 4.15. (Continued).

Table 4.2. Classification and examples of cystic lesions of the parotid gland.

Non-neoplastic cysts
  Salivary duct cyst (retention cyst)
  Lymphoepithelial cyst (branchial cleft cyst)
  HIV-associated salivary gland disease (lymphoepithelial sialadenitis)
  Dermoid cyst
  Lymphangioma

Benign tumors with macrocystic change
  Warthin tumor
  Metaplastic Warthin tumor
  Cystadenoma
  Pleomorphic adenoma
  Basal cell adenoma
  Intraparotid facial nerve schwannoma

Malignant tumors with macrocystic change
  Acinic cell carcinoma (papillary cystic variant)

Source: Adapted from: Takita et al. (2017).

Of diagnostic and therapeutic dilemma is that fine needle aspiration biopsy of cysts is occasionally nondiagnostic as the aspirate may only liberate paucicellular cyst fluid. Arriving at an accurate diagnosis from an aspirated cystic salivary gland lesion is also difficult due to the broad differential diagnosis, the possibility of sampling error, morphologic heterogeneity, and overlapping cytology of cystic entities (Pantanowitz et al. 2018). Cystic salivary gland neoplasms with mucinous features include low-grade mucoepidermoid carcinoma, papillary cystadenocarinoma, Warthin tumor, and pleomorphic adenoma with mucinous metaplasia. Cystic neoplasms without mucinous features include basal cell adenoma, canalicular adenoma, oncocytoma, sebaceous adenoma, intraductal papilloma, epithelial-myoepithelial carcinoma, intraductal carcinoma, acinic cell carcinoma, squamous cell carcinoma, and secretory carcinoma (Figure 4.16).

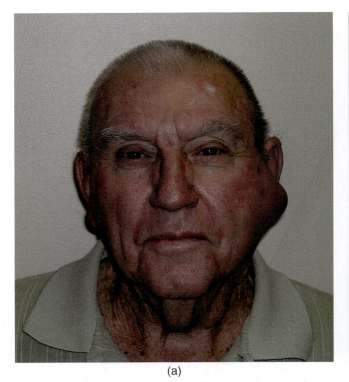
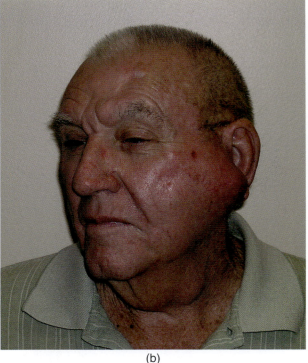

(a)   (b)

Figure 4.16. A 79-year-old man was referred with a six-month history of a mass of the left parotid gland (a and b). He had been subjected to drainage of this mass on three occasions prior to referral. One drainage procedure provided material for cytologic analysis and a diagnosis of cyst was offered. CT scans were obtained that identified a heterogeneously enhancing 4.6 cm mass of the left parotid gland with central non-enhancing cystic/necrotic components with thick enhancing internal septations. The mass was noted to be abutting the skin surface with associated overlying skin thickening (c and d). The patient underwent skin-sacrificing left superficial parotidectomy through a modified Blair incision (e) and the specimen is noted (f and g). Final pathology identified a high-grade mucoepidermoid carcinoma (h and i). The resultant defect and facial nerve preservation are noted (j).

Cysts and Cyst-Like Lesions of the Salivary Glands 137

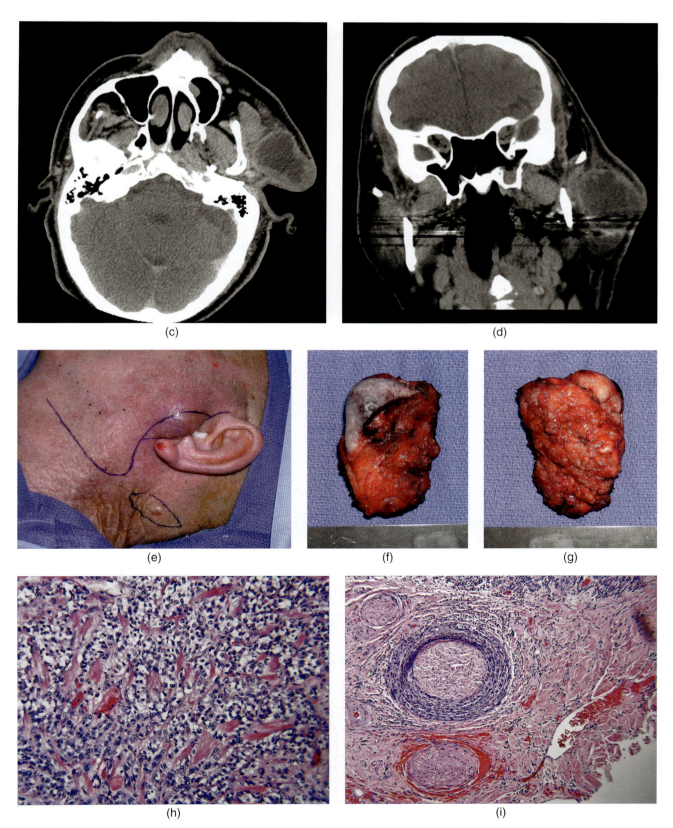

Figure 4.16. (Continued).

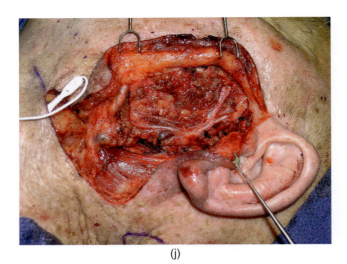

Figure 4.16. (*Continued*).

Boursiquot et al. (2020) retrospectively reviewed 677 patients who had undergone parotidectomy. Of those, 388 patients satisfied inclusion criteria, and 27 (8.8%) of those patients had parotid lesions that were classified as cystic based on preoperative imaging studies. The remaining 281 patients had solid or mixed (partially solid and partially cystic) masses. Cystic lesions were classified as complex ($n = 22$) when they were lobulated in shape, possessed a thick and/or irregular cyst wall, had internal septations, and internal density that was different than the density of water. The presence of one or more of these features led to a diagnosis of complex cyst. Cysts without any of these features were classified as simple ($n = 5$). Compared to solid or mixed lesions, cystic masses were less likely to be neoplastic (44 vs. 97%) on univariate analysis. There was no difference, however, in the risk of malignancy between cystic and solid/mixed masses (22 vs. 26%). Compared to simple cysts, there was a greater frequency of neoplasm (50 vs. 20%) and malignancy (27 vs. 0%) for complex cysts but the results were not statistically significant. Final pathology revealed five (23%) of the complex cysts to be benign neoplasms, including two pleomorphic adenomas, two Warthin tumors, and one canalicular adenoma. Six (27%) of the complex cysts were malignant, including three mucoepidermoid carcinomas, two acinic cell carcinomas, and one squamous cell carcinoma. One of the simple cysts demonstrated a benign neoplasm, pleomorphic adenoma, and there were no cases of malignancy. Overall, 12 of the 27 (44%) cystic parotid lesions were neoplastic, and 6 of 27 (22%) cystic parotid lesions were malignant. The results of this study point to the likelihood of a neoplastic diagnosis when encountering a cystic lesion of the parotid gland, as well as the possibility of a malignant diagnosis. This notwithstanding, the findings of this study should be interpreted with caution since only surgically resected parotid lesions were included. It is possible that many cystic parotid lesions did not undergo surgical removal due to the lack of suspicious findings. In the final analysis, however, it is clear that neoplastic diagnoses should be considered, including malignant diagnoses when surgeons evaluate patients with cystic parotid lesions. A sense of urgency for accurate diagnosis and treatment should be established accordingly.

Summary

- Cysts of the salivary glands may be associated with neoplasms or they may occur independently.
- While these lesions are collectively referred to as cysts, many are not actually lined by epithelium and therefore are more accurately referred to as cyst-like lesions owing to fluid-filled soft tissue lining.
- The ranula and mucocele are examples of mucous escape reactions that are not lined by epithelium.
- Severance of a salivary duct due to trauma with resultant pooling of mucous into surrounding tissues is the pathophysiology of the mucous escape reaction.
- Excision of the salivary gland with or without the associated mucous escape reaction represents curative therapy for this process.
- The mucous escape reaction is most commonly seen in the minor salivary glands.
- Mucous retention cysts are lined by epithelium, but are very rare.
- When mucous retention cysts do occur, they seem to be most common in the major salivary glands, particularly the parotid gland. Simple excision may be the treatment of choice if a cyst is definitively diagnosed preoperatively. More commonly, fine needle aspiration biopsies of cystic lesions are equivocal such that patients undergo excision of the

gland and cystic lesion en bloc. This is particularly the case with cystic lesions of the parotid gland.
- As many as 5–10% of patients with HIV-1 infection have been reported to have parotid swelling with the incidence increasing to approximately 20% in AIDS patients. Lymphoepithelial cysts account for most of these swellings.
- A radiographically appearing cystic lesion of the parotid gland should be addressed by the development of a differential diagnosis that includes mucous retention cysts as well as cystic neoplasms, particularly mucoepidermoid carcinoma. A focused and expedient workup is therefore required.

Case Presentation - *Down Yonder*

A 15-year-old girl presented with a seven-month history of a painless right neck swelling (Figure 4.17a and b) and a six-month history of a right floor of mouth swelling (Figure 4.17c). She denied pain associated with either area of swelling. A provisional clinical diagnosis of plunging ranula was established.

Past Medical History
The patient and her mother reported no contributory medical history. The patient was taking non-prescription vitamins. She reported no known drug allergies.

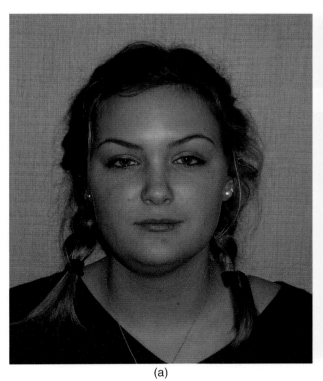
(a)

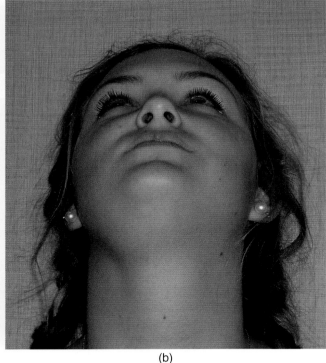
(b)

Figure 4.17. This patient presented with a seven-month history of a painless right neck swelling (a and b) and a six-month history of a right floor of mouth swelling (c). Axial (d), coronal (e), and sagittal (f) CT scans of the neck with intravenous contrast demonstrate a 4 cm homogenous lesion associated with the sublingual gland, consistent with a diagnosis of plunging ranula. The patient underwent excision of her right sublingual gland through a standard incision in the floor of mouth (g). A yellow mass was noted attached to the inferior surface of the sublingual gland as the specimen was being thoroughly isolated (h). The sublingual gland and presumed lipoma were removed en bloc (i). Final pathology identified dermoid cyst (j). The resultant defect shows the Wharton duct passing over the lingual nerve. The sublingual vein is ligated (k). The patient is noted at one year postoperatively (l and m). Her floor of mouth healed well and she was without evidence of disease.

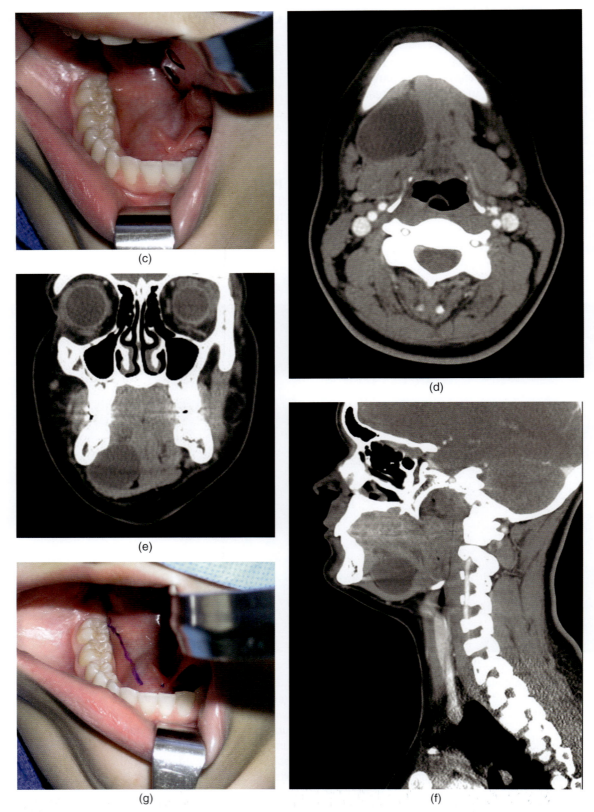

Figure 4.17. (*Continued*).

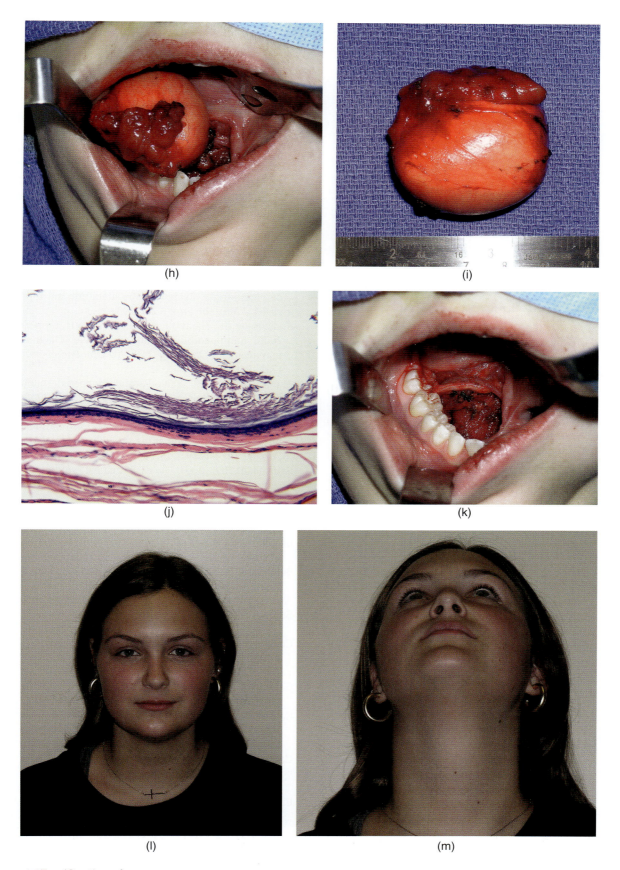

Figure 4.17. (Continued).

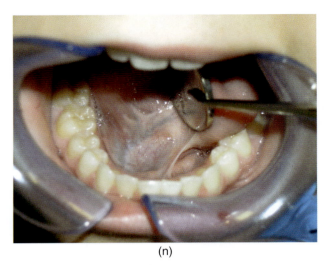

Figure 4.17. (*Continued*).

Imaging

The patient underwent a CT scan of the neck with intravenous contrast (Figure 4.17d–f) that demonstrated a 4-cm homogenous lesion associated with the sublingual gland, supportive of a diagnosis of ranula.

Surgical Procedure

The patient underwent excision of her right sublingual gland through an incision in the floor of mouth (Figure 4.17g). A thorough dissection of the sublingual gland revealed a yellow mass attached to its inferior surface that suggested a diagnosis of lipoma (Figure 4.17h). The sublingual gland and presumed lipoma were removed en bloc (Figure 4.17i). Final pathology identified dermoid cyst (Figure 4.17j). The resultant defect is noted with intact Wharton duct and underlying lingual nerve (Figure 4.17k). The patient is noted at one year postoperatively (Figure 4.17l–n). No signs of recurrent disease were appreciated, and her right Wharton duct and lingual nerve were functioning properly.

TAKE-HOME POINTS

1. A ranula is a very common diagnosis of sublingual gland pathology, especially when present in young patients, but other pathologic processes in the floor of mouth/upper neck region can masquerade as ranulas.
2. Patients with neck masses should routinely undergo CT scans with intravenous contrast, if not contraindicated.
3. When a CT scan suggests the presence of a ranula, additional entities should be entertained on a complete differential diagnosis, including a dermoid cyst.
4. A careful dissection should be undertaken of the inferior surface of the sublingual gland to investigate for other diagnoses when a clinical/radiographic diagnosis of plunging ranula is established.

References

van den Akker HP, Bays RA, Becker AE. 1978. Plunging or cervical ranula. Review of the literature and report of 4 cases. *J Max Fac Surg* 6:286-293.

Anastassov GE, Haiavy J, Solodnik P, Lee H, Lumerman H. 2000. Submandibular gland mucocele: Diagnosis and management. *Oral Surg Oral Med Oral Pathol Oral Radiol Endod* 89:159-163.

Ata N, Unverdi H. 2000. Parotid mucoepidermoid carcinoma mimicking a large mucocele. *J Craniofac Surg* 29:e295-e296.

Baurmash HD. 1992. Marsupialization for treatment of oral ranula: A second look at the procedure. *J Oral Maxillofac Surg* 50:1274-1279.

Baurmash HD. 2007. A case against sublingual gland removal as primary treatment of ranulas. *J Oral Maxillofac Surg* 65:117-121.

Bhaskar SN, Bolden TE, Weinmann JP. 1956a. Pathogenesis of mucoceles. *J Dent Res* 35:863-874.

Bhaskar SN, Bolden TE, Weinmann JP. 1956b. Experimental obstructive adenitis in the mouse. *J Dent Res* 35:852-862.

Boursiquot BC, Fischbein NJ, Sirjani D, Megwalu U. 2020. Risks of neoplasia and malignancy in surgically resected cystic parotid lesions. *Otolaryngol Head Neck Surg* 162:79-86.

Braun TW, Sotereanos GC. 1982. Cervical ranula due to an ectopic sublingual gland. *J Max Fac Surg* 10:56-58.

Carlson ER. 2015. Diagnosis and management of salivary lesions of the neck. *Atlas Oral Maxillofacial Surg Clin N Am* 23:49-61.

Cataldo E, Mosadomi A. 1970. Mucoceles of the oral mucous membrane. *Arch Otolaryngol* 91:360-365.

Catone GA. 1995. Sublingual gland mucous escape. Pseudocysts of the oral-cervical region. *Oral Maxillofac Surg Clin N Am* 7:431-477.

Catone GA, Merrill RG, Henny FA. 1969. Sublingual gland mucus-escape phenomenon – treatment by excision of sublingual gland. *J Oral Surg* 27:774-786.

Colebunders R, Francis H, Mann JM et al. 1988. Parotid swelling during human immunodeficiency virus infection. *Arch Otolaryngol Head Neck Surg* 114:330-332.

Dardick I. 1996. Mucocele and sialocysts. In: *Color Atlas/Text of Salivary Gland Tumor Pathology*. New York, Igaku-Shoin Medical Publishers, Inc., Chapter 14, pp. 131-141.

Eversole LR. 1987. Oral sialocysts. *Arch Otolaryngol Head Neck Surg* 113:51-56.

Ferraro FJ, Rush BF, Ruark D, Oleske J. 1993. Enucleation of parotid lymphoepithelial cyst in patients who are human immunodeficiency virus positive. *Surg Gynecol Obstet* 177:525-527.

Harrison JD. 2010. Modern management and pathophysiology of ranula: Literature review. *Head Neck* 32:1310-1320.

Harrison JD, Kim A, Al-Ali S, Morton RP. 2013. Postmortem investigation of mylohyoid hiatus and hernia: Aetiological factors of plunging ranula. *Clin Anat* 26:693-699.

Hze-Khoong EP, Xu L, Shen S, Yin X, Wang L, Zhang C. 2012. Submandibular gland mucocele associated with a mixed ranula. *Oral Surg Oral Med Oral Pathol Oral Radiol* 113:e6-e9.

Kokong D, Iduh A, Chukwu I, Mugu J, Nuhu S, Augustine S. 2017. Ranula: Current concept of pathophysiologic basis and surgical management options. *World J Surg* 41:1476-1481.

Koudelka BM. 1991. Obstructive Disorders. In: Ellis GL, Auclair PL, Gnepp DR (eds.) *Surgical Pathology of the Salivary Glands*. Philadelphia, WB Saunders, Chapter 3, pp. 26-38.

Lesperance MM. 2013. When do ranulas require a cervical approach? *Laryngoscope* 123:1826-1827.

Marcussen DC, Sooy CD. 1985. Otolaryngologic and head and neck manifestations of acquired immunodeficiency syndrome (AIDS). *Laryngoscope* 95:401-405.

McClatchey KD, Appelblatt NH, Zarbo RJ, Merrel DM. 1984. Plunging ranula. *Oral Surg* 57:408-412.

McGurk M. 2007. Management of the ranula. *J Oral Maxillofac Surg* 65:115-116.

McGurk M, Eyeson J, Thomas B, Harrison JD. 2008. Conservative treatment of oral ranula by excision with minimal excision of the sublingual gland: Histological support for a traumatic etiology. *J Oral Maxillofac Surg* 66:2050-2057.

Morton RP, Ahmad Z, Jain P. 2010. Plunging ranula: Congenital or acquired? *Otolaryngol Head Neck Surg* 142:104-107.

Mulligan R, Navazesh M, Komaroff E et al. 2000. Salivary gland disease in human immunodeficiency virus-positive women from the WIHS study. *Oral Surg Oral Med Oral Pathol Oral Radiol Endod* 89:702-709.

Owotade FJ, Fatusi OA, Adebiyi KE et al. 2005. Clinical experience with parotid gland enlargement in HIV infection: A report of five cases in Nigeria. *J Contemp Dent Pract* 15:136-145.

Ozturk K, Yaman H, Arbag H, Koroglu D, Toy H. 2005. Submandibular gland mucocele: Report of two cases. *Oral Surg Oral Med Oral Pathol Oral Radiol Endod* 100:732-735.

Pantanowitz L, Thompson LEF, Rossi ED. 2018. Diagnostic approach to fine needle aspirations of cystic lesions of the salivary gland. *Head Neck Pathol* 12:548-561.

Patel MR, Deal AM, Shockley WW. 2009. Oral and plunging ranulas: What is the most effective treatment? *Laryngoscope* 119:1501-1509.

Ryan JR, Ioachim HL, Marmer J et al. 1985. Acquired immune deficiency syndrome – Related lymphadenopathics presenting in the salivary gland lymph nodes. *Arch Otolaryngol Head Neck Surg* 111:554-556.

Sekikawa Y, Hongo I. 2017. HIV-associated benign lymphoepithelial cysts of the parotid glands confirmed by HIV-1 p24 antigen immunostaining. *BMJ Case Rep*.

Shaha AR, Webber C, DiMaio T et al. 1993. Benign lymphoepithelial lesions of the parotid. *Am J Surg* 166:403-406.

Sigismund PE, Bozzato A, Schumann M, Koch M, Iro H, Zenk J. 2013. Management of ranula: 9 years' clinical experience in pediatric and adult patients. *J Oral Maxillofac Surg* 71:538-544.

Sperling NM, Lin P, Lucente FE. 1990. Cystic parotid masses in HIV infection. *Head Neck* 12:137-341.

Suresh BV, Vora SK. 2012. Huge plunging ranula. *J Maxillofac Oral Surg* 11:487-490.

Takita H, Takeshita T, Shimono T et al. 2017. Cystic lesions of the parotoid gland: Radiologic-pathologic correlation according to the lastest World Health Organization 2017 classification of head and neck tumours. *Jpn J Radiol* 35:629-647.

Thoma KH. 1950. Cysts and Tumors of the Salivary and Mucous Glands. In: *Oral Pathology. A Histological, Roentgenological, and Clinical Study of the Diseases of the Teeth, Jaws, and Mouth*, 3rd edn. St. Louis, C.V. Mosby Co., pp. 1260-1265.

Work WP. 1977. Cysts and congenital lesions of the parotid gland. *Otlaryngol Clin North Am* 10:339-343.

Yoshimura Y, Obara S, Kondoh T, Naitoh S. 1995. A comparison of three methods used for treatment of ranula. *J Oral Maxillofac Surg* 53:280-282.

Zhao YF, Jia Y, Chen XM, Zhang WF. 2004. Clinical review of 580 ranulas. *Oral Surg Oral Med Oral Pathol Oral Radiol Endod* 98:281-287.

Zhao YF, Jia J, Jia Y. 2005. Complications associated with surgical management of ranulas. *J Oral Maxillofac Surg* 63:51-54.

Chapter 5
Sialolithiasis

Outline

Introduction
Pathophysiology of Sialolithiasis
Clinical Features of Sialolithiasis
  Multiple Sialoliths
  Bilateral Sialoliths
Differential Diagnosis and Diagnosis of Sialolithiasis
Treatment of Sialolithiasis
  Submandibular Sialolithiasis
  Parotid Sialolithiasis
  Treatment of Multiple Sialoliths and Bilateral (Multiple Gland) Sialoliths
Sialolithiasis of the Sublingual Gland and Minor Salivary Glands
The Relationship of Salivary Lithiasis to Nephrolithiasis, Cholelithiasis, Primary Hyperparathyroidism, and Gout
Summary
Case Presentation – *Stoneorama*
References

Introduction

Sialolithiasis is a relatively common disorder of the salivary glands characterized by the development of calculi. Sialolithiasis is thought to affect approximately 1% of the population based on autopsy studies (Williams 1999). It has been estimated to represent more than 50% of major salivary gland disease and is the most common cause of acute and chronic salivary gland infections (Escudier 1998). Sialadenitis (see Chapter 3) and sialolithiasis are disorders of the salivary glands that go hand in hand. Some consider sialolithiasis to be both a consequence and cause of sialadenitis (Berry 1995). For example, in some cases, the presence of a sialolith may cause obstruction such that the salivary gland is predisposed to retrograde infection. In other cases, the presence of sialadenitis may result in a change in the characteristics of the saliva, thereby favoring the deposition of calcium and subsequent formation of a sialolith. In addition, the development of edema within a salivary duct can exacerbate existing obstruction when a small sialolith is present. As such, sialadenitis and sialolithiasis should be considered together. Which of these pathologic processes is the instigating causative factor, however, is unknown (Williams 1999). This chapter will therefore discuss sialolithiasis and review some important concepts of sialadenitis previously discussed in Chapter 3.

Pathophysiology of Sialolithiasis

Sialolithiasis results from the deposition of calcium salts within the ductal system of salivary glands. The salivary stones are comprised primarily of calcium phosphate with traces of magnesium and ammonia with an organic matrix consisting of carbohydrates and amino acids. Kraaij et al. (2018) examined 155 salivary stones removed from sialendoscopy. Most of the stones contained phosphate (88.4%), calcium (87.0%), and magnesium (68.1%). Carbonate and oxalate were present in approximately one-third of the stones. Ammonium, cysteine, and urate were rarely detected (<3%). Historically, it has been taught that salivary stones develop around a central nidus of any number of elements, including desquamated epithelial cells, foreign bodies, microorganisms, and mucous plugs

(Bodner 1993). Progression occurs once the nidus becomes lodged within the salivary ductal system. Stagnation of saliva enhances the development of the sialolith and occurs secondary to either the nidus itself, or due to the tortuosity of the ductal system. The nidus subsequently becomes bathed in a solution supersaturated with respect to calcium and phosphate and slowly calcifies. This pathophysiologic mechanism has been empirically accepted for decades, yet a paucity of evidence exists on the specific cause of sialolith formation.

Kao et al. (2020) evaluated five salivary stones retrieved by sialendoscopy with the hypothesis that bacteria form a core biofilm around which layers of calcium phosphate and hydroxyapatite are deposited. They proposed that biofilm formation within a single salivary gland or duct promotes local ductal injury that results in the activation of the host immune response that interacts with the biofilm and calcium nanoparticles, thereby creating a scaffold upon which further calcium deposition occurs. Kasaboglu et al. (2004) analyzed the chemical composition and micromorphology of sialoliths using X-ray diffraction analysis (EDX) and scanning electron microscopy (SEM) (Kasaboglu et al. 2004). In their six cases reported, X-ray diffraction analysis determined that the sialoliths were comprised completely of multiple and polymorphous hydroxyapatite crystals. In their SEM evaluation, no foreign body or organic material and no signs of microorganism-dependent core formation were detected.

The development of infection of salivary stones related to biofilm formation has been studied by Perez-Tanoira et al. (2019). These authors prospectively studied 55 salivary stones and examined for biofilm formation using fluorescence microscopy and sonication. Biofilm formation was confirmed on the surface of 39 (71%) of stones. A total of 96 microorganisms were isolated from 45 (81.8%) salivary stones. Two or more organisms were isolated in 33 (73.3%) of cases. The primary isolates were *Streptococcus mitis/oralis* ($n = 27$; 28.1%), *Streptococcus anginosus* ($n = 10$; 9.6%), *Rothia* species ($n = 8$; 8.3%), *Streptococcus constellatus* ($n = 7$; 7.3%), and *Streptococcus gordonii* ($n = 6$; 6.2%). All patients demonstrated the presence of a biofilm who showed preoperative (12 cases) or perioperative (three cases) drainage of pus. The authors concluded their study by stating that bacterial biofilm was related to more severe cases of sialadenitis.

There are several reasons for sialolithiasis being observed most commonly in the submandibular system. First, the submandibular gland lies inferior to Wharton duct such that the flow of saliva must travel against the forces of gravity. The physical characteristics of Wharton duct, specifically its length and two acute bends, also theoretically predispose the ductal system to the development of sialolithiasis. The relatively long duct increases the transit time of saliva in the ductal system. The first bend occurs as the gland courses posterior to the mylohyoid muscle, and the second occurs just proximal to the exit of the duct superiorly into the anterior floor of mouth. While the anatomic nature of Wharton duct has been thought to be etiologic in the genesis of sialoliths in this system, the angle of the genu of the duct has been investigated as to whether it represents a significant contributory factor (Drage et al. 2002). Specifically, these researchers retrospectively studied this issue using sialograms in 23 patients with sialadenitis, 61 patients with sialolithiasis, and a control group of 18 patients. There were no statistical differences in the angle of the genu in three groups suggesting that the difference in the angle of the genu of the submandibular duct in the sagittal plane is not of etiologic significance in the formation of sialoliths. The authors indicated that the *length* of the duct might be of significance in the formation of stones; however, that parameter was not investigated in their study. One final issue related to submandibular sialolithiasis is the alkaline nature of the saliva, its viscosity, and relatively high content of calcium salts, specifically phosphates, carbonates, and oxalates that make the submandibular saliva more prone to sialolithiasis than the other major glands (see Table 5.1). Collectively, these features contribute to salivary stasis, crystallization of precipitated calcium salts with calculus formation, obstruction to salivary flow, and infection. Interestingly, *partial* obstruction appears to be of great importance in the development of sialoliths. A completely obstructed gland, although possessing salivary stagnation, does not result in an increase in stone formation (Williams 1999). In completely obstructed glands, the calcium secretory granules in the acini become depleted and the saliva is less likely to produce stones. Baurmash has stated that salivary stasis and salivary viscosity, rather than the calcium content of the salivary secretion, determine the development of sialoliths (Baurmash 2004).

Table 5.1. Composition of normal adult saliva.

	Submandibular gland	Parotid gland
Calcium	3.6 mEq/l	2.0 mEq/l
Phosphate	4.5 mEq/l	6.0 mEq/l
Bicarbonate	18 mEq/l	20 mEq/l
Sodium	21 mEq/l	23 mEq/l
Potassium	17 mEq/l	20 mEq/l
Chloride	20 mEq/l	23 mEq/l
Magnesium	0.3 mEq/l	0.2 mEq/l
Urea	7.0 mEq/l	15 mEq/l
Proteins	150 mg/dl	250 mg/dl
Amino acids	<1 mg/dl	1.5 mg/dl
Fatty acids	<1 mg/dl	1 mg/dl
Glucose	<1 mg/dl	<1 mg/dl

Clinical Features of Sialolithiasis

Miloro (1998) reported that approximately 85% of sialoliths occur in the submandibular gland, 10% in the parotid gland, 5% in the sublingual gland, and the incidence of this pathology is extremely rare in the minor salivary glands. In their retrospective review of 2322 patients with 2.959 salivary stones, Sigismund et al. (2015) identified 2378 (80.4%) submandibular stones and 581 (19.6%) parotid stones. Only 50 children (2.2%) demonstrated sialoliths in this study. There were no cases of sublingual stones or minor salivary gland stones. When involved, minor salivary gland sialoliths occur in the buccal mucosa or upper lip, forming an indurated nodule that may mimic a neoplastic process. Sialolithiasis occurs more often in males (Sigismund et al. 2015), with a peak age of occurrence between 20 and 50 years of age (Lustmann et al. 1990). Other studies identify sialolithiasis in children comprising only 3% of cases (Liu and Rawal 2013) with the youngest documented age being two years (Kim et al. 2013).

The left submandibular gland is more often affected than the right gland, and bilateral involvement in the absence of another systemic disorder is rare. Historically, stone formation has not been highly associated with systemic abnormalities of calcium metabolism (King et al. 1990). Gout is the main systemic disease thought to predispose to salivary stone formation (Blatt et al. 1958; Williams 1999; Moghe et al. 2012; Kraaij et al. 2014). The single case report of a uric acid sialolith of the parotid gland published by Blatt et al. (1958) has perpetually been quoted in the literature thereafter with a suggested cause and effect relationship between gout and sialolithiasis. The single published case involved a patient with known tophaceous gout and the partial removal of a sialolith of her Stensen duct and microscopic examination of the stone. Uric acid crystals were identified in the sialolith and the authors concluded that uric acid sialolithiasis should be included in the list of potential complications of gout. In the final analysis, one published case of uric acid sialolithiasis is insufficient to support the declaration of gout as a predisposing systemic disease for sialolithiasis. It is possible that the presence of a uric acid sialolith was casual in this case rather than being indicative of gout representing a genuine risk factor for sialolithiasis.

At least one report suggests an association between primary hyperparathyroidism and sialolithiasis (Stack and Norman 2008). These stones are primarily made up of uric acid. Theoretical associations also exist between urolithiasis and cholelithiasis, and will be discussed later in this chapter. Multiple sialolith formation independent of systemic illness in the same gland, however, is common.

While salivary stones are single in 70–80% of cases (Figure 5.1), two calculi occur in 20% of cases, and more than two calculi occur in 5% of cases (Williams 1999; Miloro and Goldberg 2002) (Figure 5.2). Sigismund et al. (2015) found multiple stones in 16.9% of patients, with 86.6% of parotid cases involving a single stone and 81.9% of submandibular cases involving a single stone. Jauregui et al. (2016) retrospectively reviewed 133 patients with chronic parotitis and identified 13 patients (10%) with multiple sialoliths. Greater

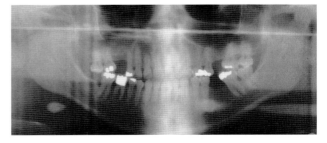

Figure 5.1. A single sialolith noted within the right submandibular gland. Isolated stones are most common in the submandibular system.

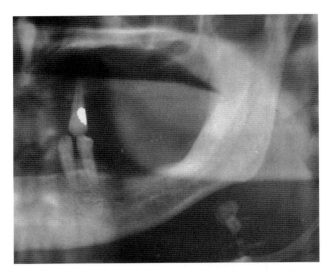

Figure 5.2. This panoramic radiograph close-up shows two sialoliths within the left submandibular gland.

than half of these patients (54%) with multiple parotid calcifications were diagnosed with autoimmune parotitis or HIV. The authors therefore recommended a workup for immune-mediated disease should be considered in patients with multiple parotid sialoliths.

Sialolithiasis of the parotid gland is rare. When stones occur in the parotid gland, they are smaller than submandibular gland stones, and more often multiple (Figure 5.3). Regarding location, submandibular stones are found in the duct in 75–85% of cases, while parotid stones are located in the hilum or gland parenchyma in at least half of cases (Williams 1999). Sigismund et al. (2015) found most of their 2378 submandibular stones located at the hilum or in the proximal duct (53%), while 37% were located in the distal 2/3 distal duct system, and 10% located in the intraglandular duct. Regarding their 581 parotid stones, 83% were found in the distal Stensen duct, and 17% were found in the intraglandular duct. Submandibular stones located within the gland are commonly oval in shape (Figure 5.4) and commonly elongated in shape when they occur in the duct. When present for long periods of time, these stones may become quite large (Figure 5.5). Bilateral salivary stones are quite rare; however, they have been observed (Lutcavage and Schaberg 1991) (Figure 5.6).

Sialolithiasis most commonly presents with painful swelling, although painless swelling or pain only are occasionally reported as symptoms.

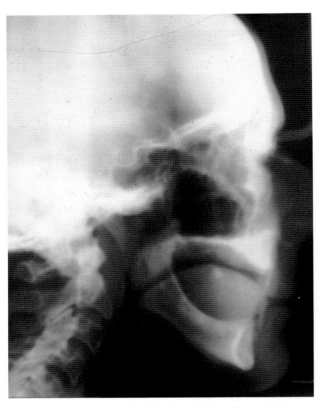

Figure 5.3. This lateral cephalometric radiograph shows a single stone located within Stensen duct.

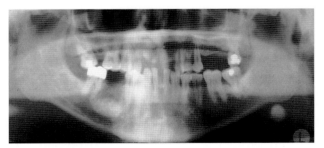

Figure 5.4. This panoramic radiograph shows an oval sialolith of the left submandibular gland.

Lustmann's study showed swelling to be present in 94% of their 245 cases of sialolithiasis, while pain occurred in 65.2%, pus secretion in 15.5%, and an absence of symptoms in 2.4% of their patients (Lustmann et al. 1990). Sigismund et al. (2015) reported on 61 (2.6%) incidentally discovered stones related to ultrasound evaluation for other diagnoses in the head and neck. When symptoms do occur, their magnitude seems to vary by the gland involved and the location and size of the

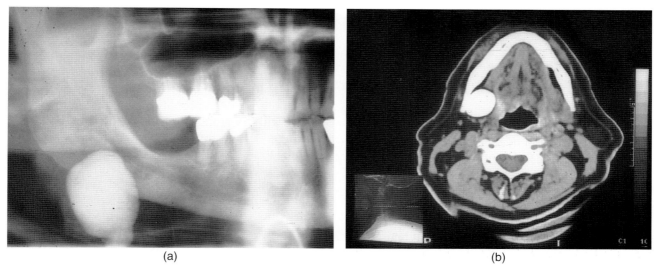

Figure 5.5. This very large sialolith is associated with the right submandibular gland as seen on panoramic radiograph (a). Due to its size, it might be confused with an osteoma of the mandible such that computerized tomograms help to identify its presence within the submandibular gland (b).

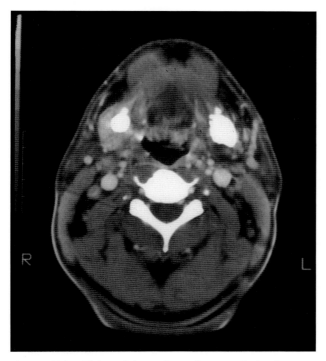

Figure 5.6. This axial section of computerized tomograms shows the presence of bilateral sialoliths of the submandibular glands.

sialolith. A small sialolith may be asymptomatic and serendipitously discovered during routine dental radiographic examination. Once the stone increases in size, salivary flow will be impaired, and spasmodic pain occurs during eating. Purulent infection may accompany sialolithiasis.

MULTIPLE SIALOLITHS

It has long been believed that multiple stones of the salivary glands represent an uncommon occurrence. With the increasing sophistication and resolution of imaging studies and the increasing use of sialendoscopy, however, it has become apparent that multiple sialoliths are uncommon but not rare as once believed (Ardekian et al. 2014). In their study of 530 consecutive cases of sialolithiasis, Ardekian et al. (2014) identified multiple calculi in 37 of 530 (7%) of these cases. The mean number of sialoliths per patient was 3.4 with 16 sialoliths being the largest number present in one patient in this series. The submandibular gland was affected in 33 cases (90%), and the parotid gland was affected in the remaining 4 cases (10%). Preoperative imaging identified a solitary sialolith in 3 of the 37 cases (8%) of multiple sialoliths where additional sialoliths were discovered by sialendoscopy. Stated differently, 92% of the cases of multiple sialoliths were correctly identified by preoperative imaging. Of the multiple submandibular sialoliths, 40% were found in the proximal aspect of the duct and 60% were located distally.

The multiple parotid sialoliths were found in the duct and were typically smaller than those located in the submandibular system.

BILATERAL SIALOLITHS

Simultaneous sialolithiasis of more than one salivary gland is less common than multiple sialoliths and is estimated to occur in fewer than 3% of cases of sialolithiasis (Sunder et al. 2014). This notwithstanding, surgeons must be vigilant in terms of investigating for the possibility of multiple gland involvement when preparing a patient for surgery related to a diagnosis of sialolithiasis. A review of the literature indicates that when multiple sialoliths occur, they occur in a bilateral same gland fashion rather than involving two different salivary glands.

Differential Diagnosis and Diagnosis of Sialolithiasis

Patients with sialolithiasis most commonly present with clinical and historical evidence of salivary calculi. A history of submandibular swelling, prandial pain, and bouts of sialadenitis are highly suggestive of a diagnosis of sialolithiasis. This notwithstanding, many patients are asymptomatic such that only a panoramic radiograph may allow for the diagnosis of submandibular sialolithiasis as it may reveal calcifications within the submandibular triangle. It has been observed that submandibular stones located anteriorly are more often symptomatic than those lodged in the intraglandular portion of the duct (Karas 1998). While such calcifications may lead to a diagnosis of submandibular sialolithiasis, it is important for the clinician to consider other diagnoses that present with submandibular calcifications, particularly when pain is absent. Among these are calcified lymph nodes associated with mycobacterial adenitis (scrofula) (Figure 5.7), phleboliths associated with oral/facial hemangiomas (Figure 5.8), and a mandibular osteoma as might occur in Gardner's syndrome (Figure 5.9). Collectively, these calcifications may, at first glance, appear consistent with a diagnosis of submandibular sialolithiasis. Close examination of panoramic radiographs may, however, allow for the clinician to establish a radiographic diagnosis other than submandibular sialolithiasis (Mandel 2006). Most submandibular calculi contain smooth borders when they exist within the gland. Calcified lymph nodes generally show irregular borders, and osteomas of the mandible are larger than most salivary gland stones, and are intimately associated with the mandible. Phleboliths are commonly multiple in number, and exist within the neck outside of the submandibular triangle. They are scattered, and have a classic lamellated appearance with a lucent core. Finally, phleboliths are smaller than sialoliths and demonstrate an oval shape, compared to the sialolith whose elliptical shape has been created by a salivary duct (Mandel and Surattanont 2004). One further entity worthy of mention is calcified atheromas of the carotid artery, which is sufficiently distant from the submandibular triangle to not be confused with a submandibular sialolith. These are most commonly located inferior and posterior to the mandibular angle adjacent to the intervertebral space between cervical vertebrae three and four (Friedlander and Freymiller 2003).

While the diagnosis of sialolithiasis is frequently confirmed radiographically, it is important for the clinician to not obtain radiographs prior to performing a physical examination. Bimanual palpation of the floor of mouth may reveal evidence of a stone in many patients. Similar palpation of the gland may also permit detection of a stone as well as the degree of fibrosis present within the gland. Examining the opening of Wharton duct for the flow of saliva or pus is an important aspect of the evaluation. It has been estimated that approximately one-quarter of symptomatic submandibular glands that harbor stones are nonfunctional or hypofunctional. Radiographs should be obtained, and may reveal the presence of a stone. It has been reported that 80% of submandibular stones are radio-opaque, 40% of parotid stones are radio-opaque, and 20% of sublingual gland stones are radio-opaque (Miloro 1998).

Treatment of Sialolithiasis

General principles of management of patients with sialolithiasis include conservative measures such as effective hydration, the use of heat, gland massage, and sialagogues that might result in flushing a small stone out of the duct. A course of oral antibiotics may also be beneficial. These measures may be particularly appropriate since some patients

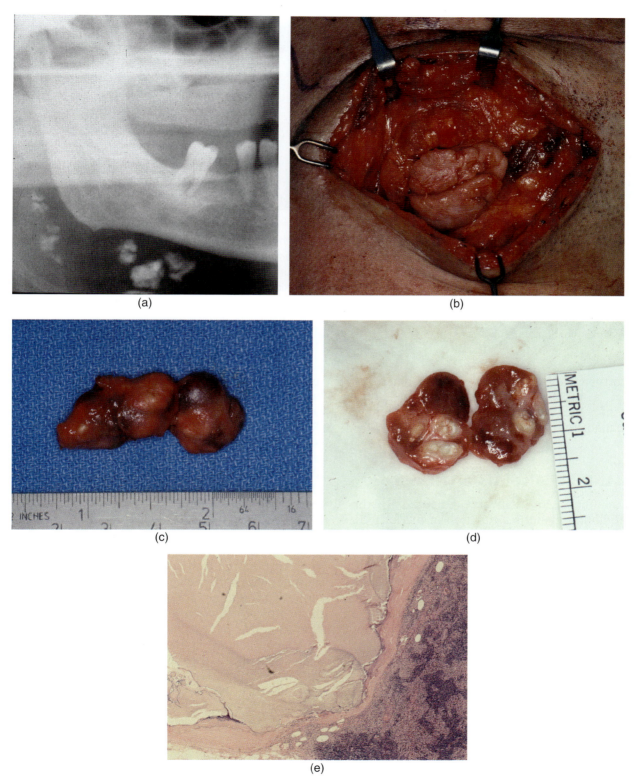

Figure 5.7. A close-up of a panoramic radiograph obtained in a patient with a chief complaint of right submandibular pain (a). The calcifications noted on this radiograph are located in the retromandibular region as well as the submandibular gland area. Exploration of the neck showed indurated lymph nodes present in association with the right submandibular gland, but clearly not sialoliths (b). The lymph nodes were removed (c) and bisected, showing macroscopic (d) and microscopic evidence of caseous necrosis (e). A diagnosis of tuberculous adenitis was therefore established. The patient was subjected to a purified protein derivative (PPD) skin test that was positive.

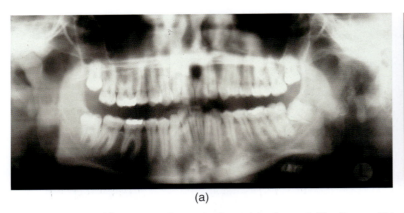
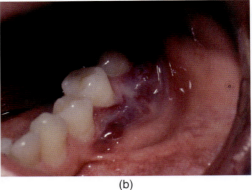

Figure 5.8. A panoramic radiograph demonstrating calcifications within the left submandibular region (a). At first glance of the radiograph, submandibular sialolithiasis is a reasonable consideration. Close examination of the radiograph reveals multicentric lamellated calcifications in the submandibular and preauricular regions, as well as a calcification superimposed on the left mandibular second molar roots. A complete physical examination revealed signs consistent with a hemangioma associated with the left mandibular gingiva (b). As such, the calcifications are presumed to represent phleboliths, and are not removed. It is important, therefore, to diagnose sialolithiasis based on a review of a radiograph as well as a physical examination.

may carry a clinical diagnosis of sialadenitis in case of a radiolucent sialolith. As such, the treatment is the same in the initial management of both diagnoses.

SUBMANDIBULAR SIALOLITHIASIS

The treatment of salivary calculi of the submandibular gland is a function of the location and size of the sialolith (Figure 5.10). For example, sialoliths present within the duct may often be retrieved with a transoral sialolithotomy procedure and sialodochoplasty. In general terms, if the stone can be palpated transorally, it can probably be removed transorally. A review of 172 patients who underwent intraoral sialolithotomy of a submandibular stone assessed results as to complete removal, partial removal, and failure (Park et al. 2006). The effect of location, size, presence of infection, and palpability of the calculi on the results was assessed. Univariate analysis showed that palpability and the presence of infection were statistically significant factors affecting transoral sialolithotomy. Palpability was the only significant factor after multivariate analysis. This study provides scientific evidence supporting intraoral removal of extraglandular submandibular gland stones regardless of location, size, presence of infection, or recurrence of calculi provided the calculi are palpable. This procedure involves excising Wharton's duct overlying the stone, thereby permitting its retrieval (Figure 5.11). Reconstruction of the duct in the form of a sialodochoplasty permits shortening of the duct and enlargement of salivary outflow, thereby preventing recurrence and allowing for healing of the gland (Rontal and Rontal 1987). A properly performed sialodochoplasty ensures effective flow of saliva from the gland in hopes of maintaining the health of the salivary gland. This procedure involves suturing the edges of the duct's mucosa to the surrounding oral mucosa (Figure 5.11). The number of sutures placed is arbitrary; however, numerous sutures are required to stabilize the reconstructed duct to the floor of mouth. Proper postoperative hydration of the patient with freeflowing saliva maintains patency of the sialodochoplasty, thereby enhancing the potential for reversal or stabilization of the underlying sialadenitis. Chronic submandibular obstructive sialolithiasis clearly leads to chronic sialadenitis with presumed parenchymal destruction. After removal of the sialolith, however, the apparent resiliency of the submandibular gland usually results in no adverse symptoms (Baurmash 2004). As such, the ability to effectively retrieve a sialolith usually refutes the need to also remove the affected salivary gland. Sialoliths located within the submandibular gland or its hilum are most commonly managed

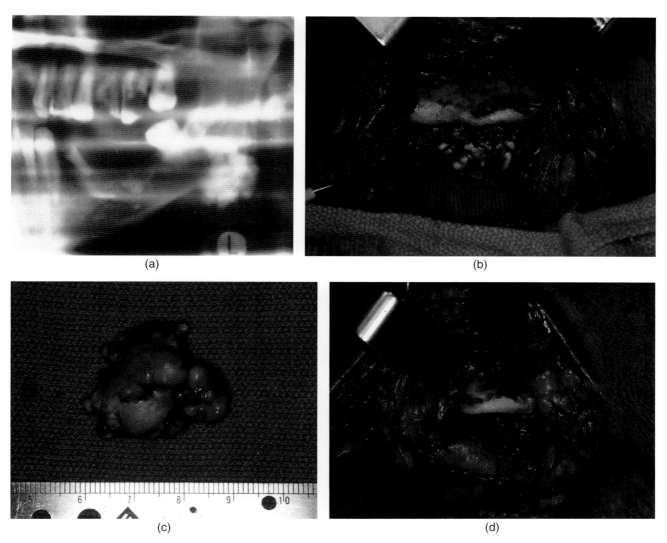

Figure 5.9. This panoramic radiographic close-up shows an irregular mass associated with the left submandibular region (a). Computerized tomograms were not obtained preoperatively, and a differential diagnosis of submandibular sialolithiasis was established. The calcification, however, does not show typical radiographic signs of a sialolith, including its irregular borders. The patient underwent exploration of the left submandibular region, whereupon the calcified mass was identified as a distinct entity from the left submandibular gland (b). The mass was removed (c) and the left submandibular gland remained in the tissue bed (d). A histopathologic diagnosis of osteoma was made. A subsequent diagnosis of Gardner's syndrome was made, and the patient underwent colectomy when a diagnosis of adenocarcinoma of the colon was established.

with submandibular gland excision (Figure 5.12). This controversial statement is made based on the relative difficulty to retrieve stones from this anatomic region of the gland, rather than based on the assumption that proximal stones cause permanent structural damage to the gland that results in the need for removal of the gland. To this end, a study examined a series of 55 consecutive patients who underwent transoral removal of stones from the hilum of the submandibular gland (McGurk et al. 2004). Stones were retrieved in 54 patients (98%), but four glands (8%) required subsequent removal due to recurrent obstruction. The authors emphasized that it was necessary for the stone to be palpable and no limitation of oral opening should exist for patients to undergo their

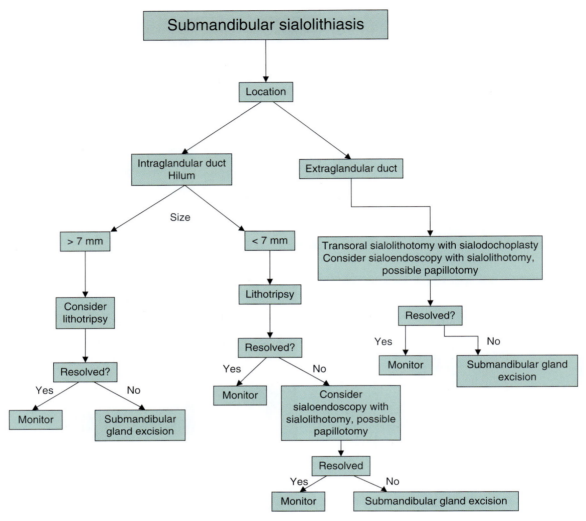

Figure 5.10. Algorithm for management of submandibular sialolithiasis.

technique. They reported an acceptable incidence of complications associated with their technique, although they lamented that it remained to be seen if the asymptomatic nature of their patients would be maintained over time.

Shock wave lithotripsy has been reported as a primary form of treatment for submandibular salivary gland stones. Salivary stone lithotripsy requires a gland to be functional by production of saliva to permit the stone fragments to be eliminated from the duct. Some authors have implemented a sour gum test prior to performing extracorporeal lithotripsy (Williams 1999). This test involves the patient chewing sour gum, whereby the clinician looks for swelling of the gland. The development of swelling indicates that the gland is functional such that extracorporeal lithotripsy may be attempted. In the absence of swelling, extracorporeal lithotripsy is contraindicated, and the gland is planned for removal. Two techniques of salivary lithotripsy have been developed, including extracorporeal, sonographically controlled lithotripsy, and intracorporeal endoscopically guided lithotripsy (Escudier 1998). Extracorporeal shock wave lithotripsy was first used to treat renal stones in the early 1980s. The shock waves can be generated by electromagnetic, piezoelectric, and electrohydraulic mechanisms and the resultant waves are brought to a focus through acoustic lenses. They then pass through a water-filled cushion to the stone where stress and cavitation act to fracture the stone. At the

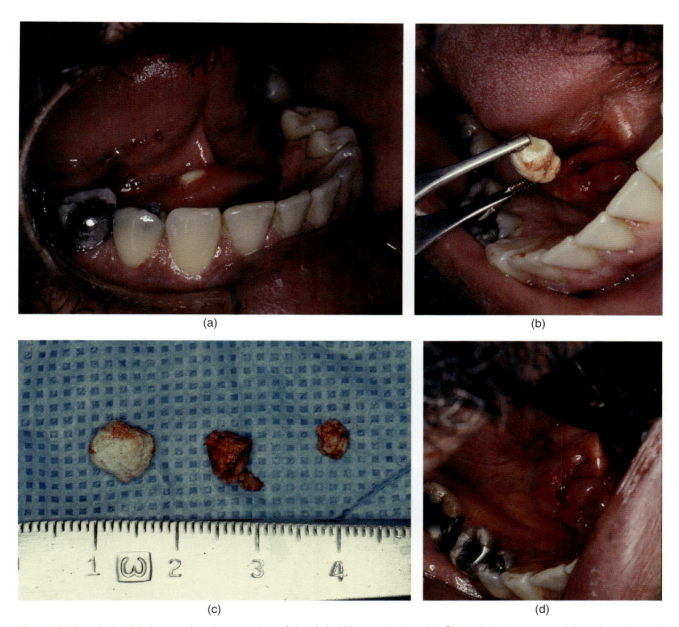

Figure 5.11. A sialolith is noted at the opening of the right Wharton's duct (a). Since this stone was able to be palpated on oral examination, it was removed transorally without necessitating the removal of the right submandibular gland. The main stone was removed (b), after which time exploration of the proximal duct revealed two additional stones that were also removed (c). A sialodochoplasty was performed to widen and shorten the right Wharton's duct (d). A sialodochoplasty performed near the papilla of Wharton's duct is termed a papillotomy.

sialolith–water interface, a compressive wave is propagated through the stone, thereby subjecting it to stress. Cavitation occurs when reflected energy at the sialolith–water interface results in a rebounding tensile or expansion wave, which induces bubbles. When these bubbles collapse, a jet of water is projected through the bubble onto the stone's surface. This force is sufficient to pit the stone and break it. Extracorporeal lithotripsy for submandibular gland stones is somewhat less successful than that of parotid stones (Williams 1999). Ottaviani and his group evaluated the results of 52 patients treated with electromagnetic extracorporeal lithotripsy for calculi of the submandibular gland

(n = 36 patients) and parotid gland (n = 16 patients). Complete disintegration was achieved in 46.1% of patients, including 15 with submandibular sialolithiasis and 9 with parotid sialolithiasis. Elimination of the stones was confirmed by sonogram. Residual concrements were detected by ultrasound in 30.8% of patients, including nine with submandibular stones, and seven with parotid stones. Four patients with residual submandibular stones required surgical retrieval. The authors concluded by indicating that if hilar and intraglandular duct stones are smaller than 7 mm in size, they may be successfully treated with lithotripsy (Williams 1999). The surgeon should proceed with submandibular gland excision if this trial of lithotripsy is not successful, or if stones larger than 7 mm are identified.

Capaccio et al. (2004) reviewed 322 consecutive symptomatic patients with sialolithiasis of the submandibular gland (234 patients) and parotid

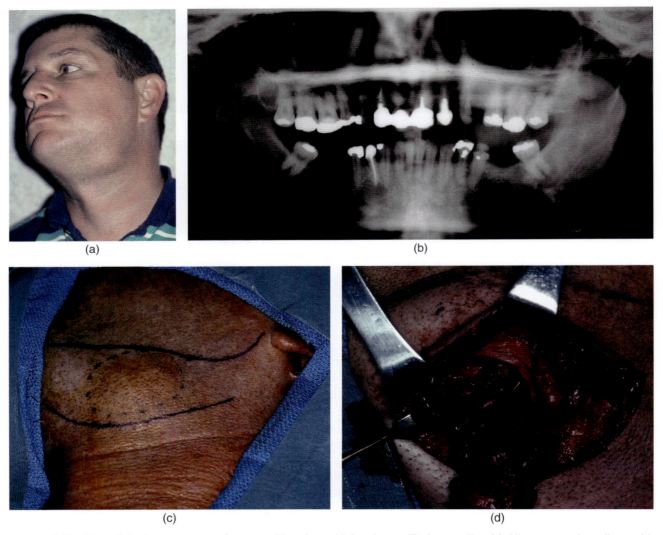

Figure 5.12. The clinical appearance of a man with pain and left submandibular swelling (a). His panoramic radiographic (b) shows a sialolith in the left submandibular gland. A standard transcutaneous approach was followed to submandibular gland excision (c). A subfascial dissection of the gland was performed. Inferior retraction on the gland allowed for preservation of the marginal mandibular branch of the facial nerve (d). Superior and anterior retraction of the gland allowed for identification of the sialolith that was located at the hilum of the gland (e). The excised gland (f) was bisected (g) and demonstrated significant scar tissue formation.

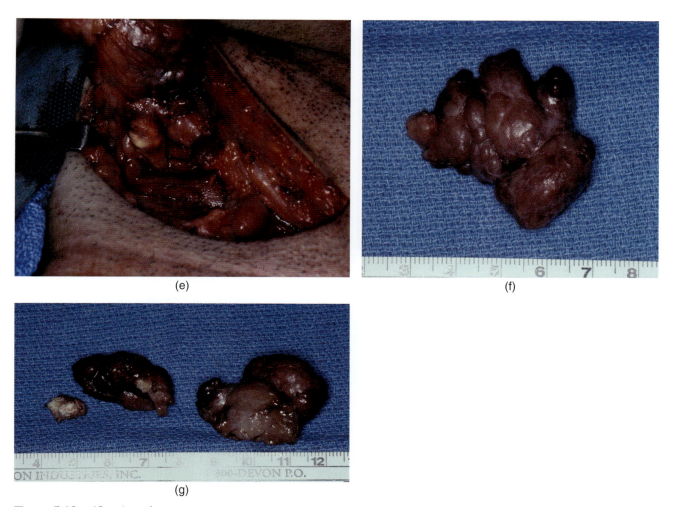

Figure 5.12. (Continued).

gland (88 patients) who underwent extracorporeal lithotripsy. Complete elimination of the stones was achieved in 45% of patients. By ultrasound, residual fragments smaller than 2 mm were detected in 27% of patients. Gland excision was required in 3% of patients, all with refractory submandibular stones. Univariate analysis showed that favorable treatment outcomes were achieved in patients younger than 46 years of age, parotid stones, stones smaller than 7 mm, and six or fewer therapeutic sessions.

Intracorporeal lithotripsy techniques are now used in which a miniature endoscope is utilized to manipulate the stone under direct vision. In this technique, shock waves are applied directly to the surface of the stone under endoscopic guidance. The shock wave may be derived from an electrohydraulic source, a pneumoballistic source, or from a laser. Pneumoballistic energy has been shown to produce calculus fragmentation with greater efficiency than lasertripsy (Arzoz et al. 1996). The disadvantage of these techniques is that the size of the endoscope and probe requires that the duct be incised to facilitate entry.

Finally, interventional sialendoscopy has been developed that may permit the use of a fine sialendoscope to retrieve salivary stones (Nakayama et al. 2003) (Figure 5.13). The size of some sialoliths, however, is such that an incision of the papilla may be necessary for their delivery. Interventional sialendoscopy may be used with lithotripsy to fragment large stones to achieve a completely noninvasive therapeutic sialendoscopy.

McGurk et al. (2004) assessed the efficacy of extracorporeal shock wave lithotripsy, basket retrieval as part of interventional sialendoscopy, and

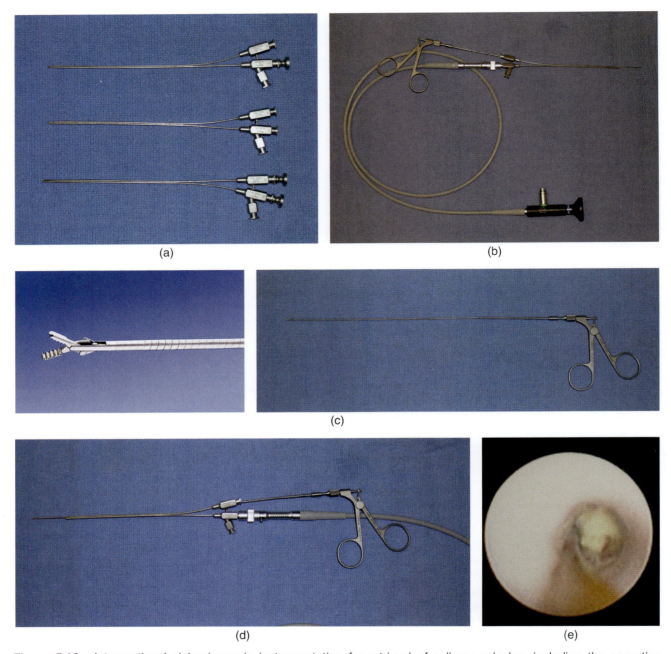

Figure 5.13. Interventional sialendoscopic instrumentation for retrieval of salivary calculus, including the operating sheaths (a) that accept the miniature endoscope in the *telescope* channel (b). The grasping forceps (c) are placed within the *working* channel of the operating sheaths (d), and can retrieve stones that may be identified on diagnostic sialendoscopy (e). Source: Courtesy of Dr. Maria Troulis, Boston, Massachusetts.

intraoral surgical removal of salivary calculi. Three hundred twenty-three patients with submandibular calculi were managed. Extracorporeal shock wave lithotripsy was successful in 43 of 131 (32.8%) patients, basket retrieval was successful in 80 of 109 (73.4%) patients, and surgical removal was successful in 137 of 143 (95.8%) patients with submandibular stones.

PAROTID SIALOLITHIASIS

Sialoliths of the parotid gland are divided anatomically into those that are located within the intraglandular duct and the extraglandular duct (Figure 5.14). Extraglandular duct sialoliths may be removed surgically through and intraoral approach (Figure 5.15). In this procedure, a C-shaped incision is made anterior to Stensen papilla. Dissection is performed deep (lateral) to the duct such that it is included in the mucosal flap such that the duct is separated from the more lateral soft tissues. A retraction suture may be placed at the anterior aspect of the mucosal aspect of the flap. The duct is dissected from anterior to posterior to identify the stone within the duct. Once the stone is located, the duct is incised longitudinally, thereby allowing for retrieval of the sialolith. The mucosal flap is reapproximated; however, the incision in the duct is not sutured. These longitudinal incisions placed in the duct do not appear to result in the formation of strictures, although transverse incisions in the duct may result in stricture formation (Seward 1968; Berry 1995). Strictures in the parotid duct will respond favorably to intermittent dilation; however, submandibular duct strictures usually require surgical intervention.

Parotid sialoliths located within the intraglandular portion of the ductal system may be addressed through an extraoral approach. Two options exist, one involving a traditional parotidectomy approach (without performing a parotidectomy) with a curvilinear skin incision in the preauricular and upper neck regions (Berry 1995) and the other involving a horizontal incision over the duct in the cheek region (Baurmash and Dechiara 1991). In the former approach, the skin flap is elevated superficial to the parotid fascia, and the duct is identified at the point where it exits the anterior border of the gland. The placement of a lacrimal probe within Stensen duct may permit accurate identification of

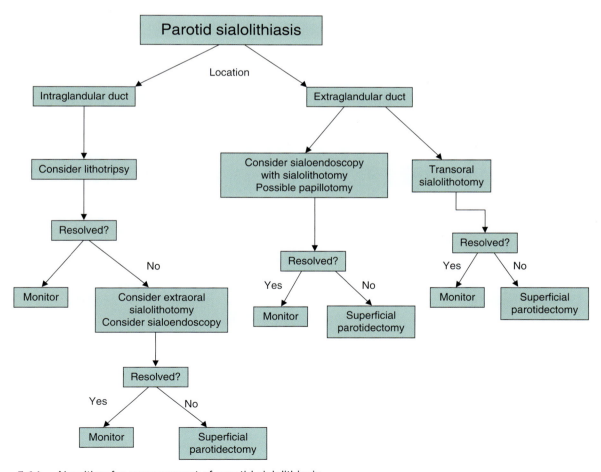

Figure 5.14. Algorithm for management of parotid sialolithiasis.

the duct. Once the duct is located, it is dissected posteriorly into the gland and the stone is identified. A longitudinal incision is made over the duct and the stone is retrieved (Figure 5.16). As in the case of a transoral sialolithotomy, the incision in the Stensen duct is not closed at the conclusion of the surgery. Sialolithotomy performed with a transcutaneous approach in the cheek may also be accomplished for a diagnosis of parotid sialolithiasis (Figure 5.17).

Extracorporeal lithotripsy seems to be quite effective for the treatment of intraparotid stones. With three outpatient treatments, 50% of patients have been reported to be rendered free of calculus (Williams 1999). Half of the remaining patients may be rendered free of symptoms, but having

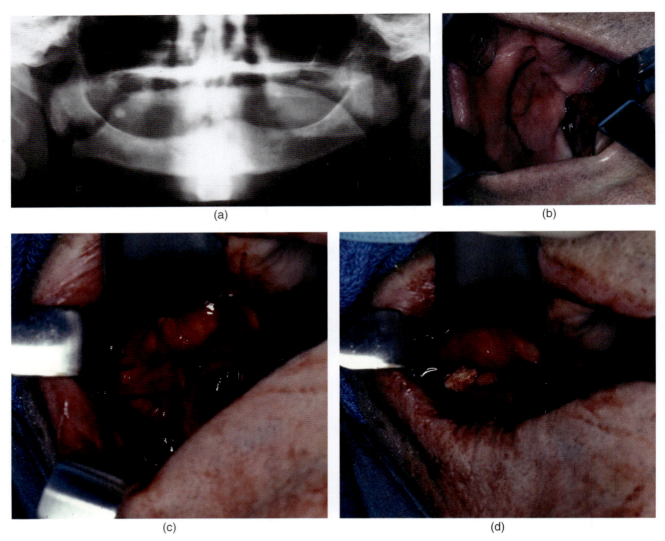

Figure 5.15. Management of an extraglandular parotid duct sialolith. The panoramic radiograph demonstrates a small sialolith in the right Stensen duct (a). The approach for this transoral sialolithotomy involved a mucosal incision anterior to Stensen papilla (b). A mucosal flap was developed that included Stensen duct such that the dissection occurred lateral to the duct (c). Continued dissection allowed for palpation of the sialolith within the duct. The duct was longitudinally incised over the sialolith (d), such that the stone could be removed (e). The mucosal flap was sutured without reapproximating the incision in Stensen duct (f). Patent salivary flow was re-established as noted two months postoperatively (g). No further treatment of the gland was required.

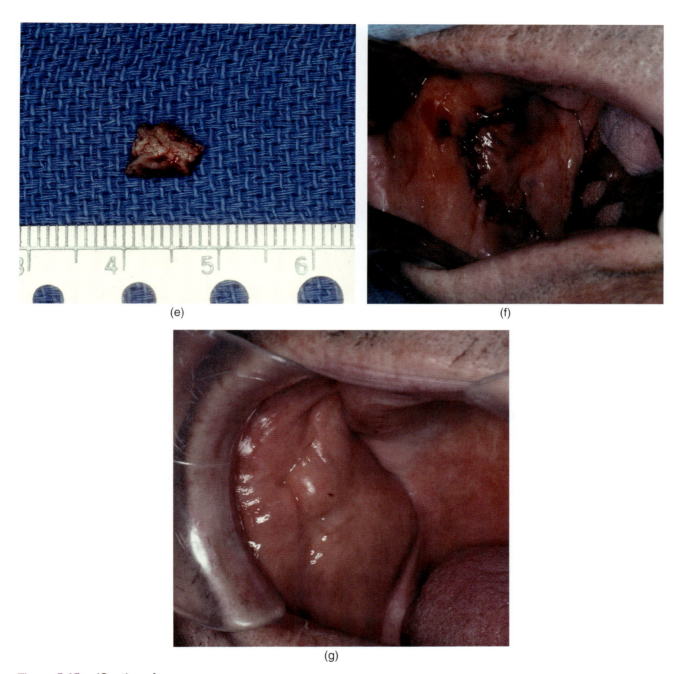

Figure 5.15. *(Continued).*

small fragments left in the ductal system. In Ottaviani's cohort of 16 patients with parotid stones, all were relieved of their symptoms with extracorporeal lithotripsy (Ottaviani 1996). Nine of their 16 patients experienced complete disintegration and elimination of stones, and 7 patients showed residual stone fragments that could be flushed out spontaneously or with salivation induced by citric acid (Ottaviani 1996).

McGurk et al. (2004) found extracorporeal shock wave lithotripsy to be successful in 44 of 90 (48.9%) patients with parotid sialoliths, and basket retrieval was successful in 44 of 57 (77.2%) of patients with parotid sialoliths. Interestingly, no

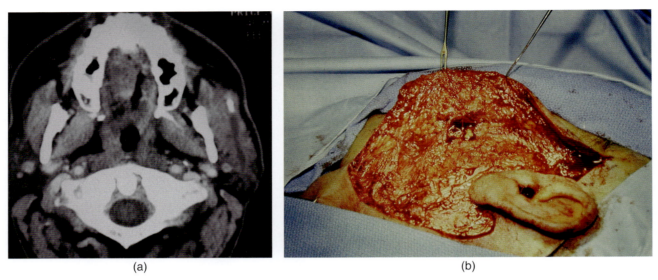

Figure 5.16. Axial CT scan demonstrating a parotid sialolith at the hilum with proximal dilatation of the duct due to obstruction of salivary flow (a). A parotidectomy approach to stone retrieval was performed without parotidectomy (b).

patients with parotid stones underwent transoral surgical removal.

TREATMENT OF MULTIPLE SIALOLITHS AND BILATERAL (MULTIPLE GLAND) SIALOLITHS

While rare, the incidence of multiple sialoliths within one salivary gland and synchronous multiple gland sialoliths requires that all patients undergo CT imaging when a diagnosis of sialolithiasis has been made (Figure 5.18). In so doing, a review of these CT scans should rule out multiple gland involvement and the presence of multiple sialoliths. When the review of the CT scan reveals multiple sialoliths in a single gland system, the count must be verified at the time of surgery. When multiple salivary glands are involved with the sialolithiasis, the surgeon should treat each gland according to standard, single gland protocols discussed in this chapter.

Sialolithiasis of the Sublingual Gland and Minor Salivary Glands

The incidence of sialolithiasis of the sublingual gland and the minor salivary glands is very low. In McGurk et al.'s (2004) study of 455 cases of salivary calculi, no cases were present in the sublingual gland or minor salivary glands. Similarly, none of the 2959 salivary stones in the study by Sigismund et al. (2015) were found in the sublingual gland or minor salivary glands. As such, swellings of these glands are most likely to engender a clinical diagnosis of neoplastic disease, with the diagnosis of sialolithiasis made only after final histopathologic analysis of the gland occurs (Figure 5.19). One report examining sialolithiasis of the minor salivary glands found that only 20% of cases were correctly clinically diagnosed as sialolithiasis (Anneroth and Hansen 1983). The paucity of accurate diagnosis may also stem from the frequent spontaneous resolution of the problem due to ejection of the calculus (Lagha et al. 2005). Two stages of minor salivary gland sialolithiasis have been described including an acute stage characterized by inflamed overlying soft tissue, whereby the most common clinical diagnosis is cellulitis of the soft tissue. The chronic stage follows and calls to mind a differential diagnosis of neoplasm, irritation fibroma, or foreign body. An anatomic distribution of 126 cases of sialolithiasis of the minor salivary glands identified a significant majority occurring in either the upper lip or the buccal mucosa. As such, sialolithiasis should be included on the differential diagnosis of an indurated submucosal nodule of the upper lip or buccal mucosa, and surgical excision should be performed.

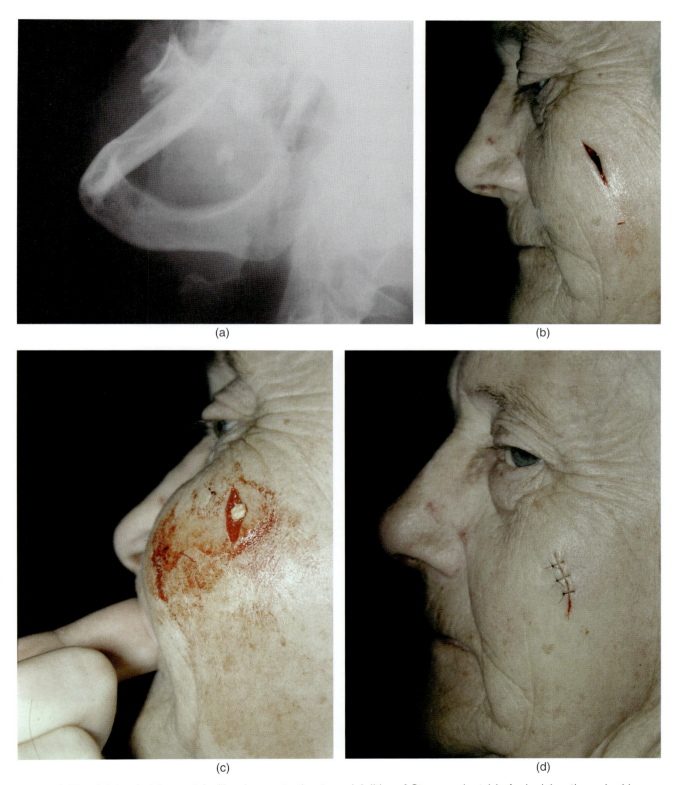

Figure 5.17. A lateral oblique plain film demonstrating two sialoliths of Stensen duct (a). An incision through skin was placed in a resting tension line of the cheek (b). A finger was inserted in the oral cavity to create better access to the duct, thereby permitting stone retrieval (c). A primary closure was obtained (d). Source: Reprinted with permission from Ord RA: Salivary Gland Disease, in: Fonseca R (ed.): volume 5, chapter 10, New York, Elsevier, pp. 273–293.

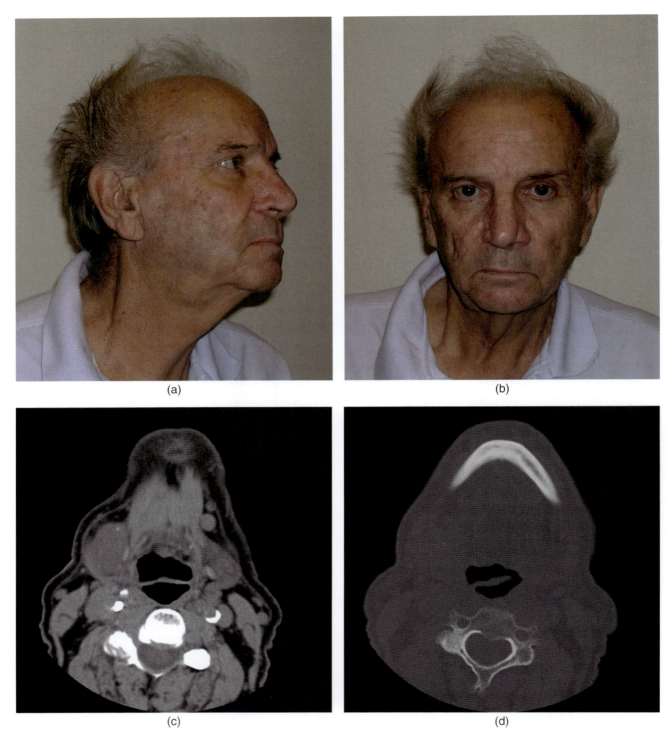

Figure 5.18. A 72-year-old man with pain and swelling of one month's duration in the right submandibular gland (a). Physical examination was significant for a tender right submandibular gland but no symptoms associated with the left submandibular gland (b). The patient underwent CT scanning that demonstrated an enlarged right submandibular gland with the presence of a single intraglandular sialolith (c and d). Thorough evaluation of the CT scans also identified five extraglandular right submandibular stones and two extraglandular left submandibular stones (e and f). The patient underwent right submandibular gland excision in a standard fashion (g and h) with exploration of the bilateral Wharton ducts to remove five right extraglandular stones and two left extraglandular stones (i). A left Wharton sialodochoplasty was performed. The patient is noted at one year postoperatively (j and k).

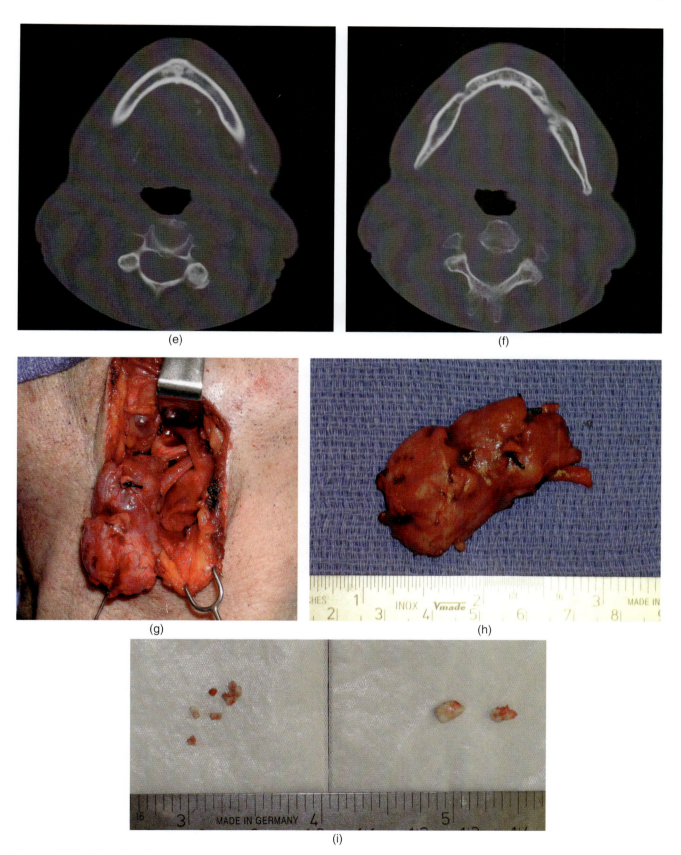

Figure 5.18. (Continued).

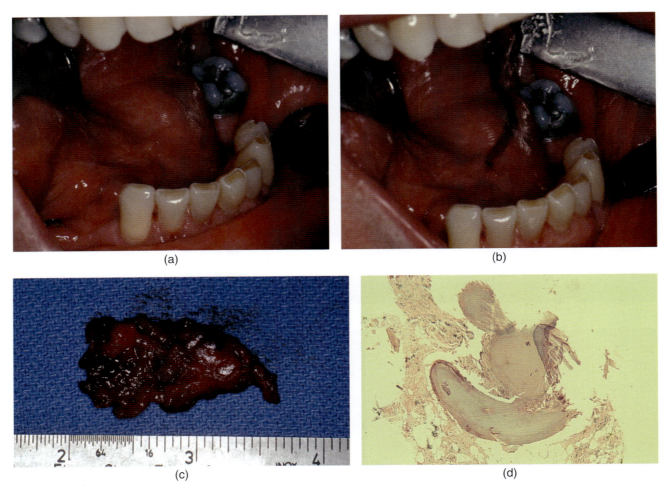

Figure 5.19. Floor of mouth swelling present in a 55-year-old woman (a). A diffuse mass is noted beneath the surface mucosa that is smooth and of normal color. A presumptive diagnosis of ranula vs. neoplasm was established. A left sublingual gland excision was performed in the standard fashion (b). The specimen (c) exhibited mild induration without signs of ranula, such that a neoplastic process was favored while the possibility of a mucous escape reaction was discarded. Final histopathology showed a sialolith (d) in the background of sialadenitis (e). The tissue bed is noted (f), particularly the lingual nerve (retracted with the vessel loop) and Wharton's duct. A six-month postoperative evaluation showed acceptable healing (g).

The Relationship of Salivary Lithiasis to Nephrolithiasis, Cholelithiasis, Primary Hyperparathyroidism, and Gout

Nephrolithiasis, defined as one or more stones in the kidney, affects more than 6% of the general population (Choi et al. 2018). Various risk factors have been proposed, including chronic kidney disease, poor hydration, increasing age, obesity, diabetes, warm climate, and a high animal protein intake. Cholelithiasis is the process of gallstone formation, and its prevalence in the United States is 5.5% in men and 8.6% in women. Gallstones are categorized as pigment stones, cholesterol stones, or mixed stones. Age, ethnicity, female gender, obesity, diabetes, and Western diet are risk factors for cholelithiasis (Kim et al. 2019).

Patients with nephrolithiasis and sialolithiasis are not routinely examined for stones in other organs. This notwithstanding, due to the composition

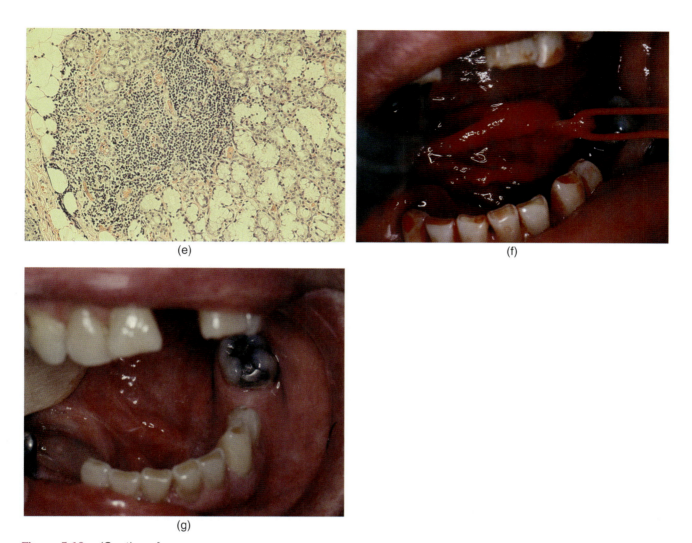

Figure 5.19. (Continued).

of salivary and kidney stones being primarily calcium carbonates and calcium phosphates, intuition suggests that there could be concordance in patients with both kidney and salivary stones. Choi et al. (2018) therefore studied nephrolithiasis as a risk factor for sialolithiasis by using data from the national cohort study from the Korean Health Insurance Review and Assessment Service. In doing so, they selected 24 038 patients with nephrolithiasis and a control group of 96 152 patients without nephrolithiasis. The incidence of sialolithiasis in the two groups was compared with a 12-year follow-up period. The overall incidence of sialolithiasis among the nephrolithiasis patients was 0.08% (19 24 038) and 0.1% (92/96 152) in the control group. The adjusted hazard ratios (HRs) of nephrolithiasis for sialolithiasis were not statistically significant. The adjusted HR of nephrolithiasis for sialolithiasis was 0.81. This study therefore found no evidence that nephrolithiasis is associated with an increased risk of sialolithiasis after adjusting for age, gender, income, region of residence, hypertension, diabetes, and dyslipidemia.

Kim et al. (2019) evaluated the association between cholelithiasis and sialolithiasis using a national sample cohort of the Korean population and two study designs. In study 1, the authors examined 21 170 cholelithiasis patients and 84 680 control patients without cholelithiasis and measured the occurrence of sialolithiasis. In study 1,

761 sialolithiasis patients were matched with 3044 control patients with sialolithiasis and the occurrence of cholelithiasis was measured. The hazard ratio for sialolithiasis was 1.49 (95% CI = 0.88–2.52) in the cholelithiasis group and the hazard ratio for cholelithiasis was 1.18 (95% CI = 0.53–2.59) in the sialolithiasis group. These results are perhaps intuitive since the stone composition is very different between gallstones and salivary stones, and the risk factors for respective stone development are also different. The authors concluded that there is no association between sialolithiasis and cholelithiasis.

Stack and Norman (2008) performed a retrospective analysis of 3000 primary hyperparathyroidism patients and identified a total of 18 patients (0.6%) with documented sialolithiasis prior to parathyroid surgery. Sialolithiasis was the first presenting symptom in six patients that led to the diagnosis of primary hyperparathyroidism. The remaining 12 patients had kidney stones as their first presenting symptom ($n = 5$) or hypercalcemia ($n = 7$). Based on a reported incidence of sialolithiasis of 0.45% in the United Kingdom, the authors interpreted their 0.6% incidence of sialolithiasis in their primary hyperparathyroidism cohort as significantly different and therefore relevant. Nonetheless, these authors are from the United States where the incidence of sialolithiasis is approximately 1%. It is unclear why they chose the incidence of sialolithiasis in the United Kingdom to compare their United States cohort of patients in whom sialolithiasis was noted. The authors offered conclusions that parathyroid surgeons should be aware of the possible existence of sialolithiasis in their patients and salivary gland surgeons should be aware of the possible existence of primary hyperparathyroidism in their patients.

Kraaij et al. (2015) performed a retrospective case control study of 208 patients (112 males, 96 females) with salivary gland stones and a control group of 208 patients (112 males, 96 females). The submandibular gland was affected in 85.6% of patients, the parotid gland in 9.6%, and the sublingual gland in 2.4%. When evaluating for the presence of cholelithiasis, nephrolithiasis, and gout, no relationship was identified between sialolithiasis and the presence of systemic disease. Interestingly, there was a higher incidence of cholelithiasis in the control group than in the sialolithiasis group. The incidence of nephrolithiasis and gout was equal in both groups.

Summary

- Sialoliths are calcium phosphate stones that develop within the ductal system of salivary glands.
- Sialolithiasis is thought to affect approximately 1% of the population based on autopsy studies.
- Sialolithiasis has been estimated to represent more than 50% of major salivary gland disease and is the most common cause of acute and chronic salivary gland infections.
- Approximately 80–85% of sialolithiasis occurs in the submandibular gland and 10–20% in the parotid gland. The incidence of this pathology is rare in the sublingual gland and minor salivary glands.
- Eighty percent of submandibular sialoliths are radio-opaque, while 40% of sialoliths of the parotid gland are radio-opaque.
- Approximately 7% of sialoliths are bilateral.
- Approximately 3% of cases of sialolithiasis occur simultaneously in multiple glands.
- Systemic stone forming disorders such as gout, cholelithiasis, and nephrolithiasis do not seem to represent predisposing factors to sialolithiasis.
- Around 75–90% of submandibular stones are located in the extraglandular duct with 10% of stones located in the intraglandular duct. Parotid stones are located in the extraglandular duct in approximately 83% of cases and in the intraglandular duct in approximately 17% of cases.
- Several "great imitators" of submandibular sialolithiasis exist, including scrofula, phleboliths, osteomas, and occasionally carotid plaques.
- Numerous techniques are available to treat sialolithiasis including surgical sialolithotomy with or without sialodochoplasty, sialendoscopy with sialolithotomy, intracorporeal or extracorporeal lithotripsy, or gland removal.

Case Presentation – *Stoneorama*

A 54-year-old man (Figure 5.20a and b) was referred with a long history of prandial swelling and pain associated with his bilateral submandibular glands. A clinical diagnosis of bilateral submandibular sialadenitis was established and his panoramic radiograph (Figure 5.20c) did not identify sialoliths.

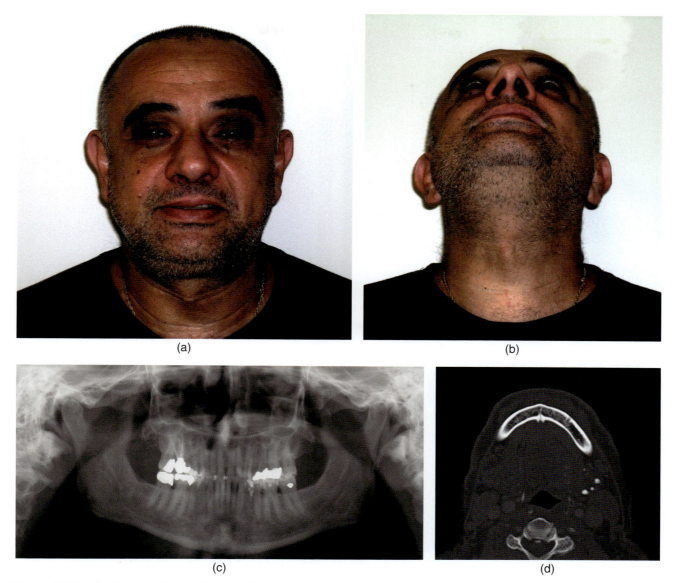

Figure 5.20. A 54-year-old man (a and b) with a long history of prandial swelling and pain associated with bilateral submandibular glands. He demonstrates mild submandibular swelling. A panoramic radiograph (c) was obtained due to a clinical diagnosis of bilateral submandibular sialadenitis with the intention of ruling out sialolithiasis. No stones were identified. CT scans identified numerous intraglandular sialoliths with those of the left submandibular gland being greater than the right (d–g). The patient underwent excision of his left submandibular gland through a traditional approach in the neck (h). The left submandibular gland specimen (i) and its radiograph (j) are noted. Thirteen sialoliths of varying size and density were identified on the specimen radiograph. The bivalved specimen (k) demonstrates clinical evidence of numerous sialoliths. Histopathology (l and m) identified chronic obstructive sialadenitis and extensive sialolithiasis of the left submandibular gland (l = hematoxylin and eosin, original magnification ×20; m = hematoxylin and eosin, original magnification ×100). (n) The resultant tissue bed from the left submandibular gland excision. (o and p) The patient appeared well at five years postoperatively and was asymptomatic related to the retained right submandibular gland.

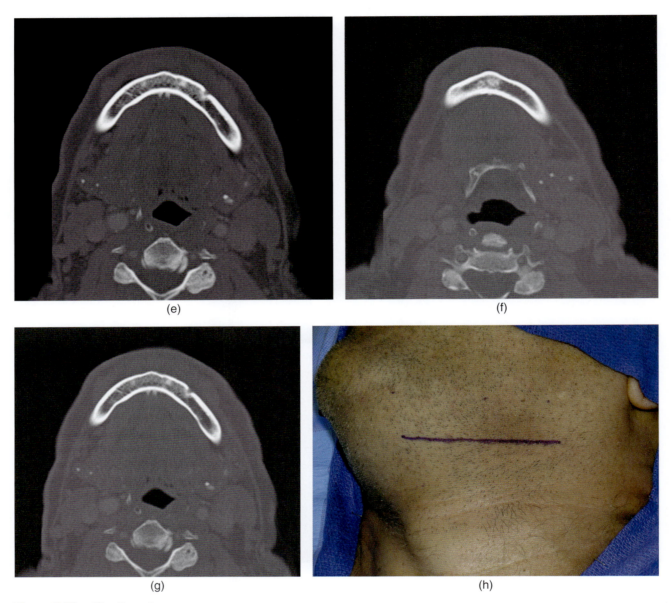

Figure 5.20. (Continued).

Past Medical History
The patient endorsed a history of hyperlipidemia, hypertension, and hepatitis C infection. He was taking no medications at the time of evaluation and he reported no known drug allergies.

Imaging
CT scans (Figure 5.20d–g) identified numerous intraglandular sialoliths with those of the left submandibular gland being greater than the right.

Diagnosis
Bilateral submandibular sialolithiasis and sialadenitis.

Surgical Intervention
The patient was advised to undergo bilateral submandibular gland excisions but opted only for the left due to its more advanced sialolithiasis. He therefore underwent excision of his left submandibular gland through a traditional approach in the neck (Figure 5.20h). The specimen (Figure 5.20i)

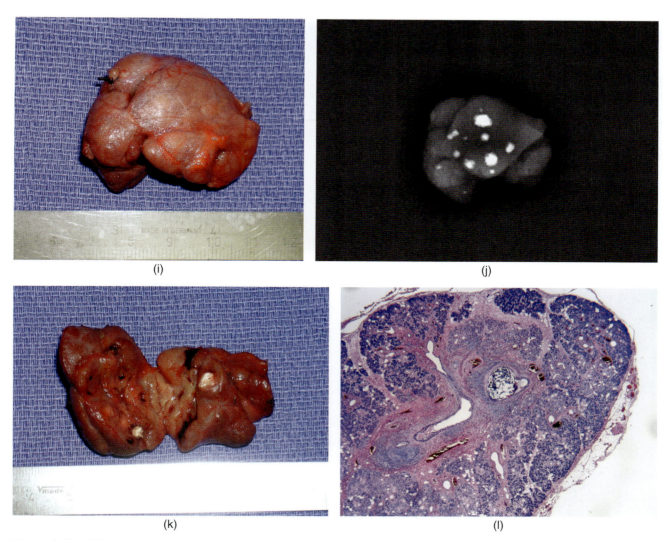

Figure 5.20. (Continued).

and its radiograph (Figure 5.20j) are noted. The bivalved specimen demonstrates numerous sialoliths (Figure 5.20k). Histopathology (Figure 5.20l and m) identified chronic obstructive sialadenitis and extensive sialolithiasis of the submandibular gland. The resultant tissue bed (Figure 5.20n) demonstrates the regional anatomy and proper hemostasis following removal of the gland/stones. The patient was asymptomatic at five years postoperatively (Figure 5.20o and p). He reported the passing of stones from the right Wharton duct as the right submandibular gland and its intraglandular stones remained at the patient's request.

TAKE-HOME POINTS

1. Patients should undergo panoramic radiographs investigating for sialoliths when their clinical presentation is consistent with a diagnosis of sialadenitis.
2. Sialoliths are identified on panoramic radiographs in 80% of cases of submandibular sialolithiasis.
3. CT scans are beneficial in the workup of patients with submandibular sialadenitis and may disclose the presence of sialoliths that were not identified on the panoramic radiograph.

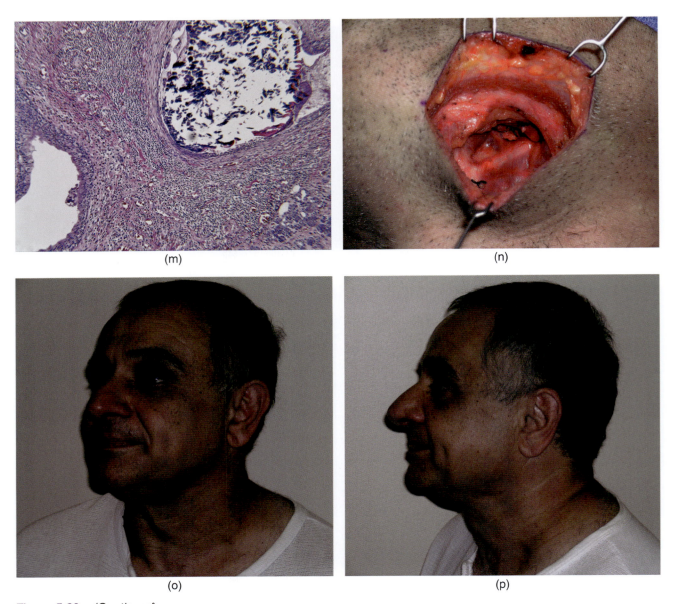

Figure 5.20. (Continued).

4. Bilateral submandibular gland excision is associated with xerostomia such that surgery should be carefully considered and executed. The xerostomia is related to the lack of non-stimulated saliva whereby patients complain of dry mouth between meals. This clinical condition is very unpleasant for patients and must be discussed when obtaining informed consent.

References

Anneroth G, Hansen LS. 1983. Minor salivary gland calculi. A clinical and histopathological study of 49 cases. *Int J Oral Maxillofac Surg* 12:80-89.

Ardekian L, Klein HH, Araydy S, Marchal F. 2014. The use of sialoendoscopy for the treatment of multiple salivary gland stones. *J Oral Maxillofac Surg* 72:89-95.

Arzoz E, Santiago A, Esnal F, Palomero R. 1996. Endoscopic intracorporeal lithotripsy for sialolithiasis. *J Oral Maxillofac Surg* 54:847-850.

Baurmash HD. 2004. Submandibular salivary stones: Current management modalities. *J Oral Maxillofac Surg* 62:369-378.

Baurmash H, Dechiara SC. 1991. Extraoral parotid sialolithotomy. *J Oral Maxillofac Surg* 49:127-132.

Berry RL. 1995. Sialadenitis and sialolithiasis. Diagnosis and management. *Oral Maxillofac Surg Clin North Am* 7:47-503.

Blatt IM, Mikkelsen WM, Denning RM. 1958. Studies in sialolithiasis II. Uric acid calculus of the parotid gland; report of a case. *Ann Otol Rhinol Laryngol* 67:1022-1032.

Bodner L. 1993. Salivary gland calculi: Diagnostic imaging and surgical management. *Compend Contin Educ Dent* 14:572-584.

Capaccio P, Ottaviani F, Manzo R, Schindler A, Cesana B. 2004. Extracorporeal lithotripsy for salivary calculi: A long-term clinical experience. *Laryngoscope* 114:1069-1073.

Choi HG, Bang W, Park B, Sim S, Tae K, Song CM. 2018. Lack of evidence that nephrolithiasis increases the risk of sialolithiasis: A longitudinal follow-up study using a national sample cohort. *PLoS One* 13:e0196659.

Drage NA, Wilson RF, McGurk M. 2002. The genu of the submandibular duct – Is the angle significant in salivary gland disease? *Dentomaxillof Radiol* 31:15-18.

Escudier MP. 1998. The current status and possible future for lithotripsy of salivary calculi. *Atlas Oral Maxillofac Surg Clin North Am* 6:117-132.

Friedlander AH, Freymiller EG. 2003. Detection of radiation-accelerated atherosclerosis of the carotid artery by panoramic radiography. *JADA* 134:1361–1313.

Jauregui EM, Kiringoda R, Ryan WR, Eisele DW, Chang JL. 2016. Chronic parotitis with multiple calcifications: Clinical and sialendoscopic findings. *Laryngoscope* 127:1565-1570.

Kao WK, Chole RA, Ogden MA. (2020). Evidence of a microbial etiology for sialoliths. *Laryngoscope* 130:69-74.

Karas ND. 1998. Surgery of the salivary ducts. *Atlas Oral Maxillofac Surg Clin North Am* 6:99-116.

Kasaboglu O, Er N, Tumer C, Akkocaoglu M. 2004. Micromorphology of sialoliths in submandibular salivary gland: A scanning electron microscope and x-ray diffraction analysis. *J Oral Maxillofac Surg* 62:1253-1258.

Kim DH, Song WS, Kim YJ, Kim WD. 2013. Parotid sialolithiasis in a two-year old boy. *Korean J Pediatr* 56:451-455.

Kim SY, Kim HJ, Lim H et al. 2019. Association between cholelithiasis and sialolithiasis. Two longitudinal follow-up studies. *Medicine* 98:e16153.

King CA, Ridgley GV, Kabasela K. 1990. Sialolithiasis of the submandibular gland: A case report. *Compend Contin Educ Dent* 11:262-264.

Kraaij S, Karagozoglu KH, Forouzanfar T, Veerman ECI, Brand HS. 2014. Salivary stones: Symptoms, aetiology, biochemical composition and treatment. *Br Dent J* 217:e23.

Kraaij S, Karagozoglu KH, Kenter YAG, Pjipe J, Gilijamse M, Brand HS. 2015. Systemic diseases and the risk of developing salivary stones: A case control study. *Oral Surg Oral Med Oral Pathol Oral Radiol* 119:539-543.

Kraaij S, Brand HS, van der Meij EH, de Visscher JG. (2018). Biochemical composition of salivary stones in relation to stone- and patient-related factors. *Med Oral Patol Oral Cir Bucal* 23:e540-544.

Lagha NB, Alantar A, Samson J et al. 2005. Lithiasis of minor salivary glands: Current data. *Oral Surg Oral Med Oral Pathol* 100:345-348.

Liu NM, Rawal J. 2013. Submandibular sialolithiasis in a child. *Arch Dis Child* 98:407.

Lustmann J, Regev E, Melamed Y. 1990. Sialolithiasis. A survey on 245 patients and a review of the literature. *Int J Oral Maxillofac Surg* 19:135-138.

Lutcavage GJ, Schaberg SJ. 1991. Bilateral submandibular sialolithiasis and concurrent sialadenitis: A case report. *J Oral Maxillofac Surg* 49:1220-1222.

Mandel L. 2006. Tuberculous cervical node calcifications mimicking sialolithiasis: A case report. *J Oral Maxillofac Surg* 64:1439-1442.

Mandel L, Surattanont F. 2004. Clinical and imaging diagnoses of intramuscular hemangiomas: The wattle sign and case reports. *J Oral Maxillofac Surg* 62:754-758.

McGurk M, Escudier MP, Brown JE. 2004. Modern management of salivary calculi. *Br J Surg* 92:107-112.

McGurk M, Makdissi J, Brown JE. 2004. Intra-oral removal of stones from the hilum of the submandibular gland: Report of technique and morbidity. *Int J Oral Maxillofac Surg* 33:683-686.

Miloro M. 1998. The surgical management of submandibular gland disease. *Atlas Oral Maxillofac Surg Clin North Am* 6:29-50.

Miloro M, Goldberg MH. 2002. Salivary Gland Infections. In: Topazian R, Goldberg M, Hupp J (eds.) Oral and Maxillofacial Infections, 4th edn. Philadelphia, WB Saunders, pp. 279-293.

Moghe S, Pillai A, Thomas S, Nair PP. 2012. Parotid sialolithiasis. *BMJ Case Rep*, published online 14 December 2012.

Nakayama E, Yuasa K, Beppu M et al. 2003. Interventional sialendoscopy: A new procedure for noninvasive insertion and a minimally invasive sialolithectomy. *J Oral Maxillofac Surg* 61:1233-1236.

Ottaviani F, Capaccio P, Campi M et al. 1996. Extracorporeal electromagnetic shock-wave lithotripsy for salivary gland stones. *Laryngoscope* 106:761-764.

Park JS, Sohn JH, Kim JK. 2006. Factors influencing intraoral removal of submandibular calculi. *Otolaryngol Head Neck Surg* 135:704-709.

Perez-Tanloira R, Aarnisalo A, Haapaniemi A, Saarinen R, Kuusela P, Kinnari TJ. 2019. Bacterial biofilm in salivary stones. *Eur Arch Otorhinolaryngol* 276:1815-1822.

Rontal M, Rontal E. 1987. The use of sialodochoplasty in the treatment of benign inflammatory obstructive submandibular gland disease. *Laryngoscope* 97:1417-1421.

Seward GR. 1968. Anatomic surgery for salivary calculi. I Symptoms, signs, and differential diagnosis. *Oral Surg Oral Med Oral Pathol* 25:150-157.

Sigismund PE, Zenk J, Koch M, Schapher M, Rudes M, Iro H. 2015. Nearly 3,000 salivary stones: Some clinical and epidemiologic aspects. *Laryngoscope* 125:1879-1882.

Stack BC, Norman JG. 2008. Sialolithiasis and primary hyperparathyroidism. *ORL* 70:331-334.

Sunder VS, Chakravarthy C, Mikkilinine R, Mahoorkar S. 2014. Multiple bilateral submandibular gland sialolithiasis. *Niger J Clin Pract* 17:115-118.

Williams MF. 1999. Sialolithiasis. *Otolaryngol Clin North Am* 32:819-834.

Chapter 6
Systemic Diseases Affecting the Salivary Glands

Outline

Introduction
Sjögren Syndrome
  Pathophysiology of Sjögren Syndrome
  Clinical Manifestations of Sjögren Syndrome
  Lymphoma and Sjögren Syndrome
  Mikulicz Disease and the Benign Lymphoepithelial Lesion
  Diagnosis of Sjögren Syndrome with Salivary Gland Biopsy
    Histopathology of Sjögren Syndrome
Sarcoidosis
  Pathophysiology of Sarcoidosis
  Clinical Manifestations of Sarcoidosis
  Diagnosis of Sarcoidosis with Salivary Gland Biopsy
    Histopathology of Sarcoidosis
Sialosis
  Clinical Manifestations of Sialosis
  Diagnosis of Sialosis with Salivary Gland Biopsy
    Histopathology of Sialosis
IgG4-Related Disease
Summary
Case Presentation – *Esoterica*
References

Introduction

Numerous systemic diseases have the capability to infiltrate salivary gland tissue. It is estimated that approximately 5–8% of the general population is affected by any of the 80 known autoimmune diseases (Jonsson and Olofsson 2011). Among those autoimmune diseases infiltrating the salivary glands include immune-modulated or idiopathic diseases such as sarcoidosis, Sjogren disease, sialosis, and lymphoepithelial lesions. IgG4-related disease also possesses the ability to involve the salivary glands. Each of these processes involves multiple physiologic systems, and may be diagnosed based on clinical signs and symptoms, many of which are very common yet may be easily overlooked and considered as non-specific. In addition, these diseases may be diagnosed at an early stage with salivary gland biopsy. It is the purpose of this chapter to describe the clinical features of salivary gland involvement by systemic diseases.

Sjögren Syndrome

Sjögren syndrome is an inflammatory autoimmune disease that manifests as a chronic, slowly progressive disease characterized by keratoconjunctivitis sicca and xerostomia. The disease was originally named for Henrik Sjogren, a Swedish ophthalmologist whose doctoral dissertation in 1933 reported the specific clinical and microscopic findings in 19 women with xerostomia and keratoconjunctivitis sicca, 13 of whom also had arthritis (Jonsson and Olofsson 2011). Since 1965, Sjögren syndrome has been defined as a triad of dry eyes, dry mouth, and rheumatoid arthritis or other connective tissue diseases (Daniels 1991). This process may evolve from an exocrine organ-specific disorder to an extraglandular multisystem disease affecting the lungs, kidneys, blood vessels, and muscles (Table 6.1). Sjögren syndrome is believed to affect 0.2–3.0% of the population with approximately one million people diagnosed in the United States (Reksten and Jonsson 2014; Turner 2014). It predominantly occurs in women between 40 and 60 years of age with a 9:1 female: male ratio (Reksten and Jonsson 2014). Because of the insidious onset of symptoms, an average time of 10 years

---

Salivary Gland Pathology: Diagnosis and Management, Third Edition. Edited by Eric R. Carlson and Robert A. Ord.
© 2022 John Wiley & Sons, Inc. Published 2022 by John Wiley & Sons, Inc.
Companion website: www.wiley.com/go/carlson/salivary

Table 6.1. Frequency of extraglandular findings in primary Sjögren syndrome.

Clinical involvement	Percent
Arthritis	60
Kidney	9
Liver	6
Lung	14
Lymphadenopathy	14
Lymphoma	6
Myositis	1
Peripheral neuropathy	5
Raynaud phenomenon	35
Splenomegaly	3

occurs between the development of first symptoms and the diagnosis of the disease (Turner 2014). One confounder in the recognition of Sjögren syndrome is that symptoms do not typically occur concurrently such that individual symptoms might be treated independently by individual doctors, thereby delaying the diagnosis of the syndrome.

PATHOPHYSIOLOGY OF SJÖGREN SYNDROME

The pathophysiology of Sjögren syndrome is believed to be the result of activation of both the cellular and humoral immune systems with resultant inflammation and cellular infiltration of the salivary and lacrimal glands and other affected organs. While the inciting event in the development of Sjögren syndrome is still unknown, a popular hypothesis is that a viral infection initiates the cascade of autoimmunity (Turner 2014). The autoantibodies in Sjögren syndrome include those produced to the ribonucleoprotein particles SS-A/Ro and SS-B/La, and these are thought to interfere with muscarinic receptors (Garcia-Carrasco et al. 2006). One study identified IgG from patients with primary Sjögren syndrome containing autoantibodies capable of damaging salivary tissue and contributing to xerostomia (Dawson et al. 2006). Other mechanisms of glandular dysfunction include destruction of glandular elements by cell-mediated mechanisms; secretion of cytokines that activate pathways bearing the signature of type 1 and 2 interferons (IFNs); and secretion of metalloproteinases (MMPs) that interfere with the interaction of the glandular cell with its extracellular matrix (Garcia-Carrasco et al. 2006). The presence of IFN induces the expression of B-cell activating factor (BAFF) that causes a migration and infiltration of T and B lymphocytes into the salivary gland cells. In addition, increased MMP-3 and MMP-9 expression has been found to be responsible for acinar destruction in Sjögren syndrome (Perez et al. 2005). These substantial increases in MMP expression in diseased labial salivary glands may be potentiated by moderate decreases in tissue inhibitors of matrix metalloproteinases (TIMPs).

CLINICAL MANIFESTATIONS OF SJÖGREN SYNDROME

Primary Sjögren syndrome is designated when it is not associated with other connective tissue diseases. This disease is an autoimmune disorder primarily characterized by chronic inflammation of exocrine glands that leads to reduced secretion of tears and saliva, for example. This notwithstanding, evidence exists that shows genetic aggregation of autoimmune diseases in families of patients with primary Sjögren syndrome (Anaya et al. 2006). The suggestion is that autoimmune diseases in general may aggregate as a trait favoring a common immunogenetic origin for diverse autoimmune phenotypes, such that a risk factor exists for the development of primary Sjögren syndrome and other autoimmune diseases. *Secondary* Sjögren syndrome is defined when the disease is associated with other clinically expressed autoimmune processes, specifically, rheumatoid arthritis, systemic lupus erythematosus, myositis, biliary cirrhosis, systemic sclerosis, chronic hepatitis, cryoglobulinemia, thyroiditis, and vasculitis. Following rheumatoid arthritis, Sjögren syndrome is the second most common autoimmune rheumatic disorder (Moutsopoulos 1993). Eight to ten years are generally required for the disorder to progress from initial symptoms to the development of the syndrome. Although typically seen in middle-aged women, Sjögren syndrome can occur in all ages and in males. It has been estimated that 80–90% of patients are women, and that the mean age at diagnosis is 50 years (Daniels 1991). Qin et al. (2015) performed a systematic review of the epidemiology of primary Sjögren syndrome to assess the prevalence rates, the incidence rates, and to investigate possible geographic variations in this disease. Their literature search yielded 1880 related citations with 21 references fulfilling the inclusion criteria. The female/male ratio in incidence data was 9.15. The female/male ratio in prevalence data was 10.72, and the overall age of primary Sjögren syndrome patients was 56 years.

Most patients with Sjögren syndrome develop symptoms related to decreased salivary gland and lacrimal gland function. Primary Sjögren syndrome patients generally complain of dry eyes, often described as a sandy or gritty feeling under the eyelids. Other symptoms such as itching of the eyes, eye fatigue, and increased sensitivity to light can accompany the primary symptoms. Many of these symptoms are due to the destruction of corneal and bulbar conjunctival epithelium and come under the diagnosis of keratoconjunctivitis sicca. This disorder is assessed by tear flow and composition. Tear flow is measured using the Schirmer test, while tear composition can be determined by tear break-up time or tear lysozyme content. The Schirmer test is considered positive when filter paper wetting of less than 5 mm occurs in five minutes, and suggests clinically significant keratoconjunctivitis sicca (Moutsopoulos 1993). There are, nonetheless, numerous false positive and negative results, such that the predictive value is limited. The integrity of the corneal and bulbar conjunctiva may be assessed using the Rose Bengal staining procedure and slit lamp examination. Punctate corneal ulcerations and attached filaments of corneal epithelium indicative of corneal and bulbar conjunctival epithelial destruction are noted on slip lamp examination in Sjögren syndrome patients.

Xerostomia is the second principal symptom of Sjögren syndrome. Xerostomia can be documented by salivary flow measurements, parotid sialography, and salivary scintigraphy. Salivary flow measurements must be adjusted for age, time of day, gender, and concomitant medications. Patients with dry mouths complain of a burning oral discomfort and difficulty in chewing and swallowing dry foods. Xerostomia is commonly associated with changes in taste and the inability to speak continuously for longer than several minutes.

Salivary gland enlargement occurs in as many as 30% of patients with Sjögren syndrome during their illness, with the parotid gland being most often enlarged (Kulkarni 2005). It is estimated that bilateral parotid gland enlargement is found in 25–60% of patients with Sjögren syndrome (Turner 2014). Bilateral painful submandibular glands have been described as a presenting symptom of this syndrome (Kulkarni 2005). While the parotid glands are most commonly enlarged, they may be the last glands to be affected in patients with Sjögren syndrome from the standpoint of decreased saliva production (Pijpe et al. 2007a). The parotid glands have a longer-lasting secretory capacity in patients with Sjögren syndrome, and therefore are the last glands to manifest hyposalivation during the disease. In the more advanced stages of the disease, both unstimulated and stimulated submandibular, sublingual, and parotid functions fall to a low level. The accelerated development of dental caries is also noted. Enlargement of the lacrimal glands is uncommon. Even when the salivary glands are not enlarged, they always exhibit lymphohistiocyte-mediated acinar destruction (Marx 1995). When enlarged, however, they show features of the benign lymphoepithelial lesion (BLL) in almost all cases. These lesions may occur in patients who do not have Sjögren syndrome. Furthermore, they may undergo malignant transformation to lymphomas in patients with or without Sjögren syndrome (Figure 6.1).

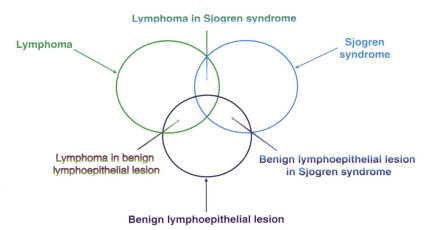

Figure 6.1. The association between the lymphoepithelial lesion, Sjögren syndrome, and lymphoma.

LYMPHOMA AND SJÖGREN SYNDROME

One of the most concerning features of Sjögren syndrome is the possible development of non-Hodgkin lymphomas (NHLs). It has been estimated that 2.7–9.8% of patients with primary Sjögren syndrome will develop lymphomas, with the most common type of NHL being the mucosa-associated lymphoid tissue (MALT) B-cell lymphoma (Alunno et al. 2018). The risk of lymphoma formation increases 2.2% per year of age with a 4.3-fold increased risk in primary Sjögren syndrome compared to the general population.

Liang et al. (2014) performed a systematic review and meta-analysis related to primary Sjögren syndrome and the risk of malignancy. Fourteen studies involving greater than 14,000 patients were included. Compared to the general population, patients with primary Sjögren syndrome had significantly increased risks of cancer overall (RR 1.53), non-Hodgkin lymphoma (RR 13.76), and thyroid cancer (RR 2.58).

The risk for NHL seems to be directly related to prolonged B-cell survival and excessive B-cell activity most likely resulting from an increased production of B-cell activating factor (BAFF). These B cells have also been noted to produce rheumatoid factor (RF). The more aggressive diffuse large B-cell lymphoma (DLBCL) is also seen in Sjögren syndrome patients, and it has been estimated that 10% of MALT lymphomas will transform into DLBCL. Clinical suspicion of NHL in patients with Sjögren syndrome should occur in symptomatic unilateral or bilateral parotid enlargement, palpable purpura, splenomegaly, and lymphadenopathy (Figure 6.2).

Patients with diagnosed MALT lymphoma of the salivary glands who have isolated, asymptomatic disease without bone marrow involvement may be managed by observation. Patients with advanced stage MALT lymphomas of the salivary glands may be managed with rituximab alone or in combination with other chemotherapeutic agents. Rituximab is a monoclonal antibody that targets the CD20 protein found on B cells, thereby resulting in their destruction. The presence of DLBCL of the salivary glands will result in treatment with rituximab and CHOP chemotherapy (cyclophosphamide, doxorubicin, vincristine, and prednisone).

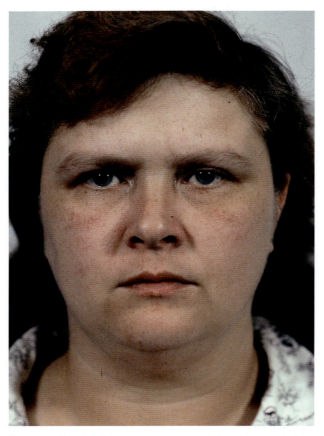

Figure 6.2. A 36-year-old woman with a known history of Sjögren syndrome associated with rheumatoid arthritis. She described a recent history of painful swelling of the right parotid gland such that an incisional parotid biopsy was recommended.

MIKULICZ DISEASE AND THE BENIGN LYMPHOEPITHELIAL LESION

The pathologic entity known as the benign lymphoepithelial lesion was once referred to as Mikulicz disease. The German surgeon, Johann von Mikulicz first described the benign lymphoepithelial lesion in 1888 in a report of a single case of lacrimal gland involvement (Daniels 1991). In 1892, Mikulicz described a patient with parotid, submandibular, and lacrimal enlargement with fibrosis and named it Mikulicz disease (Gurwale et al. 2020). The lacrimal gland enlargement was followed by enlargement of the submandibular and parotid glands, as well as minor salivary gland tissue. The term Mikulicz disease was subsequently applied to a variety of cases of bilateral salivary or lacrimal gland enlargement, including those caused by sarcoidosis, lymphoma, tuberculosis, or syphilis. The term lymphoepithelial lesion was proposed by Godwin in 1952 to describe parotid gland lesions previously called Mikulicz disease, adenolymphoma, chronic inflammation, lymphoepithelioma, or lymphocytic tumor (Godwin 1952). One year later in 1953, Morgan and Castleman observed numerous similarities of the benign lymphoepithelial lesion to the histopathology of Sjögren syndrome, and proposed that Mikulicz disease is not a distinct clinical and pathologic entity but rather one manifestation of the symptom complex of the syndrome (Morgan and Castleman 1953). They are, essentially, the same pathologic process (Jonsson and Olofsson 2011). The benign lymphoepithelial lesion may become large enough to present as a mass resembling a parotid tumor (Figure 6.3). Mikulicz disease has become known to be part of the IgG4-related diseases that will be discussed later in this chapter.

Acinar degeneration and hyperplasia and metaplasia of the ducts led to the formation of the pathognomonic epimyoepithelial islands, which define the condition. Whether myoepithelial cells or ductal basal cells are responsible for these islands has been questioned. An immunohistochemical investigation has shown that myoepithelial cells do not play a role in the formation of these islands and they should be designated lymphoepithelial metaplasia (Ihrier et al. 1999). The condition is often a manifestation of Sjögren syndrome or other immunological abnormality but may occur outside the Sjögren syndrome process. Usually, the lesion starts unilaterally but becomes bilateral in the parotids (Figure 6.4). It is less common in the submandibular and minor salivary glands (Figure 6.5).

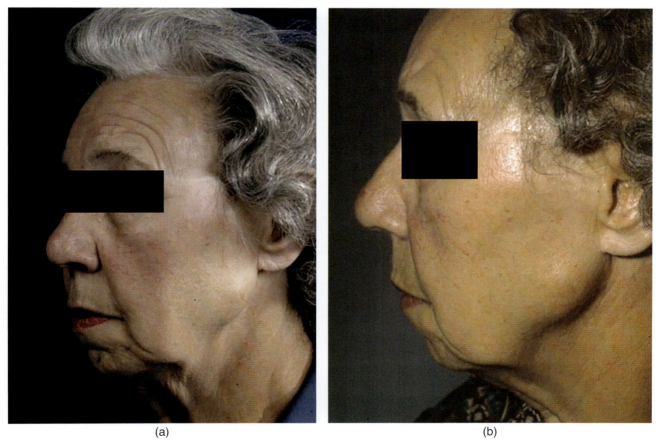

Figure 6.3. A 75-year-old woman (a and b) with a left parotid mass. Fine needle aspiration biopsy suggested lymphoma, leading to superficial parotidectomy. Histopathology identified benign lymphoepithelial lesion.

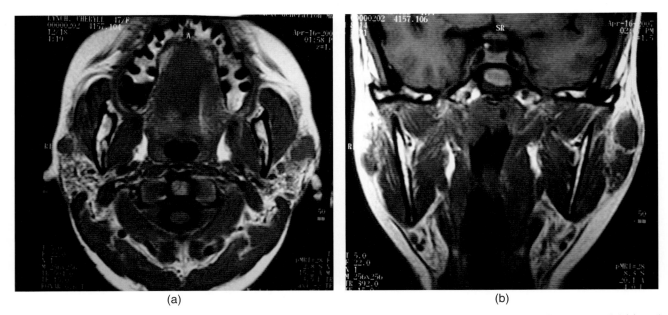

Figure 6.4. A 45-year-old woman diagnosed with Sjögren syndrome with bilateral parotid lesions shown on axial (a) and coronal images (b).

The lesion may reach a large size although it is usually asymptomatic. It may be diagnosed by fine needle aspiration if the etiology is uncertain and may require removal by parotidectomy for esthetic reasons. Sudden growth or pain may be an ominous feature as benign lymphoepithelial lesion can undergo malignant change and is perhaps not as benign as its name suggests. The lymphocytic component can undergo change to MALT lymphoma (see Chapter 15) particularly in Sjögren syndrome (Abbondanzo 2001) but also in HIV infections (Del Bono et al. 2000). Recurrent benign lymphoepithelial lesion may also undergo malignant change of its epithelial component to become an undifferentiated carcinoma with lymphoid stroma (see Chapter 8) (Cai et al. 2002).

DIAGNOSIS OF SJÖGREN SYNDROME WITH SALIVARY GLAND BIOPSY

Incisional biopsy of minor salivary glands was introduced as a clinical diagnostic procedure for Sjögren syndrome in 1966. Many studies since that time have examined the value of this biopsy procedure (Marx 1988). One study graded inflammation in labial salivary gland biopsy specimens from patients with various rheumatologic diseases and in postmortem specimens (Chisholm and Mason 1968). A grading scheme of lymphocytes and plasma cells per $4\,mm^2$ was established and has been described by numerous authors since its original description (Greenspan et al. 1974). Grade 0 referred to the absence of these cells, grade 1 showed a slight infiltrate, grade 2 showed a moderate infiltrate or less than one focus per $4\,mm^2$, grade 3 showed one focus per $4\,mm^2$, and grade 4 showed more than one focus per $4\,mm^2$. It has been noted that grade 4 (more than one focus of 50 or more lymphocytes per $4\,mm^2$ area of gland) is seen only in patients with Sjögren syndrome and was not seen in postmortem specimens. Due to the strong association with the presence of Sjögren syndrome, focal sialadenitis in a labial minor salivary gland incisional biopsy specimen with a focus score of more than one focus/$4\,mm^2$ has been proposed as the diagnostic criterion for the salivary component of this disease (Daniels et al. 1975). It has been pointed out that the focus score cannot separate early from late disease as chronicity of symptoms and focus score did not show a relationship (Greenspan et al. 1974). The highest focus score, however, was seen in patients with the sicca components of Sjögren syndrome without associated connective tissue disease. Finally, since variation

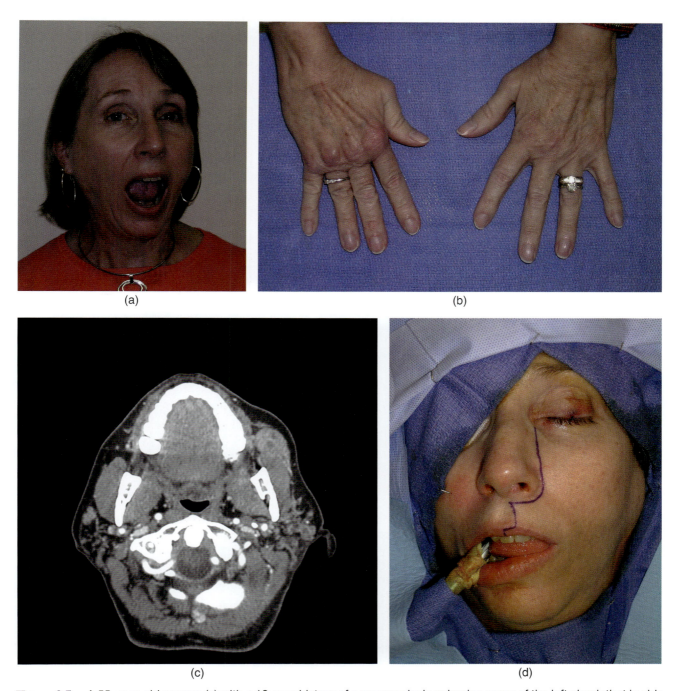

Figure 6.5. A 55-year-old woman (a) with a 10-year history of a progressively enlarging mass of the left cheek that is able to be visualized inferior to her left zygomatic buttress when she opens her mouth. She reported a history of Sjögren syndrome and rheumatoid arthritis of the hands (b). Computerized tomograms (c) identified a heterogenous mass of the left buccal region, associated with minor salivary gland tissue versus an accessory parotid gland. A salivary gland neoplasm was favored based on clinical and radiographic information. Excision was accomplished with a Weber–Ferguson incision (d) to provide access and minimize trauma to Stenson's duct and the buccal branch of the facial nerve. An incision in the buccal mucosa (e) was also utilized, which permitted effective dissection of the tissue bed (f). The specimen was removed without difficulty (g) and was diagnosed as a lymphoepithelial lesion (h, hematoxylin and eosin, original magnification ×200). She healed well and without recurrence of her lymphoepithelial lesion as noted at five years postoperatively (i).

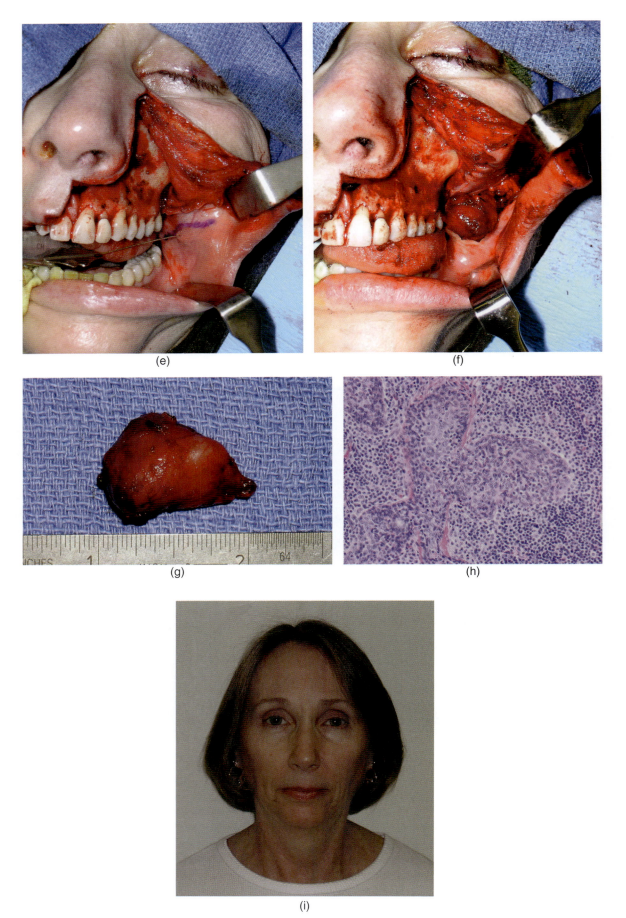

Figure 6.5. (Continued).

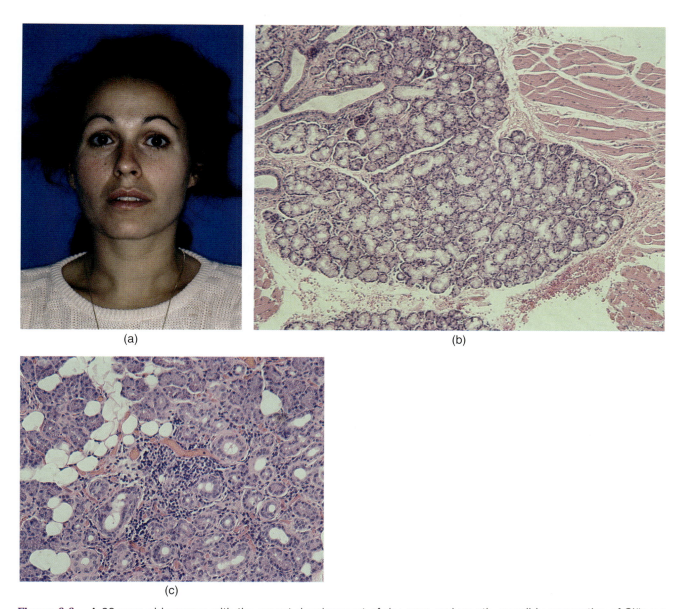

Figure 6.6. A 32-year-old woman with the recent development of dry eyes and mouth, possibly suggestive of Sjögren syndrome (a). No swelling of the parotid glands was appreciated on physical examination. An incisional biopsy of the lower lip and right parotid gland were performed. The histopathology showed a normal lower lip biopsy (b, hematoxylin and eosin, original magnification ×100) and signs consistent with Sjögren syndrome on parotid biopsy (c, hematoxylin and eosin, original magnification ×200).

of disease apparently exists from minor salivary gland lobe to lobe, at least four to seven lobes of minor salivary gland tissue should be removed and examined microscopically (Greenspan et al. 1974). Guellec et al. (2013) performed a systematic review regarding the diagnostic value of labial minor salivary gland biopsy for Sjögren syndrome. They identified 238 publications and included nine in their analysis. Minor salivary gland biopsy sensitivity ranged from 63.5 to 93.7% and specificity ranged from 61.2 to 100%. Their study indicated a lack of information about the value of minor salivary gland biopsy in the diagnosis of Sjögren syndrome.

Incisional biopsy of the parotid gland has at least theoretical benefit and justification in the diagnosis of Sjögren syndrome. Previous recommendations for major salivary gland biopsy reported potential complications of facial nerve damage, cutaneous fistula, and scarring of the facial skin when utilizing a parotid biopsy to establish or confirm a diagnosis of Sjögren syndrome. Incisional parotid biopsy may be performed without assuming any of these complications, except in very rare circumstances (Marx et al. 1988). Recent studies, in fact, point to a higher yield of diagnosis when using the parotid biopsy (Marx 1995) (Figure 6.6). In his series of 54 patients with Sjögren syndrome, 31 (58%) had a positive labial biopsy, while 54 (100%) had a positive parotid biopsy (Marx 1995). He concluded his study by stating that incisional parotid biopsy will confirm and definitively document the diagnosis of Sjögren syndrome (Figure 6.7). Pijpe et al. (2007b) assessed the value of the parotid biopsy as a diagnostic tool for primary Sjögren syndrome and compared the parotid biopsy to the labial biopsy regarding diagnostic value and morbidity. These authors studied 15 consecutive Sjögren syndrome patients and 20 controls. The sensitivity and specificity were comparable: sensitivity 78%, specificity 86%. Lymphoma was identified in one patient based on parotid biopsy whose lip biopsy was negative for lymphoma. The authors concluded that a parotid biopsy has a diagnostic potential for primary Sjögren syndrome comparable to that of a lip biopsy, and with less morbidity.

The incisional parotid biopsy will also serve to rule out the presence of lymphoma, which is observed to develop in approximately 5–10% of patients with Sjögren syndrome (Talal and Bunim 1964; Daniels 1991). Patients with Sjögren syndrome are felt to have 47 times greater incidence of lymphoma than that of an age-controlled population (Marx 1988). Ten such lymphomas were reported in Marx's study. They developed 4–12 years

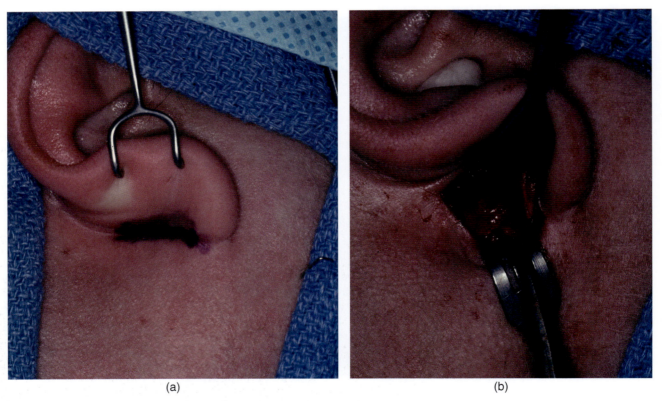

Figure 6.7. An incisional parotid biopsy was performed on the patient seen in Figure 6.1. The incision is placed behind the right ear, which enables the surgeon to procure sufficient parotid tissue to establish a diagnosis, while also providing a cosmetic scar (a). The dissection proceeds through skin and subcutaneous tissue after which time the parotid capsule is noted. This is incised and a 1 cm² specimen of parotid gland is removed (b). The closure requires a reapproximation of the parotid capsule to avoid a salivary fistula postoperatively.

after the diagnosis of Sjögren syndrome was made, with a mean of 7.2 years. In 8 of the 10 cases, a rapid change in the size of the parotid enlargement was noted, and all patients exhibited a darkening of the skin overlying the enlarged parotid gland. These changes dictated biopsy of the parotid gland in the background of the systemic disease, with the knowledge that lymphoma infrequently develops in the lower lip in patients with Sjögren syndrome.

Histopathology of Sjögren Syndrome

Abnormal salivary gland function is associated with well-defined histologic alterations including clustering of lymphocytic infiltrates as a common feature of all salivary glands and other organs affected by Sjögren syndrome (Figure 6.8). Histologic evaluation of enlarged parotid or submandibular glands usually reveals the benign lymphoepithelial lesion, with a lymphocytic infiltrate and epimyoepithelial islands. These features are not invariably noted in the major salivary glands, however (Daniels 1991). The characteristic microscopic feature of Sjögren syndrome in the minor glands is a focal lymphocytic infiltrate, and includes focal aggregates of 50 or more lymphocytes, defined as a focus, that are adjacent to normal appearing acini and the consistent presence of these foci in all or most of the glands in the specimen (Daniels 1991). Epimyoepithelial islands occur uncommonly in minor glands of patients affected by Sjögren syndrome.

Sarcoidosis

Sarcoidosis is a chronic systemic disease characterized by the production of non-caseating granulomas whose etiology is unknown. It can affect any organ system, thereby mimicking rheumatic diseases causing fever, arthritis, uveitis, myositis, and rash (Table 6.2). The peripheral blood shows a dichotomy of depressed cellular immunity and enhanced humoral immunity. Depressed cellular immunity is manifested by lymphopenia and cutaneous anergy. The enhanced humoral immunity is noted by polyclonal gammopathy and autoantibody production.

Table 6.2. Clinical involvement by sarcoidosis.

Clinical finding	Frequency in sarcoidosis (%)	Differential diagnosis
Arthritis	15	Rheumatoid arthritis
Parotid gland enlargement	5	Sjögren syndrome
Upper airway disease	3	Wegener's granulomatosis
Uveitis	18	Spondyloarthropathies
Facial nerve palsy	2	Lyme disease
Keratoconjunctivitis	5	Sjögren syndrome

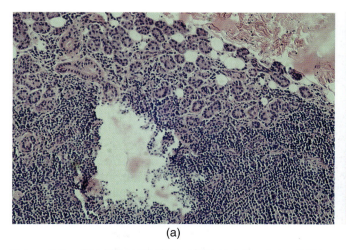
(a)

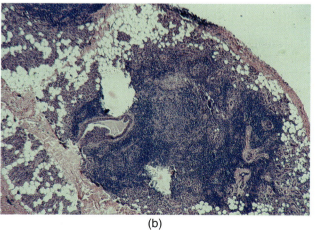
(b)

Figure 6.8. The histopathology of the incisional parotid biopsy of the patient in Figure 6.1 (a and b). Signs consistent with Sjögren syndrome were noted including an intense lymphocytic infiltrate and destruction of acinar tissue (a, hematoxylin and eosin, original magnification ×200; b, hematoxylin and eosin, original magnification ×40).

PATHOPHYSIOLOGY OF SARCOIDOSIS

The exact cause of sarcoidosis is unknown. The current hypothesis is that an alteration in the immune response occurs in genetically susceptible patients exposed to an environmental, occupation, or infectious agent. Sarcoidosis has been associated with heavy metal exposures such as beryllium and its salts, although the American Thoracic Society criteria list berylliosis as a separate entity (Heinle and Chang 2014). Firefighters who responded to the collapse of the World Trade Center have a higher incidence of sarcoid-like pulmonary disease and this may be a result of exposure to an unidentified substance (Izbicki et al. 2007). Sarcoidosis has also been linked to infectious agents such as *Propionibacterium* and *Mycobacterium*. Finally, there is a well-accepted genetic component to the pathophysiology of sarcoidosis, since certain HLA alleles appear to confer susceptibility to sarcoidosis such as HLA DR 11, 12, 14, 15, and 17, while others result in a protective effect, including HLA DR1, and DR4.

CLINICAL MANIFESTATIONS OF SARCOIDOSIS

Sarcoidosis occurs most commonly in American blacks and northern European Caucasians. It is eight times more common in American blacks than American Caucasians (Hellmann 1993). Women are affected slightly more frequently than men. An average incidence of 16.5 cases per 100 000 men and 19 cases per 1 000 000 women has been reported (Jonsson and Olofsson 2011). Onset is usually between and ages of 20 and 40, yet a second peak of disease incidence occurs in women older than 50 years (Jonsson and Olofsson 2011). Patients with sarcoidosis generally present with one of the following four problems: respiratory symptoms such as dry cough, shortness of breath, and chest pain (40–50%); constitutional symptoms such as fever, weight loss, and malaise (25%); extrathoracic inflammation such as peripheral lymphadenopathy (25%); and rheumatic symptoms such as arthritis (5–10%) (Hellmann 1993).

Respiratory symptoms are the most common presenting chief complaints including those previously mentioned. Regardless of symptoms, greater than 90% of patients with sarcoidosis have an abnormal chest radiograph. Four types of radiographic appearance have been described: type 0 is normal; type I shows enlargement of hilar, mediastinal, and occasionally paratracheal lymph nodes; type II shows the adenopathy seen in type I as well as pulmonary infiltrates (Figure 6.9). Type III demonstrates the infiltrates without the adenopathy. Type II involvement is the most common among patients with sarcoidosis who have respiratory distress.

Two patterns of arthritis are observed in sarcoidosis, and are classified as to whether the arthritis occurs within the first six months after the onset of the disease, or late in the disease. The early form of arthritis often begins in the ankles and may spread to involve the knees and other joints. The axial skeleton is typically spared. Monarthritis in the early phase is unusual. *Erythema nodosum*, a syndrome of inflammatory cutaneous nodules frequently found on the extensor surfaces of the lower extremities, occurs in about two-thirds of patients and is strikingly associated with early arthritis. *Lofgren syndrome* involves a triad of hilar lymphadenopathy, erythema nodosum, and arthritis. The late form of arthritis occurs at least six months after the onset of sarcoidosis, and is generally less dramatic than the early form. The knees are the most common joints to be involved, followed by the ankles. Monarthritis can occur in the late form of arthritis, and erythema nodosum is not commonly noted.

Other rheumatic manifestations associated with sarcoidosis include involvement of the larynx, nasal turbinates, and nasal cartilage, thereby resembling the clinical presentation of Wegener's granulomatosis (Figure 6.10). Eye involvement occurs in 22% of patients, with uveitis being most common (Hellmann 1993). The triad of anterior uveitis in conjunction with parotitis and facial nerve palsy has been referred to as *Heerfordt syndrome*, also known as uveoparotid fever.

While salivary gland involvement seems to primarily involve the parotid gland (Figure 6.11), the submandibular gland can also be involved (Werning 1991; Vairaktaris et al. 2005). Parotid gland sarcoidosis occurs in 6% of patients with sarcoidosis (James and Sharma 2000). The Armed Forces Institute of Pathology registry identified 85 cases of sarcoidosis. In the 77 cases in which a gland was specified, parotid involvement occurred in 65% of the cases, while the submandibular gland accounted for 13% of cases (Werning 1991). Submandibular gland enlargement may occur in the absence of parotid swelling, with or without

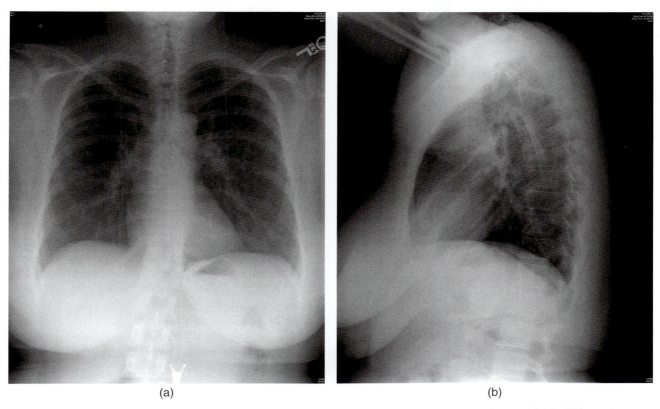

Figure 6.9. Posterior-anterior (a) and lateral (b) chest radiographs of a patient with type II sarcoidosis. This patient presented with severe shortness of breath.

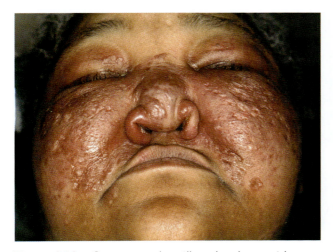

Figure 6.10. Severe nasal cartilage involvement by sarcoidosis in this elderly woman. Source: Image courtesy of Dr. James Sciubba.

clinical evidence of minor salivary gland involvement (Figure 6.12). Minor salivary gland involvement is occasionally noted histologically in the presence of clinically apparent major salivary gland swelling (Mandel, Kaynar 1994). In fact, enlargement of the major salivary glands may be the first identifiable sign of sarcoidosis (Fatahzadeh and Rinaggio 2006). When this occurs, therefore, it is important to differentiate the parotid swelling associated with sarcoidosis from that of Sjögren syndrome (Falwaczny et al. 2002). Salivary gland biopsy with histopathologic examination is one means to make this distinction.

DIAGNOSIS OF SARCOIDOSIS WITH SALIVARY GLAND BIOPSY

As with Sjögren syndrome diagnoses with salivary gland biopsies, early stage disease is perhaps more readily diagnosed with a parotid biopsy rather than a minor salivary gland biopsy. It has been pointed out that cases of sarcoidosis that do not clinically produce parotid enlargement nonetheless show involvement at the microscopic level (Marx 1995). In this review, the labial biopsy was positive in 38% of cases while 88% of parotid biopsies were positive for sarcoidosis. The lesions of sarcoidosis in labial

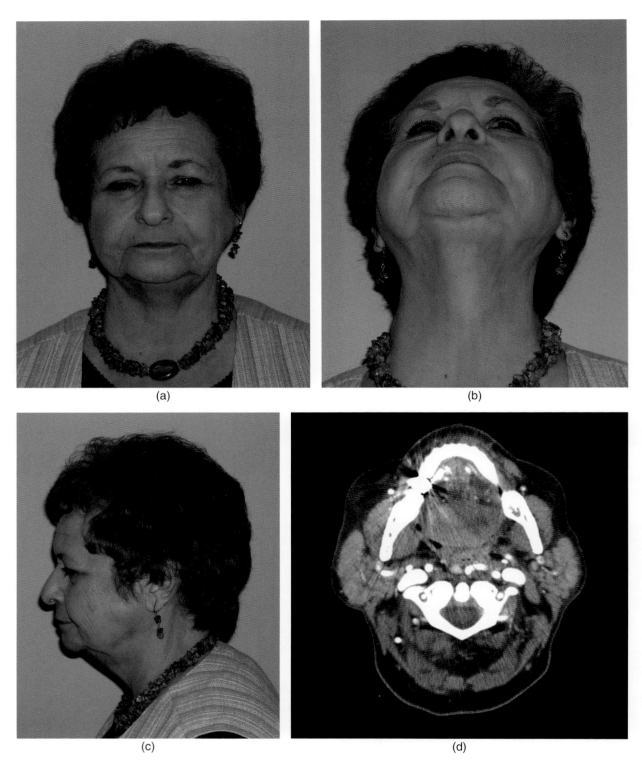

Figure 6.11. A 64-year-old woman with parotid swelling of two month's duration. The patient had been clinically diagnosed with Sjögren syndrome yet serology was negative. A fine needle aspiration biopsy of the left parotid gland swelling had been performed that suggested Warthin tumor. Physical examination identified tender swellings of the bilateral parotid glands, with the left being larger than the right (a–c). CT examination identified diffuse enlargement of the parotid glands (d) and multiple enlarged lymph nodes in the left submandibular region (e). Her chest radiograph identified bilateral interstitial prominence (f). With an equivocal diagnosis of her left parotid swelling, the patient underwent left superficial parotidectomy and removal of left submandibular lymph nodes in a standard fashion (g–i). Final histopathology (j, hematoxylin and eosin, original magnification ×100) demonstrated non-caseating granulomas consistent with a diagnosis of sarcoidosis. The excised submandibular lymph nodes showed identical histopathology. The patient was treated with a 54-week course of prednisone and methotrexate for her diagnosis of pulmonary and extrapulmonary sarcoidosis and showed a favorable response. She was doing well at her five-year postoperative evaluation (k, l).

Systemic Diseases Affecting the Salivary Glands 189

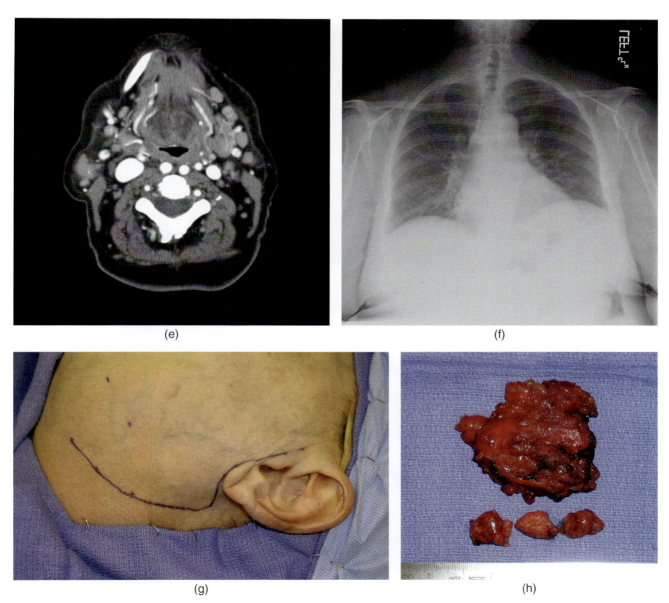

Figure 6.11. (*Continued*).

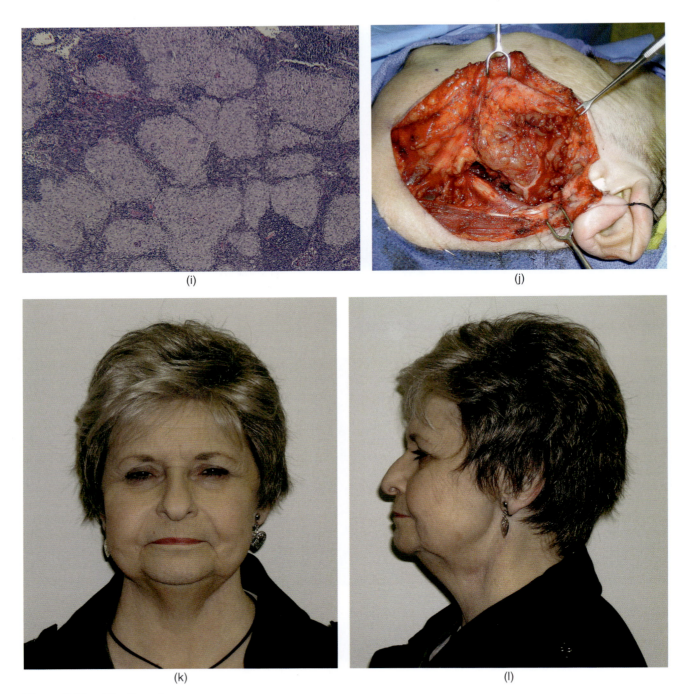

Figure 6.11. (Continued).

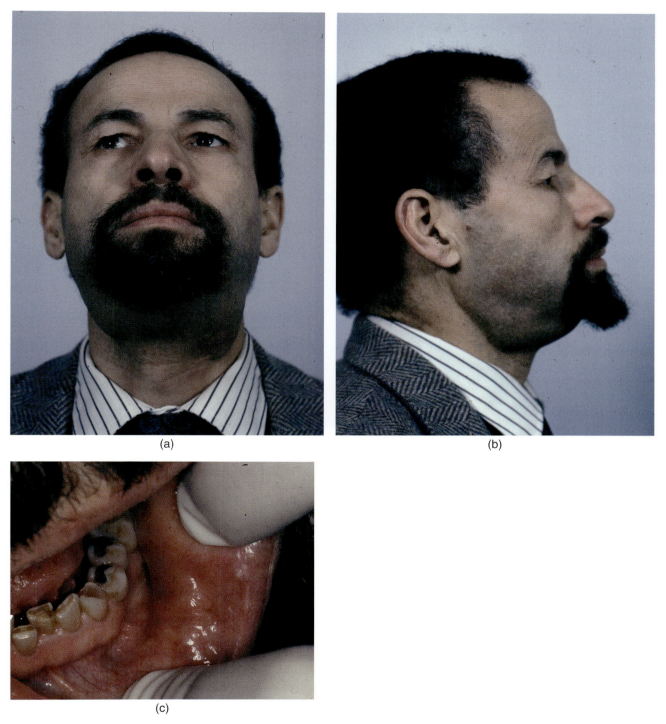

Figure 6.12. A 55-year-old man with bilateral submandibular gland swellings (a and b), as well as lower lip lesions (c). Excision of the left submandibular gland and biopsy of the lower lip swelling identified non-caseating granulomas. Additional workup identified signs consistent with sarcoidosis.

salivary gland biopsies tend to be sparse such that multiple labial glands require excision for microscopic analysis. Another report investigated the yield of minor salivary gland biopsy in the diagnosis of sarcoidosis (Nessan and Jacoway 1979). In this study of 75 patients, non-caseating granulomas were present in minor salivary gland biopsies in 44 patients (58%). There was no correlation with minor salivary gland biopsy yield and stage of the disease. The highest yield for diagnosis of sarcoidosis was found in transbronchial lung biopsies (93%). Nonetheless, the diagnosis of sarcoidosis is one of exclusion, owing to an absence of a diagnostic gold standard. As such, a compatible clinical picture is established based on the patient's symptoms, physical and radiographic findings. The biopsy of salivary gland tissue or other tissue identifies the presence of non-caseating granulomas such that a provisional diagnosis of sarcoidosis is made. It then becomes necessary to exclude other sources of granulomatous inflammation, such as Crohn's disease, deep fungal infections, and others (Critchlow and Chang 2014). It is important to point out that there are no pathognomonic diagnostic tests for sarcoidosis. Rather, the salivary biopsy must be considered with an elevated angiotensin converting enzyme (ACE) and lysozyme result, and an altered ratio of CD4/CD8 cells, among others to offer a diagnosis of sarcoidosis (Kasamatsu et al. 2007).

Histopathology of Sarcoidosis

Numerous granulomas may be seen in the salivary gland biopsy. The typical sarcoid granuloma is non-caseating and consists of a tightly packed central focus of histiocytes that is surrounded by lymphocytes and fibroblasts at its periphery (Figure 6.13). The histiocytes may be epithelioid and may join to form multinucleated giant cells, frequently of the Langhans type.

Sialosis

Sialosis, also known as sialadenosis represents a bilateral enlargement of the parotid gland that is multifactorial in its etiology (Table 6.3). It is not commonly associated with an autoimmune phenomenon as is the case for Sjögren syndrome and sarcoidosis, although it can easily be confused with these two pathologic processes due to its clinical presentation (Figure 6.14). Quite commonly,

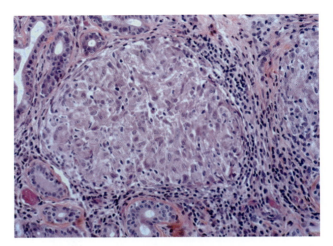

Figure 6.13 Histopathology of sarcoidosis (hematoxylin and eosin, original magnification ×200). Source: Image courtesy of Dr. Joseph A. Regezi.

Table 6.3. Classification of sialosis.

Malnutritional sialosis
   Achalasia
   Bulemia
   Alcoholism

Hormonal sialosis
   Sex hormonal sialosis
   Diabetic sialosis
   Thyroid sialosis
   Pituitary and adrenocortical disorders

Neurohumoral sialosis
   Peripheral neurohumoral sialosis
   Central neurogenous sialosis

Dysenzymatic sialosis
   Hepatogenic sialosis
   Pancreatogenic (exocrine) sialosis
   Nephrogenic sialosis
   Dysproteinemic sialosis

Mucoviscidosis

Drug-induced sialosis

Source: Werning (1991) (p.55)/Elsevier.

sialosis is caused by nutritional disturbances such as alcoholism, bulimia, or in the rare case of achalasia (Figure 6.15). Chronic alcoholism, with or without cirrhosis, results in asymptomatic enlargement of the parotid glands in 30–80% of these patients (Regezi et al. 2003). In such cases,

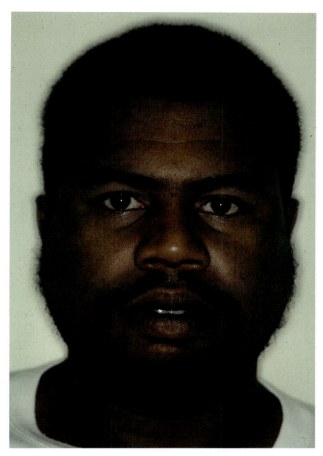

Figure 6.14. A 32-year-old man with a chronic history of bilateral parotid swellings. He gave a history of achalasia. The history suggested that the parotid swellings were consistent with a diagnosis of sialosis. There were no physical or historical findings suggestive of another diagnosis.

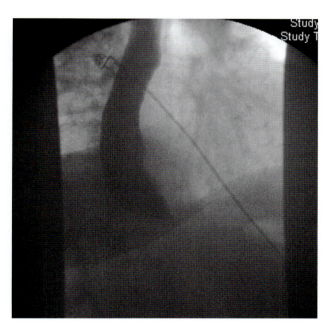

Figure 6.15. The fluoroscopic images of the barium swallow performed in the patient in Figure 6.14. The characteristic "bird's beak" deformity is noted, reflective of failure of the lower esophageal sphincter to relax. This is diagnostic of achalasia.

parotid enlargement has been attributed to protein deficiency. In diabetes mellitus, the mechanism of acinar hypertrophy associated with this condition is unknown. Due to the numerous causes of sialosis, as well as numerous diagnoses that can clinically resemble sialosis, the patient's history is paramount in such cases to properly initiate the diagnostic process. In addition, the treatment for these disorders differs significantly.

CLINICAL MANIFESTATIONS OF SIALOSIS

Sialosis is characterized by chronic, afebrile salivary enlargement. The enlargement is described by patients as slowly evolving, and recurrent. A thorough history will most frequently divulge symptoms associated with comorbid disease such as diabetes mellitus, achalasia, alcoholism, or others (Scully et al. 2008).

DIAGNOSIS OF SIALOSIS WITH SALIVARY GLAND BIOPSY

The role of salivary gland biopsy in a patient suspected as having sialosis is to rule out Sjögren syndrome, sarcoidosis, and lymphoma. Sialosis is a disease limited to the major salivary glands such that an incisional biopsy of parotid enlargement is indicated, rather than an incisional biopsy of the lip as might be considered in Sjögren syndrome or sarcoidosis. As such, a minor salivary gland biopsy is of no value in making a diagnosis of sialosis. While histopathologic confirmation of this process is valuable, it is certainly possible to make a clinical diagnosis of sialosis based on historical findings (Mandel et al. 2005). In addition, once a histopathologic diagnosis of sialosis has been established, the underlying cause of this disorder must be ascertained, if not already known preoperatively. Prompt treatment of the underlying disease process must then occur.

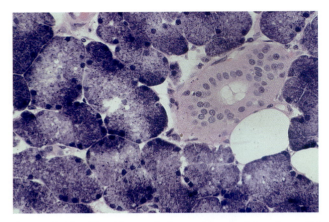

Figure 6.16. The histopathology of the incisional parotid biopsy performed on the patient in Figure 6.14 (hematoxylin and eosin, original magnification ×200). Acinar hypertrophy is noted. The physical, radiographic, and histologic information confirms a diagnosis of achalasia. He was treated with surgical myotomy of the lower esophageal sphincter.

Histopathology of Sialosis

The parotid swelling of sialosis is due to acinar enlargement (Figure 6.16). The diameter of the acinar cell tends to increase by two to three times that of normal. The nuclei tend to be basally situated, and the cytoplasm tends to the packed with granules (Carda et al. 2004). There may be no correlation between the specific clinical type of sialosis and the histologic appearance, although Carda et al. (2004) demonstrated that the structural and ultrastructural findings of parotid biopsies demonstrated that alterations are present in the salivary glands of chronic alcoholics before the terminal phase of hepatic cirrhosis. Inflammatory cells tend to be absent in sialosis. The long-standing nature of the underlying disease may ultimately lead to acinar atrophy and replacement with fat (Werning 1991; Carda et al. 2004).

IgG4-Related Disease

IgG4-related disease was designated a systemic condition in 2003 after the identification of sclerosing pancreatitis was linked to elevated serum IgG4 in 2001 (Haman et al. 2001). High levels of IgG4 were noted in patients with sclerosing pancreatitis but not in patients with conventional pancreatitis, primary biliary cirrhosis, primary sclerosing cholangitis, or Sjögren syndrome, thereby distinguishing this disorder from others of the pancreas or biliary tract. In addition, these authors indicated that if sclerosing pancreatitis is misdiagnosed, patients may be presumed to have pancreatic cancer and may undergo unnecessary treatment. The finding of a tumefactive process in IgG4 involved tissues results in the suspicion of neoplastic processes such that clinicians must consider the presence of IgG4-related disease, particularly in those tissues in which this disease process predominates (Kamisawa and Okamoto 2008; Sodavarapu et al. 2020).

IgG4-related disease has since been described in nearly every organ system and tissue including the aorta, biliary tree, breast, salivary glands, periorbital tissues, kidneys, lungs, lymph nodes, meninges, pericardium, prostate, thyroid, and skin (Stone et al. 2012), yet this process predominates in the pancreas, salivary glands, biliary system, and retroperitoneum (Figure 6.17). It has since been learned that diseases known for nearly a century such as Mikulicz disease, Kuttner tumor, inflammatory pseudotumor, and Reidel thyroiditis are part of a spectrum of IgG-4 related disease and can be replaced by a designation that is described by key pathological features (Lang et al. 2016). The two features that unite previously disparate diagnoses are a characteristic histopathological appearance and an elevated number of IgG4+ plasma cells within tissue (Deshpande et al. 2012). The diagnosis of IgG4-related disease cannot be made with certainty in the absence of an immunohistochemical stain for IgG4. The three major histopathological features associated with IgG4-related disease are:

1 *Dense lymphoplasmacytic infiltrate* – composed primarily of T cells, with scattered B cells. Plasma cells are an essential component. Eosinophils are found in mild to moderate quantities.
2 *Storiform-type fibrosis* – spindle cells, either fibroblasts or myofibroblasts, radiate from a center point, and are immersed within the lymphocytoplasmacytic infiltrate.
3 *Obliterative phlebitis* – venous channels are obliterated by the dense lymphoplasmacytic infiltrate that is seen within its wall and lumen.

Elevated IgG4 in tissue and serum assist in the diagnosis of IgG4-related disease but neither is a pathognomonic of the disease. Correlation with the three histopathological features above remains essential and misdiagnoses of IgG4-related disease

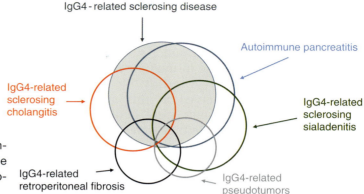

Figure 6.17. The relative incidence of the most commonly observed IgG4-related diseases occurring in the pancreas, salivary glands, biliary system, retroperitoneum, and the miscellaneous pseudotumors.

are common due to moderate elevations of serum IgG4 concentration and overreliance on the identification of IgG4-positive plasma cells in tissue (Stone et al. 2012).

The precise etiology of IgG4-related disease remains unknown and no consensus exists regarding the role of the IgG4 molecule. Nonetheless, it has been postulated that the inflammatory and fibrous processes that drive IgG4-related disease are propagated by Th2 cells and regulatory T cells (Zen and Nakanuma 2010). This is in contradistinction to most autoimmune diseases that are driven by Th1 cells and/or Th17 subsets that are responsible for the inflammatory process (Mulholland et al. 2015). The distinction of IG4-related diseases and autoimmune diseases is also seen by the former affecting mostly middle-aged males while autoimmune diseases affect mainly females (Puxeddu et al. 2018).

Zen and Nakanuma (2010) performed a cross-sectional analysis of 114 patients with IgG4-related disease and classified disease into five anatomic locations including head and neck, thoracic, hepatobiliary, retroperitoneal, and systemic. The head and neck group ($n = 23$ patients) demonstrated 17 patients with salivary gland lesions and 10 patients with lacrimal lesions; the thoracic group ($n = 16$ patients) demonstrated 11 patients with lung lesions, 5 patients with pleura lesions, and 1 patient with a breast lesion; the hepatic and pancreaticobiliary group ($n = 27$ patients) demonstrated 17 patients with pancreas lesions, 25 patients with bile duct lesions, 5 patients with gallbladder lesions, and 8 patients with liver lesions; the retroperitoneal group ($n = 13$ patients) demonstrated 6 patients with retroperitoneal fibrosis and 7 patients with aorta/artery lesions; and the systemic group ($n = 35$ patients – those patients with multiple lesions not restricted to any one of the first four groups) demonstrated 22 patients with salivary gland lesions, 4 patients with lacrimal lesions, 15 patients with lung lesions, 11 patients with pancreas lesions, 8 patients with bile duct lesions, 4 patients with gallbladder lesions, 3 patients with liver lesions, 7 patients with retroperitoneal fibrosis, 3 patients with aorta/artery lesions, 10 patients with kidney lesions, 2 patients with paravertebral lesions, 2 patients with systemic lymph node lesions, and 1 patient each with mediastinal fibrosis, prostate lesion, and peripheral nerve lesion.

The male-to-female patient ratio was almost equal in the head and neck group while male patients comprised 75–86% of the patients in the other four groups. All patients with renal lesions were in the systemic group. The serum IgG4 level was highest in the systemic group followed by the head and neck group. The number of specimen IgG4 plasma cells/high power field was highest in the head and neck group followed by the systemic group. Finally, the ratio of IgG4/IgG plasma cells was highest in the head and neck group (Zen and Nakanuma 2010).

Mulholland et al. (2015) performed a systematic review of IgG4-related diseases in the head and neck by searching Pubmed and EMBASE. Case reports, original research, and review articles published in English from 1964 to 2014 were included when their focus was IgG4-related disease. Two hundred forty-seven articles were identified and forty-three articles involving 484 patients were included in the systematic review. Three hundred eighty-four patients demonstrated disease in the orbit and 162 patients had disease in the salivary glands with 107 patients demonstrating submandibular gland disease, 29 patients demonstrating parotid disease, and 1 patient each with disease in the sublingual gland and a minor salivary gland. Many patients had disease in multiple sites in the head and neck region. A nearly 1:1 ratio of males:females was observed in this systematic review. Treatment outcomes were known in 99 patients. Of these, corticosteroids were effective for 67 patients (67.7%) in achieving a full remission. The authors concluded that a suspicion should exist for IgG4-related disease when patients display recurrent salivary and lacrimal gland swelling and lymphadenopathy in the head and neck region.

Puxeddu et al. (2018) have provided a comprehensive review of IgG4-related salivary gland disease that occurs in 27–53% of patients with IgG4-related disease. These authors pointed out that involvement of the lacrimal and salivary glands is primarily manifest by painless bilateral swelling of greater than three months. The submandibular glands are the salivary glands most commonly involved. Xerostomia is noted to be present in 30% of patients, less frequently than in Sjögren syndrome. Cervical lymphadenopathy is found in 70% of IgG4-related sialadenitis. Finally, the authors recommended the establishment of a differential diagnosis that includes solid tumors, lymphomas, and IgG4-related disease as the diagnosis is being sought. Once the diagnosis of IgG4-related disease has been established, the localization of multiple organ involvement occurs through imaging, and positron emission tomography is an emerging diagnostic option in the context of IgG4-related diseases.

Summary

- Numerous systemic diseases may infiltrate salivary gland tissue, including Sjögren syndrome, sarcoidosis, IgG4-related diseases, and sialosis.
- Sjögren syndrome and sarcoidosis are autoimmune disorders while sialosis is not.
- Sjögren syndrome is characterized by keratoconjunctivitis sicca and xerostomia, with or without association with another connective tissue disease.
- Approximately 30% of patients with Sjögren syndrome will develop salivary gland enlargement, most commonly the parotid gland.
- A salivary gland biopsy may confirm the patient's diagnosis of Sjögren syndrome. Either a labial biopsy or parotid gland biopsy may be performed. Disease may be identified more often in a parotid biopsy, even when the patient does not demonstrate parotid swelling.
- Another benefit of parotid biopsy is the identification of lymphoma that is known to develop in 5–10% of patients with Sjögren syndrome.
- Specific histologic criteria have been established for the diagnosis of Sjögren syndrome in salivary gland biopsies, specifically referred to as a focus.
- Sarcoidosis is a multisystem disease, with a predilection for involvement of the lungs.
- Erythema nodosum represents cutaneous nodules most commonly involving the extensor surfaces of the lower extremities, and occurs in about two-thirds of patients with sarcoidosis.
- Lofgren syndrome involves a triad of hilar lymphadenopathy, erythema nodosum, and arthritis.
- Approximately 5% of patients with sarcoidosis have parotid gland enlargement.
- The triad of anterior uveitis in conjunction with parotitis and facial nerve palsy has been referred to as Heerfordt syndrome.
- As with Sjögren syndrome, there is a higher yield of positive findings to make a diagnosis of sarcoidosis based on parotid biopsy compared to lip biopsy.
- Sialosis is a noninflammatory, non-neoplastic, non-autoimmune disorder with enlargement of the salivary glands, most notably the parotid gland.
- IgG4-related disease affects the salivary glands as the second most common organ system involved.
- IgG4-related sialadenitis creates a tumefactive appearance of the gland such that surgeons should approach these cases with a differential diagnosis of neoplastic disease as well as IgG4-related disease. A PET scan should be obtained to rule out systemic involvement when a diagnosis of IgG4-related disease is established.

Case Presentation – *Esoterica*

A 54-year-old man presented with a five-year history of swelling in the left neck. The swelling was not associated with prandial pain. Examination revealed a non-tender 3 cm mass of the left submandibular region. There was bilateral cervical adenopathy appreciated. There was no oral mucosal or oropharyngeal mucosal disease present.

Past Medical History
The patient denied a significant past medical history. He was taking no medications at the time of evaluation and reported no known drug allergies.

Imaging
CT scans were obtained (Figure 6.18a–d) that identified an enlarged left submandibular gland as well as a large adjacent mass, presumably a level I lymph node. Contrast enhancing enlarged lymph nodes were noted in the right neck, as well (Figure 6.18e).

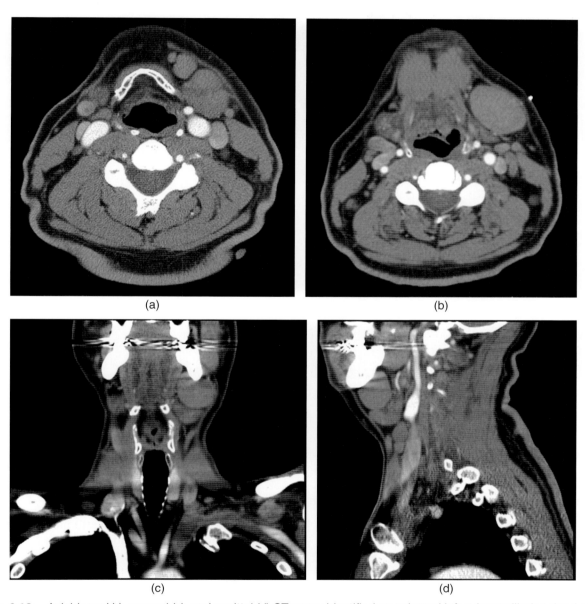

Figure 6.18. Axial (a and b), coronal (c), and sagittal (d) CT scans identified an enlarged left submandibular gland as well as a large adjacent mass, presumably a level I lymph node. Contrast enhancing enlarged lymph nodes were noted in the right neck as well (e). A Kuttner tumor of the submandibular gland and left level I lymph node was diagnosed histopathologically (f and g). A dense lymphoplasmacytic infiltrate was noted along with a storiform pattern of fibrosis and obliterative phlebitis. The IgG4 count was greater than 100/high power field in the submandibular gland specimen (f, hematoxylin and eosin, original magnification ×40; g, hematoxylin and eosin, original magnification ×200).

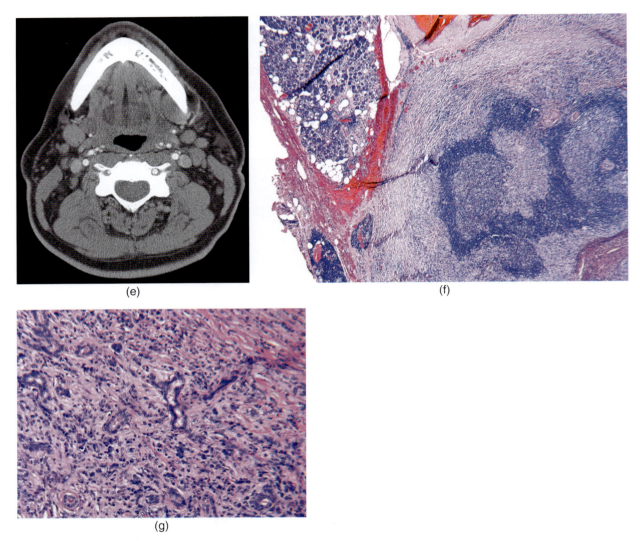

Figure 6.18. (Continued).

Cytology
A fine needle aspiration biopsy of the left submandibular mass identified polymorphous lymphocytes and no neoplasm. The results were therefore inconclusive, and necessitated tissue removal.

Surgical Intervention
The patient underwent excision of his left submandibular gland and associated enlarged level I lymph node that revealed histologic evidence of a Kuttner tumor of the submandibular gland and a preponderance of IgG4 plasma cells in the lymph node (Figure 6.18f and g). His serum IgG level was normal at 1265 mg/dl (normal 694–1618 mg/dl) and his serum IgG4 level was elevated at 197.5 mg/dl (normal 4.0–85.0 mg/dl).

Diagnosis
IgG4-related disease of the left submandibular gland and cervical lymph nodes (Kuttner tumor). Additional CT imaging of the chest, abdomen, and pelvis did not identify systemic organ involvement.

TAKE-HOME POINTS

1. Kuttner tumors should be considered when patients have cervical adenopathy and enhancing, enlarged submandibular glands.

2. Systemic imaging should be obtained when the diagnosis of IgG4-related disease is established. This imaging ideally consists of a PET scan, but CT scans of the neck, chest, abdomen, and pelvis might also be acceptable.
3. Elevated IgG4 in tissue and serum support the diagnosis of IgG4-related disease but neither is a pathognomonic of the disease.
4. The histopathological features of a dense lymphoplasmacytic infiltrate in excised tissue, a storiform fibrosis, and an obliterative phlebitis are essential to observe to establish a diagnosis of IgG4-related disease.
5. Misdiagnoses of IgG4-related disease are common due to moderate elevations of serum IgG4 concentration and overreliance on the observation of IgG4-positive plasma cells in tissue.

References

Abbondanzo SL. 2001. Extranodal marginal-zone B-cell lymphoma of the salivary gland. *Ann Diagn Pathol* 5(4):246-254.

Alunno A, Leone MC, Giacomelli R, Gerli R, Carubbi F. 2018. Lymphoma and lymphomagenesis in primary Sjogren's syndrome. *Front Med* 5:102, published 13 April.

Anaya JM, Tobon GJ, Vega P, Castiblanco J. 2006. Autoimmune disease aggregation in families with primary Sjogren's syndrome. *J Rheumatol* 33:2227-2234.

Cai YL, Wang ZH, Lu SJ. 2002. Analysis for therapy and prognosis of undifferentiated carcinoma with lymphoid stroma in the salivary gland. *Shanghai Kou Qiang Yi Xue* 11(4):310-313 (in Chinese).

Carda C, Gomez de Ferraris ME, Arriaga A, Carranza M, Peydro A. 2004. Alcoholic parotid sialosis: A structural and ultrastructural study. *Med Oral* 9:24-42.

Chisolm DM, Mason DK. 1968. Labial salivary gland biopsy in Sjogren's syndrome. *J Clin Pathol* 21:656-660.

Critchlow WA, Chang D. 2014. Cheilitis granulomatosa: A review. *Head Neck Pathol* 8:209-213.

Daniels TE. 1991. Benign Lymphoepithelial Lesion and Sjogren's Syndrome. In: Ellis GL, Auclair PL, Gnepp DR (eds.) *Surgical Pathology of the Salivary Glands*. Philadelphia, WB Saunders Co., Chapter 6, 83-106.

Daniels TE, Silverman S, Michalski JP et al. 1975. The oral component of Sjogren's syndrome. *Oral Surg Oral Med Oral Pathol* 39:875-885.

Dawson LJ, Stanbury J, Venn N. 2006. Antimuscarinic antibodies in primary Sjogren's syndrome reversibly inhibit the mechanism of fluid secretion by human submandibular salivary acinar cells. *Arthtitis Rheum* 54:1165-1173.

Del Bono V, Pretolesi F, Pontali E et al. 2000. Possible malignant transformation of benign lymphoepithelial lesions in human deficiency virus-infected patients: Report of three cases. *Clin Infect Dis* 30(6):947-949.

Deshpande V, Zen Y, Chan JKC et al. 2012. Consensus statement on the pathology of IgG4-related disease. *Mod Pathol* 25:1181-1192.

Fatahzadeh M, Rinaggio J. 2006. Diagnosis of systemic sarcoidosis prompted by orofacial manifestations. A review of the literature. *JADA* 137:54-60.

Folwaczny M, Sommer A, Sander CA, Kellner H. 2002. Parotid sarcoidosis mimicking Sjogren's syndrome: Report of a case. *J Oral Maxillofac Surg* 60:117-120.

Garcia-Carrasco M, Fuentes-Alexandro S, Escarcega RO et al. 2006. Pathophysiology of Sjogren's syndrome. *Arch Med Res* 37:921-932.

Godwin JT. 1952. Benign lymphoepithelial lesion of the parotid gland (adenolymphoma, chronic inflammation, lymphoepithelioma, lymphocytic tumor, Mikulicz disease): Report of eleven cases. *Cancer* 5:1089-1103.

Greenspan JS, Daniels TE, Talal N, Sylvester RA. 1974. The histopathology of Sjogren's syndrome in labial salivary gland biopsies. *Oral Surg Oral Med Oral Pathol* 37:217-229.

Guellec D, Cornec D, Jousse-Joulin S et al. 2013. Diagnostic value of labial minor salivary gland biopsy for Sjogren's Syndrome: A systematic review. *Autoimmun Rev* 12:416-420.

Gurwale SG, Gore CR, Gulati I, Dey I. 2020. Immunoglobulin G4-related chronic sclerosing sialadenitis: An emerging entity. *J Oral Maxillofac Pathol* 24(Suppl 1):S135-S138.

Haman H, Kawa S, Horiuchi A et al. 2001. High serum IgG4 concentrations in patients with sclerosing pancreatitis. *N Engl J Med* 344:732-738.

Heinle R, Chang C. 2014. Diagnostic criteria for sarcoidosis. *Autoimmun Rev* 13:383-387.

Hellmann DB. 1993. Sarcoidosis. In: Schumacher HR, Klippel JH, Koopman WJ (eds.) *Primer on the Rheumatic Diseases*, 10th edn. Atlanta, Arthritis Foundation, chapter 28, pp. 204-205.

Ihrler S, Zietz C, Sendelhofert A et al. 1999. Lymphoepithelial duct lesions in Sjogren-type sialadenitis. *Virchows Arch* 434(4):315-323.

Izbicki G, Chavko R, Banauch GI et al. 2007. World Trade Center "sarcoid-like" granulomatous pulmonary disease in New York City Fire Department rescue workers. *Chest* 131:1414-1423.

James DG, Sharma OP. 2000. Parotid gland sarcoidosis. *Sarcoidosis Vasc Diffuse Lung Dis* 17:27-32.

Jonsson R, Olofsson J. 2011. Autoimmune disorders, lymphoproliferaton, and granulomatous inflammation. In: Bradley PJ, Guntinas-Lichius O (eds.) *Salivary Gland Disorders and Diseases: Diagnosis and Management*. Stuggart, Thieme, chapter 16, pp. 152-166.

Kamisawa T, Okamoto A. 2008. IgG4-related sclerosing disease. *World J Gastroenterol* 14:3948-3955.

Kasamatsu A, Kanazawa H, Watanabe T, Matsuzaki O. 2007. Oral sarcoidosis: Report of a case and review of literature. *J Oral Maxillofac Surg* 65:1256-1259.

Kulkarni K. 2005. Unusual presentation of Sjogren syndrome. *South Med J* 98:1210-1211.

Lang D, Zwerina J, Pieringer H. 2016. IgG4-related disease: Current challenges and future prospects. *Therap Clin Risk Manag* 12:189-199.

Liang Y, Yang Z, Qin B, Zhong R. 2014. Primary Sjogren's Syndrome and malignancy risk: A systematic review and meta-analysis. *Ann Rheum Dis* 73:1151-1156.

Mandel L, Kaynar A. 1994. Sialadenopathy: A clinical herald of sarcoidosis. Report of two cases. *J Oral Maxillofac Surg* 52:1208-1210.

Mandel L, Vakkas J, Saqi A. 2005. Alcoholic (beer) sialosis. *J Oral Maxillofac Surg* 63:402-405.

Marx RE. 1995. Incisional parotid biopsy for diagnosis of systemic disease. *Oral Maxillofac Surg Clin North Am* 7:505-517.

Marx RE, Hartman KS, Rethman KV. 1988. A prospective study comparing incisional labial to incisional parotid biopsies in the detection and confirmation of sarcoidosis, Sjogren's disease, sialosis and lymphoma. *J Rheumatol* 15:621-629.

Morgan WS, Castleman B. 1953. A clinicopathologic study of "Mikulicz's disease" *Am J Pathol* 29:471-503.

Moutsopoulos HM. 1993. In: Schumacher HR (ed.) *Primer on the Rheumatic Diseases*, 10th edn. Atlanta, The Arthritis Foundation, Chapter 15 – Sjogren's Syndrome, 131-135.

Mulholland GB, Jeffery CC, Satija P, Cote DWJ. 2015. Immunoglobulin G4-related diseases in the head and neck: A systematic review. *J Otolaryngol Head Neck Surg* 44:24.

Nessan VJ, Jacoway JR. 1979. Biopsy of minor salivary glands in the diagnosis of sarcoidosis. *N Engl J Med* 301:922-924.

Perez P, Kwon YJ, Alliende C et al. 2005. Increased acinar damage of salivary glands of patients with Sjogren's syndrome is paralleled by simultaneous imbalance of matrix metalloproteinase 3/tissue inhibitor of metalloproteinases 1 and matrix metalloproteinase 9/tissue inhibitor of metalloproteinases 1 ratios. *Arthritis Rheum* 52:2751-2760.

Pijpe J, Kalk WWI, Bootsma H et al. 2007a. Progression of salivary gland dysfunction in patients with Sjogren's syndrome. *Ann Rheum Dis* 66:107-112.

Pijpe J. Kalk WWI, van der Wal JE et al. 2007b. Parotid gland biopsy compared with labial biopsy in the diagnosis of patients with primary Sjogren's syndrome. *Rheumatology* 46:335-341.

Puxeddu I, Capecchi R, Carta F, Tavoni AG, Migliorini P, Puxeddu R. 2018. Salivary gland pathology in IgG4-relarted disease: A comprehensive review. *J Immunol Res* 6936727.

Qin B, Wang J, Yang Z et al. 2015. Epidemiology of primary Sjogren's Syndrome: A systematic review and meta-analysis. *Ann Rheum Dis* 74:1983-1989.

Regezi JA, Sciubba JJ, Jordan RCK. 2003. Oral Pathology, Clinical Pathologic Correlations. In: Regezi JA, Sciuba JJ, Jordan RCK (eds.) *Salivary Gland Diseases*. Philadelphia, WB Saunders, Chapter 8, pp. 183-217.

Reksten TR, Jonsson MV. 2014. Sjogren's syndrome – An update on epidemiology and current insights on pathophysiology. *Oral Maxillofac Surg Clin N Am* 26:1-12.

Scully C, Bagan JV, Eveson JW, Barnard N, Turner FM. 2008. Sialosis: 35 cases of persistent parotid swelling from two countries. *Br J Oral Maxillofac Surg* 46:468-472.

Sodavarapu S, Ghotra GS, Obad N, Goyal M, Gill AS. 2020. IgG4-related diseases – Continues to be a cancer mimicker. *Cereus* 12:e6610.

Stone JH, Zen Y, Deshpande V. 2012. IgG4-related disease. *N Engl J Med* 366:539-551.

Talal N, Bunim J. 1964. The development of malignant lymphoma in the course of Sjogren's syndrome. *Am J Med* 36:529-540.

Turner MD. 2014. Salivary gland disease in Sjogren's syndrome. Sialoadenitis to lymphoma. *Oral Maxillofac Surg Clin N Am* 26:75-81.

Vairaktaris E, Vassiliou S, Yapijakis C et al. 2005. Salivary gland manifestations of sarcoidosis: Report of three cases. *J Oral Maxillofac Surg* 63:1016-1021.

Werning JT. 1991. Infectious and Systemic Diseases. In: Ellis GL, Auclair PL, Gnepp DR (eds.) *Surgical Pathology of the Salivary Glands*. Philadelphia, WB Saunders Co, pp. 39-59.

Zen Y, Nakanuma Y. 2010. IgG4-related disease. A cross-sectional study of 114 cases. *Am J Surg Pathol* 34:1812-1819.

Chapter 7
Salivary Gland Pathology in Children and Adolescents

Outline

Introduction
Nonneoplastic Salivary Gland Lesions
  Mucous Escape Reaction
  Bacterial Sialadenitis
    Acute Submandibular Sialadenitis
    Acute Suppurative Parotitis
    Chronic Juvenile Recurrent Parotitis
Neoplastic Salivary Gland Disease
  Epithelial Tumors
  Mesenchymal Tumors
    Vascular Tumors
    Lymphatic Malformations
    Neural Tumors
  Parotid Tumors
  Submandibular Gland Tumors
  Minor Salivary Gland Tumors
Summary
Case Presentation – *Size Matters*
References

Introduction

Diseases of the salivary glands are rare in the pediatric population. At the time of their 1972 study of 9983 salivary gland lesions accessioned in their system, the Armed Forces Institute of Pathology (AFIP) identified 430 salivary gland lesions in children younger than the age of 15 years, accounting for only 4.3% of the total (Krolls et al. 1972). This series included 262 nonneoplastic lesions (61%), of which there were 185 mucoceles and 67 inflammatory lesions. There were 168 cases of salivary gland tumors (39%) of which 114 were benign (68%) and 54 were malignant (32%). Sixty of the 114 (53%) benign tumors in this series were epithelial in nature and 39 (34%) represented vascular proliferations. The most common benign tumor in this series was the pleomorphic adenoma and the most common malignant tumor was the mucoepidermoid carcinoma. Ellis (1991) reviewed benign and malignant salivary gland tumors in patients under the age of 17 years and compared these numbers to patients of all ages. Children accounted for 4.5% of all patients with salivary gland lesions in their series. A total of 494 salivary gland tumors were reviewed of which 223 were malignant (45%), with 212 (95%) malignant epithelial tumors, and 11 (5%) malignant mesenchymal tumors. There were 271 total benign tumors (55%), of which 210 (78%) were benign epithelial tumors and 61 (22%) were benign mesenchymal tumors. Pleomorphic adenomas accounted for 193 cases (39%) occurring in this age group and 71% of all benign tumors in this series. The pleomorphic adenomas represented only 3.9% of these tumors occurring in all age groups, owing to the greater percentage of other benign tumors occurring in patients younger than 17 years of age. Mucoepidermoid carcinoma accounted for 123 cases (25%) occurring in this age group and 55% of all malignant tumors in this series. Similarly, the mucoepidermoid carcinomas represented only 7.7% of these tumors occurring in all age groups owing to the greater percentage of other malignant tumors occurring in patients younger than 17 years of age.

Craver and Carr (2012) reviewed their 17-year experience with 213 pediatric salivary gland lesions and identified 173 nonneoplastic lesions (81%) of

---

Salivary Gland Pathology: Diagnosis and Management, Third Edition. Edited by Eric R. Carlson and Robert A. Ord.
© 2022 John Wiley & Sons, Inc. Published 2022 by John Wiley & Sons, Inc.
Companion website: www.wiley.com/go/carlson/salivary

which there were 137 mucoceles (64% of total in series) and 26 inflammatory lesions (12% of total in series). There were 40 neoplasms of which 36 (90%) were benign and 4 (10%) were malignant.

Gellrich et al. (2020) performed a retrospective review of the salivary gland pathology of 146 children and adolescents aged 6 months to 17 years. Cases were categorized as juvenile recurrent parotitis ($n = 44$), sialolithiasis ($n = 36$), acute sialadenitis ($n = 32$), and other salivary gland disorders ($n = 34$). The other salivary gland disorders were present in 14 boys and 20 girls. They affected the submandibular gland in 10 cases, the parotid gland in 17 cases, and the sublingual gland in 7 cases. A very diverse set of diagnoses were established, including ranula ($n = 7$), lymphangioma ($n = 6$), parotid cysts ($n = 4$), stricture of the excretory duct ($n = 4$), abscess ($n = 4$), hemangioma ($n = 3$), pleomorphic adenoma ($n = 1$), acinic cell carcinoma ($n = 1$), and other disorders.

In the African pediatric population, mumps is the most common inflammatory salivary gland lesion, but in the developed world, only sporadic cases of mumps are now reported (Ajike and Lakhoo n.d.). These authors also reported that salivary gland neoplasms constituted 10% of all pediatric neoplasms. The majority are reported to be benign with the most common benign neoplasm being the pleomorphic adenoma.

In a series of 2135 patients with tumors of the major salivary glands from 1930 to 1964, 38 patients (1.7%) of 16 years of age and younger were observed to have epithelial tumors (Castro et al. 1972). Thirty-three (87%) of the tumors were in the parotid gland and five tumors (13%) were located in the submandibular gland. The most common malignant tumor was the mucoepidermoid carcinoma and the most common benign tumor was the pleomorphic adenoma. Lack and Upton (1988) reported 80 salivary gland tumors in patients of 18 years of age or younger during a 58-year period from 1928 to 1986. Twenty-five (31%) epithelial tumors were diagnosed and 55 (69%) non-epithelial tumors were diagnosed. The capillary hemangioma was the most common tumor diagnosed in this series, accounting for 27 (34%) of the 80 cases, followed by 19 cases of lymphangioma (24%), 10 cases (12.5%) of pleomorphic adenoma, and 6 cases (7.5%) of mucoepidermoid carcinoma.

Yavvari et al. (2019) probed the US-based Surveillance, Epidemiology, and End Results (SEER-18) database (1973–2014) for secondary malignant neoplasms in the pediatric population (19 years of age or younger). The database identified 99 380 cases of pediatric primary malignancies including 24 403 cases of leukemia. Secondary malignancies were identified in 1803 patients (1.81%). The most common secondary malignancies were leukemia (227 cases), thyroid cancer (217 cases), sarcomas (207 cases), and breast (203 cases). Interestingly, the secondary malignant neoplasms in pediatric leukemia survivors (251 cases) included salivary gland cancers in 18 cases (7.17%). Overall, secondary malignancies developed within 10 years after the primary diagnosis of leukemia in 109 of 251 cases (43.4%), and within 20 years of diagnosis of leukemia in 191 of 251 cases (76.1%). This study reminds the salivary gland surgeon of the possibility of identifying salivary gland cancer as a secondary malignancy in survivors of childhood leukemia.

Nonneoplastic Salivary Gland Lesions

Nonneoplastic salivary gland lesions in children are associated with a wide spectrum of etiologies (Table 7.1). Congenital abnormalities (see

Table 7.1. Inflammatory and infectious diseases of the salivary glands in children.

Bacterial infections
  Acute pyogenic infection
  Recurrent parotitis
  Intraparotid lymphadenopathy
  Mycobacterium tuberculosis
  Nontuberculous mycobacteria
  Cat-scratch disease (Bartonella henselae)
  Actinomycosis

Viral infections
  Paromyxovirus (mumps)
  Coxsackie A and B
  Echovirus
  Influenza A
  Cytomegalovirus (CMV)
  Epstein–Barr virus (EBV)
  Human immunodeficiency virus (HIV)

Noninfectious disorders
  Sarcoidosis
  Sjögren syndrome
  Pseudolymphomas

Chapter 17), acute and chronic suppurative infections and other inflammatory disorders, obstruction, neoplastic disease, and degenerative disorders should be considered as part of a differential diagnosis for a child with salivary gland swelling (Figure 7.1). These pathologic entities are less common and have a different incidence in children compared to adults (Tasca and Clarke 2011). Inflammatory disorders of the salivary glands in children may be infectious or noninfectious. Infectious disorders may involve the parenchyma of the salivary gland as a sialadenitis, or the intrasalivary gland lymph nodes as occuring in mycobacterium tuberculosis or nontuberculous mycobacteria. Noninfectious inflammatory disease tends to involve multiple salivary glands as occuring in Sjögren syndrome and sarcoidosis as a pansialadenitis. Infectious disorders more commonly involve a single gland as occuring in an acute suppurative parotitis, or a pair of major glands as most commonly occurs in mumps parotitis.

MUCOUS ESCAPE REACTION

The diagnosis and treatment of mucoceles and ranulas have been discussed in detail in Chapter 4. That notwithstanding, there are some additional comments that can be made about these lesions in pediatric patients. In terms of their peak incidence of occurrence, studies have identified that the mucocele and ranula are most commonly diagnosed in the first and second decades of life. Specifically, the report of Hayashida et al. (2010) analyzed 173 cases of mucocele and found that 132 cases (76%) occurred in the first or second decades of life with 49% of the mucoceles occurring in the second decade of life. Bhargava et al. (2014) have presented a case of a mucocele of the lower lip in an 11-month-old patient. Syebele and Butow (2010) reviewed 50 cases of mucoceles and noted that 62% were diagnosed in the first two decades of life. Of particular interest in this paper is that 48 of the 50 patients were tested for HIV infection and 33 patients (68%) were HIV-positive and 10 of these patients were younger than 10 years of age.

In terms of treatment, some authors have historically recommended a five- to six-month observation period for the ranula in pediatric patients after which time patients should undergo surgical intervention (Pandit and Park 2002; Zhi et al. 2008). Seo et al. (2010) reviewed 17 pediatric patients with symptomatic ranulas that exceeded 2 cm in diameter who underwent surgical excision of the ranula and offending sublingual gland. All patients had been observed for 3–14 months prior to being offered surgical intervention, and none of the cases underwent spontaneous resolution. In fact, in two cases, the ranula increased in size. The authors concluded that a lengthy presurgical observation period is not necessary in terms of surgical decision-making for pediatric patients with ranulas.

BACTERIAL SIALADENITIS

Bacterial sialadenitis is a relatively rare disease in children. It most frequently involves the parotid gland. Newborn children, those with preexisting immunodeficiency such as those receiving chemotherapy and children with severe dental and gingival infections are particularly at risk. Physical examination will reveal pain and swelling in the affected salivary gland. In a retrospective review of 118 patients aged 18 years and younger with parotid swellings, 75 patients (64%) had neoplasms and 43 patients (36%) had infectious or inflammatory lesions (Orvidas et al. 2000). Overall, 84% of the lesions in this series were benign. The ratio of neoplastic lesions to nonneoplastic swellings of the parotid gland of 1.74:1 in this pediatric population is noticeably different from that of most adult populations of 2.68:1 (Gallia and Johnson 1981). Parotid swellings in children, therefore, are more likely to be infectious/inflammatory compared to parotid swellings in adults that are more likely to be neoplastic.

Acute Submandibular Sialadenitis

Acute submandibular sialadenitis is a rare condition in pediatric patients (Figure 7.2). In their 30-year study of sialadenitis in patients up to 16 years of age, Kaban et al. (1978) identified 49 patients requiring 67 hospitalizations. Four distinct types of sialadenitis were diagnosed, including 18 patients with acute suppurative parotitis, 14 patients with recurrent parotitis, 9 patients with chronic parotitis, and 8 patients with acute submandibular sialadenitis. Obstruction of Wharton duct was the etiology of all eight cases of acute submandibular sialadenitis, seven of which involved sialolithiasis, and one of which involved a congenital ductal stenosis. All patients with sialolithiasis underwent submandibular gland excision, and the one patient with congenital stenosis underwent a

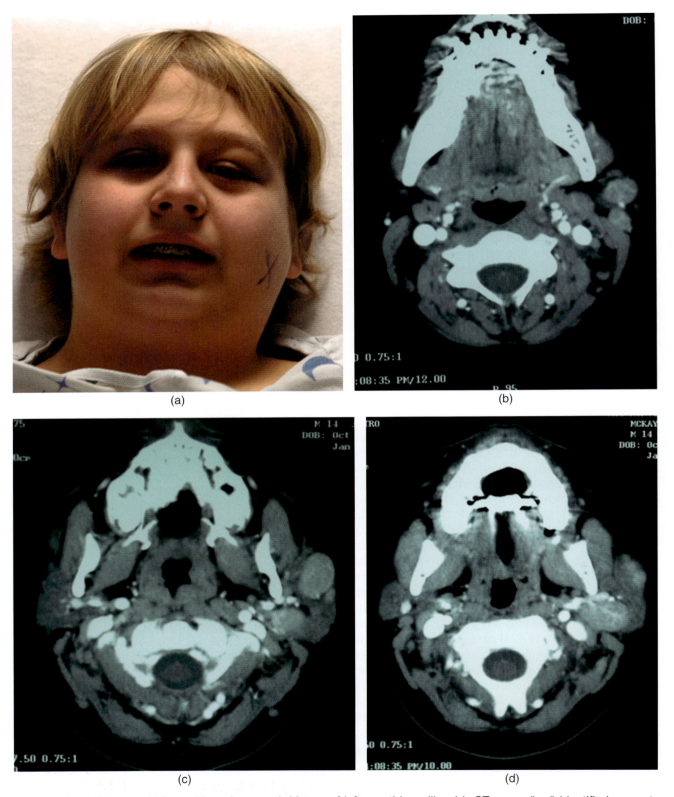

Figure 7.1. A 14-year-old boy with a nine-month history of left parotid swelling (a). CT scans (b–d) identified separate masses of the superficial and deep lobes of the left parotid gland. The patient underwent total parotidectomy with dissection and preservation of the facial nerve (e).

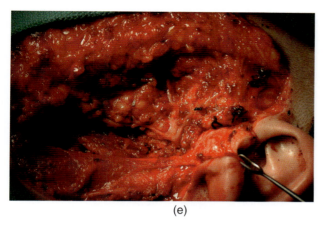

(e)

Figure 7.1 (*Continued*).

reconstructive duct procedure. As in adult patients, submandibular sialadenitis in pediatric patients should be first evaluated with radiographs to rule out the presence of a sialolith. If present, expedient removal should be undertaken. In a review of pediatric sialoliths vs. adult sialoliths, Chung et al. (2007) found that stones were more likely to be smaller and in the distal duct in children. They recommended careful bimanual palpation for diagnosis and intraoral stone removal in most children. Similar findings in radiological imaging of pediatric patients with salivary stones have been reported (Salerno et al. 2011). The long-term outcome for

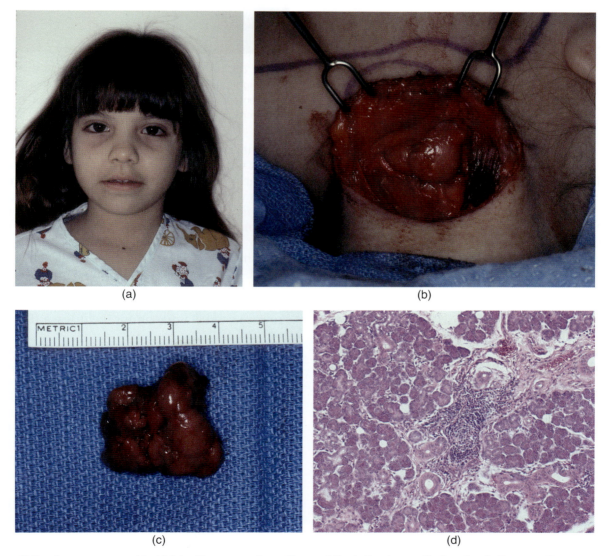

Figure 7.2. A seven-year-old girl (a) with recurrent swellings of the left submandibular gland. Conservative mseasures were undertaken initially without success. She was therefore subjected to excision of the left submandibular gland (b and c). Histopathology identified mild sialadenitis of the submandibular gland (d).

children who had intraoral stone removal is excellent with 82.4% "symptom free" (Woo et al. 2009).

An alternative to surgery is lithotripsy which has been undertaken in children with sialolithiasis. In one series of seven children, extracorporeal electromagnetic shock wave lithotripsy achieved complete stone disintegration in five cases and in two cases a residual fragment <2 mm was seen on US monitoring. The mean number of sessions to achieve this result was five (Ottaviani et al. 2001). Sialendoscopy has also been used both as a diagnostic and therapeutic procedure in children with salivary stones (Nahieli et al. 2000).

If a sialolith is not identified, medical management should be performed, including proper hydration and empiric antibiotic therapy. Severe cases of sialadenitis, those cases where questionable parental compliance exists, or immunocompromised patients will require inpatient therapy. Mild cases in otherwise healthy patients with effective parental support can be effectively managed on an outpatient basis. The development of chronic submandibular sialadenitis is not anticipated in pediatric patients as commonly occuring in adults.

Acute Suppurative Parotitis

Acute parotitis in children and infants (Figure 7.3) is primarily due to salivary stasis, and the most common responsible organisms are *Staphylococcus aureus and Streptococcus viridans*. As with adults, treatment of acute parotitis in children is primarily medical and involves hydration, sialagogues, and gentle massaging of the gland. In severe cases, intravenous antibiotics are required and surgical drainage may be necessary.

Chronic Juvenile Recurrent Parotitis

Chronic juvenile recurrent parotitis is defined as recurrent parotid inflammation and is generally associated with nonobstructive sialectasia of the parotid gland (Chitre and Premchandra 1997). Next to mumps, chronic recurrent parotitis is the most common inflammatory salivary gland disease in childhood and adolescence (Ellies and Laskawi 2010 The disease is more common in males, characterized by recurring episodes of swelling and/or pain in the parotid gland and is commonly accompanied by fever and malaise (Figure 7.4). There is typically an absence of pus

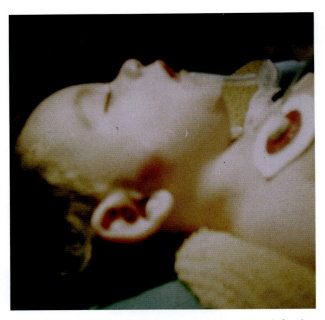

Figure 7.3. A baby with an acute suppurative infection of the right parotid gland. It was thought that this infection represented hematogenous spread of a distant infection to an intraparotid lymph node.

and the swelling lasts from several days to two weeks with spontaneous resolution. The number of attacks varies although the most common pattern is an attack every three to four months. The frequency rate peaks during the first year at school, and commonly symptoms usually subside or completely disappear after puberty (Chitre and Premchandra 1997). Clinical diagnosis can be confirmed by ultrasound that shows sialectasis or sialography showing sialectasis and ductal kinking (Nahlieli et al. 2004). In the acute phase, serum amylase can be a marker for the disease (Saarinen et al. 2013).

Treatment for this condition has historically been without universal acceptance primarily due to the uncertainty regarding its etiology as well as the rarity of the disease (Garavello et al. 2018). As such, treatment of the acute episode has been centered on relief of pain and an attempt at preventing damage to the parenchyma of the gland. Antibiotics have been found to result in rapid decrease in swelling. Sialendoscopy is also of benefit in the management of chronic recurrent parotitis in children. Hackett et al. (2012) reported on 18 pediatric patients who underwent a total of 33 sialendoscopic procedures on 27 glands. Chronic recurrent parotitis was the most frequent indication for

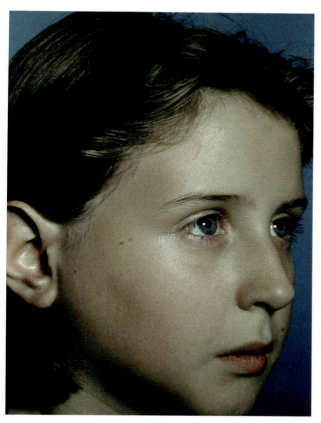

Figure 7.4. A six-year-old girl with recurrent right parotid swelling indicative of chronic recurrent parotitis.

surgery, with 12 children represented (67%) and 19 glands involved. Three patients had recurrent symptoms after the first sialendoscopy. Eight patients required only one procedure to address their symptoms, two patients required two procedures, one patient required parotidectomy, and one patient was lost to follow-up. The authors concluded that sialendoscopy is both diagnostic and therapeutic for a clinical diagnosis of chronic recurrent parotitis. Shacham et al. (2009) reported on 70 children with chronic recurrent parotitis and 5 adult patients who had chronic parotitis similar to the children in this study. All patients underwent sialendoscopy with lavage and dilatation and endoscopic injection of hydrocortisone into the gland. In 93% of patients, a single endoscopic evaluation resulted in resolution of this disease and prevented its recurrence. In a comprehensive review of the literature on the use of sialendoscopy in the management of juvenile recurrent parotitis, Canzi et al. (2013) identified 10 research series that they included in their review with a total of 179 children, average age of 7.8 years and 109 males. The most relevant diagnostic finding with sialedoscopy was white wall appearance of the duct with absent vascularity (75%). In all reports, the treatment was effective, with complete cure in 78% of cases or improvement with frequency reduction in 22%. Only 14% of children had a second or more procedures. Follow-up time for these reports was short with a range of 4–36 months. Ramakrishna et al. (2015) similarly demonstrated the effectiveness and safety of sialendoscopy for the management of juvenile recurrent parotitis in their systematic review and meta-analysis.

While the cause of chronic juvenile recurrent parotitis remains unclear, genetic, infectious (recurrent viral), allergic and immune-mediated are all possible etiologies. Maynard (1965) proposed that a low salivary flow rate due to dehydration results in a low-grade inflammation of the gland and duct epithelium. This in turn results in distortion and stricture of the distal ducts and metaplasia of the duct epithelium. Thereafter, the metaplasia results in excessive mucous secretion. These changes, along with a further reduction in salivary flow rate then predispose the gland to recurrent inflammation. A reduced salivary flow rate may result from glandular damage caused by a primary infection in the gland. That notwithstanding, the reduced salivary flow rate may be the primary factor in the pathogenesis of the disease. Maynard (1965) pointed out that the salivary flow rate was reduced in even the unaffected parotid gland in patients with unilateral disease.

Neoplastic Salivary Gland Disease

Salivary gland tumors are rare in children and include epithelial and mesenchymal, benign and malignant neoplasms. Fewer than 5% of salivary gland neoplasms develop in pediatric patients (Gontarz et al. 2018). Gontarz et al. (2018) indicated that the incidence of malignant epithelial tumors of the salivary glands in pediatric patients is 0.8 cases per 1 million children and adolescents. A review of their incidence is noted in Table 7.2 that demonstrates significant differences in the incidence and anatomic distribution of tumors in adult and pediatric populations. The 1991 AFIP data showed that children accounted for only 4.5% of all patients with salivary gland tumors. Mixed tumors, mucoepidermoid carcinomas, and acinic

Table 7.2. Comparison of the reported incidence of epithelial salivary gland neoplasms in pediatric and adult populations.

Incidence	Pediatric 3–4/million/year (%)	Adult 80/million/year (%)
• Percentage of all salivary tumors	5	90
Benign	50	80
Malignant	50	20
• Percentage of all salivary gland tumors occurring in the parotid gland	85	82
Benign	48	90
Malignant	52	10
• Percentage of all salivary gland tumors occurring in the submandibular gland	11	8
Benign	33	67
Malignant	67	33
• Percentage of all salivary gland tumors occurring in the sublingual gland	3	1
Benign	85	2
Malignant	15	98
• Percentage of all salivary gland tumors occurring in the minor salivary glands	1	8
Benign	50	60
Malignant	50	40

Source: Adapted from Bradley and Hartley (2011).

et al. 1991). The benign and malignant epithelial salivary gland tumors together account for approximately 85% of all salivary gland tumors reported in children (Ellis et al. 1991). The slight preponderance of benign tumors (55%) in pediatric patients is lower than the 63% incidence of benign salivary gland tumors in all patients in the AFIP data (Ellis et al. 1991). This observation that malignant tumors are relatively more common than benign tumors in pediatric patients suggests that the pathogenesis of salivary gland tumors in pediatric patients might be different from that of adults. A genetic predisposition for cancer may be suggested in one series in which 4 of 17 pediatric salivary cancers (23.5%) were second cancers occurring six to nine years after the first primary cancer (Chiaravali et al. 2014).

Gontarz et al. (2018) retrospectively reviewed the charts of 776 patients with salivary gland tumors, 640 of which were primary epithelial salivary gland neoplasms. Nineteen tumors developed in pediatric patients and 621 tumors were treated in adult patients older than 19 years of age. Major and minor salivary glands were affected nearly equally in pediatric patients, 52.6 and 47.7%, respectively. The distribution of major and minor salivary gland tumors in adults was 73.6 and 26.4%, respectively. Benign salivary gland tumors were noted in 10/19 pediatric patients (52.6%), while 436 of 621 tumors (70.2%) were benign in the adult patients. All pediatric benign tumors were pleomorphic adenomas and the most common benign tumor in adults was also the pleomorphic adenoma. A different distribution of malignant tumors was found when comparing the two age groups. The most common malignant tumor in pediatric patients was the mucoepidermoid carcinoma, while adenoid cystic carcinoma was the most common salivary gland malignancy in adult patients.

EPITHELIAL TUMORS

Malignant epithelial salivary gland tumors are relatively more common in children (40–60% of total) than in adults (20–30%). In the series of 494 total salivary gland tumors in children by Ellis et al. (1991), 422 (85%) were epithelial in nature and 72 (15%) were mesenchymal. This series included 271 benign tumors of which 210 (78%) were epithelial and 223 malignant tumors of which 212 cell adenocarcinomas accounted for over 92% of all epithelial tumors and about 77% of all tumors in this age group. In this series, and that of others (Krolls et al. 1972; Lack and Upton 1988; Laikui et al. 2008; Yoshida et al. 2014), mucoepidermoid carcinoma is the most common salivary gland malignancy in children. The mixed tumor is the most common benign salivary gland tumor in children in large series (Krolls et al. 1972; Ellis

(95%) were epithelial. In these pediatric patients, the pleomorphic adenoma was the most common tumor overall, accounting for 193 (39%) of the 494 pediatric tumors and 3.9% of all similar tumors occurring in all age groups owing to the greater frequency of the diagnosis of the pleomorphic adenoma in adult patients. These 193 pleomorphic adenomas represented 92% of the 210 benign epithelial tumors and 71% of the total combined benign epithelial and benign mesenchymal tumors. The Warthin tumor was the second most common benign epithelial tumor but accounted for only five cases (2.4% of benign epithelial tumors).

The mucoepidermoid carcinoma was the most common malignant tumor in the AFIP series (Ellis et al. 1991), accounting for 123 cases. These represented 58% of the 212 total number of malignant epithelial tumors and 55% of the 223 total number of malignant tumors in this series. The acinic cell adenocarcinoma was the second most common epithelial malignancy in this series (31%) and the third most common tumor overall in this series (25%).

Techavichit et al. (2016) performed a retrospective analysis of mucoepidermoid carcinoma of the salivary glands in children. They identified 14 cases that were in the submandibular gland in 4 cases, the parotid gland in 4 cases, the palate in 3 cases, and the tracheobronchial tree in 3 cases. Nine tumors were intermediate grade, three tumors were high grade, and two tumors were low grade. All patients underwent surgical treatment and three patients with major gland tumors underwent postoperative radiation therapy. One patient had cervical lymph node involvement and no patients developed distant metastases. The authors indicated that postoperative radiation therapy should be considered only in locally aggressive, high-grade tumors with incomplete resection due to the risks of craniofacial growth disturbances and the potential for secondary malignant disease.

In their series of 80 salivary gland tumors in children, Lack and Upton (1988) identified 25 epithelial tumors (31%), of which 10 were pleomorphic adenomas (40%), 6 were mucoepidermoid carcinomas (24%), and 5 were acinic cell carcinomas (20%). The pleomorphic adenomas were in the parotid gland in five cases, in the submandibular gland in four cases, and in the soft palate in one case. The mucoepidermoid carcinomas were in the parotid gland in five cases and in the premaxillary soft tissues in one case. The acinic cell carcinomas were in the parotid gland in all five cases. In China, pleomorphic adenoma was 91.45% of benign childhood tumors and mucoepidermoid carcinoma was 47.1% of malignant tumors (Fang Og et al. 2013).

Regarding survival, using SEER data (763 patients < 30 years old) and a Kaplan–Meier analysis, the relative five-year survival was 100% for < 1-year-old patients (only one patient), 50% in the 1–4-year-olds group, 87.2% in the 5–9-year-olds, 97% among the 10–14-year-olds, and 95% among 15–19-year-olds (Rutt et al. 2011). Favorable outcomes were also reported by Kuperman et al. (2010). In his series of 61 patients, 83% were parotid tumors and 46% were mucoepidermoid carcinomas. Cervical metastases were found in 37% of children and 75% underwent surgery with radiation given in 45% of cases. Overall, five-year survival rate was 93%, and 26% developed a recurrence. Predictors for poor outcome were margin status, tumor grade, and neural involvement. In a population-based study comparing adult and pediatric salivary cancers, the commonest tumor was mucoepidermoid carcinoma in each group. However, children had tumors with more favorable features and staging (76 vs. 50%), better differentiated tumors (88 vs. 49%), and a five-year overall survival of 95% ± 1.55 compared to 59% ± 0.55 for adults (Sultan et al. 2011).

Daoud et al. (2020) have described two cases of pediatric Warthin-like mucoepidermoid carcinoma. This tumor was originally described by Ishibashi et al. (2015) who identified 15 tumors that had originally been described as metaplastic Warthin tumors, among a total of 107 Warthin tumors. These authors looked for the *CRTC1–MAML2* fusion transcripts that characterize approximately 50% of mucoepidermoid carcinomas. This gene fusion occurs exclusively in mucoepidermoid carcinomas and most commonly in low- and intermediate-grade cancers with a favorable prognosis. In the study of Ishibashi et al. (2015), 5 of 15 cases of metaplastic Warthin tumor identified the *CRTC1–MAML2* fusion and designated these tumors as Warthin-like mucoepidermoid carcinomas. The authors speculated that the tumors developed de novo from normal epithelium. These five cases of Warthin-like mucoepidermoid carcinoma occurred in adult patients. In Daoud et al.'s report, the two cases of Warthin-like mucoepidermoid carcinoma occurred in teenage patients, and both tumors were in the parotid gland. The authors confirmed the presence of the *CRTC1–MAMLS2* gene fusion, thereby confirming the presence of Warthin-like mucoepidermoid carcinoma. Since the Warthin tumor is exceedingly rare in young patients, the observation of a Warthin-like appearance in a salivary gland tumor should alert the pathologist to the possible existence of a Warthin-like mucoepidermoid carcinoma.

MESENCHYMAL TUMORS

Mesenchymal salivary gland tumors are much more commonly noted in children than in adults. Ellis (1991) found 40 hemangiomas among 61 benign mesenchymal tumors (66%) and 72 benign and malignant mesenchymal tumors (56%). Lack and Upton (1988) found 27 hemangiomas in their series of 80 pediatric salivary gland tumors (34%) that represented 49% of their 55 mesenchymal tumors.

Vascular Tumors

Vascular salivary gland tumors in children typically occur in the parotid gland, are most commonly noted at or soon after birth, and are more frequent in females (Lack and Upton 1988; Ord 2004). In general, vascular tumors are classified as hemangioendotheliomas that occur in patients younger than six months of age with rapid growth and aggressive behavior (Figure 7.5). Hemangiomas are slower growing processes that occur in older children. Krolls et al. (1972) described the hemangioendothelioma as an immature hemangioma. Such tumors are characterized by a unique tripartite growth cycle of proliferation, plateau, and involution. Although most involute without intervention, many require medical or surgical treatment. Krolls et al. (1972) reported that the parotid gland was involved in 37 of their 39 vascular lesions. In Lack and Upton's (1988) series of 27 cases of hemangioma, all of which occurred in the parotid gland, 19 occurred in females, and 8 occurred in males. A decided left-side laterality was realized with a five-times-greater occurrence of the hemangioma of the left parotid gland compared to the right parotid gland. A median age of 4 months with the oldest child being 16 months of age was noted in this series. Clinical findings

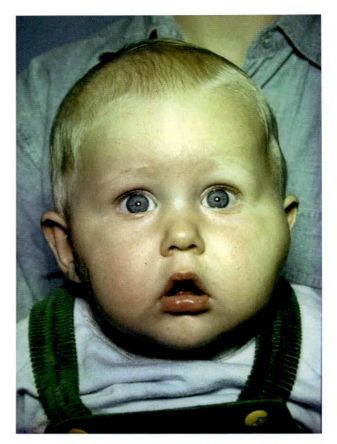

Figure 7.5. A four-month-old infant with left parotid swelling related to a hemangioendothelioma.

include a soft, compressible mass with a bluish hue to the skin. Regression and involution of rapidly growing infantile hemangioendotheliomas of the parotid gland has been reported (Scarcella et al. 1965), although parotid lesions may be associated with slower involution or scarring (Drolet et al. 1999). Following involution, phleboliths may develop and can be seen radiographically in older children (Figure 7.6).

Management of parotid hemangioendotheliomas has evolved as the natural history and behavior have become better understood. Radiation therapy was once used successfully for rapidly growing tumors in infants; however, the observation of late secondary malignancies in irradiated children has resulted in the abandonment of this modality of treatment. Surgical excision became the mainstay of treatment for many years and is occasionally still required. Excision of these lesions in infants and young children incurs a high risk for

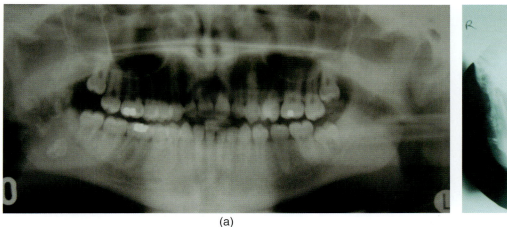
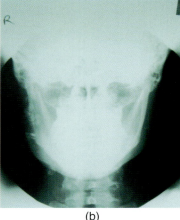

Figure 7.6. An 18-year-old patient with calcifications superimposed over the right mandibular ramus on panoramic (a) and posterior–anterior (b) radiographs. The radiographs confirm the presence of phleboliths of the right parotid gland, indicative of a hemangioma of this gland.

complications including death, facial nerve palsy, and recurrence of the tumor. As such, most authors now recommend nonoperative management for infants based on the anticipated spontaneous regression of these tumors.

In childhood hemangiomas, the efficacy of systemic corticosteroid therapy is well documented (Enjolras et al. 1990; Gangopadhyay et al. 1997) and interferon alfa-2a and alfa-2b have been used successfully (Ezekowitz et al. 1992; Soumekh et al. 1996). That said, a shift toward the use of β-blockers in infantile hemangiomas has occurred as a standard of care (Puttgen 2014). Propranolol is widely accepted to be a safer and better tolerated drug than oral corticosteroids. There is evidence that the use of propranolol is also distinguished from oral corticosteroids in its effectiveness in treating infants who are beyond the proliferative phase of growth. The proposed mechanism of action of propranolol includes rapid vasoconstriction of the lesion. Inhibition of angiogenesis by downregulation of proangiogenic growth factors such as vascular endothelial growth factor, basic fibroblast growth factor, and matrix metalloproteinases 2 and 9 seems to correspond to growth arrest. Finally, the hastening of the induction of apoptosis of endothelial cells has been proposed to result in the stimulation of regression of infantile hemangiomas. Surgical resection is reserved for those tumors that do not respond to medical therapy (Figure 7.7).

Lymphatic Malformations

Lack and Upton (1988) reported 19 children with a diagnosis of lymphangioma involving salivary glands. These presented occasionally as a primary focus of involvement, but more commonly with more extensive involvement of juxta-glandular soft tissues and secondary enclavement of the salivary gland (Figure 7.8). These 19 lymphangiomas were the second most common mesenchymal tumor in their series of which 27 cases of hemangioma were most commonly noted. The lymphangiomas were six times more common in females with a median age of six years and equal distribution on each side of the neck. In their series of 494 pediatric salivary gland tumors, Ellis (1991) identified only 5 cases of lymphangioma among 61 total benign mesenchymal tumors that also included 40 cases of hemangioma.

Treatment recommendations of the salivary lymphangioma have included observation, injection of sclerosing agents, and conservative surgery. Sclerosing agents are most successful in those lesions that have large cystic spaces. Surgical excision with the preservation of the facial nerve in the case of a parotid lymphangioma will likely not completely remove the abnormal lymphatic channels and microcysts. This notwithstanding, this debulking procedure proves to be clinically effective in controlling the disease (Ord 2004).

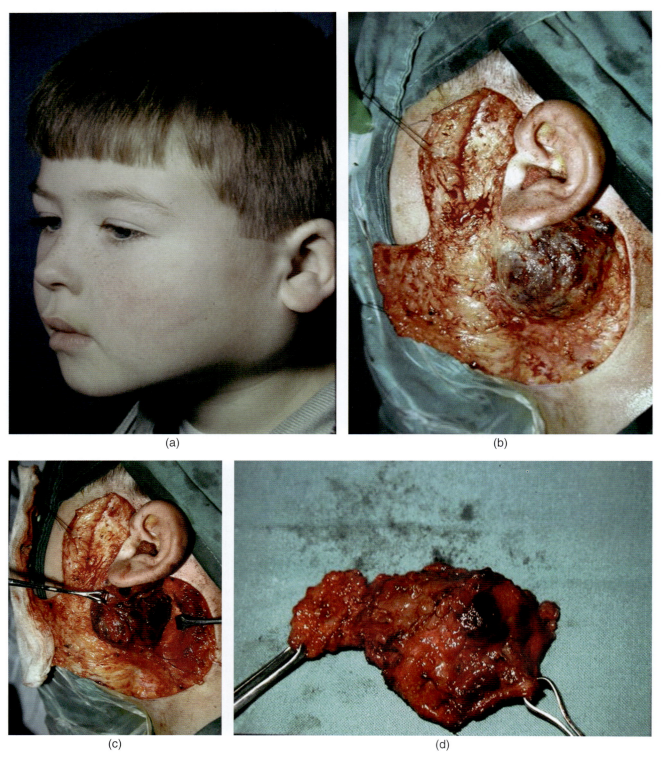

Figure 7.7. A three-year-old boy (a) with left parotid swelling that is soft and compressible. The overlying skin has a subtle blue hue, indicative of a hemangioma. The angiogram supported this diagnosis. The patient underwent left superficial parotidectomy (b and c). The specimen is noted in (d).

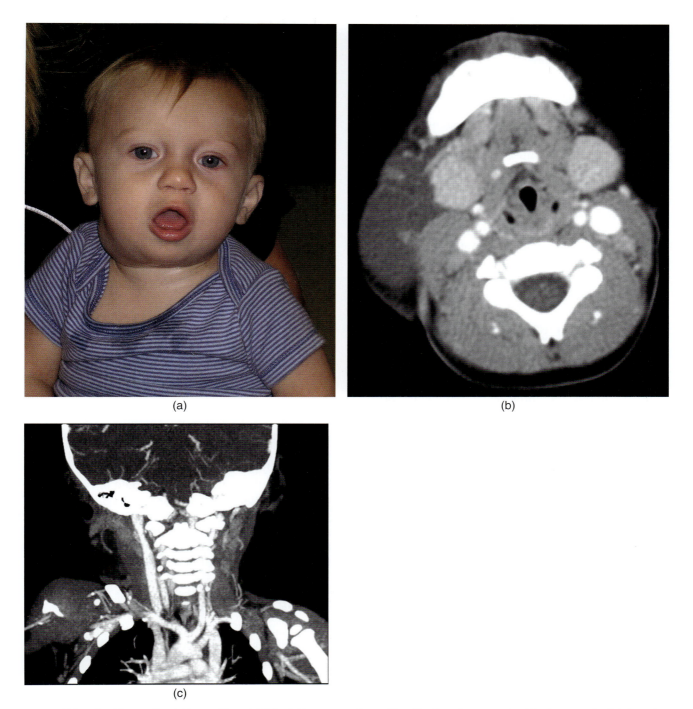

Figure 7.8. An 11-month-old boy with a right facial/upper neck swelling that has been present for two weeks (a). Imaging with CT (b and c) identified a 4-cm mass with intimate association with the submandibular and parotid glands. The patient underwent excision of the mass and lymphangioma was diagnosed.

Neural Tumors

Neural tumors of the salivary glands can be categorized as neurofibromas, neurilemmomas, and manifestations of neurofibromatosis (Ord 2004). Lack and Upton (1988) reported six patients with neural tumors involving the major salivary glands, four tumors involving the parotid gland, and one case each involving the submandibular gland and sublingual gland. The most common clinical setting was neurofibromatosis with the corresponding neural tumor being a plexiform neurofibroma. Ellis et al. (1991) reported 10 neural tumors, 7 cases of neurofibroma, and 3 cases of schwannoma. Complete removal of neurofibromas can be very difficult due to their highly infiltrative nature, such that debulking with preservation of normal anatomy is preferred (Figure 7.9).

PAROTID TUMORS

In their review of the Salivary Gland Register from 1965 to 1984 at the University of Hamburg, Seifert et al. (1986) reported on 9883 cases of salivary gland pathology including 3326 neoplasms, 80 of which occurred in children. Fifty-seven (71%) of these tumors developed in the parotid gland. Pleomorphic adenoma accounts for virtually all of the benign pediatric neoplasms occurring in the parotid gland with the Warthin's tumor representing a minor contribution at this anatomic site. In 166 children with epithelial parotid tumors, 93 (55%) were benign and 73 (45%) were malignant (Ord 2004). Of the 73 malignancies, 47 (64%) were mucoepidermoid carcinomas and 17 (23%) were acinic cell carcinomas. This relative incidence of mucoepidermoid carcinomas and acinic cell carcinomas of the parotid gland in children is distinguished from the near equal incidence of these malignancies in the parotid gland in adult patients in the AFIP data (Ellis et al. 1991). Finally, although the parotid gland is a less common site for salivary gland tumors in children compared to adults, there is a greater chance for malignancy in children.

The workup of a child with a parotid swelling does not differ significantly from that of an adult. Once inflammatory disease has been ruled out, a fine needle aspiration biopsy of a discrete parotid mass in a child is useful to establish its cytologic character (Lee et al. 2013). Structural imaging is also valuable to establish the anatomic extent of the tumor. Superficial parotidectomy or partial superficial parotidectomy with facial nerve identification and preservation are the procedures of choice for pediatric parotid tumors. Facial nerve sacrifice is only performed when preoperative palsy is noted to exist or when nerve invasion is appreciated intraoperatively. The facial nerve is more superficial in infants younger than four months of age compared to older children due to the lack of development of the mastoid process (Ord 2004). Neck dissection is performed for high-grade malignancies or when evidence of metastatic adenopathy is present.

SUBMANDIBULAR GLAND TUMORS

As in adults, submandibular gland tumors are very uncommon in pediatric patients. Of 168 salivary gland tumors in the series of Krolls et al. (1972), submandibular gland tumors included 3 lymphomas, 4 mucoepidermoid carcinomas, and 10 benign tumors. While there were 12 acinic cell carcinomas in this series, none occurred in the submandibular gland. Lack and Upton (1988) similarly identified their five cases of acinic cell carcinoma exclusively present in the parotid gland, but they identified no cases of mucoepidermoid carcinoma in the submandibular gland. These authors identified 4 of 10 cases of pleomorphic adenoma occurring in the submandibular gland. In Castro's series of 38 major salivary gland tumors, 5 were noted to occur in the submandibular gland. These included four cases of pleomorphic adenoma and one case of malignant mixed tumor. The treatment of submandibular gland tumors in children includes excision of the submandibular gland and tumor en bloc.

MINOR SALIVARY GLAND TUMORS

Minor salivary gland tumors in children are rare. Population studies have demonstrated that only 5% of minor salivary gland tumors occur in children, with a near equal distribution of benign and malignant tumors (Galer et al. 2012). In their study of 35 minor salivary gland tumors in children, Galer et al. (2012) identified 22 cases of mucoepidermoid carcinoma, 9 cases of adenoid cystic carcinoma, and 4 cases of adenocarcinoma. Thirty-one of the malignancies were low-intermediate grade. Twenty of the tumors were classified as occurring in the oral cavity and 13 were classified as occurring in the hard palate. These authors found an

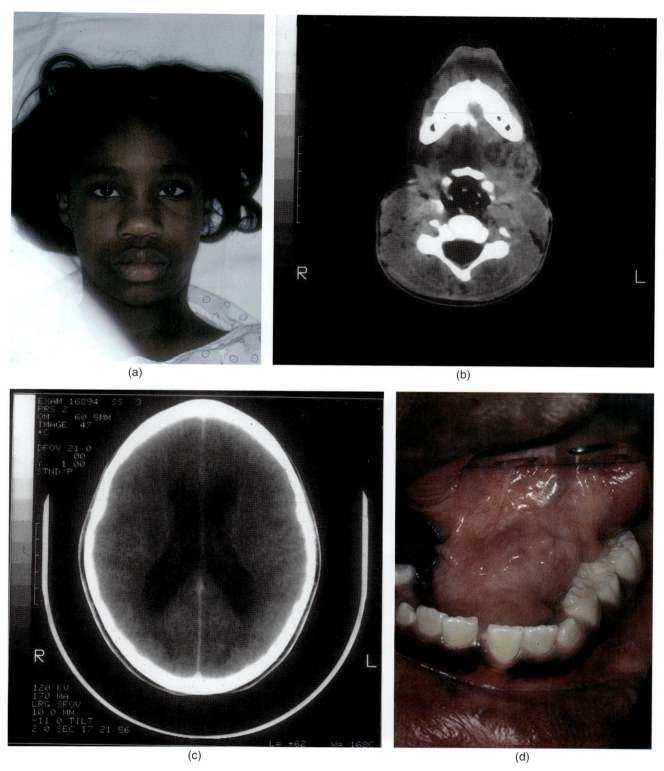

Figure 7.9. An eight-year-old girl (a) with left submandibular swelling that had been present for six months. Imaging with CT identified an ill-defined mass of the submandibular gland region (b) as well as hydrocephalus (c). Oral examination (d) showed fullness in the left sublingual space. With a differential diagnosis of neurofibroma, the patient underwent a debulking of this lesion (e and f). Histopathology identified a plexiform neurofibroma (g), indicative of neurofibromatosis. The patient did well postoperatively as noted at her two-year visit (h and i). No reaccumulation of the tumor was noted on physical examination.

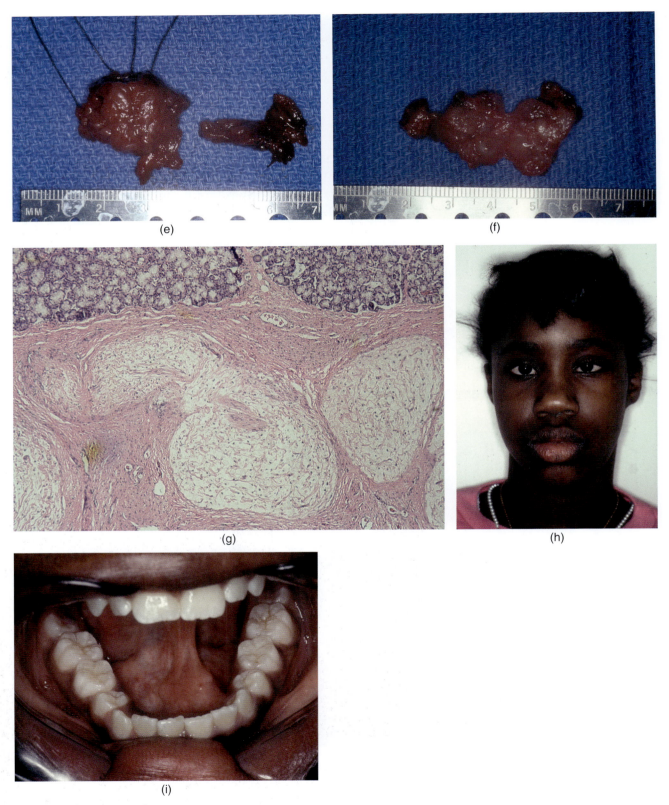

Figure 7.9. (Continued).

excellent prognosis for their patients with an overall survival of 88.4% and disease-free survival of 89.3% at five years. Preferred treatment is identical to that of adult's diagnosis for diagnosis. In the author's unpublished series of 275 minor salivary gland tumors, 12 (4.3%) were pediatric cases (age 9–19). Ten cases were malignant (83.3%), of which 7 (70%) were mucoepidermoid carcinomas and 9 of the 12 tumors were located in the palate (75%).

A mucoepidermoid carcinoma of the palate in a child should undergo structural imaging and excision of the tumor with appropriate anatomic barrier inclusion on the deep aspect of the tumor (Figure 7.10). Unless the

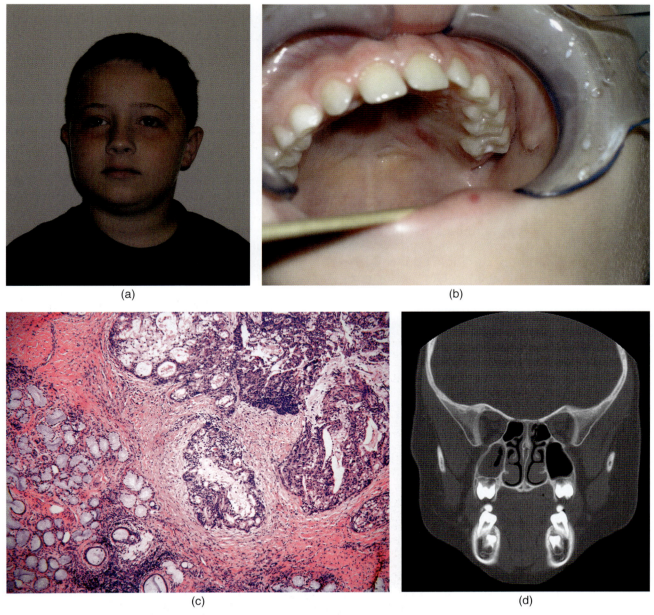

Figure 7.10. A nine-year-old boy (a) with a mass of the left hard–soft palate junction (b). Incisional biopsy identified low-grade mucoepidermoid carcinoma. Imaging with CT (c) showed no bone erosion of the hard palate, such that the patient underwent wide local excision of his cancer (d). Final histopathology (e) identified intermediate-grade mucoepidermoid carcinoma (hematoxylin and eosin, original magnification ×100).

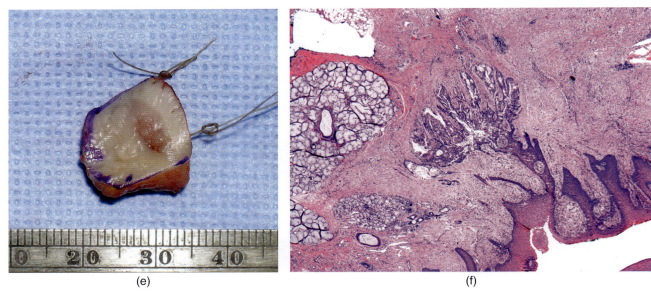

Figure 7.10. (Continued).

bone is clinically or radiologically involved, the bone does not require resection for low-grade mucoepidermoid carcinoma in children (Caccamese and Ord 2002). The periosteum appears to be an effective oncologic barrier, and its inclusion on the deep surface of the tumor permits a margin-free cancer surgery with high rates of cure.

The surgical management of benign palatal salivary gland tumors, like that of malignant salivary gland tumors, is identical to those surgeries performed in adult patients (Figure 7.11). Specifically, the inclusion of the periosteum on the deep surface of the tumor provides effective cure of these benign tumors. The superiorly located maxillary bone need not be included with the tumor specimen.

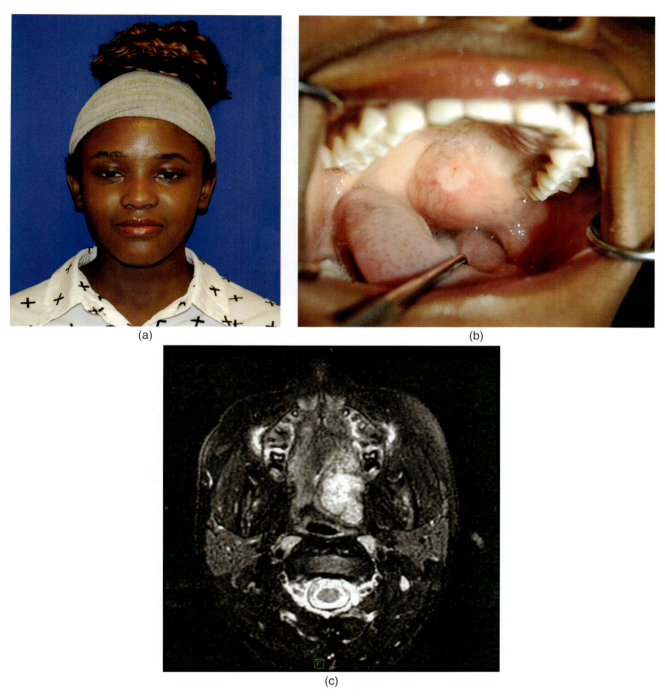

Figure 7.11. A 12-year-old girl (a) with a long history of a slowly growing mass of the palate (b). Axial T2-weighted MRI (c) identifies a hyperintense multilobulated mass consistent with a pleomorphic adenoma that was confirmed by incisional biopsy. Source: Dr John Caccamese.

Summary

- Salivary gland lesions are rare in the pediatric population that is variably defined in terms of age.
- The mucocele is the most common salivary gland lesion encountered in pediatric patients.
- Mumps has historically been the most common form of sialadenitis diagnosed in children.
- Chronic recurrent parotitis is the second most common form of sialadenitis in children.
- The pleomorphic adenoma is the most common pediatric salivary gland tumor and the most common benign tumor in children. Together with the hemangioma, these benign tumors account for nearly 90% of all benign salivary gland tumors in children.
- The mucoepidermoid carcinoma is the most common malignant pediatric salivary gland tumor. Together with the acinic cell carcinoma, these two malignant tumors account for approximately 60% of malignant salivary gland tumors in children.

Case Presentation – *Size Matters*

A 16-year-old girl was treated by her private oral surgeon for a palatal lesion in December 2004. The office notes from that time indicated that there was a "small mass with a bluish tinge in the right palate." This lesion was "excised" on December 15, 2004. The notes stated "Excisional biopsy of right posterior palate- significant amount of mucous drained. Could not identify a cystic lining." The patient healed well and the pathology was reported as a benign mucocele. The pathology report stated "The squamous mucosa is unremarkable as is a superficial minor salivary gland. Below the salivary gland though is a transected lesion consistent with a mucocele. Two fragments of tissue 1 × 0.3 × 0.3 cm and 0.8 × 0.5 × 0.2 cm."

The patient noticed another mass in the right palate in October 2009. This was not painful and the patient had not appreciated an increase in size. She saw her oral surgeon on October 24, 2009, and a biopsy of the right palate was performed that showed carcinoma ex-pleomorphic adenoma.

Past Medical History
She had a tonsillectomy as a child for a peritonsillar abscess.
She was taking an oral contraceptive.

Social History
The patient was a nonsmoker.

Examination
The patient's neck was soft with no palpable lymph nodes. On intra-oral examination, there was a 1.5 × 1.5 cm ulceration of the right palate with a crater from the biopsy. A submucosal mass was noted medial to the ulcer.

Diagnosis
T1N0 carcinoma ex-pleomorphic adenoma.

Imaging
CT scans showed erosion of the hard palate and involvement of the palatal root of the second molar. The MRI showed an enhancing mass at the posterior of the right palate as well as thickening of the antral lining in the right molar region (Figure 7.12a and b). The PET scan showed an area avid uptake in the right palate SUV 8.4, but the sinus lining had only a SUV 1.2 (Figure 7.12c).

The histopathology of the specimen (Figure 7.12d–f) confirmed a diagnosis of carcinoma ex-pleomorphic adenoma. The malignant component was an intermediate-grade mucoepidermoid carcinoma (specimen size 2 × 2 × 2 cm), with positive margins. The mucicarmine stain was positive (Figure 7.12g).

Surgical Intervention
The patient was consented for a right posterior maxillectomy and she and her family opted for an obturator reconstruction rather than a free flap. Residual intermediate-grade mucoepidermoid carcinoma was identified in the final specimen, (Figure 7.12h and i). No residual pleomorphic adenoma was seen. All margins were clear. There was no perineural invasion bone invasion was not seen, and the maxillary sinus lining was not involved. Tumor board discussion did not result in a recommendation for adjuvant radiation therapy.

One-year post-surgery, she elected to have reconstructive surgery to close the maxillectomy defect which was done with a radial forearm flap. She was most recently seen in August 2020 when clinical and MRI scans showed no evidence of recurrence 11 years and 9 months since her original surgery. Her palatal reconstruction appeared well at that time (Figure 7.12j).

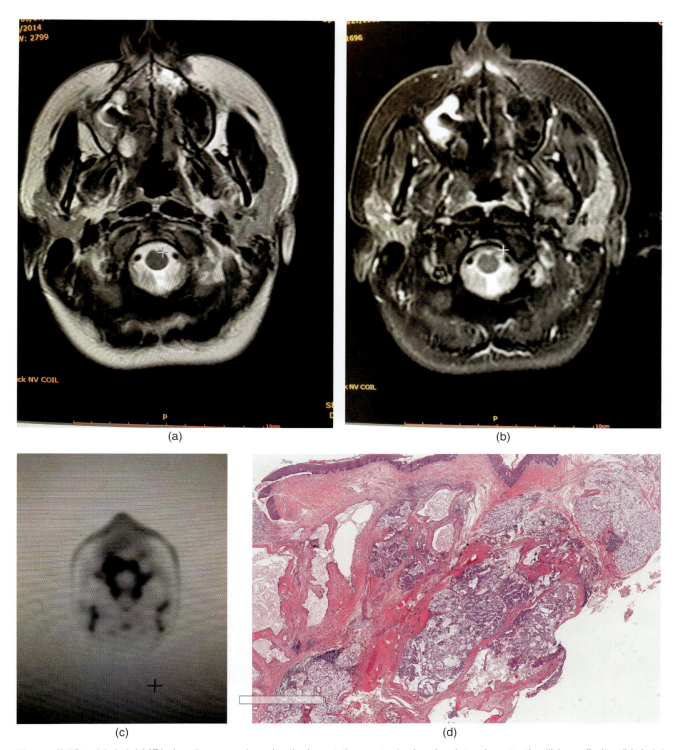

Figure 7.12. (a) Axial MRI showing an enhancing lesion at the posterior hard palate close to the "biopsy" site. (b) Axial MRI through the sinus shows the thickened enhancing sinus lining. (c) PET scan shows very intense avid uptake, "hot spot" in the right posterior hard palate. (d) Low-power view shows palatal mucosa superiorly. The tumor seems to have a thick collagenous capsule with fibrous bands. Perhaps some scarring is present from her previous biopsy. (e) Area of pleomorphic adenoma differentiation, cells in a sclerotic fibrous stroma.

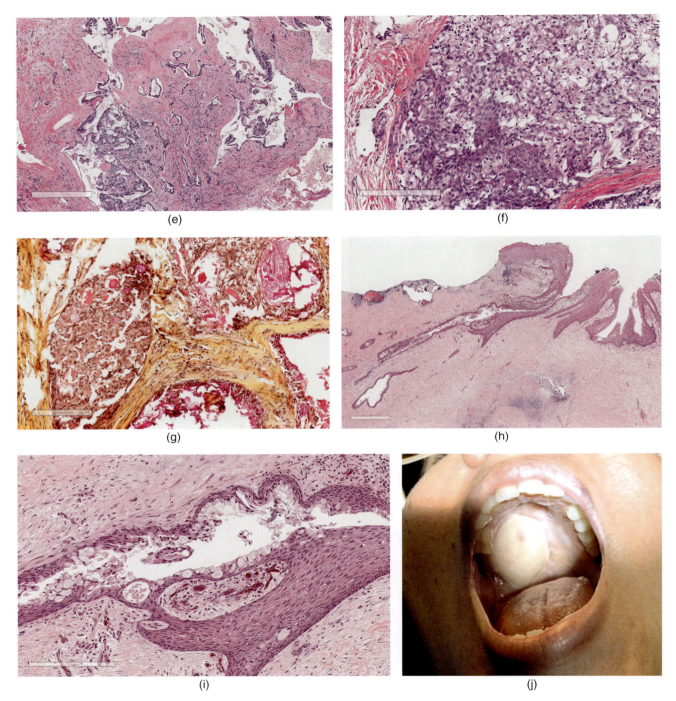

Figure 7.12. (f) High power shows mucoepidermoid carcinoma intermediate grade with foamy mucous cells and squamous cells. (g) High-power mucicarmine stain confirms the mucous cells and the diagnosis. Source: Slides provided by Dr. R. Younis Department of Oral Pathology, University of Maryland Dental School, with permission from Dr. Younis. (h) Low-power hematoxylin and eosin stain of the maxillectomy specimen shows mucoepidermoid carcinoma with a mixture of epidermoid and mucous cell lined cystic and tubular structures merging with the overlying palatal mucosa. The tumor is multifocal, "seeded into a thick collagenous scar background from the previous surgeries." Separate tumor foci are seen at the left edge of the specimen. (i) High-power view of the cystic/tubular structure. Note prominent mucous/goblet cells mixed with epidermoid cells. Source: Figure 7.12a–i by courtesy of Dr. John Papadimitriou, Professor Pathology, University of Maryland. (j) The radial forearm reconstruction of the palate is noted at 10 years, nine months following its placement.

TAKE HOME POINTS

1. The first learning points on this case are that neither of the biopsies were ideal. There is little doubt that the lesion that was "drained" as a mucocele in 2004 when the patient was 16 years was the same salivary gland tumor as that diagnosed five years later. The hard palate is not a site for mucoceles, especially in children, and it is much more likely from a clinical diagnostic view that this was a tumor, either a cystic pleomorphic or more likely a low-grade mucoepidermoid carcinoma. The fact that the specimens taken were only 2–3 mm. Deep probably means that the biopsy did not get into the substance of the tumor accounting for the negative histological result. Cystic areas can be large in mucoepidermoid carcinoma, and a sampling error probably occurred if the biopsy was too superficial.
2. In the case of the second biopsy in 2009, this was a so-called "excisional biopsy," 2 × 2 × 2 cm in dimensions. The problem is that the gross anatomic margins of the tumor have now been obliterated, with only a large ulcer remaining clinically. The margins are positive and when the patient is referred to the oncologic surgeon, he/she must now include a larger margin of normal tissue and be more radical as it is not certain where there may be microscopic residual neoplasm or where the tumor may have been seeded.
3. Although carcinoma ex-pleomorphic adenoma is an unusual malignant minor salivary gland cancer, (the authors have only seen 5 in 319 minor salivary tumors of the oral cavity), it will behave as an intermediate-grade mucoepidermoid carcinoma which usually behaves clinically more like a low-grade lesion. Salivary carcinoma appears to have a better prognosis in children as they are more often low grade and early stage.
4. Despite a delay of five years from the initial biopsy to definitive treatment, the tumor still was probably only a large T1 or early T2 in size. Low-grade mucoepidermoid carcinoma, in particular, can grow like a benign tumor and have very slow progression.

References

Ajike SO, Lakhoo K. n.d. Salivary Gland Diseases in Children and Adolescents. www.global-help.org/publicatons/books/help_pedsurgeryafrica39.pdf (accessed March 10, 2015).

Bhargava N, Agarwal P, Sharma N, Agrawal M, Sidiq M, Narain P. 2014. An unusual presentation of oral mucocele in infant and its review. *Case Rep Dent* 1–6.

Bradley PJ, Hartley B. 2011. Salivary Gland Neoplasms. In: Bradley PJ, Guntinas-Lichius O (eds.) Salivary Gland Disorders and Diseases: Diagnosis and Management. Stuttgart, Thieme, p. 94,.

Caccamese JF, Ord RA. 2002. Pediatric mucoepidermoid carcinoma of the palate. *Int J Oral Maxillofac Surg* 31(2):136-139.

Canzi P, Occhini A, Pagella F et al. 2013. Sialendoscopy in juvenile recurrent parotitis; a review of the literature *Acta Otorhinolaryngol Ital* 33(6):367-373

Castro EB, Huvos AG, Strong EW, Foote FW. 1972. Tumors of the major salivary glands in children. *Cancer* 29:312-317.

Chiaravali S, Guzzo M, Bisogno G et al. 2014. Salivary gland carcinomas in children and adolescents: The Italian TREP project experience. *Pediatr Blood Cancer* 61(11):1961-1968.

Chitre VV, Premchandra DJ. 1997. Recurrent parotitis. *Arch Dis Child* 77:359-363.

Chung MK, Jeong HS, Ko MH et al. 2007. *Int J Pediatr Otorhinolaryngol* 71(5):787-791.

Craver RD, Carr R. 2012. Paediatric salivary gland pathology. *Diagn Histopathol* 18:373-380.

Daoud EV, McLean-Holden AC, Pfeifer CM, et al. 2020. Pediatric Warthin-like mucoepidermoid carcinoma: Report of two cases with one persistent/recurrent as conventional mucoepidermoid carcinoma. *Head Neck Pathol* 14:923–928.

Drolet BA, Esterly NB, Frieden IJ. 1999. Hemangiomas in children. *N Engl J Med* 341:173-181.

Ellies M, Laskawi R. 2010. Diseases of the salivary glands in infants and adolescents. *Head Face Med* 6:1-7.

Ellis GL, Auclair PL, Gnepp DR. 1991. Surgical Pathology of the Salivary Glands. WB Saunders Co, Philadelphia, Chapter 9.

Enjolras O, Rich MC, Merland JJ, Escarde JP. 1990. Management of alarming hemangiomas in infants: A review of 25 cases. *Pediatrics* 25:491-498.

Ezekowitz RAB, Mulliken JB, Folkman J. 1992. Interferon alfa-2a therapy for life-threatening hemangiomas of infancy. *N Engl J Med* 326:1456-1463.

Fang Og, Shi S, Li ZN, Zhang X, Liu FY, Sun CE. 2013. Epithelial salivary gland tumors in children; a twenty five year experience of 122 patients. *Int J Pediatr Otorhinolaryngol* 77(8):1252-1254.

Galer C, Santillan AA, Chelius D et al. 2012. Minor salivary gland malignancies in the pediatric population. *Head Neck* 34:1648-1651.

Gallia LJ, Johnson JT. 1981. The incidence of neoplastic versus inflammatory disease in major salivary gland masses diagnosed by surgery. *Laryngoscope* 91:512-516.

Gangopadhyay AN, Sinha CK, Gopal SC et al. 1997. Role of steroids in childhood haemangioma: A 10-years review. *Int Surg* 82:49-51.

Garavello W, Redaelli M, Galluzzi F, Pignataro L. 2018. Juvenile recurrent parotitis: A systematic review of treatment studies. *Int J Pediatr Otorhinolaryngol* 112:151-157.

Gellrich D, Bichler M, Reichel CA, Schrotzlmair F, Zengel P. (2020). Salivary gland disorders in children and adolescents: A 15-year experience. *Int Arch Otorhinolaryngol* 24:e31-e37.

Gontarz M, Wyszynska-Pawelec G, Zapaa J. 2018. Primary epithelial salivary gland tumours in children and adolescents. *Int J Oral Maxillofac Surg* 47:11-15.

Hackett AM, Baranano CF, Reed M et al. 2012. Sialoendoscopy for the treatment of pediatric salivary gland disorders. *Arch Otolaryngol Head Neck Surg* 138:912-915.

Hayashida AM, Zerbinatti DCZ, Balducci I, Cabral LAG, Almeida JD. 2010. Mucus extravasation and retention phenomena: A 24-year study. *BMC Oral Health* 10:1-4.

Ishibashi K, Ito Y, Masaki A et al. 2015. *Am J Surg Pathol* 39:1479-1487.

Kaban LB, Mulliken JB, Murray JE. 1978. Sialadenitis in childhood. *Am J Surg* 135:570-576.

Krolls SO, Trodahl JN, Boyers RC. 1972. Salivary gland lesions in children. A survey of 430 cases. *Cancer* 30:459-469.

Kuperman ME, de la Graza GO, Santillan AA et al. 2010. Outcomes of pediatric patients with malignancies of the major salivary glands. *Ann Surg Oncol* 17(120:3301-3307.

Lack EE, Upton MP. 1988. Histopathologic review of salivary gland tumors in childhood. *Arch Otolaryngol Head Neck Surg* 114:898-906.

Laikui L, Hongwei L, Hongbing J, Zhixiu H. 2008. Epithelial salivary gland tumors of children and adolescents in west China population: A clinicopathologic study of 79 cases. *J Oral Pathol Med* 37:201-205.

Lee DH, Yoon TM, Lee JK, Lim SC. 2013. Clinical utility of fine needle aspiration cytology in pediatric parotid tumors. *Int J Pediatr Otorhinolaryngol* 77:1272-1275.

Maynard JD. 1965. Recurrent parotid enlargement. *Br J Surg* 52:784-789.

Nahieli O, Ekiav E, Hasson O, Zagury A, Baruchin AM. 2000. Pediatric sialolithiasis. *Oral Surg Oral Med Oral Pathol Oral Radiol Endod* 90(6):709-712.

Nahlieli O, Shacham R, Shlesinger M et al. 2004. Juvenile recurrent parotitis: A new method of diagnosis and treatment. *Pediatrics* 114:9-12.

Ord RA. 2004. Salivary Gland Tumors in Children. In: Kaban LB, Troulis MJ (eds.) Pediatric Oral and Maxillofacial Surgery. Philadelphia, Saunders.

Orvidas LJ, Kasperbauer JL, Lewis JE et al. 2000. Pediatric parotid masses. *Arch Otolaryngol Head Neck Surg* 126:177-184.

Ottaviani F, Marchisio P, Arisi E, Capaccio P. 2001. Extracorporeal shockwave lithotripsy for salivary calculi in pediatric patients. *Acta Otolaryngol* 121(7):873-876.

Pandit RT, Park AH. 2002. Management of pediatric ranula. *Otolaryngol Head Neck Surg* 127:115-118.

Puttgen KB. 2014. Diagnosis and management of infantile hemangiomas. *Pediatr Clin North Am* 61:383-402.

Ramakrishna J, Strychowsky J, Gupta M, Sommer DD. 2015. Sialendoscopy for the management of juvenile recurrent parotitis: A systematic review and meta-analysis. *Laryngoscope* 125:1472-1479.

Rutt AL, Hawkshaw MJ, Lurie D, Sataloff RT. 2011. Salivary gland cancer in patients younger than 30 years. *Ear Nose Throat J* 90(4):174-184.

Saarinen R, Kolho KL, Davidkin I, Pitkäranta A. 2013. The clinical picture of juvenile parotitis in a prospective setup. *Acta Paediatr* 102(2):177-181.

Salerno S, Giordano J, La Tona G, De Grazia E, Barresi B, Lo Casto A. 2011. Pediatric sialolithiasis distinctive characteristics in radiological imaging. *Minerva Stomatol* 60(9):435-441.

Scarcella JV, Dykes ER, Anderson R. 1965. Hemangiomas of the parotid gland. *Plast Reconstr Surg* 36:38-47.

Seifert G, Okabe H, Caselitz J. (1986). Epithelial salivary gland tumors in children and adolescents. Analysis of 80 cases (Salivary Gland Register 1965-1984). *ORL J Otorhinolaryngol Relat Spec* 48:137-149.

Seo JH, Park JJ, Kim HY et al. 2010. Surgical management of intraoral ranulas in children: An analysis of 17 pediatric cases. *Int J Pediatr Otorhinolaryngol* 74:202-205.

Shacham R, Droma EB, London D et al. 2009. Long-term experience with endoscopic diagnosis and treatment of juvenile recurrent parotitis. *J Oral Maxillofac Surg* 67:162-167.

Soumekh B, Adams GL, Shapiro RS. 1996. Treatment of head and neck hemangiomas with recombinant interferon alpha-2b. *Ann Otol Rhinol Laryngol* 105:201-206.

Sultan I, Rodruiguez-Galindo C, Al-Sharabati S, Guzzo M, Cassanova M, Ferrari A. 2011. Salivary gland carcinomas in children and adolescents: A population based study, with comparison to adult cases, *Head Neck* 33(10):1476-1481.

Syebele K, Butow KW. 2010. Oral mucoceles and ranulas may be part of initial manifestations of HIV infection. *AIDS Res Hum Retroviruses* 26:1075-1078.

Tasca RA, Clarke R. 2011. Inflammatory and Infectious Diseases of the Salivary Glands. In: Bradley PJ, Guntinas-Lichius O (eds.) Salivary Gland Disorders and Diseases: Diagnosis and Management. Stuggart, Georg Thieme Verlag, Chapter 13, pp. 110-120.

Techavichit P, Hicks MJ, Lopez-Terrada DH et al. 2016. Mucoepidermoid carcinoma in children: A single institutional experience. *Pediatr Blood Cancer* 63:27-31.

Woo SH, Jang JY, Park GY, Jeong HS. 2009. Long-term outcome of intraoral submandibular stone removal in children as compared to adults. *Laryngoscope* 119(1):116-120.

Yavvari S, Makena Y, Sukhavasi S, Makena MR. 2019. Large population analysis of secondary cancers in pediatric leukemia survivors. *Children (Bassel)* 6(12):1-7.

Yoshida EJ, Garcia J, Eisele DW, Chen AM. 2014. Salivary gland malignancies in children. *Int J Pediatr Otorhinolaryngol* 78:174-178.

Zhi K, Wen Y, Ren W, Zhang Y. 2008. Management of infant ranula. *Int J Pediatr Otorhinolaryngol* 72:823-826.

Chapter 8
Classification, Grading, and Staging of Salivary Gland Tumors

J. Michael McCoy[1] and John Sauk, DDS, MS, FAAAS, FAHNS[2]

[1] Departments of Oral and Maxillofacial Surgery, Pathology, and Radiology, University of Tennessee Graduate School of Medicine, Knoxville, TN, USA

[2] School of Dentistry, University of Louisville, Louisville, KY, USA

Outline

Introduction
Classification Systems for Salivary Gland Neoplasm
  Cellular Classification of Salivary Gland Neoplasms
    Benign Epithelial Salivary Gland Neoplasms
      Pleomorphic Adenoma (Benign Mixed Tumor)
      Warthin Tumor (Papillary Cystadenoma Lymphomatosum)
      Basal Cell Adenoma
      Canalicular Adenoma
      Oncocytoma
      Sebaceous Adenoma
      Sebaceous Lymphadenoma
      Myoepithelioma
      Cystadenoma
      Ductal Papilloma
      Sialadenoma Papilliferum
      Sclerosing Polycystic Adenoma
    Malignant Epithelial Neoplasms
      Mucoepidermoid Carcinoma
      Adenoid Cystic Carcinoma
      Acinic Cell Carcinoma
      Polymorphous Adenocarcinoma
      Adenocarcinoma NOS (Otherwise Specified)
      Basal Cell Adenocarcinoma
      Clear Cell Carcinoma
      Cystadenocarcinoma
      Sebaceous Adenocarcinoma
      Sebaceous Lymphadenocarcinoma
      Oncocytic Carcinoma
      Salivary Duct Carcinoma
      Malignant Mixed Tumors
      Carcinoma Ex-Pleomorphic Adenoma
      Salivary Carcinosarcoma
      Metastasizing Mixed Tumor
      Sialoblastoma
      Primary Squamous Cell Carcinoma
      Epithelial-Myoepithelial Carcinoma
      Poorly Differentiated Carcinomas
        Undifferentiated Carcinoma
        Small Cell Neuroendocrine Carcinoma
        Large Cell Neuroendocrine Carcinoma
        Lymphoepithelial Carcinoma
      Myoepithelial Carcinoma
      Adenosquamous Carcinoma
      Secretory Carcinoma
  Non-Epithelial Neoplasms
    Lymphomas and Benign Lymphoepithelial Lesion
    Mesenchymal Neoplasms
      Benign Mesenchymal Salivary Gland Tumors
      Malignant Mesenchymal Salivary Gland Tumors
    Malignant Secondary Neoplasms
Grading and Staging of Salivary Gland Tumors
  Molecular Systematics of Salivary Gland Neoplasms
TNM and Staging of Salivary Gland Tumors
  Extraparenchymal Extension
  TNM Descriptors
  Additional Descriptors
Summary
Case Presentation – *Reclassified*
References

Salivary Gland Pathology: Diagnosis and Management, Third Edition. Edited by Eric R. Carlson and Robert A. Ord.
© 2022 John Wiley & Sons, Inc. Published 2022 by John Wiley & Sons, Inc.
Companion website: www.wiley.com/go/carlson/salivary

Introduction

Scientific classification is a method by which researchers and clinicians categorize species of organisms. Modern classification has its roots in the work of Carolus Linnaeus, also known as Carl von Linné the Father of Taxonomy, who grouped species by shared physical characteristics. Accordingly, scientific classification belongs to the science of taxonomy or biological systematics. Molecular systematics, which uses genomic and proteomic expression data, has driven many recent revisions in these systems. In a like manner, surgeons, pathologists, and oncologists have endeavored to systematically categorize tumors based on designated characteristics to predict probable biological behavior. This in turn would help dictate appropriate therapeutic modalities to be employed and help forecast a credible prognosis. As such, the "designated characteristics" upon which tumors have been classified may be in more contemporary terms considered as "biomarkers." In like fashion, genomic and proteomic expression profiles of tumors have thrust pathology and oncology into molecular systematics to develop classifications (Uchida et al. 2010).

The role of molecular profiling or systematics for clinical decision-making and taxonomy has been recently considered and the classification of tissue or other specimens for diagnostic, prognostic, and predictive purposes based on multiple gene expression and proteomics has been noted to hold major promise for optimizing the management of patients with cancer (Ioannidis 2007). However, assay development and data analysis have been principally investigative, and there exists a lofty potential for the introduction of bias. Most troubling is that standardization of profiles has been the exception. Moreover, classifier performance is typically overinterpreted by conveying the results as p-values or multiplicative effects, whereas the absolute sensitivity and specificity of classification are modest, particularly when tested in large validation samples (Ioannidis 2007). Furthermore, validation has frequently been made with less than favorable consideration for methodology and safeguarding for bias. Most disconcerting is that the postulated classifier performance can be inflated compared to what these profiles can accomplish.

Whether traditional morphological designated characteristics or molecular systematics are employed, the aim of any classification is to demonstrate diagnostic, prognostic, and predictive performance. This can generally be accomplished for any data set by training. However, it is well known that unless training is unsupervised (no knowledge of the correct class is involved), the performance of the system being tested on the training data set is totally uninformative about its true operation (Ioannidis 2007). Cross-validation and independent validation are two methods to determine whether the proposed scheme is an accurate classifier (Allison et al. 2006). Despite the method employed, different metrics can be used to describe the classifier performance. These may include statistical testing measures, multiplicative effect measures such as likelihood ratios or hazard ratios, or absolute effect measures. Although all information has some value, absolute effect measures (sensitivity and specificity) are the most meaningful from a clinical perspective (Buyse et al. 2006).

Classification Systems for Salivary Gland Neoplasms

The classification system for salivary gland neoplasms has evolved with the accumulation of clinical experience and our understanding of the basis of neoplasia. Although a variety of classifications have been advocated, there has been some geographic variation in terminology and classification between Europeans and American authors. Historically, the first most notable classification was that put forth by Foote and Frazell (1954). Later systems reflect the recognition and description of previously unrecognized entities or the deletion of some terms that were misnomers or were considered meaningless. The succeeding classifications include those by: Thackary and Lucas (1974); Evans and Cruickshank (1970); the WHO (Thackray and Sobin 1972) (Batsakis (1979); Seifert et al. (1986b); and Ellis et al. (1991). The most recent AFIP fascicle on the subject provides a stepwise evolution of these taxonomies (Ellis and Auclair 2008).

CELLULAR CLASSIFICATION OF SALIVARY GLAND NEOPLASMS

Salivary gland neoplasms are noted for their histological variability. Reflecting the anatomy of these glands, benign and malignant salivary gland neoplasms may arise either from epithelial, mesenchymal, or lymphoid origins. The complexity of the classification and the rarity of some of these tumors, some of which display a wide spectrum of morphological patterns within the same tumor when added to the existence of hybrid lesions, challenge the surgical pathologist with a difficult task in differentiating benign from malignant tumors (Seifert and Donath 1996; Speight and Barrett 2002). Currently, the surgical pathologists often must use every available tool to properly diagnose and classify tumors arising from the major and minor salivary glands. No longer can histology alone be used for such determinations. The contemporary pathologist uses not only routine light microscopy but also immunohistochemistry, specialized imaging, and clinical characteristics of each tumor to establish the exact diagnosis. Immunohistochemistry has proved to be an excellent diagnostic adjunct to routine light microscopy.

Immunohistochemistry (IHC) is the method by which one can detect antigens in tumor cells by way of antigen/antibody testing. This method is widely used today to define the distinction between benign and malignant cells as well as the determination of exact tumor cell types (Nagao et al. 2012).

The use of IHC has become an excellent and effective manner to determine the exact cellular proteins involved with specific cell types. While still evolving, the technique of immunostaining is widely used by most if not all surgical pathology laboratories for immunophenotyping tumors. Currently, most diagnostic labs have 150–200 commercially prepared immuno markers available with many more being developed yearly. Some of the more common available markers or stains used in salivary gland pathology include: (1) various *cytokeratins* (*CK*) for determining epithelial cell origin; (2) *CD20* for the determination of B-cell lymphomas; (3) *CD3* for the identification of T-cell lymphomas; (4) *Smooth Muscle Actin* (*SMA*), *Muscle Specific Actin* (*MSA*), *and S100* for the identification of myoepithelial cells; (5) *Ki67 Index* to help distinguish malignant from benign lesions; (6) *CD117* to distinguish basal cell adenomas from pleomorphic adenomas; (7) *HMB45 and SOX-10* to identify melanin producing cells; (8) *Chromogranin and Synaptophysin* to distinguish and identify neuroendocrine cells; and (9) *S-100 and SOX-10* to distinguish various neural tissues. Many more additional immunostains are now available to aid in the determination and correct identification of salivary gland lesions.

The following cellular classification system reiterates that advocated by the National Cancer Institute of the USPHS (National Cancer Institute, www.Cancer.gov), which is derived heavily from that published by the Armed Forces Institute of Pathology (AFIP) (Ellis and Auclair 2008), (Table 8.1). Like the NCI scheme, we also include malignant non-epithelial neoplasms since these lesions embrace a sizable proportion of salivary gland neoplasms.

Table 8.1. 2017 WHO classification of salivary gland tumors.

Benign epithelial neoplasms
   Pleomorphic adenoma
   Warthin tumor
   Basal cell adenoma
   Oncocytoma
   Sebaceous adenoma
   Lymphadenoma
   Myoepithelioma
   Cystadenoma
   Ductal papillomas
   Lymphadenoma
   Sialadenoma papilliferum
   Canalicular adenoma and other ductal adenomas
Malignant epithelial neoplasms
   Mucoepidermoid carcinoma
   Adenoid cystic carcinoma
   Acinic cell carcinoma
   Polymorphous adenocarcinoma
   Clear cell carcinoma
   Basal cell adenocarcinoma
   Intraductal carcinoma
   Adenocarcinoma, NOS
   Myoepithelial carcinoma
   Secretory carcinoma
   Sebaceous adenocarcinoma
   Oncocytic carcinoma
   Salivary duct carcinoma
   Malignant mixed tumors
   Carcinoma ex-pleomorphic adenoma
   Carcinosarcoma
   Poorly differentiated carcinoma
      Undifferentiated carcinoma
      Large cell neuroendocrine carcinoma
      Small cell neuroendocrine carcinoma
   Primary squamous cell carcinoma
   Epithelial-myoepithelial carcinoma
   Lymphoepithelial carcinoma
Tumors of unknown malignant potential
   Sialoblastoma
Non-epithelial neoplasms
   Lymphomas
   Benign mesenchymal neoplasms
   Malignant mesenchymal neoplasms

Though less common, the inclusion of malignant secondary tumors is presented to be inclusive.

As noted in the introduction, statistics regarding the incidence, frequency, and prognosis have varied depending on the study. Moreover, a cursory review of the literature generally reveals that power analyses are rarely performed to access the necessary sample size for many of these studies and most rudimentary statistical measures are employed to arrive at conclusions. In large part, these deficiencies have stemmed from the general rare incidence of many salivary gland neoplasms. Although the AFIP statistics have been criticized to be biased because of the methods of case accrual as a reference service, these data are probably the most reliable especially for rare and unusual lesions.

Benign Epithelial Salivary Gland Neoplasms

Pleomorphic Adenoma (Benign Mixed Tumor)

The pleomorphic adenoma (Figure 8.1) or benign mixed tumor is the most common salivary gland neoplasm representing 35% of all salivary gland tumors. Clinically, the tumors are smooth, multilobular, and appear well-demarcated by a pseudocapsule. However, microscopically, tumor cells may be seen extending beyond the apparent pseudocapsule. The tumor is cytologically varied depending on the cellularity of the epithelial components and the mesenchymal-appearing content. The presence of both epithelial and mesenchymal-like elements arising from myoepithelial cells produces significant diversity in the appearance of these tumors. Most notable is that the stromal component may encompass myxoid, fibroid, chondroid, and even osteoid features providing the mixed appearance of these lesions (Ellis and Auclair 2008). Even with this varied histology, the pleomorphic adenoma is completely epithelial in origin with no true mesenchymal element involved. For this reason, the mesenchymal-appearing cells arising from myoepithelial cells will be immunoreactive with antibodies to smooth muscle-specific proteins such as MSA, SMA, and often S100 (Figure 8.1a and b).

Overexpression of the proto-oncogene pleomorphic adenoma gene 1 (*PLAG1*) plays a crucial role in development of pleomorphic adenomas. *PLAG1* overexpression is usually caused by chromosomal aberrations resulting in fusion genes with promoter swapping, including *CTNNB1-PLAG1*,

Table 8.2. Grading of malignant salivary gland tumors.

Low-grade
   Acinic cell carcinoma
   Basal cell adenocarcinoma
   Clear cell carcinoma
   Epithelial-myoepithelial carcinoma
   Secretory carcinoma
   Intraductal carcinoma
   Sebaceous adenocarcinoma
Low-grade, intermediate-grade, and/or high-grade
   Polymorphous adenocarcinoma
   Adenocarcinoma, NOS
   Mucoepidermoid carcinoma[a]
Intermediate- and/or high-grade
   Myoepithelial carcinoma
High-grade
   Primary squamous cell carcinoma
   Carcinosarcoma
   Salivary duct carcinoma
   Lymphoepithelial carcinoma
   Poorly differentiated carcinoma
      Undifferentiated carcinoma
      Large cell neuroendocrine carcinoma
      Small cell neuroendocrine carcinoma
   Carcinoma ex-pleomorphic adenoma
Uncertain malignant potential
   Sialoblastoma

[a]Note: The fourth edition of the World Health Organization Classification of Head and Neck Tumours is less dogmatic about the application of grading in mucoepidermoid carcinoma. In contrast to the third edition of the World Health Organization in which the AFIP grading system was featured, the fourth edition does not endorse a specific grading scheme. Given the lack of a consensus on an ideal grading criterion, only the general features of low-, intermediate-, and high-grade tumors are outlined in the fourth edition.

CHCHD7-PLAG1, *LIFR-PLAG*, and *TCEA-PLAG1* (Matsuyama et al. 2012). Recent evidence indicates that the target genes of *PLAG1* include: Bax, Fas, p53, p21, p16, Cyclin D1, EGFR, Trail-R/DR5, c-Fos, c-myc, and Igf2. *PLAG1* not only activates genes that promote cell proliferation and tumor formation but also genes that inhibit these cellular processes (Wang et al. 2013b). Although human papilloma virus (HPV) 16 and 18 have been demonstrated among some pleomorphic adenomas with p16 expression, it appears that pleomorphic adenoma of salivary glands represents a category of tumors in which the p16 positive staining is not biologically relevant to the oncogenic role of HPV infection (Hafed et al. 2012; Skalova et al. 2013a; Tarakji et al. 2013).

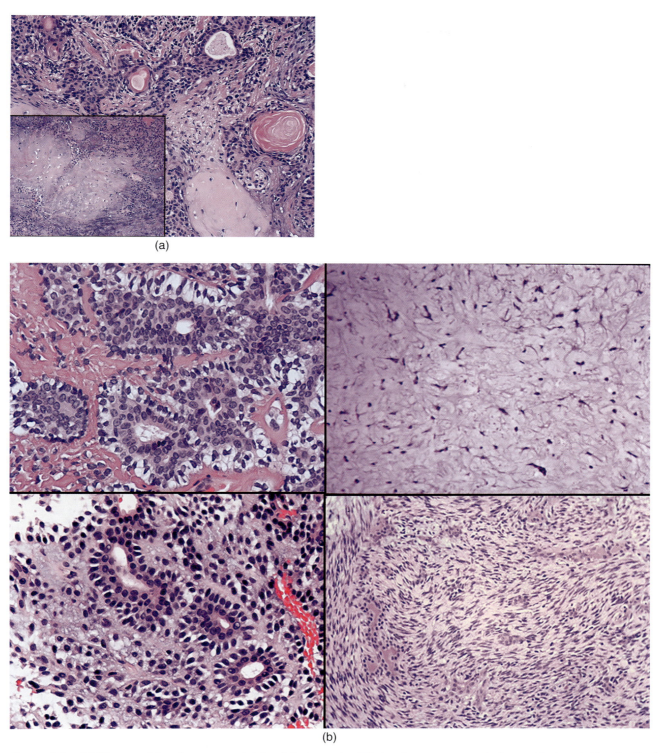

Figure 8.1. (a) Pleomorphic adenoma containing tubular and solid structures composed of round to basaloid cells. Foci of squamous metaplasia, myxoid and chondroid areas, lower left panel. H&E staining, 200×. (b) Composite figure of a pleomorphic adenoma demonstrating myxoid components (upper right), spindle-cell components (lower right), clear ductal cells surrounded by hyaline stroma (upper left) and tubular elements surrounded by a loose basophilic stroma (lower left). H&E staining, 400×.

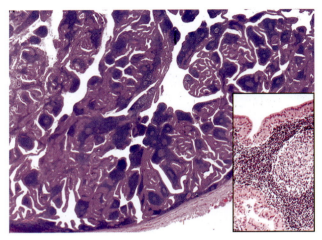

Figure 8.2. Warthin tumor with well-developed fibrous capsule delineating the lesion from normal parotid gland. The tumor is characterized by bilayered oncocytic epithelium lining cystic spaces. Closely associated with these lining cells is abundant lymphoid tissue. Lower right panel depicting the oncocytic epithelium in close proximity to a lymphoid aggregate with an associated germinal center. H&E staining, 200×/400×. Source: Courtesy of Dr. Mark Bernstein.

Warthin Tumor (Papillary Cystadenoma Lymphomatosum)

The Warthin tumor is regarded as the second most common benign salivary gland neoplasm, and as such comprises 6–10% of all parotid tumors. These tumors infrequently arise in the submandibular or minor salivary glands but are occasionally seen in these sites. Men are more commonly affected than women, with a gender ratio of 5:1. Interestingly, the prevalence increases in smokers and bilateral distribution has been noted in ∼12% of cases (Ellis and Auclair 2008).

The Warthin tumor is characterized by oncocytic epithelium arranged in a papillary configuration while being accompanied by diffuse aggregates of lymphocytes (Figure 8.2). Quite often, follicular centers are seen within the lymphocyte aggregates. These microscopic characteristics are unique within the groupings of benign salivary gland tumors and are unlike those of any other primary salivary neoplasm. Immunostaining has been of little help in determining the exact origin of Warthin tumor.

Early studies have indicated that the *CRTC1-MAML2* fusion was not exclusive to mucoepidermoid carcinoma and could be found in Warthin tumors. More recent studies have indicated that neither *CRTC1-MAML2* nor *CRTC3-MAML2* fusions

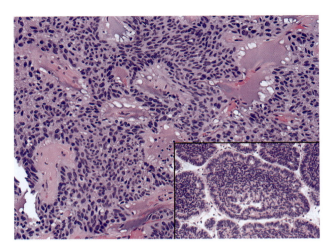

Figure 8.3. Basal cell adenoma consisting of monotonous sheets of basaloid cells lacking any myxochondroid tissues, spindled or plasmacytoid cells observed in pleomorphic adenomas. Lower right panel depicting palisaded basaloid cells surrounding a tumor cell nest. H&E staining, 200×. Source: Courtesy of Dr. Mark Bernstein.

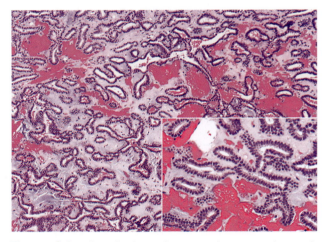

Figure 8.4. Canalicular adenoma demonstrating columns of columnar cells lining canaliculi forming interconnecting tubules and microcysts. Lower right panel showing higher magnification detail. H&E staining, 100×/200×. Source: Courtesy of Dr. Mark Bernstein.

could be detected in metaplastic Warthin tumor or metaplastic pleomorphic adenoma (Skalova et al. 2013a).

Basal Cell Adenoma

Once termed a form of monomorphic adenoma, the basal cell adenoma is a lesion characterized by a monomorphous uniform basaloid epithelial pattern, and the lack of any myxochondroid features typical of pleomorphic adenomas (Figure 8.3). The basal cell adenoma comprises between 5 and 10% of all benign salivary gland tumors with most cases arising within the parotid gland. A simultaneous occurrence of the basal cell adenoma and the relatively rare benign eccrine cylindroma of skin had been identified. Both ductal cells and myoepithelial cells can be identified by IHC means.

Canalicular Adenoma

Once described as a form of monomorphic adenoma, the canalicular adenoma (Figure 8.4) is a benign salivary gland tumor composed of interconnecting and branching cords of columnar cells manifesting as single or double rows of cells. These tumors are usually small with a well-defined capsule. A unique feature of the canalicular adenoma is that it quite often is multifocal with tumor nodules seen throughout the surrounding salivary tissue. Unlike any other salivary gland tumors, the canalicular adenoma has a significant predilection to occur in the minor salivary glands of the upper lip. This tumor comprises less than 5% of all benign salivary tumors although it makes up at least 10% of all such lesions arising within minor glands. As the canalicular adenoma is comprised only of ductal cells without a myoepithelial component, only the IHC stains for ductal cells (CD117, CK7, CK8) are positive while the common myoepithelial immunostains (SMA, MSA, S100) are negative.

Oncocytoma

The oncocytoma is a rare benign salivary gland neoplasm composed of large, polyhedral, eosinophilic granular cells (oncocytes) containing numerous atypical mitochondria (Figure 8.5). It was often considered a form of a monomorphic adenoma in prior classification schemes. Oncocytic cells are found not only in salivary tissue but also in thyroid, breast, and kidney. Although most oncocytomas are solid, a few demonstrate a papillary appearance. Most oncocytomas arise in the parotid gland though a few have been described in minor glands. In addition, most of these lesions occur in older individuals with the peak incidence in the seventh and eighth decade of life. No myoepithelial component is identified by means of IHC staining. Recognition is unremarkable although there is a clear cell variant that must be distinguished from mucoepidermoid carcinoma and other clear cell malignancies. Occasionally, the oncocytoma is demonstrated as a positive finding with technetium bone scans and PET imaging.

Oncocytosis, also known as oncocytic metaplasia, is relatively common in all major and minor salivary glands. This non-neoplastic entity is often multifocal and occurs in salivary gland lobules. Histologically, oncocytosis appears as well-defined aggregates composed of pure oncocytes located with normal salivary gland tissue. When present, these oncocytes do not distort or alter the natural morphology of the salivary gland in which they are found.

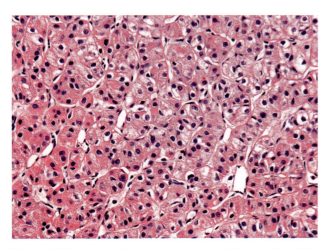

Figure 8.5. Oncocytoma characterized by eosinophilic, granular cytoplasm, with stippled nuclei. H&E staining, 400×.

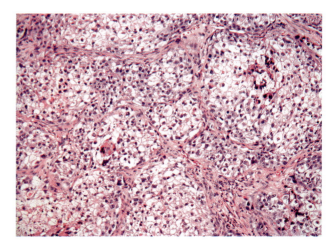

Figure 8.6. Sebaceous adenoma demonstrating numerous islands of tumor cells exhibiting both squamous and sebaceous differentiation. H&E staining, 200×.

Sebaceous Adenoma

Sebaceous cells are naturally found not only in the parotid gland but also in the minor glands of the buccal mucosa. These cells are also relatively common in lymph nodes of the head and neck area. These ectopic sebaceous glands are morphologically identical to those found in the skin although these glands when residing in salivary gland rarely produce neoplastic sebaceous tumors as they do in the skin.

The sebaceous adenoma is a rare benign salivary gland neoplasm that demonstrates sebaceous differentiation (Figure 8.6). This lesion has been identified in both the major and minor salivary glands with the buccal mucosa being the most common area of minor gland occurrence. These tumors are usually encapsulated and are comprised of nests of squamous cells demonstrating well-defined sebaceous metaplasia.

Sebaceous Lymphadenoma

The sebaceous lymphadenoma is believed by some to be a variant of the sebaceous adenoma, but which contains sebaceous glands that are surrounded by lymphoid elements. The lymphoid makeup of this tumor is histologically quite similar to that of the Warthin tumor. As with the sebaceous adenoma, the neoplastic part of this lesion is comprised of squamous cells which undergo sebaceous metaplasia. Classically, the neoplastic islands of the sebaceous lymphadenoma are much smaller than in the sebaceous adenoma.

Myoepithelioma

Myoepitheliomas are tumors that demonstrate pure myoepithelial differentiation and are believed to represent a spectrum of mixed tumors which lack epithelial features. Histologically, the myoepithelioma demonstrates only myoepithelial elements with no evidence of ductal or glandular formation identified (Figure 8.7). Various cell types are seen within the myoepithelioma including plasmacytoid, epithelioid, and spindle cells. The myoepitheliomas make up between 1 and 2% of all benign salivary gland tumors and usually involve either the parotid gland or the palate although they have been identified in other salivary glands. Though there is significant staining variability, the myoepithelial cells are immunoreactive with MSA, SMA, S100, and CK5/6 as are most myoepithelial cells. In addition, IHC is extremely helpful in distinguishing the myoepithelioma from true mesenchymal tumors such as the leiomyosarcoma, synovial sarcoma, and solitary fibrous tumor occurring in the same anatomical area.

Cystadenoma

The cystadenoma is a rare benign tumor characterized by unicystic or polycystic growths that contain regions of overgrowth that may at times be papillary in character. These benign lesions occur in both the major and the minor salivary glands with the minor gland variety more common and usually presenting much smaller in size. The cystadenoma occurs in all age groups although quite rare in children. The epithelial lining of these lesions ranges

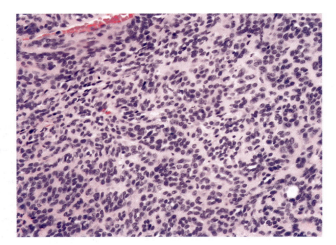

Figure 8.7. One morphologic pattern of myoepithelioma demonstrating a monotonous population of myoepithelial cells with uniform nuclei. H&E staining, 200×.

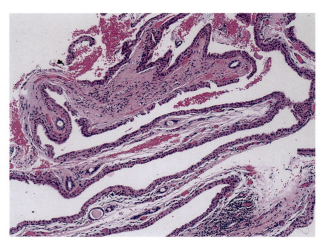

Figure 8.8. Cystadenoma characterized by tortuous cystic spaces lined by cuboidal epithelium. H&E staining, 100×.

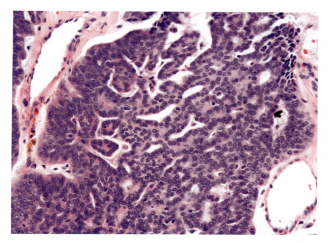

Figure 8.9. Sialadenoma papilliferum demonstrating papillary stalks composed of uniform cuboidal epithelium. H&E staining, 200×.

from cuboidal to columnar with occasional oncocytic and mucous cell types identified (Figure 8.8). The cystadenoma is often confused microscopically with a low-grade mucoepidermoid carcinoma with invasion of the surrounding soft tissue being one of the only significant microscopic differences between the two.

Ductal Papilloma

Ductal papillomas are categorized by WHO into three morphological types. These include: (1) intraductal papillomas, which are luminal papillary lesions that often result in cystic dilatation of a duct; (2) inverted ductal papillomas, which represent a papillary epithelial proliferation that occurs at the junction of salivary duct and mucosal surface; and (3) sialadenoma papilliferum, an exophytic growth involving both the mucosal surface and salivary ductal structures (Figure 8.9).

Collectively, these papillomas arise in the sixth to eighth decade of life with a slight male predominance. Evidence suggests that inverted ductal papillomas arise from superficial excretory ducts, while intraductal papillomas evolve from deeper excretory ducts. Sialadenoma papilliferum appears to have a biphasic growth pattern, suggesting origins from the exophytic and endophytic elements. Currently, there is strong support to regard these three entities as distinct based on clinical and histological parameters (Brannon et al. 2001).

Sialadenoma Papilliferum

The sialadenoma papilliferum (SP) is unique among salivary gland tumors in that it has both an exophytic and endophytic derivation. A portion of this tumor arises from the mucosal epithelium while the deeper portion appears to be contiguous with the underlying ductal epithelium of minor salivary gland (Figure 8.9). Although originally described in the late 1970s, it has proven to be quite rare in the dental and medical literature since that time (McCoy and Eckert 1980). In fact, it appears this neoplastic lesion makes up only 0.5% of all salivary gland neoplasms. Clinically, the lesion clinically presents as an exophytic mass appearing much like a squamous papilloma. On careful examination, one can discern the papillary mass growing below the mucosal surface as well. Approximately 80% of these lesions occur on the soft palate while the remainder are usually found involving the buccal mucosa. The SP evolves to no great size (1–2 cm) and has no ability to metastasize. An excisional biopsy will suffice for the removal of this benign salivary gland neoplasm.

Sclerosing Polycystic Adenoma

The sclerosing polycystic adenoma is a rare, benign process, and possibly an inflammatory lesion of salivary gland. This lesion is likely confused both histologically and clinically with salivary gland metaplasia. In fact, recent literature describes it to be a clonal proliferation and as such many authorities now consider this salivary lesion to be an adenoma (Skalova

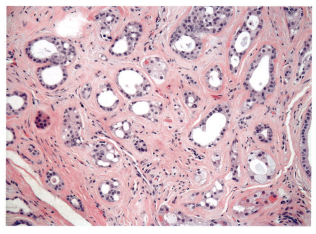

Figure 8.10. Polycystic sclerosing adenoma composed of numerous tubuloacinar structures within a dense sclerotic stroma. H&E staining, 200×.

et al. 2017). Most cases have been described within the major glands, particularly the parotid but are also seen in the minor glands. Clinically, the lesions are firm and often nodular. Microscopically, these lesions are always well circumscribed but not encapsulated. There is cystic dilation of the ducts with prominent fibrosis within each lobule (Figure 8.10). Tuboloacinar hyperplasia in a nodular pattern is a distinctive pattern. All of these features are quite similar to fibrocystic disease of the breast although the two entities do not appear to be related.

Malignant Epithelial Neoplasms
Mucoepidermoid Carcinoma

There still exists some conjecture whether mucoepidermoid carcinoma (MEC) exists as only low-grade and high-grade neoplasms rather than the three categories that are classically discussed (Spiro et al. 1978). The presence of mucoepidermoid carcinoma in the parotid gland is usually asymptomatic and generally presents as a solitary, painless mass. Occasionally, symptoms include pain, drainage from the ipsilateral ear, dysphagia, trismus, and often facial paralysis (Ellis and Auclair 2008). On rare occasion, mucoepidermoid carcinoma may occur within the bony mandible or maxilla (3:1) (Brookstone and Huvos 1992). These intra-bony tumors are referred to as central mucoepidermoid carcinomas and make up less than 4% of all mucoepidermoid carcinomas (Ellis and Auclair 2008).

Mucoepidermoid carcinomas (Figure 8.11) consist of diverse proportions of mucous, epidermoid, intermediate, columnar, and clear cells, and are often cystic in pattern. These tumors constitute 29–34% of all salivary gland malignancies and thus the MEC represents the most common malignant salivary neoplasm found in both major and minor salivary glands (Spiro et al. 1978; Spitz and Batsakis 1984; Eveson and Cawson 1985; Speight and Barrett 2002; Ellis and Auclair 2008). The best evidence to date indicates that 45% of these neoplasms initiate within the parotid glands (Goode et al. 1998; Guzzo et al. 2002). Among the minor salivary glands, mucoepidermoid carcinoma has an affinity for the buccal mucosa and the palate (Ellis and Auclair 2008). Unlike other salivary gland tumors, the MECs occur more often in the lower lip than in the upper. Generally, the mean age for these carcinomas is 47 years; however, there exists a broad age range of 8–92 years. The MEC is one of the few salivary gland malignancies occurring in childhood (Ellis and Auclair 2008). As with most other salivary gland tumors, the MEC is more common in the female population. Notably, previous exposure to ionizing radiation has been suggested to significantly increase the risk of mucoepidermoid carcinomas of the major salivary glands (Guzzo et al. 2002; Ellis and Auclair 2008).

The level of microscopic grading of mucoepidermoid is of paramount importance in establishing the treatment and prognosis (Auclair et al. 1992; Goode et al. 1998; Speight and Barrett 2002). The classic literature describes these tumors graded as

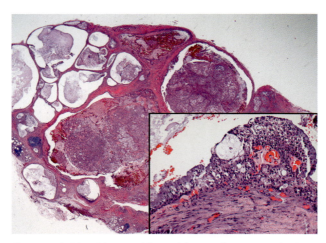

Figure 8.11. Mucoepidermoid carcinoma exhibiting large cystic spaces containing mucin and solid tumor elements. Lower right panel depicting epidermoid, intermediate and mucous cells. H&E staining, 100×/200×. Source: Courtesy of Dr. Mark Bernstein.

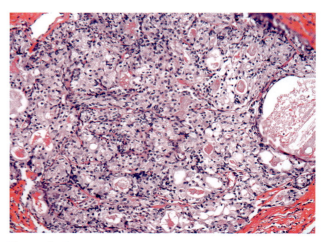

Figure 8.12. Intermediate-grade mucoepidermoid carcinoma with mostly solid features and few mucous cells. H&E staining, 200×.

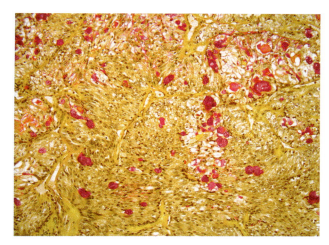

Figure 8.13. Intermediate-grade mucoepidermoid carcinoma from Figure 8.12 demonstrating numerous areas of mucin production/deposition. Mucicarmine stain, 200×.

1 Intracystic component (+2)
2 Neural invasion present (+2)
3 Necrosis present (+3)
4 Mitosis (≥4 per 10 high-power field (+3)
5 Anaplasia present (+4).

Retrospective reviews of mucoepidermoid carcinoma of the major salivary glands have revealed a statistical correlation between this point-based grading system and outcome for parotid tumors; however, similar rigor was not deemed useful for tumors of the submandibular glands, (Goode et al. 1998) or minor salivary glands (Guzzo et al. 2002). Nevertheless, when more emphasis on features of tumor invasion is employed, better correlation is obtained, indicating that tumor staging with adjunctive invasive patterns may be a better indicator of prognosis (Ellis and Auclair 2008). These results reinforce the need for analyses that encompass absolute effect measures (Brandwein et al. 2001). Of final note regarding grading is that the 2017 World Health Organization classification of salivary gland tumors does not endorse a specific grading scheme of mucoepidermoid carcinoma in contrast to the third edition in which grading was paramount in classifying this malignancy (Seethala and Stenman 2017).

low grade, intermediate grade, or high grade depending upon their cellular differentiation. Recent literature combines the low and intermediate grade, thus leaving only two grades, high and low (Cipriani et al. 2019). The classic grading of the MEC is ascertained as a sum of five microscopic parameters. Sums that are 0–4 are regarded as low-grade, those that are 5–6 are considered intermediate-grade, and sums 7–14 are regarded as high-grade cancers. The five microscopic parameters (Figures 8.12 and 8.13) considered are:

Cytokeratin immunostains usually react with the intermediate and large cells of the MEC as does EMA. The smaller cells and the pure mucous cells do not demonstrate the same staining qualities. As

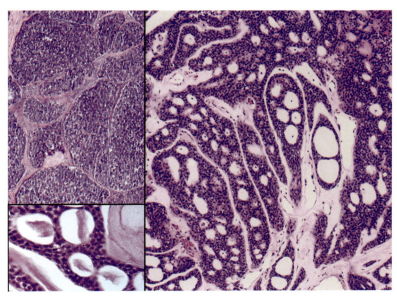

Figure 8.14. Adenoid cystic carcinoma manifesting cribriform and tubular patterns, right panel and lower left panel. Solid pattern of growth shown in upper left panel. H&E staining, 200×/400×. Source: Courtesy of Dr. Mark Bernstein.

one would expect, none of the MEC cell types react with myoepithelial immunostains. There appears to be no correlation between immunostaining and tumor grade.

A chromosomal translocation $t(11;19)$ generates a fusion oncogene, which consists of the mucoepidermoid carcinoma translocated gene (*Mect*)-1 (or *Crtc1*, or *Torc1*) fused to the mastermind-like gene family (*Maml*)-2 and is present in 38–81% of mucoepidermoid carcinomas (Warner et al. 2013). The resulting fusion protein has been generally associated with low/intermediate-grade mucoepidermoid carcinomas and correlated with clinical outcomes. The tumorigenetic effect of the *Crtc1-Maml2* fusion involves activation of the Notch and/or cAMP-responsive element binding protein (CREB) signaling pathways (Kaye 2006). Recently, there has been speculation that MECT1-*MAML2* fusion protein may promote sustained E6/E7 overexpression in the increased numbers of HR-HPV subjects manifesting mucoepidermoid after 2001 (Isayeva et al. 2013).

Adenoid Cystic Carcinoma

Adenoid cystic carcinoma (ACC) is a slow-growing yet biologically aggressive neoplasm with a notable capacity for recurrence (Brookstone and Huvos 1992; Kuhel et al. 1992). In earlier times, the ACC was known as the cylindroma or adenocystic carcinoma. To avoid confusion with similar eccrine tumors, these other designations are no longer in use. These malignant salivary tumors apparently arise from both myoepithelial and ductal cells. Three growth patterns have been acknowledged: cribriform, tubular, and a solid (basaloid) pattern (Figure 8.14). The tumors are classified according to the predominant pattern (Batsakis et al. 1990; Brookstone and Huvos 1992; Ellis and Auclair 2008). The cribriform pattern is the most common, while the solid pattern is the least (Perzin et al. 1978). Solid adenoid cystic carcinoma is a high-grade lesion with reported recurrence rates of as much as 100% compared with 50–80% for the tubular and cribriform variants (Ellis and Auclair 2008). In addition, the solid type appears to exhibit the worst long-term prognosis.

These malignant neoplasms characteristically progress as slow-growing lesions in the palate, parotid gland, and submandibular gland. Not infrequently, pain and facial paralysis are noted with progressive growth of the tumors, which may be attributed to their propensity to invade nerves (Figure 8.15) (Ellis and Auclair 2008). Adenoid cystic carcinomas tend to exhibit an extended course, resulting in a poor clinical result. The 10-year survival for these tumors (stages I–IV) is less than 50% (Speight and Barrett 2002). In that these carcinomas characteristically recur repeatedly and spur late distant metastases, clinical staging of the ACC appears to be a superior prognostic indicator than does histologic grade (Fu et al. 1977; Hamper et al. 1990; Speight and Barrett 2002; Friedrich and Bleckmann 2003). As one would expect, larger tumors with local/regional metastases demonstrate the worst prognostic pattern.

Microscopically, the ACC is histomorphologically diverse with the three major morphologic patterns, quite often all being present within a single tumor. The most common cribriform pattern demonstrates a "Swiss-cheese" appearance with numerous cyst-like structures of varying size being characteristic. Both duct and myoepithelial cells comprise this pattern. As the histologic pattern becomes more solid, the ductal cells decrease while the myoepithelial cells then predominate. Immunologically, the expression of cytokeratins, SMA, MSA, S100, and vimentin by the tumor cells substantiates the premise of a dual-cell population.

Adenoid cystic carcinomas characteristically possess a recurrent $t(6;9)(q2-23;p23-24)$ translocation that results in a novel fusion of the *MYB* proto-oncogene with the transcription factor gene *NFIB* (Chen et al. 2007). *MYB* is a hallmark of adenoid cystic carcinomas and is observed in adenoid cystic

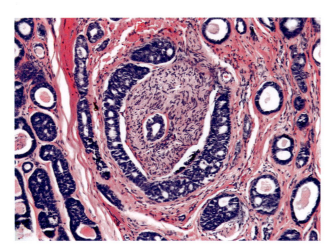

Figure 8.15. Adenoid cystic carcinoma demonstrating classic nerve invasion pattern. H&E staining, 400×.

carcinomas from a variety of sites including: salivary gland, sinonasal cavity, tracheobronchial tree, larynx, breast, and vulva (Brill et al. 2011). Moreover, copy number alterations have included losses involving 12q, 6q, 9p, 11q, 14q, 1p, and 5q and gains involving 1q, 9p, and 22q. Losses of 1p, 6q, and 15q have been associated with high-grade tumors, whereas, losses of 14q have been observed in Grade I tumors (Kasamatsu et al. 2005). The *t*(6;9) rearrangements have been associated with a complex pattern of break points, deletions, insertions, inversions, and for 9p gains (Persson et al. 2012a).

Acinic Cell Carcinoma

The acinic cell carcinoma, once described as an acinic cell tumor has also been referred to as an acinic cell adenocarcinoma. It is a malignant epithelial neoplasm in which the tumor cells convey serous or serous-like acinar differentiation as opposed to mucous acinar cells (Ellis and Auclair 2008). AFIP data have indicated that acinic cell carcinoma is the third most common salivary gland epithelial neoplasm after mucoepidermoid carcinoma and adenocarcinoma, NOS. Moreover, acinic cell carcinoma comprised 17% of primary malignant salivary gland tumors with more than 80% occurring in the parotid gland. However, others have reported a 0–19% frequency of acinic cell carcinoma among malignant salivary gland neoplasms (Ellis and Auclair 2008). When arising in minor glands, the acinic cell carcinoma is commonly seen in the upper lip or buccal mucosa. The acinic cell carcinoma is the most common malignant salivary gland tumor that occurs bilaterally. Women are generally more affected more than males, with a mean age of 44 years. Patients usually present with a slowly increasing mass in the parotid. Pain is a symptom in approximately 33% of patients. Again, staging appears to be a better prognostic predictor than histologic grading (Ellis and Auclair 2008).

Acinic cell carcinomas demonstrate various histological patterns (Figure 8.16). The present architectural classification characterizes them as solid, microcystic, papillary-cystic, and follicular (Figure 8.17). The majority of large tumors present as a spectrum of these features. Most acinic cell carcinomas are reactive with cytokeratin and other immunostains for epithelial cells while they are rarely reactive with immunostains for myoepithelial cells.

Polymorphous Adenocarcinoma

Polymorphous adenocarcinoma (PMAC) is a malignant tumor that is predominately restricted to minor salivary glands and as such represents the second most common malignancy of minor glands. Previously, the PMAC was referred to as a polymorphous low-grade adenocarcinoma (PLGA) but the 2017 WHO classification designates this tumor as polymorphous adenocarcinoma (Seethala and Stenman 2017; Poorten et al. 2018).

These tumors are distinguished by bland, uniform nuclear features, varied but distinctive

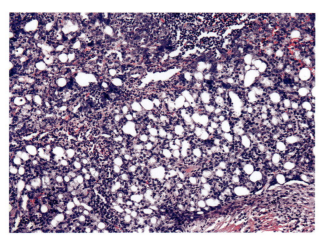

Figure 8.16. Microcystic type of acinic cell carcinoma. Note the numerous small cystic spaces. H&E staining, 200×.

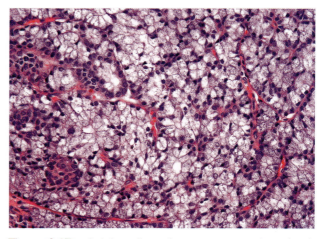

Figure 8.17. Acinic cell carcinoma composed predominately of acinar cells. H&E staining, 200×.

architecture, invasive growth, and perineural infiltration (Ellis and Auclair 2008). The PMAC has been reported to represent approximately 11% of all tumors of salivary glands and ~26% of malignant salivary neoplasms. These malignant tumors characteristically emerge as solid, nontender swellings of the mucosa of the hard and soft palates, buccal mucosa, or upper lip with the palate being the most common site. Soreness, hemorrhage, telangiectasia, or ulceration has been associated with these lesions (Ellis and Auclair 2008). Clinically, the PMAC is a slowly growing, progressive salivary gland neoplasm with an apparent survival approaching 80% at 25 years (Evans and Luna 2000). Noteworthy is that since some of these tumors may behave capriciously that the prior qualifying term, low grade, is deceptive and that the term polymorphous adenocarcinoma is now in general use (Speight and Barrett 2002).

The average age of patients has been 59 years with most cases occurring between the ages of 50 and 79 years. The gender predisposition is in favor of females in a ratio of ~2:1. The AFIP series indicates that >60% of PMACs occur in the mucosa of either the soft or the hard palates, the next most frequent sites being buccal mucosa (16%) and the upper lip (12%). The copy number alterations in polymorphous carcinomas is low indicating that these tumors are genetically stable and supporting the notion that the PMAC is a slow-growing, low-grade carcinoma with low metastatic potential (Persson et al. 2012b).

This salivary gland malignancy demonstrates a quite variable microscopic pattern as the name implies. This tumor is usually well circumscribed but not encapsulated. The PMAC is usually solid and lobulated but the periphery often demonstrates single columns or rows of tumor cells extending into the surrounding connective tissue (Figure 8.18). Often, the cells of the PMAC appear arranged in concentric circles much like paper targets (Figure 8.19). The PMAC demonstrates perineural invasion more commonly than any other salivary gland tumor including the adenoid cystic carcinoma. The tumor cells for the most part react with both antibodies to epithelial cells as well as myoepithelial cells. Often, immunostaining is utilized to distinguish the PMAC from the pleomorphic adenoma as well as from the cells of the adenoid cystic carcinoma.

Collectively, PMAC demonstrates a local recurrence rate of 10–33%, regional metastases of 9–15%, and very rare distant metastases (Seethala and Stenman 2017). This notwithstanding, the papillary variant of this malignancy has historically been noted to be more aggressive with a greater capacity for cervical lymph node metastases and distant spread. Additionally, more aggressive biologic behavior is associated with this tumor when located at the base of tongue with distinct papillary or cribriform architecture (Kennedy 2018). These features have resulted in the designation of cribriform adenocarcinoma of minor salivary gland (CAMSG). The CAMSG has a metastatic rate of 70–100% that exceeds that of PMAC. The histology

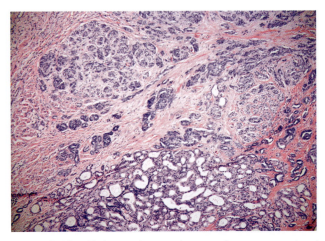

Figure 8.18. Polymorphous adenocarcinoma comprised of both small- and intermediate-size tumor cells. H&E staining, 100×.

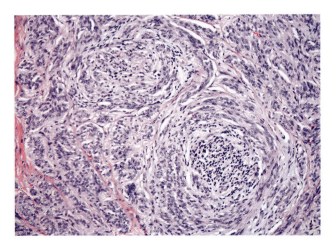

Figure 8.19. Polymorphous adenocarcinoma arranged in a concentric pattern. Near the center of the mass is peripheral nerve infiltration. H&E staining, 200×.

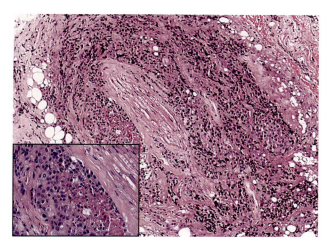

Figure 8.20. Adenocarcinoma, NOS demonstrating infiltrative growth of neoplastic epithelium, which is forming islands, cords, and dense cell sheets invading a peripheral nerve. H&E staining, 200×/400×.

of CAMSG can overlap with that of PMAC such that the WHO has not separated the CAMSG from the PMAC (Seethala and Stenman 2017; Kennedy 2018).

Adenocarcinoma, NOS (Otherwise Specified)

Adenocarcinoma, NOS demonstrates glandular or ductal differentiation but does not have any of the distinct morphologic features that typify the other, more explicit carcinoma types. The microscopic diagnosis of adenocarcinoma, NOS, is fundamentally one of elimination. Adenocarcinoma, NOS, has been suggested to be only second to mucoepidermoid carcinoma in frequency among malignant salivary gland neoplasms (Ellis and Auclair 2008). However, reports have shown a varied incidence from 4 to 10% (Speight and Barrett 2002). The AFIP reports the mean patient age of 58 years with approximately 40 and 60% of tumors occurring in the major and minor salivary glands, correspondingly, with 90% of major gland tumors occurring in the parotid gland (Ellis and Auclair 2008). Adenocarcinoma, NOS is graded according to the degree of differentiation as low-grade, intermediate-grade, and high-grade tumor (Ellis and Auclair 2008; Speight and Barrett 2002). Some reports have indicated that survival is superior for patients with tumors of the oral cavity than for those with tumors of the major glands (Matsuba et al. 1988; Ellis and Auclair 2008).

Adenocarcinoma, NOS demonstrates an extensive range of histologic features, many of which occur within the same tumor. These tumors can be formed by cords, sheets, rows, or islands of tumor cells, but either ducts or glands will be evident in every individual tumor (Figure 8.20). Often, a small aggregate of a specific type of salivary gland malignancy such as acinic cell carcinoma will be identified within the larger tumor mass.

Basal Cell Adenocarcinoma

Basal cell adenocarcinoma also known as basaloid salivary carcinoma, carcinoma ex-monomorphic adenoma, malignant basal cell adenoma, malignant basal cell tumor, and basal cell carcinoma. This low-grade malignancy is an epithelial neoplasm that is cytologically similar to the basal cell adenoma but is infiltrative and has a small potential for metastasis (Ellis and Auclair 2008). In AFIP case files spanning almost 11 years, basal cell adenocarcinoma comprised 1.6% of all salivary gland neoplasms and 2.9% of salivary gland malignancies (Ellis and Auclair 2008). Nearly 90% of tumors occurred in the parotid gland (Muller and Barnes 1996). The average age of patients is reported to be 60 years (Ellis and Auclair 2008).

Like most salivary gland neoplasms, swelling is typically the only sign or symptom experienced (Muller and Barnes 1996). A sudden increase in size may occur in a few patients (Ellis and Auclair 2008). Basal cell carcinomas are low-grade carcinomas that are infiltrative, locally destructive,

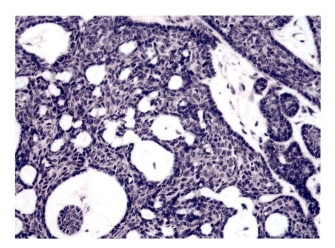

Figure 8.21. Basal cell adenocarcinoma arranged much like a basal cell adenoma but with atypical cellular features. H&E staining, 200×.

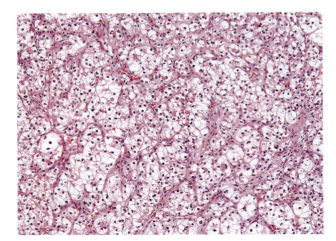

Figure 8.22. Primary clear cell carcinoma arising within the parotid gland. H&E staining, 100×.

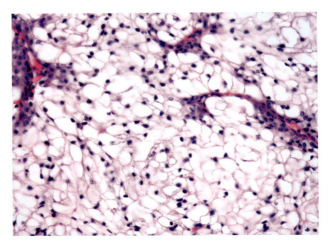

Figure 8.24. A clear cell variant of a mucoepidermoid carcinoma. H&E staining, 200×.

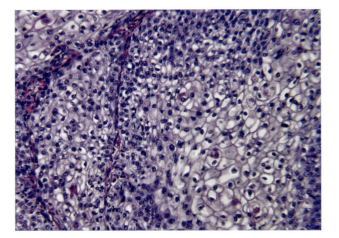

Figure 8.23. A glassy cell variant of a squamous cell carcinoma. Note the clear cell characteristics. H&E staining, 200×.

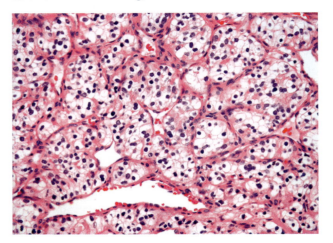

Figure 8.25. The classic clear cell variant of a renal cell carcinoma metastatic to the parotid gland. H&E staining, 200×.

and tend to recur, but only occasionally metastasize. In a retrospective series of 29 cases, there were recurrences in seven and metastases in three (Muller and Barnes 1996). In another retrospective review of 72 cases, 37% involved local recurrences (Ellis and Auclair 2008). The overall prognosis for patients with this tumor is good (Muller and Barnes 1996; Ellis and Auclair 2008; Ward et al. 2009; Jung et al. 2013).

The histologic features of the basal cell carcinoma are quite similar to its benign counterpart, the basal cell adenoma (Figure 8.21). Cytologic atypia such as the finding of atypical mitotic figures is helpful if available. Other times, this atypia is almost nonexistent. Infiltrative growth through the capsule if present or extensions into periglandular fat or muscle are very helpful findings in this type of carcinoma. Immunohistochemistry is variable from tumor to tumor but most tumors will show at least partial staining for myoepithelial cells.

Clear Cell Carcinoma

Clear cell carcinoma, also known as clear cell adenocarcinoma, is a very rare malignant epithelial neoplasm composed of a monomorphous population of cells that have optically clear cytoplasm with standard hematoxylin and eosin stains and lack features of other specific neoplasms

(Figure 8.22). Because of inconsistencies in the methods of reporting salivary gland neoplasms, meaningful incidence rates for this tumor are difficult to derive from the literature (Ellis and Auclair 2008). Most cases involve the minor salivary glands. In the AFIP case files, the mean age of patients is approximately 58 years (Ellis and Auclair 2008).

Several other types of both primary and secondary salivary gland malignancies can also demonstrate the formation of clear cells. These include the acinic cell carcinoma, the oncocytoma, the epithelial-myoepithelial carcinoma, the sebaceous carcinoma, the glassy cell squamous cell carcinoma (Figure 8.23), the mucoepidermoid carcinoma (Figure 8.24), and others. Metastasis from a clear cell malignancy is often indistinguishable from a primary clear cell salivary gland carcinoma. The most commonly encountered clear cell metastasis is a renal cell carcinoma arising from the kidney (Figure 8.25). Meticulous microscopic searching is often needed to distinguish one clear cell carcinoma from another.

In most patients, parotid swelling is the only symptom as the clear cell adenocarcinoma is a low-grade neoplasm. As of 1996, the AFIP reported that there were no deaths reported resulting from this tumor (Sicurella et al. 2004; Ellis and Auclair 2008).

Hyalinizing Clear Cell Carcinoma

Hyalinizing clear cell carcinoma (HCCC) is a unique low-grade salivary gland tumor that shows nests, cords, and trabeculae of clear and eosinophilic cells in a characteristic hyalinized stroma (Weinreb 2013). It primarily arises in the oral cavity but has been described at essentially all salivary gland and seromucous gland sites. The tumors raise a broad differential diagnosis, most of which are easily distinguished by light microscopy and immunohistochemistry. HCCC possesses a squamous line of differentiation without true myoepithelial marker expression. Mucinous differentiation, irrespective of quantity, is not an exclusion criterion and should not lead to a diagnosis of clear cell mucoepidermoid carcinoma (Weinreb 2013). Recent evidence shows that this carcinoma harbors a recurrent and consistent *EWSR1-ATF1* fusion, which also helps link this tumor to "clear cell odontogenic carcinoma" (Bilodeau et al. 2012; Weinreb 2013).

Cystadenocarcinoma

Cystadenocarcinoma, also known as malignant papillary cystadenoma, mucus-producing adenopapillary non-epidermoid carcinoma, low-grade papillary adenocarcinoma of the palate, and papillary adenocarcinoma, is a rare malignant epithelial tumor characterized histologically by prominent cystic and frequently, papillary growth but lacking features that characterize cystic variants of several more common salivary gland neoplasms. Cystadenocarcinoma is the malignant counterpart of the benign cystadenoma (Ellis and Auclair 2008).

In a review of 57 cases, the AFIP found that men and women are affected equally with the average patient age about 59 years. Approximately 65% occurred in the major salivary glands, primarily in the parotid. In addition, it is one of the most common salivary gland malignances found in the sublingual gland. Most patients present with a slowly growing asymptomatic mass. Clinically, this neoplasm is rarely associated with pain or facial paralysis. Cystadenocarcinoma is considered a low-grade neoplasm (Ellis and Auclair 2008).

A subtype of cystadenocarcinoma is known as low-grade cribriform cystadenocarcinoma (LGCCC) and is an extremely rare neoplasm of salivary gland. LGCCC usually occurs in elderly people with a female predominance. The parotid gland is the most common site of involvement. LGCCC is characterized by the papillary-cystic or cribriform proliferation pattern (Figure 8.26) and is similar to

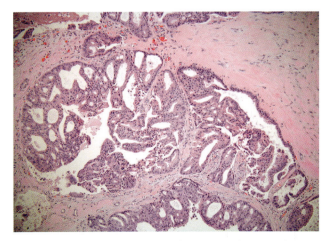

Figure 8.26. Low-grade cribriform cystadenocarcinoma, also known as the low-grade salivary duct carcinoma, is easily confused with an acinic cell carcinoma. H&E staining, 200×.

the low-grade ductal carcinoma in situ or atypical ductal hyperplasia of the breast in histology and biological features. LGCCC was originally designated as low-grade salivary duct carcinoma (LGSDC) to distinguish it from the conventional salivary duct carcinoma (SDC). In contrast with the LGCCC, conventional SDC exhibits highly aggressive malignancy and high-grade histology similar to an invasive ductal carcinoma of the breast. However, no definite association was found between LGCCC and conventional SDC; therefore, the third WHO classification regards this neoplasm as a variant of cystadenocarcinoma due to its cystic morphology (Wang et al. 2013a).

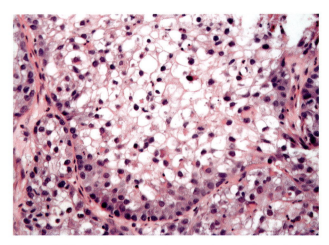

Figure 8.27. Sebaceous adenocarcinoma characterized by sebaceous differentiation within islands of squamoid cells. The histology appears similar to the sebaceous adenoma. H&E staining, 400×.

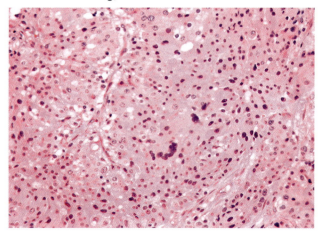

Figure 8.28. Oncocytic carcinoma demonstrating the atypical cellular features of the malignant oncocytes. H&E staining, 200×.

Histologically, LGCCC is composed of single or multiple enlarged cystic ducts accompanied by adjacent intraductal proliferation. These tumor cells are strongly positive for S100 immunostain. Based on the histological features, LGCCC should be distinguished with other common parotid tumors including papillary cystic variant of acinic cell carcinoma, conventional salivary duct carcinoma, cystadenocarcinoma, polymorphous adenocarcinoma (PMAC), carcinoma ex-pleomorphic adenoma, and mammary analogue secretory carcinoma (MASC) (Wang et al. 2013a).

Sebaceous Adenocarcinoma

Sebaceous adenocarcinoma is an uncommon malignant epithelial neoplasm that is generally regarded as an intermediate-grade neoplasm. The tumors have been noted to be comprised of islands and sheets of cells with areas of sebaceous differentiation (Figure 8.27). The cells of these tumors possess atypical nuclear morphology, and manifest an infiltrative pattern of growth (Ellis and Auclair 2008). Clinical presentation as a painless, slow-growing, asymptomatic swelling have been reported; however, lesions may be painful or result in facial nerve involvement with paralysis. Approximately one-third of these tumors has been reported to have a recurrence potential (Gnepp 1983). Most examples of this neoplasm have been limited to the parotid gland with the mean age of occurrence being 69 years (Gnepp 1983; Ellis and Auclair 2008; Wang et al. 2010).

Microscopically, the tumor is formed of sheets and islands of malignant cells, predominately of squamous and basaloid appearance. Intermittent sebaceous differentiation is always present, but it may be minimal. Perineural invasion is relatively common.

Sebaceous Lymphadenocarcinoma

Sebaceous lymphadenocarcinoma is a particularly uncommon malignant low-grade neoplasm with a good prognosis (Gnepp and Brannon 1984). These neoplasms are believed to correspond to carcinomatous transformation of sebaceous lymphadenoma. The carcinoma portion of the tumor has been reported as sebaceous adenocarcinoma; however, such a classification can lead to overtreatment as the sebaceous carcinomas are recognized as relatively aggressive tumors (Ellis and

Auclair 2008). As only four cases have been reported, all of which were associated with the parotid gland in elderly patients, there is little information available on these neoplasms (Gnepp and Brannon 1984; Ellis and Auclair 2008; Gnepp 2012).

Microscopically, this tumor consists of classic benign sebaceous lymphadenoma within lymphoid stroma. Admixed in this benign lesion are found areas of sebaceous carcinoma without the adjacent lymphoid stroma.

Oncocytic Carcinoma

Oncocytic carcinoma, also known as malignant oncocytoma or oncocytic adenocarcinoma, is a rare high-grade carcinoma, salivary neoplasm with predominantly oncocytic features. The oncocytic carcinomas constitute <1% of the cases salivary gland tumors accessioned to the AFIP files (Ellis and Auclair 2008). Most reported cases have been in the parotid gland where they present as painful lesions or associated with facial nerve paralysis (Sugimoto et al. 1993). Like other parotid gland carcinomas, tumors that are less than 2 cm have a better prognosis than larger tumors. Thus, TNM staging correlates with the prognosis (Goode et al. 1998). The AFIP series reports that the average age of patients with these neoplasms has been 63 years (Ellis and Auclair 2008; Zhou et al. 2010).

As with benign oncocytomas, the oncocytic adenocarcinoma is composed of sheets of round and polyhedral cells with fine eosinophilic cytoplasm. Ultrastructurally, these granules are composed of excessive numbers of atypical mitochondria. While many of the cells have no unusual features, and look identical to those of the benign oncocytoma, others demonstrate atypical mitotic figures and other pleomorphic features (Figure 8.28). The finding of these two cell groupings leads one to speculate that the oncocytic carcinoma arises from a pre-existing benign oncocytoma.

Salivary Duct Carcinoma

Salivary duct carcinoma, or salivary duct adenocarcinoma, is a high-grade malignant epithelial neoplasm comprised of elements that bear a resemblance to expanded salivary gland ducts. The AFIP files indicate that salivary duct carcinomas represent only <1% of all epithelial salivary gland neoplasms with 75% of cases affecting the parotid gland and with a male gender predominance of 1.5–1.0 and mean incidence occurring in the seventh and eighth decades of life (Ellis and Auclair 2008). Parotid swelling has generally been the most common presenting symptom. However, facial nerve involvement has been noted in ~25% of patients. Although a low-grade variant of this tumor has been described, the high-grade variants of this neoplasm have been regarded as one of the most aggressive types of salivary gland carcinoma. One review has revealed that one-third of patients

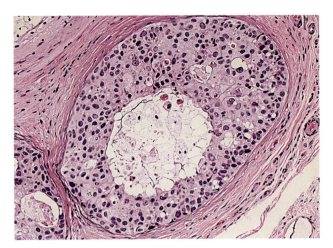

Figure 8.29. Salivary duct carcinoma containing comedonecrosis centrally within a tumor nodule surrounded by a prominent hyalinized fibrous connective tissue. H&E staining, 400×. Source: Courtesy of Dr. Mark Bernstein.

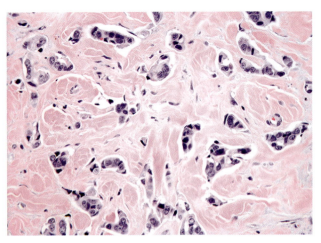

Figure 8.30. Nodules of salivary duct carcinoma embedded within a dense connective tissue stroma. H&E staining, 400×.

with these neoplasms developed rapid local recurrence and 46% developed distant metastasis (Ellis and Auclair 2008). The high-grade tumors are epitomized by local invasion, hematogenous and lymphatic metastatic spread, and a dismal prognosis (Delgado et al. 1996; Guzzo et al. 2002; Ellis and Auclair 2008).

The high-grade form of the salivary duct carcinoma is invariably composed of rounded solid or cystic nodules of tumor. While the smaller nodules are filled with additional tumor, the larger ones demonstrate a characteristic comedonecrosis rarely seen in other salivary gland tumors (Figure 8.29). The epithelial cells can be poorly differentiated although some show only a few atypical features. Dense fibrosis is a hallmark of salivary duct carcinoma. Within this dense fibrous stroma are small nests of malignant tumor cells (Figure 8.30).

The low-grade salivary duct carcinoma has recently been reclassified as low-grade cribriform cystadenocarcinoma. Even though the histology is somewhat similar to the high-grade variant, the clinical behavior is vastly different. The terminology has therefore been altered allowing the treating clinician a better understanding of the two lesions and thus decreasing the possibility of treating the patient inappropriately.

An analysis of PLAG1 and HMGA2 rearrangements in salivary duct carcinoma (SDC) has revealed that a large proportion of SDCs arise in pleomorphic adenomas (PAs), with or without residual evidence of a PA. However, a small proportion of SDCs appear to arise in low-grade cribriform cystadenocarcinoma and ductal carcinoma in situ (Bahrami et al. 2013).

Malignant Mixed Tumors

Carcinoma ex-pleomorphic adenoma, carcinosarcoma, and metastasizing mixed tumor have all been regarded as subtypes of malignant mixed tumors. The most common among these is the carcinoma ex-pleomorphic adenoma. On the other hand, the carcinosarcoma is a true malignant mixed tumor with both epithelial and mesenchymal elements cytologically malignant. However, the carcinosarcoma and the metastasizing mixed tumor, which demonstrate semantic inexactness, are extremely rare (Ellis and Auclair 2008).

Carcinoma Ex-Pleomorphic Adenoma

Carcinoma ex-pleomorphic adenoma, sometimes termed carcinoma ex. mixed tumor, is a malignant epithelial neoplasm that demonstrates evidence of malignancy arising primarily from or in a benign pleomorphic adenoma in one of the major salivary glands (Roijer et al. 2002). Thus, the diagnosis necessitates that the sample contains benign tumor as well as carcinomatous elements (LiVolsi and Perzin 1977). Only the epithelial component is malignant, not the myoepithelial as is seen in the

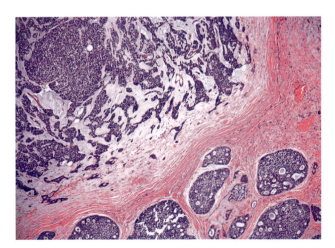

Figure 8.31. Carcinoma ex-pleomorphic adenoma. The histology demonstrates adenoid cystic carcinoma (top) arising within a basal cell adenoma (bottom). H&E staining, 100×.

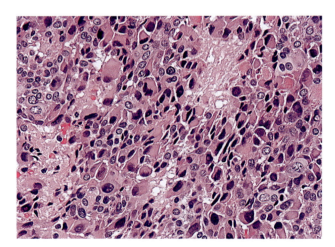

Figure 8.32. Carcinoma ex-pleomorphic adenoma exhibiting nuclear abnormalities, including pleomorphism, hyperchromatism, and large nucleoli with variations in cellularity within a pleomorphic adenoma. H&E staining, 400×. Source: Courtesy of Dr. Mark Bernstein.

carcinosarcoma. It appears that the longer a patient is afflicted with a pleomorphic adenoma, the more likely the transformation into the malignant form. AFIP files have indicated that carcinoma ex-pleomorphic adenoma encompasses 8.8% of all mixed tumors and 4.6% of all malignant salivary gland tumors, making it the sixth most common malignant salivary gland tumor (Ellis and Auclair 2008). The most common clinical symptoms have been that of a painless mass, although, one-third of patients have been noted to present with facial paralysis (Ellis and Auclair 2008). Like other major salivary gland malignancies, tumor stage, grade, and degree of invasion determine prognosis (Brandwein et al. 2002).

The benign portion of this tumor makes up a variable amount of the entire mass. The malignant portion may be completely separate from the benign element (Figure 8.31) or they may be intermingled. In most tumors, the malignant portion appears most like an adenocarcinoma (Figure 8.32) NOS but other carcinoma ex-pleomorphic adenomas demonstrate area composed of mucoepidermoid carcinoma, acinic cell carcinoma, and various others. If the malignant portion of the tumor is surrounded by benign mixed tumor, it is known as *carcinoma in situ ex-pleomorphic adenoma or noninvasive carcinoma ex-pleomorphic adenoma.*

Altered *PLAG1* or *HMGA2* genes have been detected in most case of carcinoma ex-pleomorphic adenomas (CA-ex-PA). Although PLAG1 detection was specific for carcinoma ex-pleomorphic adenoma versus other carcinomas, its use as a standalone discriminatory test is limited by variable expression (Bahrami et al. 2012).

Salivary Carcinosarcoma

Salivary carcinosarcoma has been regarded and designated a true malignant mixed tumor. Consequently, these neoplasms contain cellular elements, which are both carcinomatous and sarcomatous in nature. Either or both cellular components are expressed in metastatic lesions. Although carcinosarcomas may develop on their own, others arise in association with or within benign mixed tumors. Most of these tumors occur in the major salivary glands where they have presented clinically with swelling, pain, nerve palsy, and/or ulceration. These tumors are extremely rare with only a few cases being acknowledged by the AFIP (Ellis and Auclair 2008). Carcinosarcoma is an aggressive, high-grade malignancy with a survival of 3.6 years (Stephen et al. 1986; Taki et al. 2013).

Microscopically, carcinosarcomas always contain elements of both carcinoma and sarcoma. The sarcoma portion usually predominates over the other segment. The sarcomatous segment is usually represented by chondrosarcoma but other types such as fibrosarcoma or osteosarcoma have been identified.

Metastasizing Mixed Tumor

Metastasizing mixed tumor is an uncommon histological benign salivary gland neoplasm that enigmatically metastasizes. Reportedly, there are long intervals occuring between the diagnosis of a primary "benign" tumor and the metastases. The histological attributes of the metastatic lesions are essentially those that epitomize pleomorphic adenoma (Ellis and Auclair 2008). Most of these benign lesions occur in the major salivary glands as a single, well-defined mass. Metastases have been described in the lung, lymph nodes, and bone. Interestingly, metastases or recurrences may occur up to 26 years after excision of the primary neoplasm (Santaliz-Ruiz et al. 2012; Schneider et al. 1977).

Sialoblastoma

Sialoblastoma is an extremely rare neoplasm of major salivary glands with fewer than 20 cases identified in the literature. Tumors of the ductal or secretory epithelial cells of salivary gland are exceedingly rare in children younger than 2 years of age. The sialoblastoma has been recognized and usually presents at birth or shortly thereafter. These tumors are composed of basaloid and myoepithelial cells that resemble the developing salivary anlage. The sialoblastoma has been reported under a variety of names such as congenital basal cell adenoma, basal cell adenoma, basaloid adenocarcinoma, and congenital hybrid basal cell adenoma-adenoid cystic carcinoma (Choudhary et al. 2013). It has been suggested that these tumors be divided into benign and malignant lesions based on cytologic features and patterns of growth that include nerve and vascular invasion and necrosis. Brandwein et al. (1999) suggested caution should be used in designating aggressive (malignant) and nonaggressive (benign) sialoblastoma on the basis of histomorphology alone (Batsakis and Frankenthaler 1992; Ellis and Auclair 2008).

Primary Squamous Cell Carcinoma

Primary squamous cell carcinoma is a rare neoplasm of salivary glands. This neoplasm occurs in the parotid gland approximately nine times more frequently than in the submandibular gland, with a partiality toward males (Spitz and Batsakis 1984; Sterman et al. 1990; Gaughan et al. 1992; Ellis and Auclair 2008). Patients generally present with an asymptomatic mass in the parotid region. However, with progression, symptoms may comprise pain and/or facial nerve palsy (Shemen et al. 1987). Identification of these lesions requires segregating this primary carcinoma from metastatic disease originating from other head and neck or oral occurrences (Ellis and Auclair 2008). The diagnosis of primary disease probably cannot be made in minor salivary glands because of the size of the glands and proximity to mucosa that is vulnerable to develop squamous cell carcinoma (Ellis and Auclair 2008). Existing literature suggests that preceding exposure to ionizing radiation increases the risk for developing primary salivary squamous carcinoma; however, the sample size used in these studies was meager (Schneider et al. 1977; Spitz and Batsakis 1984; Shemen et al. 1987). The frequency of this primary salivary squamous carcinoma has ranged from 0.9 to 4.7% (Ellis and Auclair 2008). AFIP series have indicated that over a 10-year interval, primary squamous cell carcinoma comprised 2.7% of all tumors; 5.4% of malignant tumors; and 2.5% of parotid neoplasms and 2.8% of submandibular tumors; with an average age of 64 years (Ellis and Auclair 2008). Primary salivary gland squamous carcinoma is graded similar to extrasalivary squamous cell carcinomas; utilizing (low, intermediate, and high) degree of differentiation (Speight and Barrett 2002). The prognosis for these primary salivary gland cancers is dire with an 18% 10-year survival rate (Shemen et al. 1987).

The histopathology of primary squamous cell carcinoma arising in salivary gland is not unlike those arising elsewhere (Figure 8.33). These tumors are predominately keratin producing but several are poorly differentiated without keratin production (Figure 8.34). Nerve involvement is quite common. Special stains for intracellular mucin production are often needed to rule out high-grade mucoepidermoid carcinoma masquerading as a primary squamous cell lesion.

Epithelial-Myoepithelial Carcinoma

Epithelial-myoepithelial carcinoma (EMC), also designated by some as adenomyoepithelioma, clear cell adenoma, tubular solid adenoma, monomorphic clear cell tumor, glycogen-rich adenoma, glycogen-rich adenocarcinoma, clear cell carcinoma, and salivary duct carcinoma, is an uncommon, low-grade epithelial neoplasm composed of variable proportions

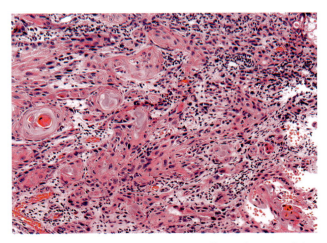

Figure 8.33. Primary squamous cell carcinoma arising within a parotid gland. Note the large amount of keratin production in this moderately differentiated tumor. H&E staining, 200×.

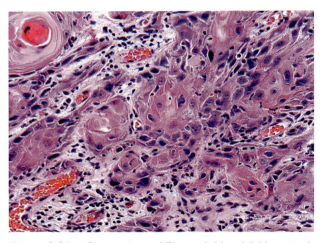

Figure 8.34. Closer view of Figure 8.33 exhibiting atypical nuclear features of the malignant squamous cells. H&E staining, 400×.

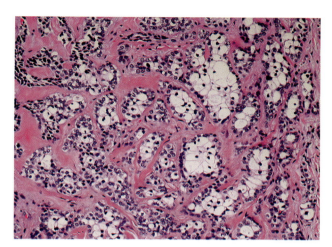

Figure 8.35. Myoepithelial carcinoma of salivary gland. Note the larger clear cells as well as the smaller epithelial cells. Surrounding each group of cells is a dense fibrous stroma. H&E staining, 200×.

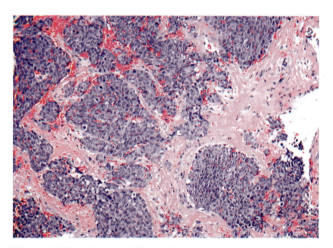

Figure 8.36. Poorly differentiated carcinoma arranged in groups. Note the lack of cellular organization. H&E staining, 200×.

of ductal and large, clear-staining, differentiated myoepithelial cells. These neoplasms make up approximately 1% of all epithelial salivary gland tumors (Batsakis et al. 1992; Ellis and Auclair 2008). Epithelial-myoepithelial carcinomas are principally limited to the parotid glands, although an occasional tumor is identified arising in oral minor salivary glands. The lesions commonly present as localized painless swellings, although larger lesions maybe associated with pain or compromise of the facial muscle tone (Daley et al. 1984; Collina et al. 1991).

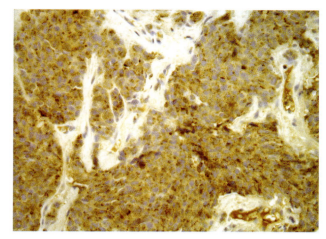

Figure 8.37. Poorly differentiated carcinoma as in Figure 8.35. This immunostain demonstrates the positive neuroendocrine features of these cells. Chromogranin immunostain, 200×.

The best current data indicate that the mean age of patients with these lesions is approximately 60 years with a gender bias of 60% toward females (Ellis and Auclair 2008). Although these tumors have a propensity to metastasize to regional parotid and cervical lymph nodes, and may on rare occasion give rise to distant metastasis and death, these tumors are generally regarded as low-grade carcinomas with a high frequency of recurrence (Collina et al. 1991; Simpson et al. 1991; Batsakis et al. 1992; Noel and Brozna 1992; Arora et al. 2013).

The histology of the epithelial-myoepithelial carcinoma is relatively unique. Most lesions are well defined and occasionally encapsulated. The tumors themselves are made of up two cell populations: large, elongated clear cells and smaller cuboidal ductal cells (Figure 8.35). Occasionally, one encounters an EMC comprised almost completely of clear cells. Immunochemically, the clear cells stain as myoepithelial cells. Most of these tumors show little in the way of atypia with only occasional pleomorphism described.

Poorly Differentiated Carcinomas

Poorly differentiated carcinomas of salivary glands are a group of rare malignant epithelial neoplasms that lack the specific light-microscopic morphologic features of other types of salivary gland carcinomas. These tumors often appear with the cells arranged as sheets, strands, and nests (Figure 8.36). The cells are slightly larger than a lymphocyte and possess oval, hyperchromatic nuclei, limited cytoplasm and generally have a high mitotic index. Rarely, pseudorosettes are encountered. Most of these tumors stain with cytokeratins and EMA (Figure 8.37). Occasionally, a small number of these also stain with chromogranin or synaptophysin, which supports their neuroendocrine origin.

These carcinomas are histologically similar to undifferentiated or poorly differentiated carcinomas that arise in other organs and tissues. Accordingly, metastatic carcinoma is a principal matter in the differential diagnosis of these tumors (Ellis and Auclair 2008). Four separate types are discussed arising within salivary gland: undifferentiated carcinoma, small cell neuroendocrine carcinoma, large cell neuroendocrine carcinoma, and lymphoepithelial carcinoma.

Undifferentiated Carcinoma

Undifferentiated carcinomas of salivary glands can have both large cells and small cells, be neuroendocrine in origin or not, and stain with similar immunostains or not. They are very similar histologically to undifferentiated carcinomas of other organ systems. For this reason alone, great care must be taken in identifying the specific tumor type as a great number of these lesions ultimately prove to be metastatic from a malignancy distant to salivary gland. As a rule, these tumors are very aggressive and offer a two-year survival of approximately 50%.

Small Cell Neuroendocrine Carcinoma

Small cell neuroendocrine carcinomas (SCNECs) have also been termed extrapulmonary oat cell carcinomas. These primary malignant tumors are comprised of undifferentiated cells that do exhibit neuroendocrine differentiation (Figure 8.38). As such, these tumors have been regarded as the undifferentiated equivalent of the anaplastic small cell carcinoma seen primarily in the lungs. Small cell carcinoma has represented approximately 1.8% of all major salivary gland malignancies in the AFIP series (Gnepp and Wick 1990). The tumors have a mean patient age of 56 years, with half of the cases presenting as asymptomatic parotid masses of only brief duration (Perez-Ordonez et al. 1998; Ellis and Auclair 2008). These are high-grade neoplasms with an estimated survival rate at two and five years of 70 and 46%, respectively (Gnepp et al. 1986).

Some authorities differentiate between small cell undifferentiated carcinomas with neuroendocrine features versus those without these features (de Vicente Rodriquez et al. (2004). Immunostaining is the most effective means to distinguish one from another. Chromogranin, synaptophysin, and NSE will generally be reactive on those tumors with neuroendocrine features.

Large Cell Neuroendocrine Carcinoma

Large cell neuroendocrine carcinoma (LCNEC) is a malignant neoplasm that lacks all features of

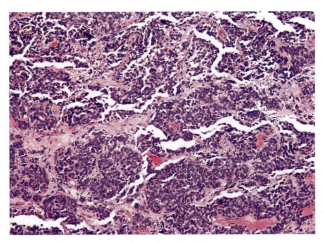

Figure 8.38. Small cell undifferentiated carcinoma of minor salivary gland. Note the complete lack of cell orientation. The cells are slightly larger than mature lymphocytes. H&E staining, 200×.

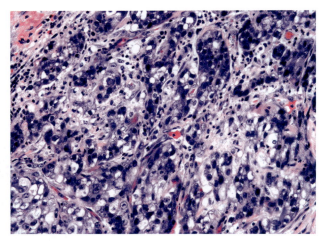

Figure 8.39. Large cell undifferentiated carcinoma of the submandibular gland. The entire tumor is composed of large, pleomorphic cells with no specific orientation. H&E staining, 200×.

differentiation. However, in rare instances, poorly formed duct-like structures have been described. Rapid growth of a parotid swelling is a common clinical presentation (Gaughan et al. 1992). These tumors are high-grade lesions that commonly metastasize. Tumors that are T3 or greater in size have been noted to have a dismal prognosis (Batsakis and Luna 1991). These neoplasms comprise approximately 1% of all epithelial salivary gland tumors, with most cases occurring in the parotid glands of elderly patients (Hui et al. 1990; Batsakis and Luna 1991; Ellis and Auclair 2008).

Microscopically, these tumors lack features of acinar, ductal, or myoepithelial differentiation. The cells are commonly arranged in sheets separated by fibrous septae. In general, the cells of the LCNEC are quite pleomorphic with many atypical mitotic figures seen (Figure 8.39). The cells of most LCNEC react with cytokeratin immunostains as well as the majority neuroendocrine stains.

Lymphoepithelial Carcinoma

Lymphoepithelial carcinoma, which is also known as undifferentiated carcinoma with lymphoid stroma and carcinoma ex lymphoepithelial lesion, is an undifferentiated tumor coupled with a dense lymphoid stroma. Notably, these cancers have commonly been linked with Epstein-Barr virus infection (Leung et al. 1995). Moreover, an unusually high incidence of these tumors has been identified most often in the parotid glands and to a less extent in the submandibular gland of Eskimo and Inuit populations (Bosch et al. 1988; Ellis and Auclair 2008). Pain is a common presenting symptom; however, in 20% of patients, facial nerve involvement has been recorded (Borg et al. 1993). Cervical lymph node metastasis has been a common finding at initial presentation, and 20% of patients develop distant metastases within a three-year period (Bosch et al. 1988; Borg et al. 1993).

Microscopically, this malignancy is comprised of dense, cytologically benign lymphoid aggregates, often with germinal centers. Among the lymphocytes are inconspicuous collections of large malignant epithelioid cells, many of which are arranged in a syncytial pattern (Figure 8.40). Immunochemically, these large malignant cells stain with cytokeratins and EMA but not with myoepithelial stains (Figure 8.41). Over half the cases are also EBV reactive.

Myoepithelial Carcinoma

Myoepithelial carcinoma is a very rare, malignant salivary gland neoplasm that almost entirely manifests myoepithelial differentiation. This tumor represents the malignant complement of benign myoepithelioma (Ellis and Auclair 2008; Kane and Bagwan 2010). Most patients, mean age 55 years, present with a painless mass generally within the parotid gland (66%) (Ellis and Auclair 2008).

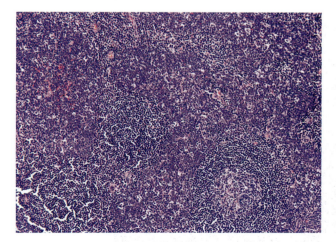

Figure 8.40. Lymphoepithelial carcinoma is composed of large malignant cells imbedded within a lymphoid stroma. Often, it is difficult to microscopically discern the malignant cells in this dense stroma. H&E staining, 100×.

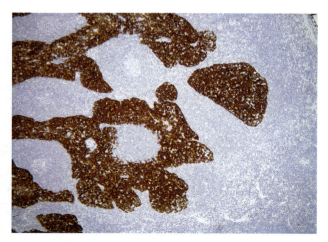

Figure 8.41. Immunohistochemistry is a great help in determining the exact tumor type in the same lesion as in Figure 8.39. Note the ease with which stain depicts these large malignant cells within the lymphoid stroma. Pan cytokeratin (pan CK) immunostain, 100×.

The tumors are often intermediate-grade or high-grade carcinomas (Savera et al. 2000; Ellis and Auclair 2008). Interestingly, the histological grade of these neoplasms does not appear to correlate in a good way with clinical behavior. As such, some tumors manifesting with a low-grade histologic pattern may behave in an aggressive manner (Savera et al. 2000).

Myoepithelial carcinoma is composed of the same type cells as its benign counterpart. The cells range from clear cells to spindle cells to plasmacytoid cells and beyond. Unlike the benign variant, the malignant myoepithelioma demonstrates an invasive growth pattern, which for the most part is the one distinguishing feature that is diagnostic. Most immunochemical stains used for myoepithelial cells are also reactive with the malignant variant, at least the better differentiated type.

Adenosquamous Carcinoma

Adenosquamous carcinoma (ASC) is an extremely uncommon malignant neoplasm that emerges concurrently from surface mucosa and salivary gland ductal epithelium. Although relatively common in other organs such as the uterus and cervix, the ASC is rare arising from salivary gland. These tumors possess histopathologic characteristics of squamous cell carcinoma and of adenocarcinoma. Analysis of the few cases reported seems to indicate that this is an extremely aggressive malignancy with a dismal prognosis (Ellis and Auclair 2008; Kusafuka et al. 2013).

This diagnosis of adenosquamous carcinoma requires both well-defined surface squamous cell carcinoma and adenocarcinoma deeper within the specimen. These two elements do not intermingle or arise from one another but separately. This type of cancer is easily confused microscopically with mucoepidermoid carcinoma. Other varieties of squamous cell carcinoma such as the adenoid squamous or the pseudo-glandular variants can also be in the differential.

Secretory Carcinoma

Mammary analogue secretory carcinoma (2017 WHO terminology: secretory carcinoma of salivary gland) of salivary gland origin resembles secretory carcinoma of the breast. This tumor is characterized immunohistochemically by strong S-100 protein, mammaglobin, and vimentin immunoexpression. Secretory carcinomas generally are solitary, unencapsulated but well-circumscribed tumors of the parotid gland. Patients of all ages are affected including children and young adults. These tumors may possess a prominent fluid-containing cystic component. These lesions are considered a low-grade malignancy, although high-grade transformation and aggressive clinical behavior have been uncommonly described. Secretory carcinomas are not highly infiltrative, perineural invasion is uncommon, and lymphovascular invasion has not been described. These cancers often exhibit a lobulated growth pattern and are frequently composed of microcystic, tubular, and solid structures with abundant eosinophilic homogenous or bubbly secretions (Figures 8.42 and 8.43).

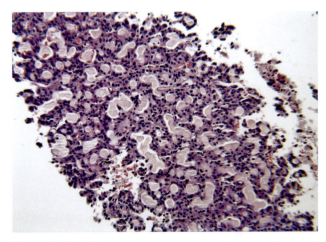

Figure 8.42. Mammary analogue secretory carcinoma of salivary gland. Note the tubular architecture. H&E staining, 200×.

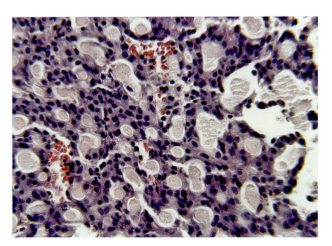

Figure 8.43. Mammary analogue secretory carcinoma of salivary gland. Note the microcystic spaces quite similar to those of an acinic cell carcinoma. H&E staining, 400×.

With these histological features, confusion with the microcystic form of acinic cell carcinoma (ACC) is quite common (Bissinger et al. 2017). Colloid-like material stains positively for periodic acid-Schiff with and without diastase as well as for Alcian Blue (Hung et al. 2019). Secretory carcinoma has been shown to harbor a *t*(12;15) (p13;q25) translocation, resulting in *ETV6-NTRK3* fusion product. Analysis for the presence of the *ETV6-NTRK3* fusion transcript has revealed positivity in both HG and low-grade components of secretory carcinoma in a limited number of cases. Analysis of *TP53* and *CTNNB1* gene mutations in the HG component of MASCs as well as detection of copy number aberration of *EGFR* and *CCND1* gene has not revealed any abnormalities. Recognizing HG-transformed MASC and testing for *ETV6* rearrangement may be of potential value in patient treatment, because the presence of the *ETV6-NTRK3* translocation may represent a therapeutic target in MASC (Skalova et al. 2010, 2014; Bishop 2013). Secretory carcinoma mimics acinic cell carcinomas (ACCs) histologically. Many non-parotid ACCs have retrospectively demonstrated to actually represent secretory carcinoma. However, the impact of diagnostic error is mitigated by the low-grade and nonaggressive nature of secretory carcinoma (Bishop et al. 2013).

Non-Epithelial Neoplasms
Lymphomas and Benign Lymphoepithelial Lesion

Lymphomas of the major salivary glands are typically non-Hodgkin lymphomas. AFIP reviews have indicated that non-Hodgkin lymphomas constituted 16.3% of all malignant tumors that arise in the major salivary glands. Moreover, non-Hodgkin lymphomas of the parotid gland comprised 80% of all cases (Ellis and Auclair 2008; Dispenza et al. 2011; Shum et al. 2014).

Patients with benign lymphoepithelial lesions, now designated lymphoepithelial sialadenitis (LESA), as well as patients with Sjögren syndrome (Figure 8.44) are considered at an increased risk for development of non-Hodgkin lymphoma (Ihrler et al. 2000; Abbondanzo 2001; Bernatsky et al. 2006). The benign lymphoepithelial lesion is clinically distinguished by unilateral and occasionally bilateral enlargement of the salivary glands (Figure 8.45). In affected salivary glands, the lesion is composed of parenchymal atrophy, as well as foci of distinctive myoepithelial islands bounded by a diffuse infiltration of lymphocytes, that can possess germinal centers (Ellis and Auclair 2008). It should be noted that these histologic changes do not occur in minor salivary glands. In minor glands, such as those in the lip, the changes seen involve destruction of glandular tissue and replacement with small, discrete islands of lymphocytes. Because of these histologic features, minor gland biopsies often serve as surrogates for parotid biopsies when Sjögren syndrome is considered. Immunophenotypically and genotypically, the lymphocytic component consists of polyclonal B-lymphocytes and/or T-lymphocytes.

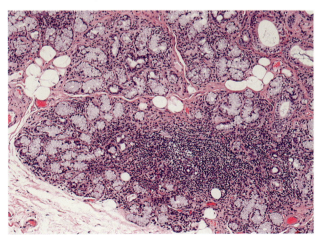

Figure 8.44. Lymphoid aggregate in mucous minor salivary gland often seen in Sjögren syndrome. H&E staining, 100×. Source: Courtesy of Dr. Mark Bernstein.

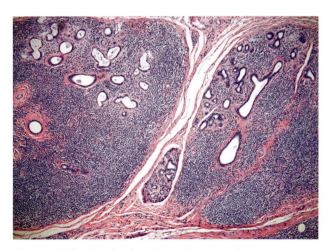

Figure 8.45. Benign lymphoepithelial lesion, now designated as lymphoepithelial sialadenitis (LESA), of the submandibular gland taken from a patient with Sjögren syndrome. Note the obliteration of normal glandular architecture by the lymphocytes. H&E staining, 100×.

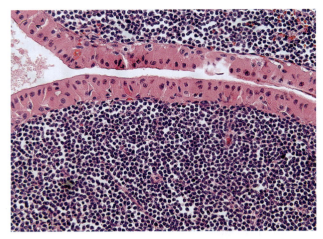

Figure 8.46. Small B-cell lymphoma arising within a Warthin tumor from the parotid gland. Note the diffuse lymphocyte pattern without germinal centers. H&E staining, 200×.

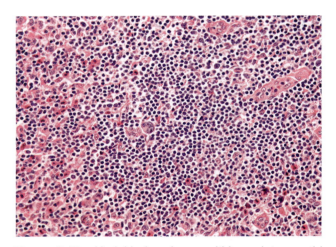

Figure 8.47. Hodgkin lymphoma within an intraparotid node. Note the classic Reed Sternberg cell in the middle of the field. H&E staining, 200×.

The B-cell lymphocytic component has been noted to result in clonal expansion and may progress to a non-Hodgkin lymphoma. Most of the non-Hodgkin lymphomas arising within benign lymphoepithelial lesions are marginal zone lymphomas of mucosa-associated lymphoid tissue (MALT) (Ihrler et al. 2000; Abbondanzo 2001). MALT lymphomas of the salivary glands, like their complement in other sites, are for the most part clinically indolent lesions (Harris 1991; Ellis and Auclair 2008). Occasionally, such low-grade lymphomas can also arise in other salivary gland tumors (Figure 8.46).

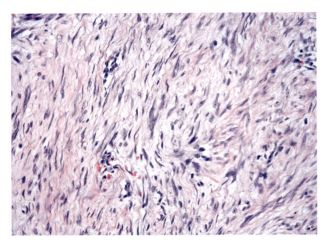

Figure 8.48. Benign spindle cell tumor of the parotid gland. After immunostaining, this lesion was determined to be an aggressive fibromatosis. H&E staining, 400×.

It is notable that primary non-MALT lymphomas of the salivary glands have been described and have a prognosis comparable to nodal lymphomas of the same types (Salhany and Pietra 1993). In contrast to non-Hodgkin lymphomas, Hodgkin lymphomas of the major salivary glands are most unusual. If present, Hodgkin lymphoma of salivary glands is usually contained only within the intraglandular nodes unlike non-Hodgkin lymphoma, which can efface an entire salivary gland with its malignant lymphoid cells (Figure 8.46). Most Hodgkin lymphomas of salivary gland arise in the parotid gland (Figure 8.47), and manifest as either nodular-sclerosing or lymphocyte-predominant variants (Gleeson et al. 1986; Ellis and Auclair 2008).

Mesenchymal Neoplasms

Benign and malignant mesenchymal neoplasms comprise 2–5% of all neoplasms that occur within the major salivary glands (Seifert and Oehne 1986). In patients younger than 18 years of age, a great number of parotid lesions are represented by benign vascular tumors.

Benign Mesenchymal Salivary Gland Tumors

The most common varieties of benign mesenchymal salivary gland neoplasms include hemangiomas, lipomas, lymphangiomas, and benign fibroblastic or myofibroblastic tumors (Figure 8.48). The histology of these lesions is identical to their presentation in

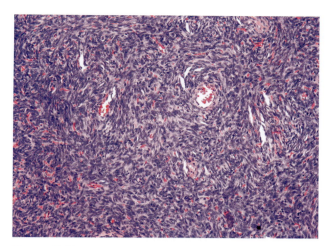

Figure 8.49. Another spindle cell tumor of the parotid gland determined to represent a malignant solitary fibrous tumor (hemangiopericytoma). Note the high degree of cellularity. H&E staining, 200×.

other organ systems. Treatment varies with the tumor type. Many of the vascular tumors found in the major salivary glands of infants will involute by the time the patient is 8–10 years old.

Malignant Mesenchymal Salivary Gland Tumors

Malignant mesenchymal salivary gland sarcomas include: malignant peripheral nerve sheath tumors, angiosarcomas, malignant solitary fibrous tumor (Figure 8.49), pleomorphic undifferentiated sarcomas, rhabdomyosarcomas, and myxofibrosarcomas, as well as many other rarer types. These sarcomas account for approximately 1.5% of all malignant tumors of the major salivary glands (Seifert and Oehne 1986; Luna et al. 1991). Primary salivary gland sarcomas behave like soft-tissue sarcomas in other locations; however, prognosis is governed by cell of origin, histological grade, tumor size, and stage (Auclair et al. 1986; Luna et al. 1991; Weiss 2001). The necessity to establish a primary salivary gland origin by excluding the likelihood of metastasis and direct extension from other adjacent locations cannot be overemphasized. Furthermore, the consideration of the very rare salivary gland carcinosarcoma should be considered when a sarcoma is identified within a major salivary gland (Ellis and Auclair 2008).

Malignant Secondary Neoplasms

Malignant neoplasms from primary sites outside the salivary glands may involve the major salivary glands by: (1) direct extension from malignancies that lie adjacent to the salivary glands; (2) hematogenous metastases from distant or regional primary tumors; and (3) lymphatic metastases to lymph nodes within the salivary gland (Ellis and Auclair 2008). It is estimated that ~80% of metastases to the major salivary glands are from primary tumors somewhere else in the head and neck. Direct extension into the parotid and submandibular glands is usually from squamous cell carcinomas of the skin and from melanomas arising from the skin of adjacent areas. Basal cell carcinoma and Merkel cell carcinoma also involve the major salivary glands in a similar fashion though not as commonly. The parotid gland is the site for most metastases to salivary gland followed by the submandibular gland (Seifert et al. 1986a). Most metastases to the major salivary glands are squamous cell carcinomas and melanomas. More rarely, carcinomas from the lung, kidney, and breast have been recognized presumably reaching these sites by a hematogenous route (Seifert et al. 1986a), (Batsakis and Bautina 1990). The peak incidence for metastatic tumors in the salivary glands is reported to be in the seventh decade of life (Ellis and Auclair 2008).

Grading and Staging of Salivary Gland Tumors

MOLECULAR SYSTEMATICS OF SALIVARY GLAND NEOPLASMS

One of the earliest attempts to use molecular systematics was to identify genes with altered expression in salivary adenoid cystic carcinoma (ACC). These studies observed expression of genes indicative of myoepithelial differentiation including those whose protein products are components of basement membranes and extracellular matrix (Frierson Jr. et al. 2002). More recent studies have indicated that the combination of copy number, gene express profiling, and identification of gene fusions and rearrangements provides an improved strategy for identification and classification of salivary neoplasms (Maruya et al. 2004; Leivo et al. 2005; Patel et al. 2006).

The greatest progress in molecular systematics has been in the identification of gene fusions and rearrangements which have led to the identification of new entities, provided insights with neoplastic entities in other organ systems, and identified potential therapeutic targets. For example, adenoid cystic carcinoma has been shown to be cytogenetically characterized by a tumor type-specific t(6;9)(q22–23;p23–24) translocation found as the anomaly in a subgroup of tumors. This translocation generates a fusion of the *MYB* proto-oncogene to the transcription factor gene *NFIB*. In the resulting *MYB-NFIB* fusion oncogene, which is highly overexpressed in adenoid cystic carcinoma, the 3′ part of *MYB*, including several target sites for negatively regulating microRNAs, is replaced by the last coding exon(s) of *NFIB*. The predicted *MYB-NFIB* fusion protein retains the DNA-binding and transactivation domains of wild type MYB, and is therefore expected to activate *MYB* target genes. Increased *MYB* expression has been reported in 17 of 20 adenoid cystic carcinomas with the *MYB-NFIB* fusion, but also in 14 of 20 fusion-negative adenoid cystic carcinomas.

Collectively, these findings indicate that *MYB* overexpression, as a result of the *MYB-NFIB* fusion or through alternative mechanisms, is a significant feature of most salivary ACCs, suggesting that *MYB* may be involved in ACC development and could be a potential target to develop novel therapeutic strategies for ACC treatment (Mitani et al. 2010). In addition, *MYBL1-NFIB* and *MYBL1-RAD51B* gene fusions resulting from t(8;9) and t(8;14) translocations and 5″*NFIB* fusions have also been described (Brayer et al. 2016; Mitani et al. 2010). Moreover, activating *NOTCH1* mutations have been reported in a group of patients with poor prognosis (Ferrarotto et al. 2017).

Pleomorphic adenomas have been cytogenetically demonstrated to harbor specific chromosomal aberrations, most of which result in fusion genes involving *PLAG1* on 8q12 or *HMGA2* on 12q13-15. Several fusion partners including *CTNNB1*, *CHCHD7*, *LIFR*, and *TCEA1* fused to *PLAG1*, and *FHIT*, *NFIB*, and *WIF1* fused to *HMGA2* have been identified. *PLAG1* is subsequently activated by the reciprocal chromosomal translocations and promoter swapping/substitution resulting in *PLAG1* protein overexpression. All pleomorphic adenomas examined have shown constant and specific immunohistochemical expression of *PLAG1* irrespective of detectable gene rearrangements, suggesting that the immunohistochemistry for *PLAG1* is diagnostically useful, and that overexpression of the *PLAG1* protein occurs by variable mechanisms (Matsuyama et al. 2012).

The belief that *PLAG1* alterations are specific for pleomorphic adenoma and carcinomas derived thereof has been supported by the demonstration that most carcinoma ex-pleomorphic adenomas (CA-ex-PA), regardless of morphologic subtype, carry altered *PLAG1* or *HMGA2* genes, and that FISH for *PLAG1*, along with immunohistochemistry for *PLAG1*, discriminate CA-ex-PA from its de novo carcinoma counterpart (Bahrami et al. 2012, 2013). Analysis of *PLAG1* and *HMGA2* rearrangements in salivary duct carcinoma (SDC) and examination of the role of precursor lesions have revealed that a large proportion of SDCs arise in pleomorphic adenomas (PAs), with or without residual evidence of a PA, while a small proportion of SDCs arise in low-grade cribriform cystadenoma (LGCCCs) or within ductal carcinoma in situ. Furthermore, utilization of *PLGA1* expression has shown that myoepithelial tumors of the salivary glands show some parallel features with pleomorphic adenoma. These morphological similarities and the known pathogenetic association of pleomorphic adenoma and malignant salivary gland tumors with myoepithelial differentiation have not implicated PLAG1 in the development of salivary myoepithelial tumors since the proportion of 8q12-alterations in these tumors is very low (Friedrich et al. 2012). However, overexpression of ERBB2 protein has been noted in a significant number of cases have demonstrated a copy number gain and/or overexpression of androgen receptors (Andersson and Stenman 2016). Salivary duct carcinoma (SDC) has been shown to possess HER2 gene amplification, mutations of TP53, PIK3CA, and HRAS and loss or mutation of PTEN. Also, a recurrent NCOA4-RET fusion has also been found in SDC and a subset of SDC with apocrine features is associated with overexpression of androgen receptors (Skálová et al. 2018).

Among mucoepidermoid carcinomas (MECs), the recognition of a chromosomal translocation t(11;19)(q21;p13) that generates a fusion oncogene has shown the *MECT1-MAML2* gene fusion is a highly specific genetic alteration in MEC with predominance in low-grade and high-grade mucoepidermoid carcinomas associated with improved survival (Miyabee et al. 2009; Skálová et al. 2018).

The gene fusion of *EWSR1-ATF1* fusion has been shown as a consistent finding in HCCC, with novel break-points described (*EWSR1* exon 11 and *ATF1* exon 3), and was the first finding of this fusion in an epithelial neoplasm. These findings allow HCCC to be distinguished from its mimics, such as epithelial-myoepithelial carcinoma and mucoepidermoid carcinoma, which have not been shown to harbor *EWSR1* (or *ATF1*) rearrangement (Antonescu et al. 2011). Furthermore, HCCC was also negative for the POU5F1 rearrangement found in SMET, and for the *PBX1* or *ZNF444* rearrangements in other SMETs (Antonescu et al. 2011; Thway and Fisher 2012).

In that HCCCs possess mucinous features reminiscent of MEC, the search for *MAML2* rearrangements led to the discovery that 82% of HCCCs carry a *EWSR1* rearrangement by FISH, suggesting that HCCC is not a salivary equivalent of SMET. Subsequently, clear cell odontogenic carcinoma (CCOC) and HCCC were examined for EWSR1 rearrangement, previously having recognized that these two tumors had extensive morphologic and immunohistochemical overlap (Bilodeau et al. 2012). Notably, a *EWSR1* rearrangement was found in 11/12 (92 %) HCCCs and 5/8 (63 %) CCOCs, suggesting that either CCOC represents a central example of HCCC or that CCOC represents an "odontogenic analogue" to HCCC (Weinreb 2013).

Polymorphous adenocarcinoma and cribriform adenocarcinoma of (minor) salivary gland origin are related entities with partly differing clinical-pathologic and genomic profiles. Polymorphous adenocarcinomas are characterized by hot spot point E710D mutations in the PRKD1 gene, whereas cribriform adenocarcinoma of (minor) salivary glands' origin is characterized by translocations involving the PRKD1-3 genes (Skálová et al. 2018).

Mammary analogue secretory carcinoma of salivary gland origin (MASC) is a tumor resembling secretory carcinoma of the breast characterized by strong S-100 protein, mammaglobin, and vimentin expression. This relationship was further substantiated by the demonstration that these salivary gland tumors possess a $t(12;15)$ (p13;q25) translocation resulting in *ETV6-NTRK3* fusion between the ETV6 gene on chromosome 12 and the *NTRK3* gene on chromosome 15. The resulting transcript encodes a chimeric oncoprotein consisting of the helix-loop-helix (HLH) protein dimerization domain of *ETV6* fused to the protein tyrosine kinase (PTK) domain of *NTRK3* (Evans and Luna 2000; Wai et al. 2000; Urano et al. 2015; Damjanov et al. 2016; Skálová et al. 2016).

Although molecular profiles of salivary neoplasms as yet are not included in the grading and staging of these tumors, these facets of neoplasia are rapidly becoming signatures, which are sure to provide reliable biomarkers, identify targets for treatment, and provide a behavioral component to a grading system.

TNM and Staging of Salivary Gland Tumors

Salivary gland tumors of the head and neck have a diverse anatomic distribution that include major salivary glands and minor salivary glands of the lip and oral cavity; pharynx; sinuses and nose. The anatomic location in part influences the definition of the three elements primary tumor (T), lymph nodes (N), and metastasis (M) that provide the basis for the American Joint Committee on Cancer (AJCC) staging (Table 8.3). It is noteworthy that minor salivary gland tumors are staged similar to squamous cell carcinoma according to the site in which they arise (e.g. oral cavity, lip, pharynx, and sinuses).

Tumors of the major salivary glands are staged according to the following criteria: (1) "T" – tumor size with or without extraparenchymal extension (EPE) and with or without facial nerve involvement (parotid only), (2) "N" – lymph node involvement and presence of metastases with or without extranodal extension (ENE), and (3) "M" – with or without distant metastatic disease (Lydiatt et al. 2017; Spiro et al. 1975; Fu et al. 1977; Levitt et al. 1981; Kuhel et al. 1992). Tumors arising in the minor salivary glands are staged according to the anatomic site of origin (e.g. oral cavity and sinuses). The American Joint Committee on Cancer (AJCC) (2017) has also designated staging of minor gland tumors by TNM classification (Gress et al. 2017).

There are no significant changes to T stage in the AJCC 8th edition for major salivary gland. Carcinomas for which the Tis (tumor in situ) designation may be applied include some intracapsular carcinomas ex-pleomorphic adenoma, and intraductal carcinomas. However, as with squamous cell carcinoma of the head and neck sites (excluding nasopharynx and human papillomavirus (HPV)-related carcinomas), N stage now incorporates extranodal extension (ENE) (Lydiatt et al. 2017).

EXTRAPARENCHYMAL EXTENSION

Extraparenchymal extension as described for salivary gland capsule involvement is clinical or macroscopic evidence of invasion of soft tissues or nerve through the gland capsule (T1, T2, T3), except those listed under T4a and 4b. Microscopic evidence alone does not constitute extraparenchymal extension for classification purposes (Lydiatt et al. 2017).

By AJCC/UICC convention, the designation "T" refers to a primary tumor that has not been previously treated. The symbol "p" refers to the pathologic classification of the TNM, as opposed to the clinical classification, and based on clinical stage information supplemented/modified by operative findings and gross and microscopic evaluation of the resected specimens (Gress et al. 2017). pT entails a resection or excisional biopsy of the primary tumor adequate to evaluate the highest pT category, pN entails removal of nodes adequate to validate lymph node metastasis, and pM implies microscopic examination of distant lesions. Clinical classification (cTNM) is usually carried out by the referring physician before treatment during initial evaluation of the patient or when pathologic classification is not possible. Imaging evaluation is also acceptable in certain instances.

Pathologic staging is usually performed after surgical resection of the primary tumor. Pathologic staging depends on pathologic documentation of the anatomic extent of disease, whether or not the primary tumor has been completely removed. If a biopsied tumor is not resected for any reason (e.g. when technically unfeasible) and if the highest T and N categories or the M1 category of the tumor can be confirmed microscopically, the criteria for pathologic classification and staging have been satisfied without total removal of the primary cancer.

TNM DESCRIPTORS

For identification of special cases of TNM or pTNM classifications, the "m" suffix and "y," "r," and "a" prefixes are used. Although they do not affect the stage grouping, they indicate cases needing separate analysis.

The "m" suffix indicates the presence of multiple primary tumors in a single site and is recorded in parentheses: pT(m)NM.

The "y" prefix indicates those cases in which classification is performed during or following initial multimodality therapy (i.e. neoadjuvant chemotherapy, radiation therapy, or both chemotherapy and radiation therapy). The cTNM or pTNM category is identified by a "y" prefix. The ycTNM or ypTNM categorizes the extent of tumor present at the time of that examination. The "y" categorization is not an estimate of tumor prior to multimodality therapy (i.e. before initiation of neoadjuvant therapy).

The "r" prefix indicates a recurrent tumor when staged after a documented disease-free interval, and is identified by the "r" prefix: rTNM.

The "a" prefix designates the stage determined at autopsy: aTNM.

ADDITIONAL DESCRIPTORS

Residual Tumor (R)

Tumor remaining in a patient after therapy with curative intent (e.g. surgical resection for cure) is categorized by a system known as R classification, shown below.

RX Presence of residual tumor cannot be assessed
R0 No residual tumor
R1 Microscopic residual tumor
R2 Macroscopic residual tumor

Summary

- The classification of salivary gland tumors accounts for their cellular derivation from epithelial, mesenchymal, or lymphoid origins.
- The rarity of some of these tumors, some of which display a wide spectrum of morphological patterns within the same tumor, as well as the existence of hybrid tumors results in a difficult task of differentiating benign from malignant tumors.
- For the most part, salivary gland tumors exist as benign or malignant neoplasms, with anticipated biologic behavior.
- The pleomorphic adenoma distinguishes itself as a benign tumor that may take on malignant characteristics and behavior.
- Some low-grade salivary gland malignancies represent highly curable neoplasms.
- Gene expression profiles may be used to predict biologic behavior of salivary gland malignancies. This notwithstanding, histologic grading and clinical staging remain the two most important considerations in determining the treatment of these neoplasms and their prognosis.
- Major salivary gland staging occurs according to size, extraparenchymal extension, lymph node involvement, the presence of metastases, and whether the facial nerve is involved as may occur in parotid tumors.

Table 8.3. Staging of malignant salivary gland tumors.

TNM definitions
MAJOR SALIVARY GLANDS

Primary tumor (pT)

- pTX: Primary tumor cannot be assessed
- pT0: No evidence of primary tumor
- pTis: Carcinoma in situ
- pT1: Tumor 2 cm or smaller in greatest dimension *without extraparenchymal extension*[a]
- pT2: Tumor 2 cm but not larger than 4 cm in greatest dimension *without extraparenchymal* extension[a]
- pT3: Tumor larger than 4 cm and/or tumor *having extraparenchymal extension*[a]
- pT4: Moderately advanced or very advanced disease
- pT4a: Moderately advanced disease. Tumor invades skin, mandible, ear canal, and/or facial nerve
- pT4b: Very advanced disease. Tumor invades skull base and/or pterygoid plates and/or encases carotid artery

Regional lymph nodes (N)

- pNX: Regional lymph nodes cannot be assessed
- pN0: No regional lymph node metastasis
- pN1: Metastasis in a single ipsilateral lymph node, 3 cm or smaller in greatest dimension and ENE (−)
- pN2: Metastasis in a single ipsilateral lymph node, 3 cm or smaller in greatest dimension and ENE(+); *or* larger than 3 cm but not larger than 6 cm in greatest dimension and ENE (−)
- pN2a: Metastasis in a single ipsilateral lymph node 3 cm or smaller in greatest dimension and ENE(+); *or* a single ipsilateral node larger than 3 cm but not larger than 6 cm in greatest dimension and ENE(−)
- pN2b: Metastasis in multiple ipsilateral lymph nodes, none larger than 6 cm in greatest dimension and ENE(−)
- pN2c: Metastasis in bilateral or contralateral lymph nodes, none larger than 6 cm in greatest dimension and ENE(−)
- pN3: Metastasis in a lymph node larger than 6 cm in greatest dimension and ENE(−); *or* in a single ipsilateral node larger than 3 cm in greatest dimension and ENE(+); *or* multiple ipsilateral, contralateral, or bilateral nodes and with ENE(+); *or* a single contralateral node 3 cm or smaller ENE(+)
- pN3a: Metastasis in a lymph node larger than 6 cm in greatest dimension and ENE(−)
- pN3b: Metastasis in a single ipsilateral node larger than 3 cm in greatest dimension and ENE(+); *or* multiple ipsilateral, contralateral, or bilateral nodes and with ENE(+)

Note: Extra Nodal Extension should by recorded as ENE(−) or ENE(+).

Distant metastasis (M)

- pMX: Distant metastasis cannot be assessed
- pM0: No distant metastasis
- pM1: Distant metastasis

AJCC stage groupings

When T is...	And N is...	And M is...	Stage group is...
Tis	N0	M0	0
T1	N0	M0	I
T2	N0	M0	II
T3	N0	M0	III
T0, T1, T2, T3	N1	M0	III

T4a	N0, N1	M0	IVA
T0, T1, T2, T3, T4a	N2	M0	IVA
Any T	N3	M0	IVB
T4b	Any N	M0	IVB
Any T	Any N	M1	IVC

Residual Tumor (R)
Tumor in a patient after therapy with curative intent (e.g. surgical resection for cure) is categorized by a R classification.

- RX-Presence of residual tumor cannot be assessed
- R0-No residual rumor
- R1-Microscopic residual tumor
- R2-Macroscopic residual tumor

Minor salivary glands
   Lip and Oral Cavity
   Minor salivary gland tumors are staged similar to squamous cell carcinoma according to the site in which they arise (e.g. Oral cavity, lip, pharynx, sinuses, etc.)

Primary tumor (T)

- pTX: Primary tumor cannot be assessed
- pTis: Carcinoma *in situ*
- pT1: Tumor ≤ 2 cm, ≤ 5 mm depth of invasion (DOI)
- pT2: Tumor ≤ 2 cm, DOI > 5 mm and ≤ 10 mm or tumor > 2 cm but ≤ 4 cm, and ≤ 10 mm DOI
- pT3: Tumor > 4 cm or any tumor > 10 mm DOI
- pT4: Moderately advanced or very advanced local disease
- pT4a Moderately advanced local disease (Lip, etc.). Tumor invades through cortical bone (superficial erosion of cortex or tooth socket is not sufficient to classify tumor as T4), *or* involves the inferior alveolar nerve, floor of mouth, or skin of face, (i.e., chin or nose); Tumor (Oral cavity) invades adjacent structures only (e.g. through cortical bone of the mandible or maxilla, *or* invades the maxillary sinus or skin of the face)
- pT4b: Very advanced local disease. Tumor invades masticator space, pterygoid plates, *or* skull base, and/or encases the internal carotid artery

Regional Lymph Nodes (N)

- pNX: Regional lymph nodes cannot be assessed
- pN0: No regional lymph node metastasis
- pN1: Metastasis in a single ipsilateral lymph node, 3 cm or smaller in greatest dimension and ENE(−)
- pN2: Metastasis in a single ipsilateral lymph node, 3 cm or smaller in greatest dimension and ENE(+); *or* larger than 3 cm but not larger than 6 cm in greatest dimension and ENE(−); *or* metastases in multiple ipsilateral lymph nodes, none larger than 6 cm in greatest dimension and ENE(−); *or* in bilateral or contralateral lymph node(s), none larger than 6 cm in greatest dimension and ENE(−)
- pN2a: Metastasis in a single ipsilateral lymph node 3 cm or smaller in greatest dimension and ENE(+); *or* a single ipsilateral node larger than 3 cm but not larger than 6 cm in greatest dimension and ENE(−)
- pN2b: Metastasis in multiple ipsilateral lymph nodes, none larger than 6 cm in greatest dimension and ENE(−)
- pN2c: Metastasis in bilateral or contralateral lymph node(s), none than 6 cm in greatest dimension and ENE(−)
- pN3: Metastasis in a lymph node larger than 6 cm in greatest dimension and ENE(−); *or* metastasis in a single ipsilateral node larger than 3 cm in greatest dimension and ENE(+); *or* multiple ipsilateral, contralateral or bilateral nodes any with ENE(+); *or* a single contralateral node 3 cm or smaller and ENE(+)

- pN3a: Metastasis in a lymph node larger than 6 cm in greatest dimension and ENE(−)
- pN3b: Metastasis in a single ipsilateral node larger than 3 cm in greatest dimension and ENE(+); *or* a single contralateral node 3 cm or smaller and ENE(+)

Distant metastasis (M)

- MX: Distant metastasis cannot be assessed
- M0: No distant metastasis
- M1: Distant metastasis

AJCC stage groupings for all cancers except mucosal melanoma

When T is...	And N is...	And M is...	Stage group is...
Tis	N0	M0	0
T1	N0	M0	I
T2	N0	M0	II
T3	N0	M0	III
T1, T2, T3	N1	M0	III
T4a	N0, N1	M0	IVA
T1, T2, T3, T4a	N2	M0	IVA
Any T	N3	M0	IVB
T4b	Any N	M0	IVB
Any T	Any N	M1	IVC

Residual Tumor (R)

- RX-Presence of residual tumor cannot be assessed
- R0-No residual rumor
- R1-Microscopic residual tumor
- R2-Macroscopic residual tumor

[a] Extraparenchymal extension is clinical or macroscopic evidence of invasion of soft tissues. Microscopic evidence alone does not constitute extraparenchymal extension for classification purposes.

Case Presentation – *Reclassified*

A 28-year-old man was referred with a three-month history of a lesion of his left soft palate (Figure 8.50). He denied pain, dysphagia, and odynophagia. He reported slow yet progressive growth of the lesion.

Past medical history

The patient denied a contributory past medical history. He was taking no medications and reported no known drug allergies at the time of evaluation.

Physical examination

The patient demonstrated a 1.5 cm mass of the left lateral soft palate based on the picture supplied by the referring surgeon. The lesion was indurated and nontender by report.

Diagnosis

A large incisional biopsy was performed prior to referral that identified mammary analogue secretory carcinoma (Figure 8.50b and c).

Imaging

CT scans were obtained that identified a minimal burden of disease isolated to the soft palate (Figure 8.50d–f).

Surgical intervention

The patient was taken to the operating room for a soft palate resection, observing 1 cm linear margins (Figure 8.50g). The specimen was delivered (Figure 8.50h) and final pathology confirmed the diagnosis of secretory carcinoma, the reclassified mammary analogue secretory carcinoma

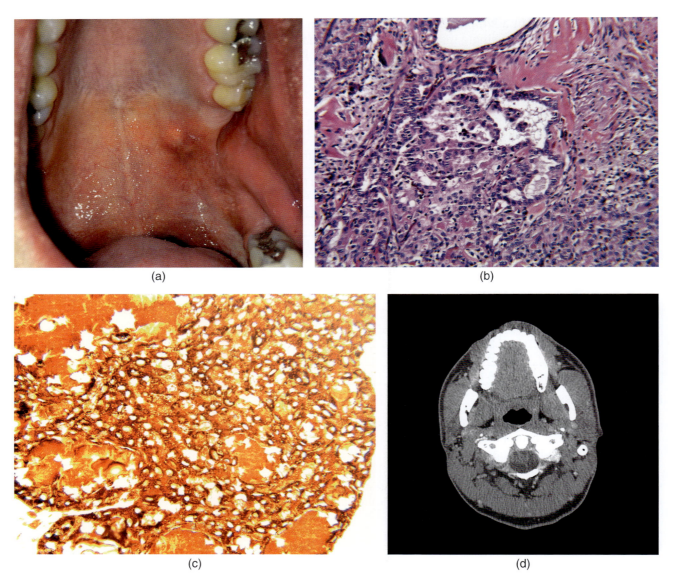

Figure 8.50. (a) A mass of the left soft palate that conjures numerous benign and malignant entities on its differential diagnosis. (b) Incisional biopsy resulted in a diagnosis of secretory carcinoma, the reclassified mammary analogue secretory carcinoma. Hematoxylin and eosin, original magnification × 100. (c) Mammaglobin stain, original magnification × 400. This intense staining pattern is diagnostic of the secretory carcinoma. Axial (d), coronal (e), and sagittal (f) CT scans demonstrate an insignificant burden of tumor remaining in the left soft palate. (g) The patient's tumor is definitively excised with 1 cm linear margins. (h) The oral mucosal side of the specimen. (i) Final pathology confirmed the incisional biopsy diagnosis of secretory carcinoma. Hematoxylin and eosin, original magnification × 200. (j) The defect of the soft palate following definitive tumor excision. A very small area of full-thickness sacrifice of the soft palate is noted. (k) The immediate surgical obturator device provides postoperative function.

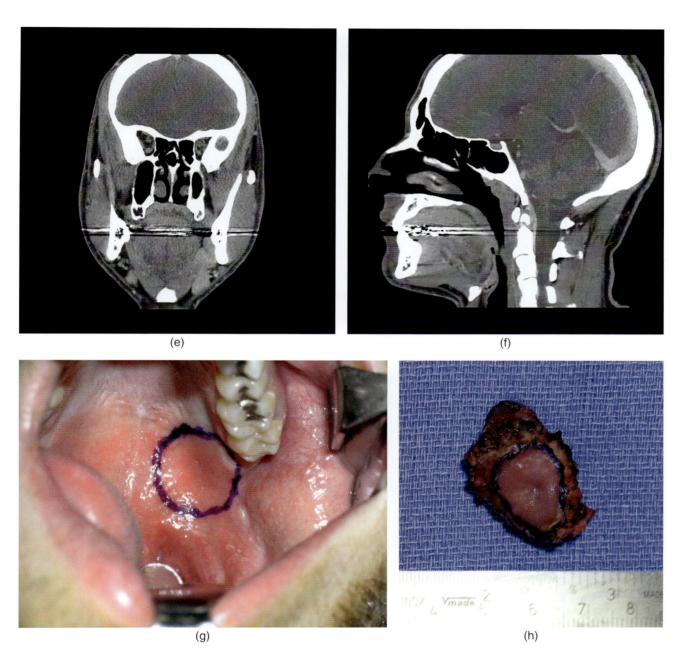

Figure 8.50. (Continued).

(Figure 8.50i) offered by the incisional biopsy. Due to the limited burden of disease clinically and radiographically, the excision of the tumor maintained most of the integrity of the soft palate (Figure 8.50j). An immediate surgical obturator (Figure 8.50k) was placed to permit unimpeded function postoperatively. The patient remains free of disease five years postoperatively.

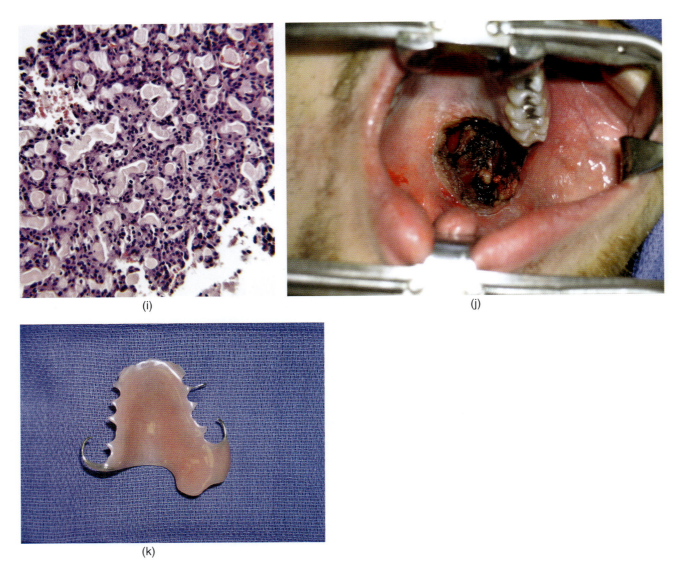

Figure 8.50. (Continued).

TAKE-HOME POINTS

1. Palatal masses should always result in a differential diagnosis that includes benign and malignant salivary gland tumors.
2. Clinical photographs are ideally obtained prior to incisional biopsy of small masses in case the biopsy results in very little disease remaining following the biopsy.
3. The incisional biopsy of a palatal tumor should be procured from the center of the mass.
4. A malignant incisional biopsy diagnosis of a palatal tumor should be followed by obtaining CT scans prior to performing definitive cancer surgery.
5. The 2017 World Health Organization reclassified the mucinous analogue secretory carcinoma as a secretory carcinoma. These tumors are most common in the parotid gland but can be diagnosed elsewhere in head and neck salivary gland tissue.

References

Abbondanzo SL. 2001. Extranodal marginal-zone B-cell lymphoma of the salivary gland. *Ann Diagn Pathol* 5(4):246–254.

Allison DB, Cui X, Page GP, Sabripour M. 2006. Microarray data analysis: From disarray to consolidation and consensus. *Nat Rev Genet* 7(1):55–65.

American Joint Committee on Cancer. 2017. Major Salivary Glands AJCC Cancer Staging Manual, 8th edn. Switzerland, Springer Nature, pp. 95–102.

Andersson MK, Stenman G. 2016. The landscape of gene fusions and somatic mutations in salivary gland neoplasms – implications for diagnosis and therapy. *Oral Oncol* 57:63–69.

Antonescu CR, Katabi N, Zhang L, et al. 2011. EWSR1-ATF1 fusion is a novel and consistent finding in hyalinizing clear-cell carcinoma of salivary gland. *Genes Chromosom Cancer* 50(7):559–70.

Arora SK, Sharma N, Bhardwaj M. 2013. Epithelial myoepithelial carcinoma of the head and neck region. *Indian J Otolaryngol Head Neck Surg* 65(Suppl 1):163–166.

Auclair PL, Goode RK, Ellis GL. 1992. Mucoepidermoid carcinoma of intraoral salivary glands. Evaluation and application of grading criteria in 143 cases. *Cancer* 69(8):2021–2030.

Auclair PL, Langloss JM, Weiss SW, Corio RL. 1986. Sarcomas and sarcomatoid neoplasms of the major salivary gland regions. A clinicopathologic and immunohistochemical study of 67 cases and review of the literature. *Cancer* 58(6):1305–1315.

Bahrami A, Dalton JD, Shivakumar B, Krane JF. 2012. PLAG1 alterations in carcinoma ex-pleomorphic adenoma: Immunohistochemical and fluorescence in situ hybridization studies of 22 cases. *Head Neck Pathol* 6:328–335.

Bahrami A, Perez-Ordonez B, Dalton JD, Weinreb I. 2013. An analysis of PLAG1 and HMGA2 rearrangements in salivary duct carcinoma and examination of the role of precursor lesions. *Histopathology* 63:250–262.

Batsakis JG. 1979. Tumors of the Head and Neck: Clinical and Pathological Considerations. Baltimore, MD, Williams & Wilkins, p. 9.

Batsakis JG, Bautina E. 1990. Metastases to major salivary glands. *Ann Otol Rhinol Laryngol* 99(6 Pt 1):501–503.

Batsakis JG, el-Naggar AK, Luna MA. 1992. Epithelial-myoepithelial carcinoma of salivary glands. *Ann Otol Rhinol Laryngol* 101(6):540–542.

Batsakis JG, Frankenthaler R. 1992. Embryoma (sialoblastoma) of salivary glands. *Ann Otol Rhinol Laryngol* 101(11):958–960.

Batsakis JG, Luna MA. 1991. Undifferentiated carcinomas of salivary glands. *Ann Otol Rhinol Laryngol* 100(1):82–84.

Batsakis JG, Luna MA, el-Naggar A. 1990. Histopathologic grading of salivary gland neoplasms: III. Adenoid cystic carcinomas. *Ann Otol Rhinol Laryngol* 99(12):1007–1009.

Bernatsky S, Ramsey-Goldman R, Clarke A. 2006. Malignancy and autoimmunity. *Curr Opin Rheumatol* 18(2):129–134.

Bilodeau EA, Weinreb I, Antonescu CR, et al. 2012. Clear cell odontogenic carcinomas show EWSR1 rearrangements: A novel finding and biologic link to salivary clear cell carcinomas. *Mod Pathol* 25(Supplement 2s):1001–1005.

Bishop JA. 2013. Unmasking MASC: Bringing to light the unique morphologic, immunohistochemical and genetic features of the newly recognized mammary analogue secretory carcinoma of salivary glands. *Head Neck Pathol* 7:35–39.

Bishop JA, Yonescu R, Batista D, et al. 2013. Most non-parotid "acinic cell carcinomas" represent mammary analog secretory carcinomas. *Am J Surg Pathol* 37(7):1053–1057.

Bissinger, O, Gotz C, Kolk A, Bier H, et al. 2017. Mammary analogue secretory carcinoma of salivary glands: Diagnostic pitfall with distinct immunohistochemical profile and molecular features. *Rare Tumors* 9(7162):89–92.

Borg MF, Benjamin CS, Morton RP, Llewellyn HR. 1993. Malignant lympho-epithelial lesion of the salivary gland: A case report and review of the literature. *Australas Radiol* 37(3):288–291.

Bosch JD, Kudryk WH, Johnson GH. 1988. The malignant lymphoepithelial lesion of the salivary glands. *J Otolaryngol* 17(4):187–190.

Brandwein M, Al-Naeif NS, Manwani D, et al. 1999. Sialoblastoma: Clinicopathological/immunohistochemical study. *Am J Surg Pathol* 23(3):342–348.

Brandwein MS, Ferlito A, Bradley PJ, et al. 2002. Diagnosis and classification of salivary neoplasms: Pathologic challenges and relevance to clinical outcomes. *Acta Otolaryngol* 122(7):758–764.

Brandwein MS, Ivanov K, Wallace DI, et al. 2001. Mucoepidermoid carcinoma: A clinicopathologic study of 80 patients with special reference to histological grading. *Am J Surg Pathol* 25(7):835–845.

Brannon RB, Sciubba JJ, Giulani M. 2001. Ductal papillomas of salivary gland origin: A report of 19 cases and a review of the literature. *Oral Surg Oral Med Oral Pathol* 92 (1):68–77.

Brayer KJ, Frerich CA, Kang H, Ness SA. 2016. Recurrent fusions in MYB and MYBL1 define a common, transcription factor-driven oncogenic pathway in salivary gland adenoid cystic carcinoma. *Cancer Discov* 6:176–187.

Brill LB, Kanner WA, Fehr A, et al. 2011. Analysis of MYB expression and MYB-NFIB gene fusions in adenoid cystic carcinoma and other salivary neoplasms. *Mod Pathol* 24:1169–1176.

Brookstone MS, Huvos AG. 1992. Central salivary gland tumors of the maxilla and mandible: A clinicopathologic study of 11 cases with an analysis of the literature. *J Oral Maxillofac Surg* 50(3):229–236.

Buyse M, Loi S, van't Veer L, et al. 2006. Validation and clinical utility of a 70-gene prognostic signature for women with node-negative breast cancer. *J Natl Cancer Inst* 98(17):1183–1192.

Chen W, Zhang HL, Shao XJ, et al. 2007. Gene expression profile of salivary adenoid cystic carcinoma associated with perineural invasion. *Tohoku J Exp Med* 212(3):319–334.

Choudhary K, Panda S, Beena VT, et al. 2013. Sialoblastoma: A literature review from 1966 to 2011. *Natl J Maxillofac Surg* 4(1):13–18.

Cipriani N, Lusardi J, McElherne J, et al. 2019. Mucoepidermoid carcinoma a Comparison of histologic grading systems and relationship to MAML2 rearrangement and prognosis. *Am J Surg Pathol*:43(7):885–897.

Collina G, Gale N, Visona A, et al. 1991. Epithelial-myoepithelial carcinoma of the parotid gland: A clinico-pathologic and immunohistochemical study of seven cases. *Tumori* 77(3):257–263.

Daley TD, Wysocki GP, Smout MS, Slinger RP. 1984. Epithelial-myoepithelial carcinoma of salivary glands. *Oral Surg Oral Med Oral Pathol* 57(5):512–519.

Damjanov I, Skenderi F, Vranic S, 2016. Mammary analogue secretory carcinoma (MASC) of the salivary gland: A new tumor entity. *Bosn J Basic Med Sci* 16(3):237–238.

de Vicente Rodriquez JC, Fresno Forcelledo MF, Junquera Gutierrez LM, et al. 2004. Small cell undifferentiated carcinoma of the submandibular gland with neuroendocrine features. *Ann Otol Rhinol Laryngol* 113(1):55–59.

Delgado R, Klimstra D, Albores-Saavedra J 1996. Low-grade salivary duct carcinoma. A distinctive variant with a low-grade histology and a predominant intraductal growth pattern. *Cancer* 78(5):958–967.

Dispenza F, Cicero G, Mortellaro G, et al. 2011. Primary non-Hodgkin's lymphoma of the parotid gland. *Braz J Otorhinolarygol* 77: 639–644.

Ellis GL, Auclair P. 2008. Tumors of the Salivary Glands. Atlas of Tumor Pathology, 4th Series Fascicle 9. Washington, DC, Armed Forces Institute of Pathology, pp. 368–372.

Ellis, GL, Auclair PL, Gnepp, DR. 1991. Surgical Pathology of Salivary Glands, 1st edn. Philadelphia, W.B. Saunders, p. 129.

Evans HL, Luna MA. 2000. Polymorphous low-grade adenocarcinoma: A study of 40 cases with long-term follow up and an evaluation of the importance of papillary areas. *Am J Surg Pathol* 24(10):1319–1328.

Evans RW, Cruickshank AH. 1970. Epithelial Tumors of Salivary Glands. Philadelphia, Saunders, p. 19.

Eveson JW, Cawson RA. 1985. Salivary gland tumours. A review of 2410 cases with particular reference to histological types, site, age and sex distribution. *J Pathol* 146(1):51–58.

Ferrarotto R, Mitani Y, Diao L, et al. 2017 Activating NOTCH1 mutations define a distinct subgroup of patients with adenoid cystic carcinoma who have poor prognosis, propensity to bone and liver metastasis, and potential responsiveness to Notch1 inhibitors. *J Clin Oncol* 35:352–360.

Foote FW, Frazell EL. 1954. Tumors of Major Salivary Glands, 1st edn. Washington, DC, Armed Forces Institute of Pathology, p. 8.

Friedrich RE, Bleckmann V. 2003. Adenoid cystic carcinoma of salivary and lacrimal gland origin: Localization, classification, clinical pathological correlation, treatment results and long-term follow-up control in 84 patients. *Anticancer Res* 23(2A):931–940.

Friedrich RE, Dilcher J, Jaehne M, Loning T. 2012. Chromosomal rearrangements in *PLAG1* of myoepithelial salivary gland tumours. *Anticancer Res* 32(5): 1977–1981.

Frierson HF, Jr., El-Naggar AK, Welsh JB, et al. 2002. Large scale molecular analysis identifies genes with altered expression in salivary adenoid cystic carcinoma. *Am J Pathol* 161(4):1315–1323.

Fu KK, Leibel SA, Levine ML, et al. 1977. Carcinoma of the major and minor salivary glands: Analysis of treatment results and sites and causes of failures. *Cancer* 40(6):2882–2890.

Gaughan RK, Olsen KD, Lewis JE. 1992. Primary squamous cell carcinoma of the parotid gland. *Arch Otolaryngol Head Neck Surg* 118(8):798–801.

Gleeson MJ, Bennett MH, Cawson RA. 1986. Lymphomas of salivary glands. *Cancer* 58(3):699–704.

Gnepp DR. 1983. Sebaceous neoplasms of salivary gland origin: A review. *Pathol Annu* 18(Pt 1):71–102.

Gnepp DR. 2012. My journey into the World of salivary gland sebaceous neoplasms *Head Neck Pathol* 6(1):101–110.

Gnepp DR, Brannon R. 1984. Sebaceous neoplasms of salivary gland origin. Report of 21 cases. *Cancer* 53(10):2155–2170.

Gnepp DR, Corio RL, Brannon RB. 1986. Small cell carcinoma of the major salivary glands. *Cancer* 58(3):705–714.

Gnepp DR, Wick MR. 1990. Small cell carcinoma of the major salivary glands. An immunohistochemical study. *Cancer* 66(1):185–192.

Goode RK, Auclair PL, Ellis GL. 1998. Mucoepidermoid carcinoma of the major salivary glands: Clinical and histopathologic analysis of 234 cases with evaluation of grading criteria. *Cancer* 82(7):1217–1224.

Gress DM, Edge SB, Greene FL, et al. 2017. Principles of cancer staging. In: Amin MB (ed.), AJCC Cancer Staging Manual, 8th edn. New York, NY, Springer, pp. 3–30.

Guzzo M, Andreola S, Sirizzotti G, Cantu G. 2002. Mucoepidermoid carcinoma of the salivary glands: Clinicopathologic review of 108 patients treated at the

National Cancer Institute of Milan. *Ann Surg Oncol* 9(7):688–695.

Hafed L, Farag H, Shaker O, El-Rouby D. 2012. Is human papilloma virus associated with salivary gland neoplasms? An in situ-hybridridization study. *Arch Oral Biol* 57(9):1194–1199.

Hamper K, Lazar F, Dietel M, et al. 1990. Prognostic factors for adenoid cystic carcinoma of the head and neck: A retrospective evaluation of 96 cases. *J Oral Pathol Med* 19(3):101–107.

Harris NL. 1991. Extranodal lymphoid infiltrates and mucosa-associated lymphoid tissue (MALT). A unifying concept. *Am J Surg Pathol* 15(9):879–884.

Hui KK, Luna MA, Batsakis JG, et al. 1990. Undifferentiated carcinomas of the major salivary glands. *Oral Surg Oral Med Oral Pathol* 69(1):76–83.

Hung YP, Jo VY, Hornick JL. 2019. Immunohistochemisry with a pan-TRK antibody distinguishes secretory carcinoma of the salivary gland from acinic cell carcinoma. *Histopathology* 75:54–62.

Ihrler S, Baretton GB, Menauer F, et al. 2000. Sjogren's syndrome and MALT lymphomas of salivary glands: A DNA-cytometric and interphase-cytogenetic study. *Mod Pathol* 13(1):4–12.

Ioannidis JP. 2007. Is molecular profiling ready for use in clinical decision making? *Oncologist* 12(3):301–311.

Isayeva T, Said-Al-Naisef N, Ren Z, et al. 2013. Salivary mucoepidermoid carcinoma: Demonstration of transcriptionally active human papillomavirus 16/18. *Head Neck* 7:135–148.

Jung MJ, Roh J-L, Choi S-H, et al. 2013. Basal cell adenocarcinoma of the salivary gland: A morphological and immunohistochemical comparison with basal cell adenoma with and without capsular invasion. *Diagn Pathol* 8:171.

Kane SV, Bagwan IN. 2010. Myoepithelial carcinoma of the salivary glands clinicopathologic study of 51 cases in a tertiary cancer center. *Arch Otolaryngol Head Neck Surg* 136(7):702–712.

Kasamatsu A, Endo Y, Uzawa K, et al. 2005. Identification of candidate genes associated with salivary adenoid cystic carcinomas using combined comparative genomic hybridization and oligonucleotide microarray analyses. *Int J Biochem Cell Biol* 37(9):1869–1880.

Kaye F. 2006. Emerging biology of malignant salivary gland tumors offers new insights into classification and treatment of mucoepidermoid cancer. *Clin Cancer Res* 12:3878–3881.

Kennedy, RA. 2018. WHO is in and WHO is out of the mouth, salivary glands, and jaws sections of the 4th edition of the WHO classification of head and neck tumours. *Br J Oral Maxillofac Surg* 56:90–95.

Kuhel W, Goepfert H, Luna M, et al. 1992. Adenoid cystic carcinoma of the palate. *Arch Otolaryngol Head Neck Surg* 118(3):243–247.

Kusafuka K, Miki T, Nakajima T. 2013. Adenosquamous carcinoma of the parotid gland. *Histopathology* 63(4):593–595.

Leivo I, Jee KJ, Heikinheimo K, et al. 2005. Characterization of gene expression in major types of salivary gland carcinomas with epithelial differentiation. *Cancer Genet Cytogenet* 156(2):104–113.

Leung SY, Chung LP, Yuen ST, et al. 1995. Lymphoepithelial carcinoma of the salivary gland: In situ detection of Epstein-Barr virus. *J Clin Pathol* 48(11):1022–1027.

Levitt SH, McHugh RB, Gomez-Marin O, et al. 1981. Clinical staging system for cancer of the salivary gland: A retrospective study. *Cancer* 47(11):2712–2724.

LiVolsi VA, Perzin KH. 1977. Malignant mixed tumors arising in salivary glands. I. Carcinomas arising in benign mixed tumors: A clinicopathologic study. *Cancer* 39(5):2209–2230.

Luna MA, Tortoledo ME, Ordonez NG, et al. 1991. Primary sarcomas of the major salivary glands. *Arch Otolaryngol Head Neck Surg* 117(3):302–306.

Lydiatt WM, Mukherji SK, O'Sullivan B, et al. 2017. Major salivary glands. In: Amin MB (ed.), AJCC Cancer Staging Manual, 8th edn. New York, NY, Springer, pp. 95–101.

Maruya S, Kim HW, Weber RS, et al. 2004. Gene expression screening of salivary gland neoplasms: Molecular markers of potential histogenetic and clinical significance. *J Mol Diagn* 6(3):180–190.

Matsuba HM, Mauney M, Simpson JR, et al. 1988. Adenocarcinomas of major and minor salivary gland origin: A histopathologic review of treatment failure patterns. *Laryngoscope* 98(7):784–788.

Matsuyama A, Hisaoka M, Hashimoto H. 2012. PLAG1 expression in mesenchymal tumors: An immunohistochemical study with special emphasis on the pathological distinction between soft tissue myoepithelioma and pleomorphic adenoma of the salivary gland. *Pathol Int* 62:1–7.

McCoy, JM, Eckert, EF. 1980. Sialoadenoma papilliferm. *J Oral Surg* 69(9):691–693.

Mitani Y, Li J, Rao PH, et al. 2010. Comprehensive analysis of the *MYB-NFIB* gene fusion in salivary adenoid cystic carcinoma: Incidence, variability, and clinicopathologic significance. *Clin Cancer Res* 16:4722–4731.

Miyabee S, Okabe M, Nagatsuka H, et al. 2009. Prognostic significance of p27^{Kip1}, Ki-67, and *CRTC1-MAML2* fusion transcript in mucoepidermoid carcinoma: A molecular and clinicopathologic study of 101 cases. *J Oral Maxillofac Surg* 67(7):1432–1441.

Muller S, Barnes L. 1996. Basal cell adenocarcinoma of the salivary glands. Report of seven cases and review of the literature. *Cancer* 78(12):2471–2477.

Nagao, T, Sato, E, Inoue, R, et al. 2012. Immunohistochemical analysis of salivary gland tumors: Application for pathology practice. *Acta Histochem Cytochem* 45(5):269–282.

Noel S, Brozna JP. 1992. Epithelial-myoepithelial carcinoma of salivary gland with metastasis to lung: Report of a case and review of the literature. *Head Neck* 14(5):401–406.

Patel KJ, Pambuccian SE, Ondrey FG, et al. 2006. Genes associated with early development, apoptosis and cell cycle regulation define a gene expression profile of adenoid cystic carcinoma. *Oral Oncol* 42(10):994–1004.

Perez-Ordonez B, Caruana SM, Huvos AG, Shah JP. 1998. Small cell neuroendocrine carcinoma of the nasal cavity and paranasal sinuses. *Hum Pathol* 29(8):826–832.

Persson F, Fehr A, Sundelin K, et al. 2012a. Studies of genomic imbalances and the MYB-NFIB gene fusion in polymorphous low-grade adenocarcinoma of the head and neck. *Int J Oncol* 40:80–84.

Persson M, Andren Y, Moskaluk CA, et al. 2012b. Clinically significant copy number alterations and complex rearrangements of MYB and NFIB in head and neck adenoid cystic carcinoma. *Genes Chromosom Cancer* 51:805–817.

Perzin KH, Gullane P, Clairmont AC. 1978. Adenoid cystic carcinomas arising in salivary glands: A correlation of histologic features and clinical course. *Cancer* 42(1):265–282.

Poorten V, Triantafyllou A, Skalova A, et al. 2018. Polymorphous adenocarcinoma of the salivary glands: Reappraisal and update. *Eur Arch Otorhinolaryngol* 275:1681–1695.

Roijer E, Nordkvist A, Strom AK, et al. 2002. Translocation, deletion/amplification, and expression of HMGIC and MDM2 in a carcinoma ex pleomorphic adenoma. *Am J Pathol* 160(2):433–440.

Salhany KE, Pietra GG. 1993. Extranodal lymphoid disorders. *Am J Clin Pathol* 99(4):472–485.

Santaliz-Ruiz LE, Morales G, Santini H, et al. 2012. Metastasizing pleomorphic adenoma: A fascinating enigma. *Case Rep Med* 2012:148103.

Savera AT, Sloman A, Huvos AG, Klimstra DS. 2000. Myoepithelial carcinoma of the salivary glands: A clinicopathologic study of 25 patients. *Am J Surg Pathol* 24(6):761–774.

Schneider AB, Favus MJ, Stachura ME, et al. 1977. Salivary gland neoplasms as a late consequence of head and neck irradiation. *Ann Intern Med* 87(2):160–164.

Seethala RR, Stenman G. 2017. Update from the 4th edition of the World Health Organization classification of head and neck tumours: Tumors of the salivary gland. *Head Neck Pathol* 11:55–67.

Seifert G, Donath K. 1996. Hybrid tumours of salivary glands. Definition and classification of five rare cases. *Eur J Cancer B Oral Oncol* 32B(4):251–259.

Seifert G, Hennings K, Caselitz J. 1986a. Metastatic tumors to the parotid and submandibular glands – analysis and differential diagnosis of 108 cases. *Pathol Res Pract* 181(6):684–692.

Seifert G, Miehlke, A., Haubrich, J., Chilla, R. 1986b. Diseases of the Salivary Glands: Pathology-Diagnosis-Treatment-Facial Nerve Surgery. Stuttgart, George Thieme Verlag, p. 171.

Seifert G, Oehne H. 1986. Mesenchymal (non-epithelial) salivary gland tumors. Analysis of 167 tumor cases of the salivary gland register. *Laryngol Rhinol Otol (Stuttg)* 65(9):485–491.

Shemen LJ, Huvos AG, Spiro RH. 1987. Squamous cell carcinoma of salivary gland origin. *Head Neck Surg* 9(4):235–240.

Shum JW, Emmerling M, Lubek JE, Ord RA. 2014. Parotid lymphoma: A review of clinical presentation and management. *Oral Surg Oral Med Oral Pathol Oral Radiol* 118:e1–e5.

Sicurella F, Gregorio A, Stival P, Brenna A. 2004. Clear cell carcinoma of minor salivary gland of the tongue. *Acta Otorhinolaryngol Ital* 24:157–160.

Simpson RH, Clarke TJ, Sarsfield PT, Gluckman PG. 1991. Epithelial-myoepithelial carcinoma of salivary glands. *J Clin Pathol* 44(5):419–423.

Skalova A, Kaspirkova J, Andrle P, et al. 2013a. Human papillomaviruses are not involved in the etiopathogenesis of salivary gland tumors. *Ces-slov Pathol* 49(2):72–75.

Skalova A, Michal M, Simpson RHW. 2017. Newly described salivary gland tumors. *Mod Pathol* 30, S217-S43.

Skálová A, Stenman G, Simpson RHW, et al. 2018. The role of molecular resting in the differential diagnosis of salivary gland carcinomas. *Am J Surg Pathol* 42(2):e11–e27.

Skalova A, Vanecek T, Majewska H, et al. 2014. Mammary analogue secretory carcinoma of salivary glands with high-grade transformation *Am J Surg Pathol* 38(1):23–33.

Skalova A, Vanecek T, Sima R, et al. 2010. Mammary analogue secretory carcinoma of salivary glands, containing the ETV6-NTRK3 fusion gene: A hitherto undescribed salivary gland tumor entity. *Am J Surg Pathol* 34(5):599–608.

Skálová A, Vanecek T, Simpson RH, et al. 2016. Mammary analogue secretory carcinoma of salivary glands: Molecular analysis of 25 ETV6 gene rearranged tumors with lack of detection of classical ETV6-NTRK3 fusion transcript by standard RT-PCR: Report of 4 cases harboring ETV6-X gene fusion. *Am J Surg Pathol* 40(1):3–13.

Skalova A, Vanecek T, Simpson RHW, et al. 2013b. CRTC1-MAML2 and CRTC3-MAML2 fusions were not detected in metaplastic Warthin tumor and metaplastic pleomorphic adenoma of salivary glands. *Am J Surg Pathol* 37(17)1743-1750.

Speight PM, Barrett AW 2002. Salivary gland tumours. *Oral Dis* 8(5):229–240.

Spiro RH, Huvos AG, Berk R, Strong EW. 1978. Mucoepidermoid carcinoma of salivary gland origin. A clinicopathologic study of 367 cases. *Am J Surg* 136(4):461–468.

Spiro RH, Huvos AG, Strong EW. 1975. Cancer of the parotid gland. A clinicopathologic study of 288 primary cases. *Am J Surg* 130(4):452–459.

Spitz MR, Batsakis JG. 1984. Major salivary gland carcinoma. Descriptive epidemiology and survival of 498 patients. *Arch Otolaryngol* 110(1):45–49.

Stephen J, Batsakis JG, Luna MA, et al. 1986. True malignant mixed tumors (carcinosarcoma) of salivary glands. *Oral Surg Oral Med Oral Pathol* 61(6):597–602.

Sterman BM, Kraus DH, Sebek BA, Tucker HM. 1990. Primary squamous cell carcinoma of the parotid gland. *Laryngoscope* 100(2 Pt 1):146–148.

Sugimoto T, Wakizono S, Uemura T, et al. 1993. Malignant oncocytoma of the parotid gland: A case report with an immunohistochemical and ultrastructural study. *J Laryngol Otol* 107(1):69–74.

Taki NH, Laver N, Quinto T, Wein RO. 2013. Carcinosarcoma de novo of the parotid gland: Case report. *Head Neck* 35(5):E161–163.

Tarakji B, Baraoudi K, Darwish S, et al. 2013. Immunohistochemical expression of p16 in pleomorphic salivary gland adenoma. *Turk Patoloji Derg* 29:36–40.

Thackray AC, Lucas RB. 1974. Tumors of Major Salivary Glands, 2nd edn. Washington, DC, Armed Forces Institute of Pathology.

Thackray AC, Sobin LH. 1972. Histological Typing of Salivary Gland Tumors. Geneva, World Health Organization.

Thway K, Fisher C.2012. Tumors With EWSR1-CREB1 and EWSR1-ATF1 fusions: The current status. *Am J Surg Pathol* 36(7):e1–e11.

Uchida K, Oga A, Mano T, et al. 2010. Screening for DNA copy number aberrations in mucinous adenocarcinoma arising from the minor salivary gland: Two case reports. *Cancer Genet Cytogenet* 203(2):324–327.

Urano M, Nagao T, Miyabe S, et al. 2015. Characterization of mammary analogue secretory carcinoma of the salivary gland: Discrimination from its mimics by the presence of the ETV6-NTRK3 translocation and novel surrogate markers. *Hum Pathol* 46(1):94–103.

Wai DH, Knezevich SR, Lucas T, et al. 2000. The *ETV6-NTRK3* gene fusion encodes a chimeric protein tyrosine kinase that transforms NIH3T3 cells *Oncogene* 19(7):906–915.

Wang H, Yao J, Solomon, Axiotis CA. 2010. Sebaceous carcinoma of the oral cavity: A case report and review of the literature. *Oral Surg Oral Med Oral Pathol Oral Radiol Endod* 110:e37–e40.

Wang L, Liu Y, Lin X, et al. 2013a. Low-grade cribriform cystadenoma of salivary glands: Report of two cases and review of the literature. *Diagn Pathol* 8 (28):1–6.

Wang Y, Shang W, Lei X, et al. 2013b. Opposing functions of PLAG1 in pleomorphic adenoma: A microarray analysis of PLAG1 transgenic mice. *Biotechnol Lett* 35:1377–1385.

Ward BK, Seethala RR, Barnes EL, Y Lai SY. 2009. Basal cell adenocarcinoma of a hard palate minor salivary gland: Case report and review of the literature. *Head Neck Oncol*, 1:41

Warner KA, Adams A, Bernardi L, et al. 2013. Characterization of tumorigenic cell lines from the recurrence and lymph node metastasis of a human salivary mucoepidermoid carcinoma. *Oral Oncol* 49:1059–1066.

Weinreb I. 2013. Hyalinizing clear cell carcinoma of salivary gland: A review and update. *Head Neck Pathol* 7(1):20–29.

Weiss S, Goldblum J. 2001. Weiss's Soft Tissue Tumors, 4th edn. St. Louis, Mo, Mosby.

Zhou C-X, Shi D-Y, Ma D-Q, et al. 2010. Primary oncocytic carcinoma of the salivary glands: A clinicopathologic and immunohistochemical study of 12 cases. *Oral Oncol*, 46(10):773–778.

Chapter 9
The Molecular Biology of Benign and Malignant Salivary Gland Tumors

Randy Todd, DMD, MD, DSc
Private Practice of Oral and Maxillofacial Surgery, Peabody, MA, USA

Outline

Introduction: The Puzzle and the Promise
Salivary Gland Tumor Cell Biology
Molecular Biology of Salivary Gland Neoplasms
    Protein Dysregulation and Salivary Gland Neoplasm Phenotypes
    Enhanced Proliferation
    Evasion of Apoptosis
    Immortalization
    Neovascularization
    Invasion and Metastasis
    Nucleic Acid Dysregulation and Salivary Gland Neoplasms
    Genetic Alterations in Salivary Gland Tumors
    Epigenetic Alterations of Gene Expression in Salivary Gland Tumors
Summary and Clinical Applications
    Diagnostic Applications
    Therapeutic Applications
Summary
References

Introduction: The Puzzle and the Promise

At present, the molecular biology of head and neck neoplasms is poorly understood. The vast majority of malignancies in this region originate from the squamous epithelium; therefore, the primary research focus has been squamous cell carcinoma. Far less is known regarding the molecular mechanisms governing benign and malignant salivary gland tumors (Kaye 2006; Lin et al. 2018). Salivary gland tumors account for 0.4–13.5 cases per 100 000 (1–3% of head and neck carcinomas and 0.3% of all malignancies) in the United States (Eveson et al. 2005; Vander Poorten et al. 2012; Lin et al. 2018). Proposed risk factors include diet, history of radiation, genetic predisposition, nickel, tobacco use (Warthin tumor), and certain occupational exposures (rubber manufacturing, beauty shop workers (Carlson et al. 2013; Lin et al. 2018). How these risk factors translate into the molecular events that govern salivary gland tumor progression largely remains unclear. However, themes from the hallmarks of neoplasia found with tumors at other anatomic sites are proving true in salivary gland tumors. Therefore, by identifying molecular events observed in other tumors that are common in salivary gland neoplasms, we can begin to unravel some of the puzzle of these complex lesions and appreciate the promise of translating benchwork success into novel, biologically based diagnostic and therapeutic strategies.

What are some of the challenges of studying the molecular biology of benign and malignant salivary gland tumors? First, salivary gland tumors are relatively uncommon. As stated earlier, salivary gland tumors account for a small percentage of head and neck neoplasms (Bansal et al. 2012). Squamous epithelial lesions account for greater than 90% of tumors in this region. Second, a great deal of heterogeneity exists in the origin (by location and histology) of salivary gland tumors. Location is associated with certain predilections (Fonseca et al. 2016). The majority of tumors occur

---

Salivary Gland Pathology: Diagnosis and Management, Third Edition. Edited by Eric R. Carlson and Robert A. Ord.
© 2022 John Wiley & Sons, Inc. Published 2022 by John Wiley & Sons, Inc.
Companion website: www.wiley.com/go/carlson/salivary

in the major salivary glands (parotid, submandibular and sublingual) (Prenen et al. 2008). Seventy percent of salivary gland tumors occur in the parotid gland, with 85% of those tumors being benign (Adelstein et al. 2012; Ochal-Choinska and Osuch-Wojikiewicz, 2016). Yet 50–90% of minor salivary gland tumors are malignant (Lopes et al. 1998; Hellquist et al. 2019). How certain salivary glands are more predisposed to malignant transformation is unclear. In addition to location, the cellular etiology of salivary gland neoplasms varies greatly. Salivary gland tumors are the most complex and diverse of all tumors (Bell and Hanna 2012). There is a great overlap in cell/tissue types (as well as variety in production/distribution of extracellular material) involved, leading to constant reclassification of these tumors (Adelstein et al. 2012) (Figure 9.1). Furthermore, there is a great deal of heterogeneity with respect to clinical behavior. Aggressive behavior is inversely correlated with the fraction of myoepithelial cells (Batsakis et al. 1989). High-grade lesions have a greater tendency for lymphatic spread. Distant hematogenous metastases (primarily to the lungs, bones or liver) are more common in adenoid cystic carcinoma, adenocarcinoma not otherwise specified, carcinoma ex pleomorphic adenoma, small cell carcinoma, and ductal carcinoma than other salivary gland cancers (Huang et al. 2018). Adenoid cystic carcinoma and polymorphous adenocarcinoma have a higher predilection for neurotropism. Third, salivary gland tumors tend to be very indolent: adenoid cystic carcinoma patients can live 10–20 years after diagnosis (Prenen et al. 2008; Dillon et al. 2016). Therefore, salivary tumors represent a significant challenge to study at the molecular level. Because they are uncommon, salivary gland tumors are very difficult to collect in sufficient numbers to validate target molecule findings. In addition, the histologic spectrum in the etiology of these tumors clouds direct comparisons: do tumor specimens within the same study set have similar clonal origin? As a result of being so rare and complex, understanding the molecular basis of these tumors suffers from lack of databases, materials, cell lines, and animal models, as well as robust clinical studies (Bell and Hanna 2012). However, understanding the precise molecular underpinnings of salivary gland tumor progression promises novel, powerful modalities for patient management.

Advances in our understanding of the molecular events that govern human disease promise a personalized approach to medicine (Keller et al. 2017; Lassche et al. 2019). Individual tumor biology will allow disease progression/response to be better predicted and offer novel treatment targets with fewer side effects (Dietel et al. 2013). Diagnostic information will be obtainable not only from biopsy tissue, but blood and saliva (Sidranski 2002; Yoshizawa et al. 2013). Molecular

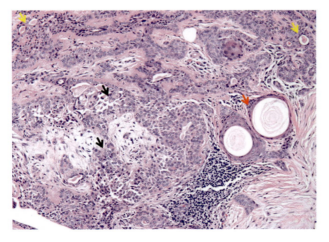

Figure 9.1. **Why are salivary gland tumors so hard to study?** Among the most important characteristics that make salivary gland tumors extremely difficult to study at the molecular level is the heterogeneity of the cellular and extracellular matrix composition and distribution. For example, pleomorphic adenoma, the most common benign salivary gland tumor, shows a wide array of normal and neoplastic cell types, as well as variety of cell products. In this view, the tumor is composed of a proliferation of glandular epithelium and myoepithelial cells (black arrows) within a variably hyalinized and myxoid stroma. Discrete ductal elements cuffed by myoepithelial cells are appreciated throughout (yellow arrows). Focal squamous differentiation/cystic degeneration is also appreciated (red arrow). Understanding the role and interactions of each cell type in the biology of the developing tumor is a complex task. Source: Figure courtesy of Dr. Vikki Noonan, Division of Oral Pathology, Boston University Henry M. Goldman School of Dental Medicine, Boston, MA 02118.

markers will be able to better diagnose and differentiate between salivary gland tumors (Dietel et al. 2013). Identification of the molecular determinants of salivary gland tumor progression will better guide existing treatment protocols by ensuring prediction of treatment response and prognosis will be more reliable (Lassche et al. 2019). Therapeutic options for salivary gland tumor patients will also be improved. Molecular events underlying disease progression will serve as novel therapeutic targets, alone or in combination. Both conventional and biologically based treatment protocols will also be improved by reducing side effects, earlier identification of recurrent disease and reducing recurrent disease (Sidranski 2002; Kolch et al. 2005; Taube et al. 2005; Wang et al. 2015; Emmerson and Knox 2018). Before exploring these exciting new possibilities, a review of salivary gland tumor cellular and molecular biology is necessary.

Salivary Gland Tumor Cell Biology

Today, the most clinically significant attributes of salivary gland tumors include the stage, histologic grade, anatomic site, patient age, and adequacy of tumor margin (Zarbo 2002). Over the last half century, the diversity of salivary gland neoplasms has been more greatly appreciated (Nagao et al. 2012). Two important classification schemes have emerged to define the origin/development, identification, and behavior/prognosis of salivary gland tumors: histogenesis and morphogenesis. Both schemes explain salivary gland tumorigenesis in terms of stem cells (undifferentiated cells endowed with limitless capacity for self-renewal) and progenitor cells (stem cell daughter cells with a committed differentiation program and limited replication ability) emerging from the basic cellular framework of the salivary gland (excretory duct, striated duct, intercalated duct, and acinus) (Dardick and Burford-Mason 1993) (Figure 9.2). The newly identified salivary gland tumors (such as basal cell adenoma, polymorphous adenocarcinoma, epithelial-myoepithelial carcinoma, and salivary duct carcinoma) reflect a trend in pathology to look beyond the histogenesis of the disease and focus on morphogenesis (Zarbo 2002).

Histogenetic classification categorizes tumors based on the cell type within the normal salivary gland unit that is involved in tumor induction (Batsakis et al. 1989; Sreeja et al. 2014; Emmerson and Knox 2018). According to histogenetic classification schemes, salivary gland tumors with terminal ductal, myoepithelial, and acinar differentiation were believed to originate from distal intercalated duct reserve cells (Figure 9.2a). Salivary gland tumors with large duct, squamous or mucinous cell differentiation originate from an excretory duct reserve cell. The dichotomy between cells of origin is believed to have clinical significance: tumors derived from the main ductal segments tend to be high grade and more aggressive, whereas tumors from the terminal ductal segments are low grade or benign (Bell and Hanna 2012). Myoepithelial cells in the terminal duct have been postulated to have "tumor suppressor" effects, leading to indolent and protracted behavior (Dardick et al. 1982). Loss of myoepithelial cells coincides with more aggressive behavior. Several theories have been proposed as to the role of stem cells and progenitor cells: basal reserve theory, pluripotent unicellular theory, semipluripotent bicellular reserve cell theory, and the multicellular theory (Cheuk and Chan 2007). Central to all the histogenetic classification schemes is (1) tumorigenesis does not originate in the acinus and (2) salivary gland tumor cell biologic behavior arises from either dedifferentiation (loss of specialized features) or transdifferentiation (acquisition of another differentiated cell phenotype) (Dardick and Burford-Mason 1993). Due to difficulties in clinically classifying certain tumors, as well as some inconsistencies with current cellular and molecular biology findings, an alternative classification scheme has been proposed (Dardick and Burford-Mason 1993).

Morphogenetic classification, a newer approach to salivary gland neoplasm classification, explains tumor anatomy based on three primary criteria: types of cell differentiation, patterns of tumor cell organization, and synthesis/distribution of extracellular materials (Dardick et al. 1982; Dardick and Burford-Mason 1993; Sreeja et al. 2014) (Figure 9.2b). Two models exist in the morphogenesis classification scheme. The linear model proposes that stem cells give rise to two distinct progenitors: epithelial and myoepithelial. The stochastic model is a bidirectional pathway where two separate epithelial and myoepithelial progenitors are generated (Bell and Hanna 2012). In the salivary gland tumor, three morphogenetic tumor

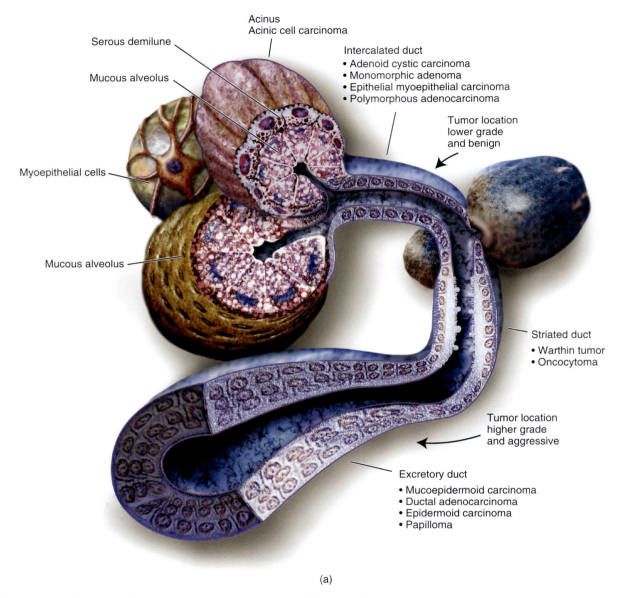

(a)

Figure 9.2. Histogenetic versus morphogenetic classification: How do salivary gland tumors arise? (a) Based on related histology between normal salivary gland development and salivary gland tumors, histogenetic classification proposes that heterogeneity is dependent on the location of the stem/progenitor cells. Tumors originating more proximal to the acini tend to be low grade and benign while those arising nearer the excretory ducts tend to be more high grade and aggressive. Histogenic classification has proven an imperfect means of predicting tumor biology. (b) Morphogenetic classification is based on (1) cell type (luminal cells, myoepithelial-like cells, basal-like cells), (2) type and distribution of extracellular material, and (3) pattern of cellular organization. Morphogenic classification may prove a sounder basis for the molecular study of salivary gland tumors. Both schemes are important attempts at understanding the biology of salivary gland tumor development to better identify and predict the behavior of this heterogeneous group of neoplasms.

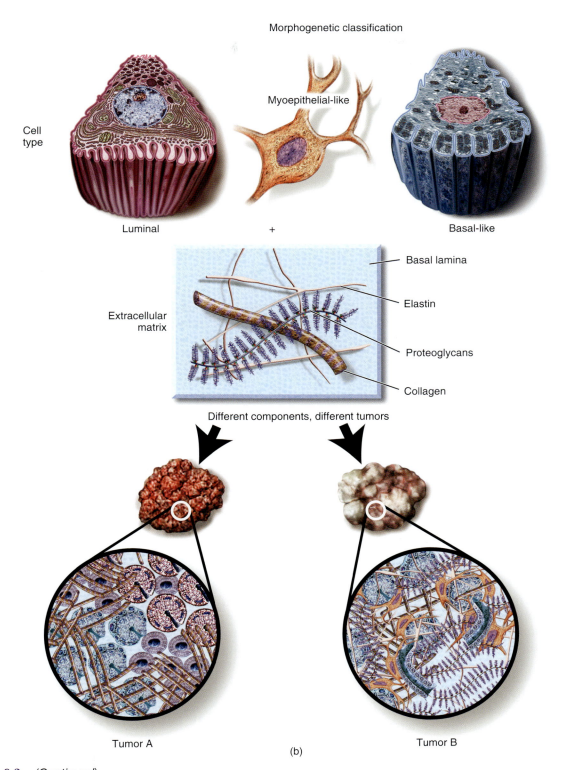

Figure 9.2. (*Continued*).

forms arise: luminal and myoepithelial cells; only luminal cells; only myoepithelial/basal cells (Dardick and Burford-Mason 1993). Salivary gland tumors differ based on variations of cell type (cuboidal/columnar sheets, islands and duct-like structures), myoepithelial cell type (spindle, plasmacytoid, clear), ductal: myoepithelial cell ratio and presence/absence/type of extracellular material (Sreeja et al. 2014). While histogenetic classification suggests dedifferentiation occurs, morphogenesis classification proposes stem cell/progenitor cell inhibition of differentiation. In addition to the clinical importance of these two theories, the application of the histogenetic and morphogenetic models has important implications into the molecular events governing salivary gland tumorigenesis. The histogenetic classification is a more taxonomic approach. The morphogenetic approach is a more working classification that seeks to unravel overlapping histologic patterns using the biologic feature of the tumor (Dardick et al. 1985).

While hematoxylin–eosin staining remains the gold standard for salivary gland tumor diagnosis, immunohistochemistry (IHC) is more commonly being used to better understand the morphogenesis of the disease and enhance diagnostic accuracy (Nagao et al. 2012). While few tumor type-specific markers are available, IHC marker panels can support and enhance the histological assessment. At present, most IHC markers target differentiation-related proteins (Nagao et al. 2012). For example, markers of luminal/acinar epithelial differentiation might include the epithelial membrane antigen, carcinoembryonic antigen, and low-molecular weight keratins. Myoepithelial IHC markers include S-100, GFAF, vimentin, and high-molecular weight keratins. More specific myoepithelial markers include calponin, caldesmon, and alpha-smooth muscle actin. Tumor matrix production can be assessed by IHC detection of amylase, type IV collagen and laminin. Organelle IHC staining can also help identify certain tumor types: mitochondria staining of oncocytic tumors and lysozyme staining for tumors with acinar differentiation. Differential diagnosis of salivary gland tumors with certain structural/architectural histological patterns can be aided by IHC examination using these marker panels (Zarbo 2002). Several salivary gland tumors exhibit a cribriform pattern. Clear cell salivary gland tumors not only can be distinguished from each other using EMA and calpontin, but from metastatic tumors such as renal cell carcinoma (by RCC or CD10) and melanoma (by Malan-A). Specimens with limited sample can be differentiated as either benign or malignant using proliferation markers such as Ki-67 and certain tumor-related proteins (discussed below). Lastly, salivary "undifferentiated carcinoma" (small cell carcinoma, large cell carcinoma, and lymphoepithelial carcinoma) can be distinguished from lymphoma if they stain positive for pan-CK and negative for leukocyte common antigen.

Central to the concept of these classification schemes is the existence of a subset of tumorigenic cells with stem cell-like characteristics (Adams et al. 2013). Like stem cells in normal tissues, tumor stem cells undergo self-renewal and demonstrate multi-lineage differentiation. Interestingly, cancer stem cells may play an important role in resistance to chemotherapy and radiation therapy (Adams et al. 2015). There are two hypotheses regarding the origin of tumor stem cells. First, a normal stem cell may undergo an initiating change at the molecular level. A second hypothesis (known as the tumor initiation cell theory) states that normal differentiated cells acquire a mutation (or mutations) that supports tumor growth by allowing the altered cell to act like a stem cell (Adams et al. 2013). While playing a pivotal role in tumor progression, the biology of stem cells or tumor initiating cells in salivary gland tumorigenesis remains incompletely understood (Emmerson and Knox 2018).

While a more accurate classification of salivary gland tumors may improve diagnosis and provide a more precise therapeutic protocol, many biomarkers today target differentiation proteins that are usually used to separate one cell type from another. However, in addition to considering the biology of salivary gland cell types, it is important to view salivary gland tumor biology in the context of general tumor biology and identify/exploit and consider disease-specific biomarkers to improve patient management.

Molecular Biology of Salivary Gland Neoplasms

While identifying certain differentiation- and matrix-associated molecules has aided in the classification and diagnosis of salivary gland tumors, the molecular mechanisms underlying salivary gland tumor progression are poorly understood. However, like in neoplasms at other anatomic sites, an understanding of the biologic determinants governing salivary gland tumors can better direct the classification, diagnosis, and management of the disease. Therefore, several lines of investigation regarding salivary gland tumor molecular biology are best appreciated in the general context of cancer molecular and tumor biology.

The fundamental paradigm of molecular biology is that deoxyribonucleic acid (DNA) is transcribed into messenger ribonucleic acid (mRNA), which is translated into protein (Figure 9.3a). Genes are the coding units within chromosomal DNA. The code is transferred from the nucleus to the cytoplasm via mRNA. There, the mRNA is used as a template to create proteins that are responsible for cellular structure and function. Therefore, while "disease genes" do refer to chromosomal DNA regions that are associated with a pathologic process, it is the alteration of the protein function that is the primary molecular/biochemical determinant. In cancer, "oncogenes" are normal genes altered that support tumorigenesis; "tumor suppressor genes" are inactivated regulatory genes that would block tumor formation. However, it is really the overactive oncoproteins and inhibited tumor suppressor proteins that ultimately lead to tumor development. DNA, mRNA, and proteins associated with tumor progression can also serve as diagnostic and therapeutic targets. The following sections will consider the contribution DNA, mRNA, and proteins identified to be altered during tumorigenesis in general and salivary gland neoplasms, as well as how these events might be exploited clinically.

PROTEIN DYSREGULATION AND SALIVARY GLAND NEOPLASM PHENOTYPES

Proteins associated with tumor development are dysregulated through two primary mechanisms. First, a structurally intact ("normal" or "wild type") protein can be produced in altered quantities (or temporally and/or anatomically ectopic production or reduced/absent product). Second, an altered protein can be produced that may be overactive (or constituently active), inactive, or abnormally interact with/sequester other proteins. With regard to tumor development, qualitatively or quantitatively altered proteins are often growth factors/extracellular ligands, cell surface receptors, cytoplasmic/nuclear secondary messengers, and transcription factors. Each of these proteins forms interconnecting signal transduction networks that control function in both heath and disease.

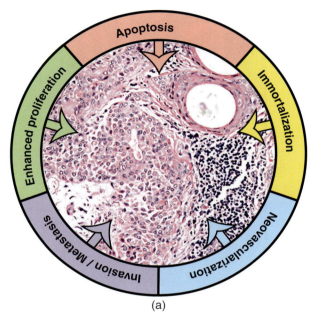

(a)

Figure 9.3. Paradigms in tumor biology: What are the cellular and molecular alterations of a cancer cell? (a) Neoplastic cells acquire several phenotypes that provide a selective advantage to their normal counterparts. These important characteristics include enhanced proliferation (due to overactive growth promoters and inactivated/suppressed growth inhibitors), failure to undergo apoptosis, immortalization, neovascularization (allowing tumors to increase in size and spread), and invasion/metastasis (allowing malignant cells to grow at sites remote from the primary tumor). These phenotypes are regulated by networks of signal transduction pathways. (b) Deregulation of these cell traits can occur through alterations in the fundamental molecular mechanisms governing the cell. Elements of signal transduction pathways include protein ligands (cytokines, growth factors, matrix molecules), cell surface ligand receptors, cytoplasmic secondary messengers, and nuclear transcription factors (left). Large-scale and small-scale damage to chromosomal DNA (as well as epigenetic alterations) can lead to quantitative or qualitative changes in messenger RNA, which carries the blueprint of the signal transduction proteins for production. Synthesis of quantitatively or qualitatively altered regulatory proteins can, in turn, lead to the phenotypes observed in tumor cells.

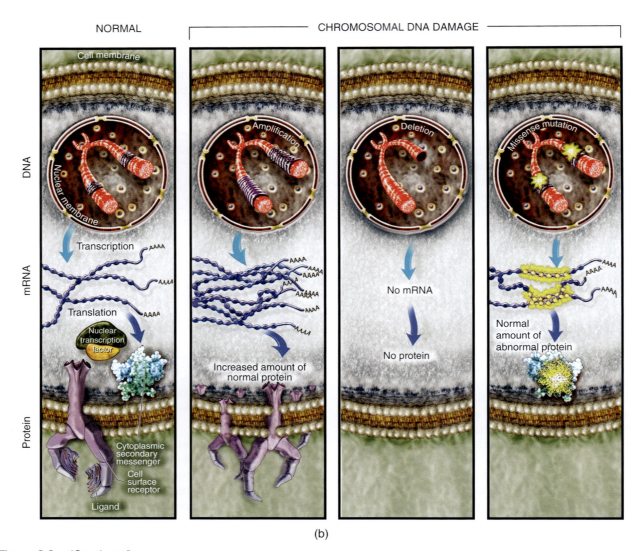

Figure 9.3. (*Continued*).

Tumor cells share several traits or phenotypes. Each contributes to a behavior that allows the tumor cell to outcompete its normal counterpart. These phenotypes do not appear simultaneously but accumulate in a preferred, but not absolute, order over time (Vogelstein and Kinzler 1998). Cellular behaviors commonly seen in tumor cells include enhanced proliferation, escape of apoptosis, immortalization, neovascularization, and, in the case of malignant tumors, invasion/metastasis (Figure 9.3b). While the mechanisms contributing to these phenotypes are much less defined than tumors at other anatomic sites, certain themes are emerging.

Enhanced Proliferation

Salivary gland tumor cells can divide faster than their normal counterparts (Catalano et al. 2013). Two fundamental mechanisms support this phenotype. First, tumor cells do not have to wait for a signal to start cell division due to the overactivity of growth promoting networks. Second, growth constraints are bypassed or inactivated in a tumor cell (to be discussed later). Growth signals are overactivated in a tumor cell by generating its own proliferation signals through several different mechanisms, including production of its own growth factors, amplification of extracellular signals using overexpressed (or constituently active) cell surface receptors, dependence on overactive intracellular messengers, or alteration of transcription factors that regulate the production other proteins (Black and Dinney 2008; Grandal and Madshus 2008; Lee and Muller 2010; Smith et al. 2010; Brognard and Hunter 2011).

Proliferation-associated proteins, which include extracellular ligands/ligand receptors, constituently functioning secondary messengers and nuclear transcription factors, have been shown to be overactive in various salivary gland neoplasms (Skalova and Leivo 1996) (Figure 9.4). Extracellular ligands and their receptors, such as the epidermal growth factor (EGF) and its receptor (EGFR), are aberrantly expressed in a variety of salivary gland cancers, such as adenoid cystic carcinoma and high-grade mucoepidermoid carcinoma (Liu et al. 2012; Ach et al. 2013; Cros et al. 2013; Nakano et al. 2013; Goyal et al. 2015; Keller et al. 2017). Part of the human epidermal growth factor receptor (HER) superfamily, EGFR (or HER-1) is joined by HER-2/NEU and HER-3 as receptors commonly overexpressed by adenoid cystic carcinomas (Todd and Wong 1999; Gibbons et al. 2001; Can et al. 2018). Expression of HER-4 in salivary gland tumors is less clear. A secondary messenger pathway downstream from EGF-EGFR binding, the PI3K-AKT pathway, is also dysregulated in acinic cell carcinoma (Diegel et al. 2010; Zboray et al. 2018). The Wnt/β-catenin pathway is also overactive due either to direct alteration of factors within the cascade or indirectly through loss of pathway inhibitors (WNT inhibitory factor-1) (Liu et al. 2012; Ishibashi et al. 2018). The SOX 4 transcription factor is also highly overexpressed in adenoid cystic carcinoma (Frierson et al. 2002). In short, aberrantly expressed/active growth promoters appear to contribute to salivary gland neoplastic progression. While the important proliferation pathways are not fully defined for any particular salivary tumor, these pathways appear to be able to be disrupted by signals appearing in the microenvironment, at the cell surface, within the cytoplasmic signaling cascades, as well as through transcription factors that regulate other growth promoting molecules.

The second fundamental mechanism supporting enhanced proliferation is the loss of proteins that inhibit cell division (Lee and Muller 2010; Blanpain 2013). Proliferation is governed by an internal cell cycle clock that runs through four phases: a G1 or gap phase, S-phase where the cell duplicates its genetic material, a second gap phase (or G2), then an M phase where the cell divides (Vermeulen et al. 2003). While each phase is tightly regulated, the primary checkpoint where the cell commits to cell division is at the restriction (or R) point at the end of G1 (Vermeulen et al. 2003). Cells that do not pass R-point enter differentiation/senescence programs (Chandler and Peters 2013; Seethala 2017). The key regulator of R-point is the retinoblastoma protein (pRb) (Henley and Dick 2012; Anderson et al. 2017). Cells that pass through R-point move irreversibly toward S-phase due to the activity of the transcription factor E2F (Classon and Harlow 2002). Cell cycle progression is blocked at R-point when pRb binds E2F, thereby preventing the activation of the E2F-mediated pathways that ultimately lead to cell division (Dyson 1998). Loss of pRB activity allows progression through R-point/activation of E2F pathways unhindered. Many tumor cells suffer a reduction or loss of pRb (Manning and Dyson 2012). Neoplastic cells that have normal pRB levels frequently have a disruption upstream or downstream of pRb. In salivary gland tumors, the presence of pRB is variable. As expected, pRb is present in higher levels in normal versus benign and malignant salivary gland tumors (Liu et al. 2005). However, downregulation of pRb appears to be more important in some salivary gland neoplasms more than others: pRb is infrequently altered in adenoid cystic carcinoma but abnormally expressed in acinic cell carcinoma, as well as many benign and malignant myoepithelial tumors (Yamamoto et al. 1996; Shintani et al. 2000; Etges et al. 2004; Liu et al. 2005; Vekony et al. 2008).

Unregulated proliferation is not enough to generate a tumor. Other cellular checkpoints exist that inhibit rapid cellular division. A rapidly expanding cell mass can quickly outgrow its nutrient supply. Cells also have an inherent limit to the number of times it can divide, independent of the rate of that division. Lastly, the cell has a program to eliminate aberrant cells: apoptosis.

Evasion of Apoptosis

An important mechanism to remove damaged cells is apoptosis (Hanahan and Weinberg 2011). Key triggers of apoptosis include growth factor

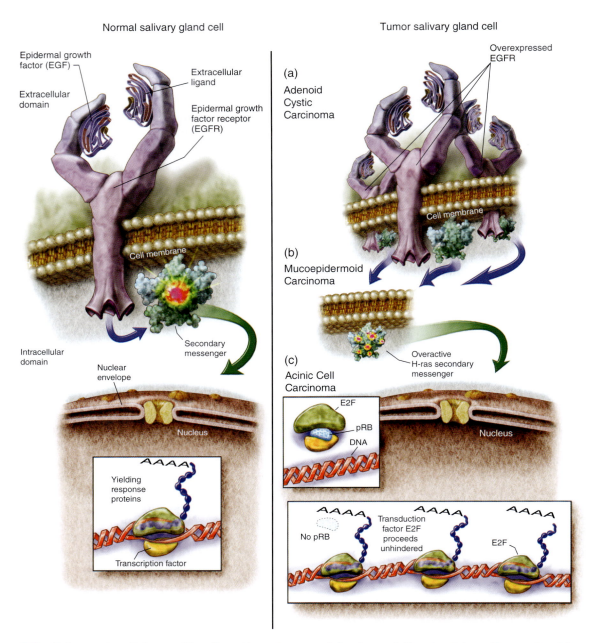

Figure 9.4. Enhanced cellular proliferation: How does protein deregulation lead to salivary gland tumor cell behavior? Important signal transduction pathways that regulate cellular proliferation are abrogated in salivary gland tumors. In normal cells, extracellular ligands bind to cell surface receptors. Ligand–receptor binding activates secondary messengers that regulate several functions, including the production of response proteins via nuclear transcription factors. (a) In adenoid cystic carcinoma, the epidermal growth factor receptor (EGFR) is overexpressed, leading to hypersensitivity of the cell to the many ligands that bind to EGFR. (b) The secondary messenger H-ras is constitutively active (or activated independent of upstream stimuli) in mucoepidermoid carcinomas. (c) The cell cycle regulator pRb is downregulated in acinic cell carcinoma. Without pRb, the transcription factor E2F proceeds unhindered, thereby enhancing cellular proliferation programs. While there are many regulators within each signal transduction pathway, only one element needs to be altered to potentially change a phenotype-like enhanced proliferation. However, networks of other pathways may limit some alterations from causing an overall cellular change.

withdrawal, ionizing radiation, chemotherapy cytokine exposure, high calcium concentrations, nitric oxide, or oxidative stress (Fadeel and Orrenius 2005). An apoptotic cell is dismantled, condensed, and eventually eliminated by phagocytosis. Apoptosis can be initiated through external stimuli, as well as internal factors (Ouyang et al. 2012). Cells with damaged proliferative regulatory pathways would normally be eliminated through apoptosis. Therefore, the pathways leading to apoptosis also have to be inactivated during salivary gland tumorigenesis (Flores et al. 2017; Da Silva et al. 2019).

A major regulator of apoptosis is p53. In response to extracellular (such as UV radiation, ionizing radiation, hypoxia) and intracellular insults (such as DNA damage, oncogene signaling, transcriptional abnormalities), p53 induces cell growth arrest and DNA repair (Golubovskaya and Cance 2013). If the damage is too profound, p53 initiates apoptosis (Vogelstein and Kinzler 1992). Tumor cells can evade apoptosis by eliminating p53 function, either by reducing p53 quantitatively or altering p53 structure. Mutated p53 acts in a dominant negative manner, sequestering wild type (or normal) p53 (Nag et al. 2013). Like pRb, most human cancers subvert p53 directly or by abrogating upstream or downstream mediators in its pathway (Vogelstein and Kinzler 1992). Salivary gland tumor cells, particularly malignancies, do subvert apoptosis (Ben-Izhak et al. 2007). In fact, in many cases, apoptosis assays, as well as specific apoptosis mediators, are believed to be useful in separating salivary gland cancers from their benign counterparts, (Nagao et al. 1998; Weber et al. 2002) though this is not a universal finding (Karja et al. 1997; Rosa et al. 1997). While mutated p53 has been identified in a wide variety of salivary gland neoplasms, variations in findings are likely the result of varied experimental approach and specimen procurement (Deguchi et al. 1993; Felix et al. 1996; Yin et al. 2000; Kiyoshima et al. 2001; Nagler et al. 2003; Marques et al. 2008; Ben-Izhak et al. 2009; Faur et al. 2015; Ochal-Choinska and Osuch-Wojicikiewicz 2016; Goulart-Fihlo et al. 2019). Like the pRb pathway, upstream and downstream elements of the p53 pathway, including c-MYC, MDM2, pAKT and BCL-2, have been shown to be altered in various salivary gland neoplasms (Deguchi et al. 1993; Rosa et al. 1997; Nagao et al. 1998, 2003; Marques et al. 2008; Jin et al. 2012).

Immortalization

Cells that can rapidly proliferate without being cleared through apoptosis still face another challenge: senescence. Under normal conditions, cells can divide a fixed number of times before they stop or senesce (Hayflick 1965). The major underlying mechanism for the halt is that chromosome caps or telomeres are exhausted. Loss of telomeres leads the ends of the chromosomes to stick to adjacent chromosomes if the cell is allowed to divide; therefore, cell division is halted (Shay and Wright 2005). The majority of tumor cells avoid senescence by synthesizing the enzyme telomerase that restores the chromosomal cap (Xu et al. 2013). Initial reports suggest that malignant salivary gland cells exhibit telomerase activity, whereas expression in their benign counterparts is variable (Shigeishi et al. 2011). EGFR may be an upstream positive regulator of telomerase in these tumors (Sowa et al. 2018). Overexpression of pleomorphic adenoma gene-1 (PLAG-1) in salivary gland tumors also leads to a capacity for limitless cellular replication via the IGF-2 pathway (Declercq et al. 2008; Escalente et al. 2016).

Neovascularization

Cells require nutrients to fuel growth and a means to eliminate waste. Both processes cannot cross a gradient greater than three to four cell layers thick (Folkman 2006). Therefore, even cells with enhanced proliferative capability, absent apoptotic activity, and immortality will remain dormant unless a new blood supply arises to support that growth (Gimbrone et al. 1972). Tumor cells must develop an "angiogenic switch" that supports new endothelial growth (Gimbrone et al. 1972). Few incipient tumor masses develop this switch (Auguste et al. 2005).

Like tumors at other anatomic sites, angiogenesis appears to be an important event in salivary gland tumor progression (Theocharis et al. 2015; Koochek-Dezfuli et al. 2019). Microvascular density appears to increase in association with salivary gland tumors, though some controversy remains whether neovascularization is greater in malignant versus benign disease (Vidal et al. 2013; Shieh et al. 2009). Increased densities of mast cells and tumor-associated macrophages appear to be a cellular source of pro-angiogenic factors in salivary gland neoplasms (Shieh et al. 2009; Vidal et al. 2013). Vascular endothelial growth factor (VEGF) and

NOTCH are important signaling pathways that support neovascularization in salivary gland tumors (Liu et al. 2012; Andisheh Tadbir et al. 2013; Margaritescu et al. 2013 Bell et al. 2014; Blockowiak et al. 2018; Bell et al. 2015). A significant number of salivary gland carcinomas (65%) express VEGF (Lim et al. 2003; Wang et al. 2015). Tumor hypoxia leads to HIFα-HIFβ dimerization that, in turn, induces VEGF overexpression (Lim et al. 2003). The activity of angiogenesis inhibitors is less defined. Thrombospondin-1 appears to be downregulated in salivary gland carcinomas while TIMP-2 is highly active in the stroma of pleomorphic adenomas (Kishi et al. 2003; Zhang et al. 2009b). Fusion proteins also support angiogenesis in salivary gland tumors (Ono and Okada 2018). Factors supporting angiogenesis, such as VEGF, are believed to correlate with tumor aggressiveness (Demasi et al. 2012). In fact, angiogenesis and another important tumor phenotype, invasion and metastasis, share many overlapping cellular and molecular mechanisms of disease (Lequerica-Fernandez et al. 2007; de Faria et al. 2011).

Invasion and Metastasis

Tumor invasion is the primary phenotype that demarks benign from malignant disease (Comoglio and Trusolino 2002). While locally aggressive benign tumors may displace or destroy surrounding tissue, invasion marks the escape of the cancer cell into the surrounding "normal" stroma. Invasion is instigated by the cancer cell but is supported by underlying stromal cells (Talmadge and Fidler 2010). At the lead edge of invasion, enzymes are released to break down the basement membrane (Willis et al. 2013). In the early stages of invasion, the cancer cell undergoes an epithelial-mesenchymal transition (EMT). Several cellular phenotypes are lost during EMT, including cell proliferation, certain differentiation genetic pathways, and altered E-cadherin expression (Cavallaro and Christofori 2004; Berx and van Roy 2009). However, EMT cells gain other phenotypes, such as increased mobility, a fibroblast-like morphology, upregulation of stem cell-like programs, and expression of N-cadherin (Mani et al. 2008). Tumor-stimulated neovasculature not only helps support cancer cell growth, but allows escape routes for the tumor to spread to remote sites (Samples et al. 2013). Metastasis involves the intravasation of the cancer cell into the blood or lymphatic vessels; thereafter, the cancer cell extravasates into a distant organ site (Klymkowsky and Savagner 2009). The disseminated cancer cell then undergoes a second transformation, a mesenchymal-epithelial transition (MET), reverting the cell back to more static cellular programs leading to basement membrane synthesis, a return of cell polarity and restoration of differentiated functions (Ahmad and Hart 1996). The cascade(s) leading to the timing, mechanisms, and tropism of metastasis are poorly understood (Hanahan and Weinberg 2011).

Invasion and metastasis are important (but very variable) themes in salivary gland tumor biology (Wang et al. 2017). Neoplasms like adenoid cystic carcinoma are not only locally invasive, but have a tropism for neural spread and a predisposition for late metastasis. Mucoepidermoid carcinoma tends to be locally invasive alone. Pathways leading to these invasion/metastatic phenotypic variations between salivary gland neoplasms are beginning to emerge (Huang et al. 2018). Like other cancers, matrix metalloproteinases appear to be an important event contributing to basement membrane destruction and invasion in a variety of salivary gland cancers (Nagel et al. 2004; Luukkaa et al. 2008, 2010a, 2010b; Yang et al. 2012). Transforming growth factor-β and E-cadherin alterations contribute to EMT in the early stages of salivary gland cancer invasion (Prabhu et al. 2009; Ghahhari et al. 2012; Jia et al. 2012; Sun et al. 2012; Dong et al. 2013; Zhao et al. 2013; Cao et al. 2018). Perineural invasion appears to be supported by nerve growth factor, brain-derived neurotropic factor, EMMPRIN, and tyrosine kinase A (Wang et al. 2006; Shang et al. 2007; Liu et al. 2012; Yang et al. 2012). The tyrosine kinase receptor pathway c-KIT and an associated factor SLUG appear to regulate important cellular phenotypes of the invasive cell (Jeng et al. 2000; Andreadis et al. 2006; El-Nagdy et al. 2013; Lee et al. 2012; Liu et al. 2012; Yin and Ha 2016). Ultimately, the salivary gland cancer cell is allowed to escape via vascular channels induced by factors such as VEGF (Jia et al. 2012). Lastly, N-cadherin appears to be an important extracellular molecule contributing to both perineural invasion and metastasis (Jia et al. 2012). Factors inhibiting invasion and metastasis, such as maspin and MCM2, are also suppressed during salivary gland carcinogenesis (Martins et al. 2005; Ghazy et al. 2011).

NUCLEIC ACID DYSREGULATION IN SALIVARY GLAND NEOPLASMS

Thus far, the genesis of salivary gland neoplastic cellular behavior has been presented in terms of aberrant protein function. Enhanced proliferation, apoptosis evasion, immortalization, angiogenesis, and invasion/metastasis have been explained by upregulated proteins, absent inhibitory protein function, and altered function (such as constituent activation and dominant-negative sequestration). These changes occur at the cell surface, the cytoplasm, and the nucleus. Behind the alteration of these regulatory proteins are often important aberrant nucleic acid activities. Both major and subtle changes in the structure of chromosomal DNA can lead to important changes in these regulatory proteins. Furthermore, epigenetic activity can also result in perturbations in gene expression (or mRNA levels) that can also disrupt these important regulatory pathways.

Genetic Alterations in Salivary Gland Tumors

Abrogation of key cellular regulatory pathways often begins with altered gene activity encoding factor[s] that govern those pathways. Genes are coding regions within the cell's chromosomal DNA (Todd et al. 2000). Structurally, genes are composed of promoter/enhancer regions (that control the timing and amount of gene activity), introns and exons (that carry the protein code separated by "spacers"), and a termination codon (that stops transcription) (Kim et al. 2002b). Chromosomal DNA is composed of protein (principally histone proteins) and four nucleic acids (adenine, thymine, guanine, and cytosine) (Todd et al. 2000; Kim et al. 2002a). The integrity of these regions is closely protected by structural and chemical elements (Chao and Lipkin 2006). Neoplastic cells suffer from genomic instability and errors in DNA repair that can lead to up- or downregulation of genetic activity, as well as alterations of the genetic code (Abbas et al. 2013). Many tumor phenotypes support the generation of genetic errors: enhanced proliferation increases the rate of genetic errors; evasion of apoptosis protects cells harboring mutations from being eliminated; and immortalization allows genetic errors to be inherited for a longer period of time. Cancer itself is considered a genetic disease resulting from an accumulation of mutations that occur in a preferred but not absolute order (Vogelstein and Kinzler 1998). These genomic alterations occur at vastly different scales, from whole chromosomes to a single nucleotide.

Important genome guardian pathways are altered in salivary gland tumors. The MDM2-p14^{ARF}-p53 regulatory pathway functions to protect the genome from environmental mutagens, such as radiation and various chemical agents. This pathway has been found to be altered in salivary gland carcinoma (Jin et al. 2012; Kang et al. 2017). In fact, it has been suggested that p53 mutation may be an important early event in the transition from benign to malignant salivary gland disease (Ohki et al. 2001). Other mismatch repair systems, such as hMSH1/2, have not been found to be important to salivary gland tumor progression (Ohki et al. 2001; Castrilli et al. 2002).

Some genetic alterations are so large that they can be observed directly under a microscope. Many tumor cells have an abnormal chromosome number (aneuploidy). Other damage involves large chromosomal regions. Translocation results in two chromosomes swapping DNA regions (Todd and Munger 2003). If these breaks occur near a gene promoter, a quantitative alteration of gene expression can result. If the break occurs in a coding region, a protein with altered function might be generated. Gene amplification occurs when DNA region is duplicated multiple times, often 50–100 fold (Todd and Munger 2003). Chromosomal deletion results in the complete loss of genetic material (Todd and Munger 2003). The loss of several key regulatory proteins has been associated with deletion of one or both gene copies.

Large-scale chromosomal alterations occur both in benign and malignant salivary gland tumors (Giefing et al. 2008; Gouveris et al. 2011; Escalente et al. 2016). As in hematologic malignancies and sarcomas, several chromosomal translocations have been observed in salivary gland tumors, some appearing to be tumor-specific (Stenman 2005; Bhaijee et al. 2011). A fusion protein of the MYB oncogene and NFIB transcription factor through a translocation between chromosomes 6 and 9 (t[6;9] [q22–23;pq23–24]) (Brill et al. 2011; Yin and Ha 2016) (Figure 9.5). Approximately 80% of adenoid cystic carcinomas share the MYB-NFIB gene fusion oncoprotein (Persson et al. 2009; Dillon et al. 2016; Wysocki et al. 2016). The fusion product results in an overactive MYB fusion protein that targets genes

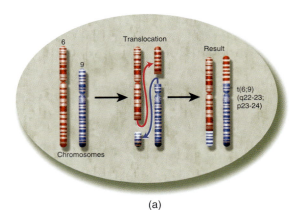

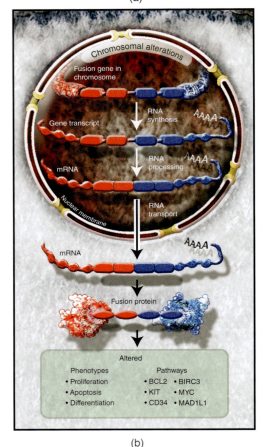

Figure 9.5. How chromosomal alterations lead to phenotypes in salivary gland tumors: The MYB-NFIB gene fusion is a molecular hallmark of adenoid cystic carcinoma. (a) A translocation of genetic material occurs between chromosomes 6 and 9 (t[6;9][q22–23;p23–24]). (b) The fusion of genetic material leads to a modification of both genes. This fused gene is then transcribed into modified mRNA that is later translated into a highly overexpressed fusion protein that leads to the deregulation of several signal pathways involved in cell proliferation, apoptosis, and differentiation, including BCL2, KIT, CD34 BIRC3, MYC, and MAD1L1.

involved in apoptosis, cell cycle regulation and cell adhesion in adenoid cystic carcinoma (Liu et al. 2012; Wysocki et al. 2016). The translocation between chromosomes 11 and 19 (t[11;19][q21–22;p13]) results in the CRTC1/MAML2 fusion gene frequently observed in mucoepidermoid carcinoma (Adelstein et al. 2012; Lin et al. 2018). The fusion oncoprotein replaces the NOTCH binding domain of MAML2 with the CREB-binding domain of CRTC1, creating a mutant transcription factor that activates several growth promoting signal pathways. Tumors harboring this translocation tend to be less aggressive (Behboudi et al. 2006; Adelstein et al. 2012). Gene fusion between PLAG1 and CTNNB1 appears to be specific for pleomorphic adenoma (t[3;8][p21;q12]) (Matsuyama et al. 2011; Stenman 2013; Escalente et al. 2016; El Hallani et al. 2018). This translocation results in β-catenin promoter swapping, thereby deregulating PLAG-1 target genes via the IGF2/IGF1R mitogenic pathway (Declercq et al. 2008). Lastly, mammary analog secretory carcinoma of the salivary glands harbors the ETV6-NTRK3 gene fusion (t[12;15][p13;q25]) (Skalova et al. 2010). ETV6-NTRK3-induced transformation appears to be mediated through the IGF1R pathway (Fehr et al. 2011). Currently, almost 400 gene fusions have been identified in about 20% of human cancers (Bell and Hanna 2012).

Other large-scale chromosomal alterations include gene amplification and deletions. Several genes are amplified in salivary gland tumors. MET, an important gene for invasion and metastasis, is amplified in salivary gland carcinomas and has been found as a predictor of poor prognosis (Ach et al. 2013; Bell et al. 2014; Gutschenritter et al. 2017). The HER-2/NEU gene amplification has been associated with high-grade transformation in several salivary gland carcinoma, including acinic cell carcinoma, adenoid cystic carcinoma, myoepithelial carcinoma, salivary duct carcinoma, and mucoepidermoid carcinoma (Glisson et al. 2004; Cornolti et al. 2007; Hashimoto et al. 2012; Nagao 2013). In a subset of adenoid cystic carcinoma, the c-KIT oncogene is amplified in a sucentromeric region of chromosome 4q (Rao et al. 2008; Yin and Ha 2016). Adenoid cystic carcinoma can also harbor several gene amplifications, including ERB-B1, CCND1, and PIK3CA (Sequeiros-Santiago et al. 2009). Amplification patters of these oncogenes have clinicopathologic correlations: CCND1 (advanced tumor stage); ERBB1 (distant metastasis); ERTT1/CCND1/

PIK3CA (reduced survival) (Sequeiros-Santiago et al. 2009; Santana et al. 2019). Amplification of the HER2, MDM2, and HMGA2 genes are believed to be important in the malignant transformation of pleomorphic adenoma (Carlson et al. 2013). Several chromosomal deletions have been associated with salivary gland tumors. Activity of the tumor suppressor gene PTEN is reduced due to a chromosomal deletion (often in association with amplification of the EGFR and HER2 genes) (Ettl et al. 2012a; Saintigny et al. 2018). Deletion of a portion of the short arm of chromosome 1 (1p32–p36) is one of the most frequent genomic alterations in adenoid cystic carcinoma, though which gene at this locus is important for disease progression is unclear (Rao et al. 2008). Furthermore, a loss of genetic material at the end of chromosome 6q is frequently combined with a reciprocal translocation between chromosome 6q and chromosome 9p (or some other chromosome) in adenoid cystic carcinoma (El-Naggar et al. 1999). The deleted portion of chromosome 6q is believed to harbor a tumor suppressor gene. The combination of an activated oncogene and inhibition of a tumor suppressor supports the hypothesis of a multistep accumulation of genetic alterations during tumorigenesis.

Small-scale changes in the nucleotide sequence of DNA can have profound changes to the proteins they encode (Arana and Kunkel 2010; Kim and Mirkin 2013). Single nucleotide changes are referred to as point mutations (Kim et al. 2002a). These changes can result in the alteration of a protein structure/function (missense mutation) or failure to the protein to synthesize (nonsense mutation). Furthermore, addition or subtraction of nucleotide(s) leads to frame shift mutations, which can alter how an entire protein is translated (Kim et al. 2002a). Point mutations in a number of regions of c-KIT have led to overactivity in adenoid cystic carcinoma (Vila et al. 2009). In animal and human studies, altered function of p53 has been attributed, in part, to point mutations that cause mutated p53 to sequester and inactivate wild type p53 (Papadaki et al. 1996; Turgut et al. 2006; Jiang et al. 2015). Activating point mutations in the RAS oncogene have been found in benign and malignant salivary gland tumors, including pleomorphic adenoma, carcinoma ex pleomorphic adenoma, adenocarcinoma, and mucoepidermoid carcinoma (Milasin et al. 1993; Okutsu et al. 1993; Yoo and Robinson 2000; Schneider et al. 2016; Yue et al. 2017).

Epigenetic Alteration of Gene Expression in Salivary Gland Tumors

While large- and small-scale structural alterations and lead to gene expression changes (as well as quantitative and/or qualitative gene product alterations), nonstructural regulatory mechanisms can be abrogated in salivary gland tumorigenesis. Gene expression is, in part, regulated by conformational changes in the DNA. Acetylation of the histone proteins in the chromosomal DNA can lead to the activation or suppression of gene expression (Verdone et al. 2005). Addition or removal of methyl groups within the gene promoter can also activate or suppress gene activity (Baylin 2005). Furthermore, mRNA already transcribed can be further regulated. For example, micro RNAs, usually 22 nucleotides in length, can sequester mRNA, thereby blocking translation and promoting degradation (Bora et al. 2012).

Methylation/demethylation of a gene promoter can activate or suppress gene activity. Therefore, aberrant promoter methylation can lead to overexpressed oncogenes or inactivation of tumor suppressor genes without an alteration in the genetic code (Kishi et al. 2005; Williams et al. 2006; Yin and Ha 2016). In the case of tumor suppressor genes, one gene may be structurally altered while the other suffers an alteration in the methylation status of its promoter. For example, in salivary gland carcinoma, $p16^{INK4a}$ and $p14^{ARF}$ often suffer a deletion in one gene copy and hypermethylation of the promoter in the other (Suzuki and Fujioka 1998; Nishimine et al. 2003; Li et al. 2005; Guo et al. 2007; Ochal-Choińska and Osuch-Wójcikiewicz 2016). Over 40 genes, including MYB, E-cadherin, suprabasin, PTEN, have been shown to be up- or down regulated during salivary gland tumorigenesis based on promoter methylation (Zhang et al. 2007; Lee et al. 2008; Fan et al. 2010; Bell et al. 2011; Shao et al. 2011a; Shao et al. 2012). Though there is a great deal of heterogeneity in promoter methylation, the methylation status of several genes has been correlated with several clinical observations, including transformation of benign to malignant, diagnosis of specific tumors, local/perineural invasion, and metastatic spread (Williams et al. 2006; Lee et al. 2008; Durr et al. 2010; Fan et al. 2010; Schache et al. 2010; Hu et al. 2011; Shao et al. 2011b; Shao et al. 2012; Dos Santos et al. 2019; Xu et al. 2019). Large-scale or high throughput gene expression analysis can uncover pathways/pathway elements leading to certain tumor phenotypes. For example, the overexpression of SOX-4, the most significantly overexpressed oncogene in adenoid cystic carcinoma, likely contributes to malignant progression by downregulating NFκB inhibitors (such as IκB) and upregulating apoptosis inhibitors (such as survivin) (Pramoonjago et al. 2006).

Recently, altered post-transcriptional activity in salivary gland tumors has been shown to result from changes in long noncoding RNAs (lnc-RNAs) and micro-RNAs. Exceeding 200 nucleotides in length, lnc-RNAs do not translate into a protein but regulate genes by interfering with mRNA translation (Liu et al. 2019). For example, upregulation of lncRNA ADAMTS9-AS2 promotes adenoid cystic carcinoma metastasis by interfering with microRNAs that inhibit the PI3K/Akt and MEK/Erk signaling pathways (Xie et al. 2018). MicroRNAs are small (~22 nucleotides) noncoding RNAs that also bind mRNA and lead to degradation and/or translation inhibition (Denaro et al. 2019). Certain profiles of microRNAs may provide a means of differentiating salivary gland tumors (Cinpolat et al. 2017). MicroRNA signatures have also been associated with a number of clinical characteristics in salivary gland tumors, including growth and invasion, cell cycle deregulation, and aggressiveness/poor outcome (Zhang et al. 2009a; He et al. 2013; Liu et al. 2013; Mitani et al. 2013; Shin et al. 2013; Boštjančič et al. 2017). Recently, evidence that mutations in SPEN, an RNA binding protein, contributes to transcriptional reprogramming in adenoid cystic carcinoma has been demonstrated (Frierson and Moskaluk 2013).

Summary and Clinical Applications

Our understanding of the molecular determinants governing salivary gland neoplasia is very preliminary. Salivary gland tumors are uncommon lesions that are composed of over 30 different pathologic entities, many with several subtypes according to the fourth edition of the World Health Organization Histological Classification of Salivary Gland Tumors in 2017 (Seethala and Stenman 2017). Furthermore, within each lesion, there is a vast histologic heterogeneity with each "normal" and neoplastic cell type contributing to disease progression. Chromosomal large-scale (translocations, amplifications, deletions) and small-scale (point mutations) alterations, as well as epigenetic changes (such as methylation changes in gene promoters) lead to quantitative and qualitative changes in gene expression. These alterations in gene expression result in important changes in the quantity and/or activity of important regulatory proteins. These proteins, extracellular ligands, receptors, secondary messengers, and transcription factors, serve in a network of signal transduction pathways that control critical cellular functions such as proliferation, apoptosis, senescence/differentiation, angiogenesis, and invasion/metastasis. The abrogation of these regulatory pathways is not completely understood for any salivary gland tumor. However, with the data available, translation of these benchtop findings into the clinical setting has begun.

DIAGNOSTIC APPLICATIONS

At present, diagnosis of salivary gland tumors involves physical examination, imaging and fine needle aspiration cytology (FNAC) (Carlson et al. 2013; Griffith et al. 2017). The sensitivity of FNAC of benign and malignant salivary neoplasms ranges from 73 to 86%, whereas the specificity is 97% for benign tumors and 85% for malignant tumors (Schindler et al. 2001; Carlson et al. 2013; Turk and Wenig 2014; Tyagi and Dey 2015). When possible, immunohistochemistry can further refine the diagnosis (Nagao et al. 2012). While treatment of salivary gland neoplasms almost always involves surgical excision, an accurate preoperative diagnosis will aid therapeutic planning (Schindler et al. 2001). At present, primary clinicopathologic parameters (such as patient age, histiotyping, grade, and disease stage) guide treatment (Vander Poorten et al. 2012). There is often a poor correlation between tumor histology and biological aggressiveness (Leivo 2006). Along with histiotyping, optical grading and clinical staging are currently the primary determinants in treatment planning (Vander Poorten et al. 2012). Low-grade/low-stage tumors are treated with excision alone while high-grade/high-stage tumors may include neck dissection and radiation/chemoradiation (Bell and Hanna 2012). However, grading schemes have a great deal of variability and poor reproducibility, leading to difficulties in treatment planning and determination of patient prognosis (Seethala 2011). Therefore, exploiting molecular biomarkers of neoplastic progression promises a more personalized management.

Advances in diagnostic methods promise a better understanding of the disease (Pusztaszeri and Faquin 2015; Seethala and Griffith 2016) (Figure 9.6a). Molecular markers not only target FNAC and open biopsy samples, but other specimens such as blood/serum and saliva. Furthermore, not only is the gene product a potential marker, but DNA and mRNA as well (Sidranski 2002; Yoshizawa et al. 2013). DNA, a stable and easily detectable molecule, only contributes to neoplastic phenotypes if a gene is active. Today, several robust single and high throughput analyses exist to identify tumor-associated DNA alterations (Liu et al. 2012; Watson et al. 2013). While lacking the stability of DNA, mRNA is a direct reflection of gene activity. Analytic techniques are available allow for detection of mRNA in small quantities, as well as high throughput detection of gene expression signatures (Golub et al. 1999; Buckhaults 2006). In addition to immunohistochemistry, novel proteomic approaches allow identification of protein targets in multiple samples, as well as multiple modifications of the same protein target (Donadio et al. 2013; Ellis et al. 2013; Paiva-Fonseca et al. 2013). DNA, mRNA, and protein biomarkers can target either the result of a signal transduction network, such as the tumor phenotypes of enhanced proliferation (Ki-67 immunostaining), apoptosis (TUNEL assay), or immortalization (hTERT assay) or the specific elements of those pathways (growth factors/receptors, secondary messengers, transcription factors) (Ben-Izhak et al. 2007; Ben-Izhak et al. 2008; Bussari et al. 2018) (Figure 9.6b). While the use of individual pathway elements as biomarkers is self-evident, molecules indicating the result of a signaling network may be a direct or indirect byproduct of that pathway. For example, enhanced proliferation is a phenotype regulated by several separate pathways. Ki-67, an antiapoptotic protein, is present in the G1, S, and G2 phases of the cell cycle; therefore, counting the number of cells that stain positive for Ki-67 is an indicator of how rapidly a tumor is proliferating (Murakami et al. 1992). To date, Ki-67 may be the most important supplement to optical grading as a prognostic indicator for adenoid cystic carcinoma, acinic cell carcinoma, mucoepidermoid carcinoma, and salivary duct carcinoma (Vander Poorten et al. 2012). These biologically based markers promise earlier diagnosis, more precise disease stratification, more accurate prediction of disease response (and selection of alternative treatment), more sensitive disease monitoring, ability of predict/mitigate treatment side effects, and prevention of disease recurrence (Sidranski 2002, Fonseca et al. 2016).

While the immunohistochemical detection of protein targets is aiding diagnosis and classification of salivary gland tumor today, molecular alterations identified using fluorescent in situ hybridization, reverse transcriptase- polymerase chain reaction, and next generation sequencing are emerging as a means to more precisely define these neoplasms (Escalante et al. 2016; Fonseca et al. 2016; Skalova et al. 2018). Given the prominence of chromosomal translocations in salivary gland tumorigenesis, the resultant gene fusions serve as an attractive biomarker (Andersson and Stenman 2016). The MYB-NFIB fusion tends to appear exclusively in adenoid cystic carcinoma while the majority of mucoepidermoid carcinoma is associated with the CRTC1-MAML2 translocation (Behboudi et al. 2006; Persson et al. 2009). In fact, mucoepidermoid carcinoma harboring the CRTC1-MAML2 translocation show a significantly better survival rate (Behboudi et al. 2006; Escalante et al. 2016). Over 90% of mammary analog secretory carcinomas contain the ETV6-NTRK3 gene fusion (Skalova et al. 2010; Fehr et al. 2011). Interestingly, carcinoma ex pleomorphic adenomas contain translocations containing either PLAG1 or HMGA2, but pleomorphic adenomas do not (Persson et al. 2009). Gene amplifications have also been tested as biomarkers. Amplifications of ERBB1, CCND1, and PIK3CA in adenoid cystic carcinoma indicate reduced survival (Sequeiros-Santiago et al. 2009). HER2/NEU amplification may be an efficacy predictor for salivary gland tumors treated with lapatinib, as well as a marker for carcinoma ex pleomorphic adenoma (versus pleomorphic adenoma) (Vidal et al. 2009; Hashimoto et al. 2012). Chromosomal deletions are also being explored as biomarkers. Deletion of 1p32–p36, the most frequent genetic change in adenoid cystic carcinoma, may be an indicator of poor prognosis (Rao et al. 2008). Deletion mutations in exon 19 of EGFR appear to indicate improved clinical response when treated with the tyrosine kinase inhibitors gefitinib and erlotinib (Dahse and Kosmehl 2008). Deletion in the CDKN2A gene, combined with the MECT1-MAML2 fusion gene, indicates poor prognosis in mucoepidermoid carcinoma patients, suggesting an important step in tumorigenesis (Anzick et al. 2010).

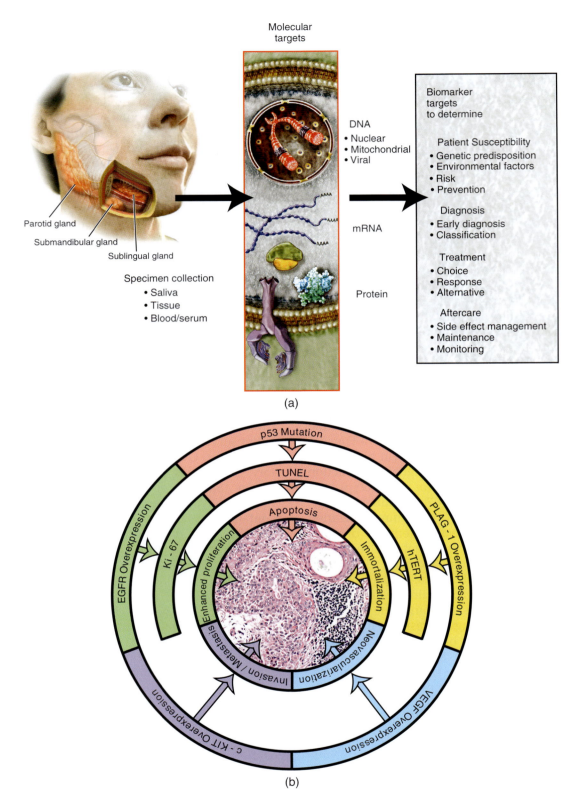

Figure 9.6. How can biomarkers aid in salivary gland tumor diagnosis? Biomarkers of neoplasia are already being explored to augment the current diagnostic workup of salivary gland tumor patients. (a) In addition to utilizing biopsy and fine needle aspiration samples, investigators are testing biomarker availability in saliva and the bloodstream. Diagnostic targets may be DNA, RNA, or proteins. The purpose of these targets would be to better understand patient risk/predisposition, identify/classify disease earlier, guide treatment choice, and improve patient monitoring. (b) Tumor biomarkers can target specific neoplastic phenotypes (outer circle) or individual molecular events (inner circle).

Deletion of the long arm of chromosome 6 is a consistent finding in adenoid cystic carcinoma (Bell and Hanna 2012).

Epigenetic alterations of gene expression have also been explored as a biomarker. Benign and malignant as well as high-grade versus low-grade tumors show distinct methylation patterns (Williams et al. 2006; Dos Santos et al. 2019). Promoter methylation of p16 correlates with the malignant transformation of pleomorphic adenoma (Schache et al. 2010; Hu et al. 2011). Hypermethylation of EN1 appears to be specific early event in adenoid cystic carcinoma development (Bell et al. 2011). The hypomethylated suprabasin gene in adenoid cystic carcinoma is associated with metastasis (Shao et al. 2012). Lastly, emerging studies support marker panels, rather than single biomarkers. Identification of multiple genetic changes, as well as alterations of gene expression and protein, has been explored as biomarkers to help direct patient treatment (Ettl et al. 2012b; Nardi et al. 2013).

DNA, mRNA, and protein biomarkers, alone and in combination, are being explored to aid in identifying clinically relevant salivary tumor phenotypes. First, as alluded to earlier, molecularly based markers are being used to identify malignant transformation (Schneider et al. 2014; Hellquist et al. 2019). Expression of hTERT/EGFR, MSF, and VEGF, as well as polymorphisms in MDM2 and p14^{ARF}, has been correlated with malignant transformation (Aljorani et al. 2011; de Faria et al. 2011; Shigeishi et al. 2011; Jin et al. 2012). Both c-KIT and SLUG expression correlates with invasion (and metastasis) of adenoid cystic carcinoma (Tang et al. 2010; Wong et al. 2016). Biomarkers have been identified demarking the malignant transformation of benign tumors. Mena (actin regulatory protein) expression is upregulated in salivary gland carcinomas but absent in normal and benign neoplastic salivary gland tissue (Gurzu et al. 2012). In addition to the studies cited above separating pleomorphic adenoma from carcinoma ex pleomorphic adenoma, aberrant expression of p53, BCL-2, and EGFR has been found to useful in distinguishing salivary basal cell adenoma from adenocarcinoma (Nagao et al. 1998).

Second, biomarkers are being used to differentiate tumors (as well as subclassify histologically similar tumors) (Donadio et al. 2013; Paiva-Fonseca et al. 2013). Given the heterogeneous (as well as overlapping) histology of salivary gland tumors and often limited tissue specimen for diagnosis, biomarkers not only might identify malignant tissue, but be able to discriminate between histologically similar salivary gland tumors and tumors from remote anatomic sites. Immunohistochemical detection of p63 can differentiate between salivary gland oncocytoma and oncocytic carcinoma from metastatic renal cell carcinoma (McHugh et al. 2007). Gene expression and immunohistochemical panels have been identified separating pleomorphic adenoma and adenoid cystic carcinoma from other salivary gland tumors, as well as histological overlap of adenoid cystic carcinoma from polymorphous adenocarcinoma (Skalovaa and Leivo 1996; Maruya et al. 2004; El-Nagdy et al. 2013). Expression signatures of microRNAs can differentiate salivary gland tumors (Denaro et al. 2019). The oncogene c-KIT is found in 100% of myoepithelial carcinomas (and lymphoepithelial carcinomas) and 80–94% of adenoid cystic carcinomas (Jeng et al. 2000; Mino et al. 2003). Lastly, p63 expression might be helpful in separating acinic cell carcinoma from mucoepidermoid carcinoma (Sams and Gnepp 2013).

Third, biomarkers are being explored as patient management guideposts (Escalante et al. 2016; Yin and Ha 2016; Lin et al. 2018). Several studies have correlated specific biomarkers with aggressive behavior and invasive phenotypes. For example, NCAM has been implicated in perineural invasion (Shang et al. 2007; Kehagias et al. 2013). In adenoid cystic carcinoma and mucoepidermoid carcinoma, mutant p53, VEGF, aniopoietins, and c-KIT/SLUG expression has been associated with aggressive/invasive growth and metastasis (Papadaki et al. 1996; Tang et al. 2010; Demasi et al. 2012). Various marker/marker panels have been explored as prognostic indicators: PTEN loss/EGFR/HER2 overexpression; BCL-2/p53/Ki-67; MMP-1/7/9/13; EBFR/p53/E-cadherin (mucoepidermoid carcinoma); and 1p32-p36 deletion (adenoid cystic carcinoma) (Yin et al. 2000; Nagler et al. 2003; Hoyek-Gebeily et al. 2007; Luukkaa et al. 2008, 2010a; Rao et al. 2008; Ettl et al. 2012a; Stenner et al. 2012). Deregulation of p16 and p53 pathways has been implicated with recurrence (Vekony et al. 2008; Byrd et al. 2013). Survival has been correlated with several marker/marker panels: p27^{Kip1}, Ki-67/CRTC1-MAML2 (mucoepidermoid carcinoma); EGFR/HER2/survivin/ pSTAT3 loss; p53/Ki-67/TUNEL; MET/EGFR/PTEN loss; and ERBB1/CCND1/PIK3CA

(Ben-Izhak et al. 2007; Ben-Izhak et al. 2008; Miyabe et al. 2009; Sequeiros-Santiago et al. 2009; Stenner et al. 2011; Ettl et al. 2012a; Ach et al. 2013). Lastly, individual markers and marker panels are being studied to determine tumor-associated alterations that might direct current therapeutic protocols (Dahse and Kosmehl 2008; Vidal et al. 2009; Nardi et al. 2013).

THERAPEUTIC APPLICATIONS

While patient assessment might improve the efficacy of current treatment protocols, novel, biologically based treatment approaches can also be developed based on molecular defects leading to salivary gland tumorigenesis (Chandana and Conley 2008; Keller et al. 2017; Lassche et al. 2019). At present, surgical excision is the primary treatment of salivary gland tumors (Wang et al. 2015). Furthermore, radiation alone or in combination with chemotherapy may play an important role in local control administered either postoperatively or as definitive treatment (Carlson et al. 2013). However, for patients where obtaining a surgical margin is impossible, perineural spread is noted or locally advanced, recurrent, or metastatic spread is discovered, the present therapeutic options are limited and often palliative (Bell and Hanna 2012; Schvartsman et al. 2019). To date, several therapeutic strategies have been developed to exploit a better understanding of how tumors develop.

The goal of a biologically based therapeutic strategy is to tailor treatment to the specific molecular defects resulting in tumor behavior (Lassche et al. 2019) (Figure 9.7a). An additional benefit of this molecular approach is to limit side effects of treatment, though associated toxicities do exist (Dy and Adjei 2013). Targets of this designer therapy can be any member of the molecular paradigm: DNA, RNA, or protein. Many DNA-based strategies simply replace damaged genes with "normal" ones. Other strategies include activation of cancer cell-clearing immune response, enhancement of DNA repair enzyme activity, drug resistance gene inactivation, or enzymatic destruction of viral/oncogenic material (Kelley and Fishel 2008; Ortiz et al. 2012). Delivery approaches of these therapeutic genes include microorganisms (principally viruses) and nanocarrier methods (Mohit and Rafati 2013; Thakor and Gambhir 2013). Gene expression or mRNA can also serve as a target. Two major approaches are RNA interference or manipulation of gene expression through changes in methylation (Morris 2006; Gallinari et al. 2007). Lastly, the gene products (proteins) themselves can serve as targets. The two principle approaches employ either monoclonal antibodies or low-molecular weight proteins (Gibbs 2000; Sliwkowski and Mellman 2013). Molecular targets, used alone or in tandem, attack aberrant neoplastic cell behavior at the very defects responsible. Experimental and clinical strategies fall primarily into three broad categories: monoclonal antibodies, small molecule inhibitors, and RNA interference.

To date, many therapeutics targeting signal transduction pathways have demonstrated prolonged disease stabilization in Phase II trials but very few have shown objective responses (Wang et al. 2017). Studies using monoclonal antibodies to EGFR gene family members have been performed with limited success (Figure 9.7b). The EGFR (HER1/ErbB1) family of transmembrane tyrosine kinase receptors has been an attractive therapeutic target for tumors at a variety of anatomic sites. Therefore, several monoclonal antibodies to EGFR family members are available. Cetuximab showed disease stabilization in 12 of 23 adenoid cystic carcinoma patients for a median of six months but no objective responses (Goyal et al. 2015. Trastuzumab targets the HER-2/NEU receptor noted in a significant portion of breast cancers. A study of three mucoepidermoid carcinoma patients administered trastuzumab showed a partial response in one patient and stabilization of the disease in two others (Haddad et al. 2003). A larger study of adenoid cystic carcinoma patients treated with gefitinib (another ErbB1 monoclonal antibody) showed disease stabilization in 53% of patients that extended for 16 weeks in 26% (Vattemi et al. 2008). Thirty salivary gland cancer patients with either recurrent or metastatic disease were treated with cetuximab, another ErbB1 antibody, and, of the 23 who were available at three months, 11 showed stabilization of the disease (Vattemi et al. 2008). Monoclonal antibodies have also been used in combination with conventional chemotherapy (Kaidar-Person et al. 2012; Caballero et al. 2013). Lastly, MECT1-MAML2 fusion positive adenoid cystic carcinoma cancer cells showed reduced proliferation when treated with EGFR inhibitors (Escalante et al. 2016).

Small molecule inhibitors are promising therapeutic targets for salivary gland tumors. In the 1960s, the gene fusion BCR-ABL in chronic myeloid leukemia led to the first-line tyrosine kinase

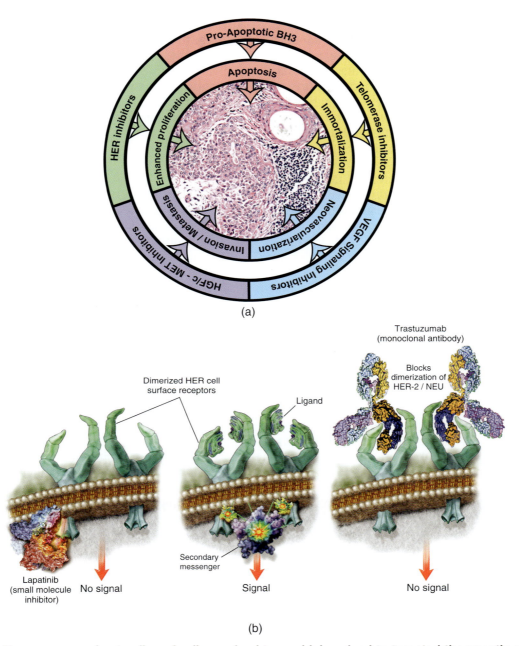

Figure 9.7. How can an understanding of salivary gland tumor biology lead to targeted therapeutic options? At present, several biologically based tumor therapies are under clinical trials. (a) The cellular phenotypes that salivary gland tumors share with other forms of neoplasia are potential targets. (b) The HER cell surface receptors are deregulated in several tumors, including salivary gland tumors. After binding a ligand, these receptors dimerize and activate secondary messengers which support cellular proliferation (middle). Aberrant activity of HER-1/EGFR secondary messaging can be blocked using the small molecule inhibitor lapatinib (left). Dimerization of HER-2/NEU can be blocked using the monoclonal antibody trastuzumab, thereby preventing any downstream signaling.

inhibitor dasatinib (Escalante et al. 2016). While salivary gland gene fusions currently lack small molecule inhibitor agents, several other molecular alterations have been targeted. A Phase II trial of dasatinib for recurrent or metastatic c-KIT positive adenoid cystic carcinoma patients was well tolerated, showed an objective response and disease stabilization (Wang et al. 2015). Lapatinib, an orally administered reversible inhibitor of ErbB1/2 tyrosine kinase activity, was tested in adenoid cystic carcinoma patients that showed expression of one or both receptors: of 14 patients, 9 had stable disease (Agulnik et al. 2007). The tyrosine kinase inhibitor imatinib mesylate, a potent blocker of c-KIT activity, was tested in two separate studies of adenoid cystic carcinoma patients; however, no objective response was noted in either study (Hotte et al. 2005; Pfeffer et al. 2007). As part of a greater study, the small molecule inhibitor of VEGF/c-KIT/PDGFR tyrosine kinase activity showed partial response in an adenoid cystic carcinoma patient after three treatment cycles (Rugo et al. 2005).

Currently, RNA interference (RNAi) targeting is in preclinical testing. In experimental models of mucoepidermoid carcinoma and adenoid cystic carcinoma, RNAi targeting the gene fusions MECT1-MAML2 and MYB-NFIB, as well as MAPK and EGFR, has shown promise in reversing important malignant phenotypes (Komiya et al. 2006; He et al. 2013; Liu et al. 2013; Stenman 2013). RNAi-mediated EMMPRIN silencing inhibited proliferation and perineural invasion of human adenoid cystic carcinoma cells in vitro and in vivo (Yang et al. 2012). In addition, RNAi blocking of lncRNA has shown promise in salivary gland tumor cells (Civenni 2017). While a powerful experimental tool, translation of RNAi from preclinical to clinical applications in salivary gland tumor patients remains untested (Crooke et al. 2018).

While not exhaustive, this survey reinforces themes discussed in this chapter that underlie the complexity of understanding, diagnosing, and treating salivary gland tumor patients. Clinical studies are undermined by the uncommon appearance and complex nature of these tumors; therefore, interpretation of clinical trials is hampered by small institutional series of extremely heterogeneous patient populations (Chau et al. 2012). Tumors with highly varied and complex composition with often protracted clinical courses render assessment of treatment response (versus prolonged tumor progression) difficult to assess (Goyal et al. 2015). Survival may be an impractical study endpoint due to the rare and often slow progression of these tumors. Change of tumor size has been proposed as a more sensitive, appropriate endpoint (Chau et al. 2012). Biologically based therapy necessitates that the study subjects carry the proper genetic defect. Furthermore, failure to respond may not be the result of conventional causes of treatment failure, such as improper dosing, but the failure to recognize the multiple genetic defects critical to address these tumors (Locati et al. 2009). Just as salivary gland tumorigenesis is a multistep accumulation of genetic errors, the successful treatment of salivary gland tumors will necessitate the identification and remedy of these critical genetic defects.

Summary

- Salivary gland tumors are complex, heterogeneous tumors.
- Neoplastic salivary gland cells share several phenotypic traits, including enhanced proliferation, evasion of apoptosis, immortalization, neovascularization, and invasion/metastasis.
- Traits of salivary gland neoplastic cells result from quantitatively or quantitatively altered signal transduction regulatory proteins. Regulatory factors include extracellular ligands, cell surface receptors, secondary messengers, and transcription factors.
- Signal transduction regulatory proteins can be altered genetically and epigenetically.
- Large-scale genetic changes include chromosomal translocations, amplifications, and deletions. Point mutations are an example of small-scale genetic changes. Large- and small-scale changes can lead to either up- or downregulation of gene expression or transcriptional errors leading to the production of proteins with altered functions.
- Epigenetic changes lead to transcriptional or post-transcriptional changes.
- The molecular alterations supporting salivary gland tumorigenesis are poorly understood. Defining universal and tumor-specific signal transduction pathway alterations will generate a fingerprint for each salivary gland tumor. These biomarkers will likely be panels of DNA, mRNA, and protein alterations. A precise understanding of the genetic makeup of individual tumors will allow personalized patient management.
- Advantages of personalized salivary gland diagnostic applications include better tumor diagnosis/classification, screening and risk assessment, identification of lifestyle modifications for risk reduction, and prognosis determination.

- Advantages of personalized salivary gland therapeutic applications include improved prediction of treatment efficacy/treatment planning, more precise dose modulations, stratification of patients for targeted therapy, better post-surgical follow-up for early detection of recurrent tumors.
- Improvements in specimen acquisition, high throughput analysis, and bioinformatics should help overcome many of the difficulties in understanding these rare, complex tumors.

References

Abbas T, Keaton MA, Dutta A. 2013. Genomic instability in cancer. *Cold Spring Harb Perspect Biol* 5:a012914.

Ach T, Zeitler K, Schwarz-Furlan S, et al. 2013. Aberrations of MET are associated with copy number gain of EGFR and loss of PTEN and predict poor outcome in patients with salivary gland cancer. *Virchows Arch* 462:65–72.

Adams A, Warner K, Nor JE. 2013. Salivary gland cancer tem cells. *Oral Oncol* 49:845–853.

Adams A, Warner K, Pearson AT, et al. 2015. ALDH/CD44 identifies uniquely tumorigenic cancer stem cells in salivary gland mucoepidermoid carcinomas. *Oncotarget* 6:26633–26650.

Adelstein DJ, Koyfman SA, El-Naggar AK, Hanna EY. 2012. Biology and management of salivary gland cancers. *Semin Radiat Oncol* 22:245–253.

Agulnik M, Cohen EW, Cohen RB, et al. 2007. Phase II study of lapatinib in recurrent or metastatic epidermal growth factor receptor and/or erbB2 expressing adenoid cystic carcinoma and non adenoid cystic carcinoma malignant tumors of the salivary glands. *J Clin Oncol* 25:3978–3984.

Ahmad, A. Hart IR. 1996. Biology of tumor micrometastasis. *J Hematother* 5:525–535.

Aljorani LE, Bankfalvi A, Carey FA, et al. 2011. Migration-stimulating factor as a novel biomarker in salivary gland tumours. *J Oral Pathol Med* 40:747–754.

Andersson MK, Stenman G. 2016. The landscape of gene fusions and somatic mutations in salivary gland neoplasms – Implications for diagnosis and therapy. *Oral Oncol* 57:63–69.

Anderson HJ, Pointdujour-Lim R, Shields CL. 2017. Treatments for retinoblastoma then and now. *JAMA Ophthalmol* 135:e164652.

Andisheh Tadbir A, Khademi B, Malekzadeh M, et al. 2013. Upregulation of serum vascular endothelial growth factor in patients with salivary gland tumor. *Patholog Res Int* 75:740582.

Andreadis D, Epivatianos A, Poulopoulos A, et al. 2006. Detection of C-KIT (CD117) molecule in benign and malignant salivary gland tumours. *Oral Oncol* 42:57–65.

Anzick SL, Chen WD, Park Y, et al. 2010. Unfavorable prognosis of CRTC1-MAML2 positive mucoepidermoid tumors with CDKN2A deletions. *Genes Chromosomes Cancer* 49:59–69.

Arana ME, Kunkel TA. 2010. Mutator phenotypes due to DNA replication infidelity. *Semin Cancer Biol* 20:304–311.

Auguste P, Lemiere S, Larrieu-Lahargue F, Bikfalvi A. 2005. Molecular mechanisms of tumor vascularization. *Crit Rev Oncol* 54:53–61.

Bansal K, Bindal R, Kapoor C, et al. 2012. Current concepts in diagnosis of unusual salivary gland tumors. *Dent Res J (Isfahan)* 9:S9–S19.

Batsakis JG, Regezi JA, Luna MA, El-Naggar A. 1989. Histogenesis of salivary gland neoplasms: A postulate with prognostic implications. *J Laryngol Otol* 103:939–944.

Baylin S. 2005. DNA methylation and gene silencing in cancer. *Nat Clin Pract Oncol* 2(Suppl 1):S4–S11.

Behboudi A, Enlund F, Winnes M, et al. 2006. Molecular classification of mucoepidermoid carcinomas-prognostic significance of the MECT1-MAML2 fusion oncogene. *Genes Chromosomes Cancer* 45:470–481.

Bell A, Bell D, Weber RS, El-Naggar AK 2011. CpG island methylation profiling in human salivary gland adenoid cystic carcinoma. *Cancer* 117:2898–2909.

Bell D, Hanna EY. 2012. Salivary gland cancers: Biology and molecular targets for therapy. *Curr Oncol Rep* 14:166–174.

Bell D, Hanna EY, Miele L, et al. 2014. Expression and significance of notch signaling pathway in salivary adenoid cystic carcinoma. *Ann Diagn Pathol* 18:10–13.

Bell D, Ferrarotto R, Fox MD, et al. 2015. Analysis and significance of c-MET expression in adenoid cystic carcinoma of the salivary gland. *Cancer Biol Ther* 16:834–838.

Ben-Izhak O, Akrish S, Nagler RM. 2008. Ki67 and salivary cancer. *Cancer Invest* 26:1015–1023.

Ben-Izhak O, Laster Z, Akrish S, et al. 2009. The salivary tip of the p53 mutagenesis iceberg: Novel insights. *Cancer Biomark* 5:23–31.

Ben-Izhak O, Laster Z, Araidy S, Nagler, RM. 2007. TUNEL – an efficient prognosis predictor of salivary malignancies. *Br J Cancer* 96:1101–1106.

Berx G, Van Roy F. 2009. Involvement of members of the cadherin superfamily in cancer. *Cold Spring Harb Perspect Biol* 1:a003129.

Bhaijee F, Pepper DJ, Pitman KT, Bell D. 2011. New developments in the molecular pathogenesis of head and neck tumors: A review of tumor-specific fusion oncogenes in mucoepidermoid carcinoma, adenoid cystic carcinoma, and NUT midline carcinoma. *Ann Diagn Pathol* 15:69–77.

Black PC, Dinney CP. 2008. Growth factors and receptors as prognostic markers in urothelial carcinoma. *Curr Urol Rep* 9:55–61.

Blanpain C. 2013. Tracing the cellular origin of cancer. *Nat Cell Biol* 15:126–134.

Błochowiak KJ, Sokalski J, Bodnar MB, et al. 2018.Expression of $VEGF_{165}b$, VEGFR1, VEGFR2 and CD34 in benign and malignant tumors of parotid glands. *Adv Clin Exp Med* 27:83–90.

Bora RS, Gupta D, Mukkur TK, Saini KS. 2012. RNA interference therapeutics for cancer: Challenges and opportunities. *Mol Med Rep* 6:9–15.

Boštjančič E, Hauptman N, Grošelj A, et al. 2017. Expression, mutation, and amplification status of EGFR and its correlation with five miRNAs in salivary gland tumours. *Biomed Res Inst* 2017:9150402.

Brill LB, 2nd, Kanner WA, Fehr A, et al. 2011. Analysis of MYB expression and MYB-NFIB gene fusions in adenoid cystic carcinoma and other salivary neoplasms. *Mod Pathol* 24:1169–76.

Brognard J, Hunter T. 2011. Protein kinase signalling networks in cancer. *Curr Opin Genet Dev* 21:4–11.

Buckhaults P. 2006. Gene expression determinants of clinical outcome. *Curr Opin Oncol* 18:57–61.

Bussari S, Ganvir SM, Sarode M, et al. 2018. Immunohistochemical detection of proliferative marker Ki-67 in benign and malignant salivary gland tumors. *Contemp Dent Pract* 19:375–383.

Byrd SA, Spector ME, Carey TE, et al. 2013. Predictors of recurrence and survival for head and neck mucoepidermoid carcinoma. *Otolaryngol Head Neck Surg* 149:402–408.

Caballero M, Tagliapietra A, Grau JJ. 2013. Metastatic adenoid cystic carcinoma of the salivary gland responding to cetuximab plus weekly paclitaxel after no response to weekly paclitaxel alone. *Head Neck* 35:E52–E54.

Can NT, Lingen MW, Mashek H, et al. 2018 Expression of hormone receptors and HER-2 in benign and malignant salivary gland tumors. *Head Neck Pathol* 12:95–104.

Cao Y, Liu H, Gao L, et al. 2018. Cooperation between Pten and Smad4 in murine salivary gland tumor formation and progression. *Neoplasia* 20:764–774.

Carlson J, Licitra L, Locati L, et al. 2013. Salivary gland cancer: An update on present and emerging therapies. *Am Soc Clin Oncol Educ Book* 33:257–263.

Castrilli G, Fabiano A, La Torre G, et al. 2002. Expression of hMSH2 and hMLH1 proteins of the human DNA mismatch repair system in salivary gland tumors. *J Oral Pathol Med* 31:234–238.

Catalano V, Turdo A, Di Franco S, et al. 2013. Tumor and its microenvironment: A synergistic interplay. *Semin Cancer Biol* 23:522–532.

Cavallaro U, Christofori G. 2004. Cell adhesion and signalling by cadherins and Ig-CAMs in cancer. *Nat Rev Cancer* 4:839–849.

Chandler H, Peters G. 2013. Stressing the cell cycle in senescence and aging. *Curr Opin Cell Biol* 25:765–771.

Chandana SR, Conley BA. 2008.Salivary gland cancers: Current treatments, molecular characteristics and new therapies. *Expert Rev Anticancer Ther* 8(4):645–652.

Chao E, Lipkin S. 2006. Molecular models for the tissue specificity of DNA mismatch repair-deficient carcinogenesis. *Nucleic Acids Res* 34:840–852.

Chau NG, Hotte SJ, Chen EX, et al. 2012. A phase II study of sunitinib in recurrent and/or metastatic adenoid cystic carcinoma (ACC) of the salivary glands: Current progress and challenges in evaluating molecularly targeted agents in ACC. *Ann Oncol* 23:1562–1570.

Cheuk W, Chan JK. 2007. Advances in salivary gland pathology. *Histopathology* 51:1–20.

Cinpolat O, Unal ZN, Ismi O, et al. 2017. Comparison of microRNA profiles between benign and malignant salivary gland tumors in tissue, blood and saliva samples: A prospective, case-control study. *Braz J Otorhinolaryngol* 83:276–284.

Civenni G. 2017. Targeting promoter-associated noncoding RNA in vivo;. *Methods Mol Biol* 1543:259–270.

Classon M, Harlow E. 2002. The retinoblastoma tumour suppresson in development and cancer. *Nat Rev Cancer* 2:910–917.

Comoglio P, Trusolino L. 2002. Invasive growth: From development to metastasis. *J Clin Invest* 109:857–862.

Cornolti G, Ungari M, Morassi ML, et al. 2007. Amplification and overexpression of HER2/neu gene and HER2/neu protein in salivary duct carcinoma of the parotid gland. *Arch Otolaryngol Head Neck Surg* 133:1031–1036.

Crooke ST, Witztum JL, Bennett CF, Baker BF. 2018. RNA-targeted therapeutics. *Cell Metab* 27:714–739.

Cros J, Sbidian E, Hans S, et al. 2013. Expression and mutational status of treatment-relevant targets and key oncogenes in 123 malignant salivary gland tumours. *Ann Oncol* 24:2624–2629.

Da Silva GM, Saavedra V, Ianez RCF, et al. 2019. Apoptotic signaling in salivary mucoepidermoid carcinoma. *Head Neck* 41:2904–2913.

Dahse R, Kosmehl H. 2008. Detection of drug-sensitizing EGFR exon 19 deletion mutations in salivary gland carcinoma. *Br J Cancer* 99:90–92.

Dardick I, Burford-Mason AP. 1993. Current status of histogenetic and morphogenetic concepts of salivary gland tumorigenesis. *Crit Rev Oral Biol Med* 4:639–677.

Dardick I, Jeans MT, Sinnott NM, et al. 1985. Salivary gland components involved in the formation of squamous metaplasia. *Am J Pathol* 119:33–43.

Dardick I, Van Nostrand AW, Phillips MJ. 1982. Histogenesis of salivary gland pleomorphic adenoma (mixed tumor) with an evaluation of the role of the myoepithelial cell. *Hum Pathol* 13:62–75.

De Faria PR, Lima RA, Dias FL, et al. 2011. Vascular endothelial growth factor and thymidine phosphorylase expression in salivary gland tumors with distinct metastatic behavior. *J Oral Pathol Med* 40:456–459.

Declercq J, Van Dyck F, Van Damme B, Van De Ven WJ. 2008. Upregulation of Igf and Wnt signalling associated genes in pleomorphic adenomas of the salivary glands in PLAG1 transgenic mice. *Int J Oncol* 32:1041–1047.

Deguchi H, Hamano H, Hayashi Y. 1993. c-myc, ras p21 and p53 expression in pleomorphic adenoma and its malignant form of the human salivary glands. *Acta Pathol Jpn* 43:413–422.

Demasi AP, Silva CA, Silva AD, et al. 2012. Expression of the vascular endothelial growth factor and angiopoietins in mucoepidermoid carcinoma of salivary gland. *Head Neck Pathol* 6:10–15.

Denaro M, Navari E, Ugolini C, et al. 2019. A microRNA signature for the differential diagnosis of salivary gland tumors. *PLoS One* 14(1):e0210968.

Diegel CR, Cho KR, El-Naggar AK, et al. 2010. Mammalian target of rapamycin-dependent acinar cell neoplasia after inactivation of Apc and Pten in the mouse salivary gland: Implications for human acinic cell carcinoma. *Cancer Res* 70:9143–9152.

Dietel M, Johrens K, Laffert M, et al. 2013. Predictive molecular pathology and its role in targeted cancer therapy: A review focussing on clinical relevance. *Cancer Gene Ther* 20:211–221.

Dillon PM, Chakraborty S, Moskaluk CA, et al. 2016. Adenoid cystic carcinoma: A review of recent advances, molecular targets, and clinical trials. *Head Neck* 38:620–627.

Donadio E, Giusti L, Seccia V, et al. 2013. New insight into benign tumours of major salivary glands by proteomic approach. *PLoS One* 8:e71874.

Dos Santos ES, Ramos JC, Normando AGC, et al. 2019. Epigenetic alterations in salivary gland tumors. *Oral Dis* 26(8):1610–1618.

Dong L, Ge XY, Wang YX, et al. 2013. Transforming growth factor-beta and epithelial-mesenchymal transition are associated with pulmonary metastasis in adenoid cystic carcinoma. *Oral Oncol* 49:1051–1058.

Durr ML, Mydlarz WK, Shao C, et al. 2010. Quantitative methylation profiles for multiple tumor suppressor gene promoters in salivary gland tumors. *PLoS One* 5:e10828.

Dy GK, Adjei AA. 2013. Understanding, recognizing, and managing toxicities of targeted anticancer therapies. *CA Cancer J Clin* 63:249–279.

Dyson N. 1998. The regulation of E2F by pRB-family proteins. *Genes Dev* 12:2245–2262.

El Hallani S, Udager AM, Bell D, et al. 2018. Epithelial-myoepithelial carcinoma: Frequent morphologic and molecular evidence of preexisting pleomorphic adenoma, common HRAS mutations in PLAG1-intact and HMGA2-intact cases, and occasional TP53, FBXW7, and SMARCB1 alterations in high-grade cases. *Am J Surg Pathol* 42:18–27.

El-Nagdy S, Salama NM, Mourad MI. 2013. Immunohistochemical clue for the histological overlap of salivary adenoid cystic carcinoma and polymorphous low-grade adenocarcinoma. *Interv Med Appl Sci* 5:131–139.

El-Naggar AK, Dinh M, Tucker SL, et al. 1999. Numerical chromosomal changes in DNA hypodiploid solid tumors: Restricted loss and gain of certain chromosomes. *Cytometry* 37:107–112.

Ellis MJ, Gillette M, Carr SA, et al. 2013. Connecting genomic alterations to cancer biology with proteomics: The NCI clinical proteomic tumor analysis consortium. *Cancer Discov* 3:1108–1112.

Emmerson E, Knox SM. 2018. Salivary gland stem cells: A review of development, regeneration and cancer. *Genesis* 56:e23211.

Escalante DA, Wang H, Fundakowski CE 2016. Fusion proteins in head and neck neoplasms: Clinical implications, genetics, and future directions for targeting *Cancer Biol Ther* 17:995–1002.

Etges A, Nunes FD, Ribeiro KC, Araujo VC. 2004. Immunohistochemical expression of retinoblastoma pathway proteins in normal salivary glands and in salivary gland tumours. *Oral Oncol* 40:326–31.

Ettl T, Baader K, Stiegler C, et al. 2012a. Loss of PTEN is associated with elevated EGFR and HER2 expression and worse prognosis in salivary gland cancer. *Br J Cancer* 106:719–726.

Ettl T, Stiegler C, Zeitler K, et al. 2012b. EGFR, HER2, survivin, and loss of pSTAT3 characterize high-grade malignancy in salivary gland cancer with impact on prognosis. *Hum Pathol* 43:921–931.

Fadeel B, Orrenius S. 2005. Apoptosis: A basic biological phenomenon with wide-ranging implications in human disease. *J Int Med* 258:479–517.

Fan X, Chen B, Xu J, et al. 2010. Methylation status of the PTEN gene in adenoid cystic carcinoma cells. *Mol Med Rep* 3:775–779.

Faur AC, Sas I, Motoc AG, et al. 2015. Ki-67 and p53 immunostaining assessment of proliferative activity in salivary tumors. *J Morphol Embryol* 56:1429–1439.

Fehr A, Loning T, Stenman G. 2011. Mammary analogue secretory carcinoma of the salivary glands with ETV6-NTRK3 gene fusion. *Am J Surg Pathol* 35:1600–1602.

Felix A, El-Naggar AK, Press MF, et al. 1996. Prognostic significance of biomarkers (c-erbB-2, p53, proliferating cell nuclear antigen, and DNA content) in salivary duct carcinoma. *Hum Pathol* 27:561–566.

Flores BC, Lourenço SV, Damascena AS, et al. 2017. Altered expression of apoptosis-regulating miRNAs in salivary gland tumors suggests their involvement in salivary gland tumorigenesis. *Virchows Arch* 470:291–299.

Folkman J. 2006. Angiogenesis. *Annu Rev Med* 57:1–18.

Fonseca FP, Sena Filho M, Altemani A, et al. 2016. Molecular signature of salivary gland tumors: Potential use as diagnostic and prognostic marker. *J Oral Pathol Med* 45:101–110.

Frierson HF, Jr, El-Naggar AK., Welsh JB, et al. 2002. Large scale molecular analysis identifies genes with altered expression in salivary adenoid cystic carcinoma *Am J Pathol* 161:1315–1323.

Frierson HF, Jr, Moskaluk CA. 2013. Mutation signature of adenoid cystic carcinoma: Evidence for transcriptional and epigenetic reprogramming. *J Clin Invest* 123:2783–2785.

Gallinari P, Di Marco S, Jones P, et al. 2007. HDACs, histone deacetylation and gene transcription: From molecular biology to cancer therapeutics. *Cell Res* 17: 195–211.

Ghahhari NM, Ghahhari HM, Kadivar M. 2012. Could a possible crosstalk between AMPK and TGF-beta signaling pathways be a key player in benign and malignant salivary gland tumors? *Onkologie* 35:770–774.

Ghazy SE, Helmy IM, Baghdadi HM. 2011. Maspin and MCM2 immunoprofiling in salivary gland carcinomas. *Diagn Pathol* 6:89.

Gibbons MD, Manne U, Carroll WR, et al. 2001. Molecular differences in mucoepidermoid carcinoma and adenoid cystic carcinoma of the major salivary glands. *Laryngoscope* 111:1373–1378.

Gibbs J. 2000. Mechanism-based target identification and drug discovery in cancer research. *Science* 287:1969–1973.

Giefing M, Wierzbicka M, Rydzanicz, M, et al. 2008. Chromosomal gains and losses indicate oncogene and tumor suppressor gene candidates in salivary gland tumors. *Neoplasma* 55:55–60.

Gimbrone MJ, Leapman S, Cotran R. 1972. Tumor dormancy in vivo; by prevention of neovascularization. *J Exp Med* 136:261–276.

Glisson B, Colevas AD, Haddad R, et al. 2004. HER2 expression in salivary gland carcinomas: Dependence on histological subtype. *Clin Cancer Res* 10:944–6.

Golub T, Slonim D, Tamayo P, et al. 1999. Molecular classification of cancer: Class discovery and class prediction by gene expression monitoring. *Science* 286:531–537.

Golubovskaya VM. Cance WG. 2013. Targeting the p53 pathway. *Surg Oncol Clin N Am* 22:747–764.

Goulart-Filho JAV, Montalli VAM, Passador-Santos F, et al. 2019. Role of apoptotic, autophagic and senescence pathways in minor salivary gland adenoid cystic carcinoma. *Diagn Pathol* 14(1):14.

Gouveris H, Lehmann CG, Heinrich UR, et al. 2011. Genomic changes in salivary gland pleomorphic adenomas detected by comparative genomic hybridization. *Neoplasma* 58:97–103.

Goyal G, Mehdi SA, Ganti AK. 2015. Salivary gland cancers: Biology and systemic therapy. *Oncology* 29:773–780.

Grandal MV, Madshus IH. 2008. Epidermal growth factor receptor and cancer: Control of oncogenic signalling by endocytosis. *J Cell Mol Med* 12:1527–1534.

Griffith CC, Schmitt AC, Little JL, Magliocca KR 2017. New Developments in salivary gland pathology: Clinically useful ancillary testing and new potentially targetable molecular alterations. *Arch Pathol Lab Med* 141:381–395.

Guo XL, Sun SZ, Wang WX, Wei FC, et al. 2007. Alterations of p16INK4a tumour suppressor gene in mucoepidermoid carcinoma of the salivary glands. *Int J Oral Maxillofac Surg* 36:350–353.

Gurzu S, Krause M, Ember I, et al. 2012. Mena, a new available marker in tumors of salivary glands? *Eur J Histochem* 56(1):e8.

Gutschenritter T, Machiorlatti M, Vesely S, et al. 2017. Outcomes and prognostic factors of resected salivary gland malignancies: Examining a single institution's 12-year experience. *Anticancer Res* 37:5019–5025.

Haddad R, Colevas AD, Krane JF, et al. 2003. Herceptin in patients with advanced or metastatic salivary gland carcinomas. A phase II study. *Oral Oncol* 39:724–727.

Hanahan D, Weinberg R. 2011. Hallmarks of cancer: The next generation. *Cell* 144:646–674.

Hashimoto K, Yamamoto H, Shiratsuchi H, et al. 2012. HER-2/neu gene amplification in carcinoma ex pleomorphic adenoma in relation to progression and prognosis: A chromogenic in-situ hybridization study. *Histopathology* 60:E131–E142.

Hayflick L. 1965. The limited in vitro life-time of human diploid cell strains. *Exp Cell Res* 37:614–636.

He Q, Zhou X, Li S, et al. 2013. MicroRNA-181a suppresses salivary adenoid cystic carcinoma metastasis by targeting MAPK-Snai2 pathway. *Biochim Biophys Acta* 1830:5258–5266.

Hellquist H, Paiva-Correia A, Vander Poorten V, et al. 2019. Analysis of the clinical relevance of histological classification of benign epithelial salivary gland tumours. *Adv Ther* 36:1950–1974.

Henley SA, Dick FA. 2012. The retinoblastoma family of proteins and their regulatory functions in the mammalian cell division cycle. *Cell Div* 7:10.

Hotte SJ, Winquist EW, Lamont E, et al. 2005. Imatinib mesylate in patients with adenoid cystic cancers of the salivary glands expressing c-kit: A Princess Margaret Hospital phase II consortium study. *J Clin Oncol* 23:585–590.

Hoyek-Gebeily J, Nehme E, Aftimos G, et al. 2007. Prognostic significance of EGFR, p53 and E-cadherin in mucoepidermoid cancer of the salivary glands: A retrospective case series. *J Med Liban* 55:83–88.

Hu YH, Zhang CY, Tian Z, et al. 2011. Aberrant protein expression and promoter methylation of p16 gene are correlated with malignant transformation of salivary pleomorphic adenoma. *Arch Pathol Lab Med* 135:882–889.

Huang XY, Gan RH, Xie J, et al. 2018. The oncogenic effects of HES1 on salivary adenoid cystic carcinoma cell growth and metastasis. *BMC Cancer* 18:436.

Ishibashi K, Ishii K, Sugiyama G, et al. 2018. Regulation of ß-catenin phosphorylation by PR55ß in adenoid cystic carcinoma. *Cancer Genomics Proteomics* 15:53–60.

Jeng YM, Lin CY, Hsu HC. 2000. Expression of the c-kit protein is associated with certain subtypes of salivary gland carcinoma. *Cancer Lett* 154:107–111.

Jia J, Zhang W, Liu JY, et al. 2012. Epithelial mesenchymal transition is required for acquisition of anoikis resistance and metastatic potential in adenoid cystic carcinoma. *PLoS One* 7:e51549.

Jiang D, Dumur CI, Massey HD, et al. 2015. Comparison of effects of p53 null and gain-of-function mutations on salivary tumors in MMTV-Hras transgenic mice. *PLoS One* 10(2):e0118029.

Jin L, Xu L, Song X, et al. 2012. Genetic variation in MDM2 and p14ARF and susceptibility to salivary gland carcinoma. *PLoS One* 7:e49361.

Kaidar-Person O, Billan S, Kuten A. 2012. Targeted therapy with trastuzumab for advanced salivary ductal carcinoma: Case report and literature review. *Med Oncol* 29:704–706.

Kang H, Tan M, Bishop JA, et al. 2017. Whole-exome sequencing of salivary gland mucoepidermoid carcinoma. *Clin Cancer Res* 23:283–288.

Karja VJ, Syrjanen KJ, Kurvinen AK, Syrjanen SM. 1997. Expression and mutations of p53 in salivary gland tumours. *J Oral Pathol Med* 26:217–223.

Kaye FJ. 2006. Emerging biology of malignant salivary gland tumors offers new insights into the classification and treatment of mucoepidermoid cancer. *Clin Cancer Res* 12:3878–3881.

Kehagias N, Epivatianos A, Sakas L, et al. 2013. Expression of N-cadherin in salivary gland tumors. *Med Princ Pract* 22:59–64.

Keller G, Steinmann D, Quaas A, et al. 2017. New concepts of personalized therapy in salivary gland carcinomas. *Oral Oncol* 68:103–113.

Kelley MR, Fishel ML. 2008. DNA repair proteins as molecular targets for cancer therapeutics. *Anticancer Agents Med Chem* 8:417–425.

Kim JC Mirkin SM. 2013. The balancing act of DNA repeat expansions. *Curr Opin Genet Dev* 23:280–288.

Kim Y, Donoff R, Wong D, Todd R. 2002a. The nucleotide: DNA sequencing and its clinical application. *J Oral Maxillofac Surg* 60:924–930.

Kim Y, Flynn T, Donoff R, et al. 2002b. The gene: The polymerase chain reaction (PCR) and its clinical application. *J Oral Maxillofac Surg* 60:808–815.

Kishi M, Nakamura M, Nishimine M, et al. 2005. Genetic and epigenetic alteration profiles for multiple genes in salivary gland carcinomas. *Oral Oncol* 41:161–169.

Kishi M, Nakamura M, Nishimine M, et al. 2003. Loss of heterozygosity on chromosome 6q correlates with decreased thrombospondin-2 expression in human salivary gland carcinomas. *Cancer Sci* 94:530–535.

Kiyoshima T, Shima K, Kobayashi I, et al. 2001. Expression of p53 tumor suppressor gene in adenoid cystic and mucoepidermoid carcinomas of the salivary glands. *Oral Oncol* 37:315–322.

Klymkowsky MW, Savagner P. 2009. Epithelial-mesenchymal transition: A cancer researcher's conceptual friend and foe. *Am J Pathol* 174:1588–1593.

Kolch W, Mischak H, Pitt A. 2005. The molecular make-up of a tumour: Proteomics in cancer research. *Clin Sci* 108:369–383.

Komiya T, Park Y, Modi S, et al. 2006. Sustained expression of Mect1-Maml2 is essential for tumor cell growth in salivary gland cancers carrying the t(11;19) translocation. *Oncogene* 25:6128–6132.

Koochek Dezfuli M, Seyedmajidi M, Nafarzadeh S, et al. 2019. Angiogenesis and lymphangiogenesis in salivary gland adenoid cystic carcinoma and mucoepidermoid carcinoma. *Asian Pac J Cancer Prev* 20:3547–3553.

Lassche G, Van Boxtel W, Ligtenberg MJL, et al. 2019. Advances and challenges in precision medicine in salivary gland cancer. *Cancer Treat Rev* 80:101906.

Lee ES, Issa JP, Roberts DB, et al. 2008. Quantitative promoter hypermethylation analysis of cancer-related genes in salivary gland carcinomas: Comparison with methylation-specific PCR technique and clinical significance. *Clin Cancer Res* 14:2664–2672.

Lee EY, Muller WJ. 2010. Oncogenes and tumor suppressor genes. *Cold Spring Harb Perspect Biol* 2:a003236.

Lee S. K, Kwon MS, Lee YS, et al. 2012. Prognostic value of expression of molecular markers in adenoid cystic cancer of the salivary glands compared with lymph node metastasis: A retrospective study. *World J Surg Oncol* 10:266.

Leivo I. 2006. Insights into a complex group of neoplastic disease: Advances in histopathologic classification and molecular pathology of salivary gland cancer. *Acta Oncol* 45:662–668.

Lequerica-Fernandez P, Astudillo A, De Vicente JC. 2007. Expression of vascular endothelial growth factor in salivary gland carcinomas correlates with lymph node metastasis. *Anticancer Res* 27:3661–3666.

Li J, El-Naggar A, Mao L. 2005. Promoter methylation of p16INK4a, RASSF1A, and DAPK is frequent in salivary adenoid cystic carcinoma. *Cancer* 104:771–776.

Lim JJ, Kang S, Lee MR, et al. 2003. Expression of vascular endothelial growth factor in salivary gland carcinomas and its relation to p53, Ki-67 and prognosis. *J Oral Pathol Med* 32:552–561.

Liu H, Luo J, Luan S, et al. 2019. Long non-coding RNAs involved in cancer metabolic reprogramming. *Cell Mol Life Sci* 76:495–504.

Liu J, Shao C, Tan ML, et al. 2012. Molecular biology of adenoid cystic carcinoma. *Head Neck* 34:1665–1677.

Liu L, Hu Y, Fu J, et al. 2013. MicroRNA155 in the growth and invasion of salivary adenoid cystic carcinoma. *J Oral Pathol Med* 42:140–147.

Liu T, Zhu E, Wang L, et al. 2005. Abnormal expression of Rb pathway-related proteins in salivary gland acinic cell carcinoma. *Hum Pathol* 36:962–970.

Lin HH, Limesand KH, Ann DK. 2018. Current state of knowledge on salivary gland cancers. *Crit Rev Oncog* 23:139–151.

Locati LD, Perrone F, Losa M, et al. 2009. Treatment relevant target immunophenotyping of 139 salivary gland carcinomas (SGCs). *Oral Oncol* 45:986–990.

Lopes MA, Santos GC, Kowalski LP. 1998. Multivariate survival analysis of 128 cases of oral cavity minor salivary gland carcinomas. *Head Neck* 20:699–706.

Luukkaa H, Klemi P, Hirsimaki P, et al. 2008. Matrix metalloproteinase (MMP)-1, −9 and −13 as prognostic factors in salivary gland cancer. *Acta Otolaryngol* 128:482–490.

Luukkaa H, Klemi P, Hirsimaki P, et al. 2010a. Matrix metalloproteinase (MMP)-7 in salivary gland cancer. *Acta Oncol* 49:85–90.

Luukkaa H, Klemi P, Leivo I, et al. 2010b. Expression of matrix metalloproteinase-1, −7, −9, −13, Ki-67, and HER-2 in epithelial-myoepithelial salivary gland cancer. *Head Neck* 32:1019–1027.

Mani SA, Guo W, Liao MJ, et al. 2008. The epithelial-mesenchymal transition generates cells with properties of stem cells. *Cell* 133:704–715.

Manning AL, Dyson NJ. 2012. RB: Mitotic implications of a tumour suppressor. *Nat Rev Cancer* 12:220–226.

Margaritescu C, Munteanu MC, Nitulescu NC, et al. 2013. Acinic cell carcinoma of the salivary glands: An immunohistochemical study of angiogenesis in 12 cases. *Rom J Morphol Embryol* 54:275–284.

Marques YM, De Limamde D, De Melo Alvessde M, Jr, et al. 2008. Mdm2, p53, p21 and pAKT protein pathways in benign neoplasms of the salivary gland. *Oral Oncol* 44:903–908.

Martins MT, Altemani A, Freitas L, Araujo VC. 2005. Maspin expression in carcinoma ex pleomorphic adenoma. *J Clin Pathol* 58:1311–1314.

Maruya S, Kim HW, Weber RS, et al. 2004. Gene expression screening of salivary gland neoplasms: Molecular markers of potential histogenetic and clinical significance. *J Mol Diagn* 6:180–190.

Matsuyama A, Hisaoka M, Nagao Y, Hashimoto H. 2011. Aberrant PLAG1 expression in pleomorphic adenomas of the salivary gland: A molecular genetic and immunohistochemical study. *Virchows Arch* 458:583–592.

Mchugh JB, Hoschar AP, Dvorakova M, et al. 2007. p63 immunohistochemistry differentiates salivary gland oncocytoma and oncocytic carcinoma from metastatic renal cell carcinoma. *Head Neck Pathol* 1:123–131.

Milasin J, Pujic N, Dedovic N, et al. 1993. H-ras gene mutations in salivary gland pleomorphic adenomas. *Int J Oral Maxillofac Surg* 22:359–361.

Mino M, Pilch BZ, Faquin WC. 2003. Expression of KIT (CD117) in neoplasms of the head and neck: An ancillary marker for adenoid cystic carcinoma. *Mod Pathol* 16:1224–1231.

Mitani Y, Roberts DB, Fatani H, et al. 2013. MicroRNA profiling of salivary adenoid cystic carcinoma: Association of miR-17-92 upregulation with poor outcome. *PLoS One* 8:e66778.

Miyabe S, Okabe M, Nagatsuka H, et al. 2009. Prognostic significance of p27Kip1, Ki-67, and CRTC1-MAML2 fusion transcript in mucoepidermoid carcinoma: A molecular and clinicopathologic study of 101 cases. *J Oral Maxillofac Surg* 67:1432–1441.

Mohit E, Rafati S. 2013. Biological delivery approaches for gene therapy: Strategies to potentiate efficacy and enhance specificity. *Mol Immunol* 56:599–611.

Morris K. 2006. Therapeutic potential of siRNA-mediated transcriptional gene silencing. *Biotechniques* (Suppl):7–13.

Murakami M, Ohtani I, Hojo H, Wakasa H. 1992. Immunohistochemical evaluation with Ki-67: An application to salivary gland tumours. *J Laryngol Otol* 106:35–38.

Nag S, Qin J, Srivenugopal KS, et al. 2013. The MDM2-p53 pathway revisited. *J Biomed Res* 27:254–271.

Nagao T. 2013. "Dedifferentiation" and high-grade transformation in salivary gland carcinomas. *Head Neck Pathol* 7 (Suppl 1):S37–S47.

Nagao T, Sato E, Inoue R, et al. 2012. Immunohistochemical analysis of salivary gland tumors: Application for surgical pathology practice. *Acta Histochem Cytochem* 45:269–282.

Nagao T, Sugano I, Ishida Y, et al. 1998. Basal cell adenocarcinoma of the salivary glands: Comparison with basal cell adenoma through assessment of cell proliferation, apoptosis, and expression of p53 and bcl-2. *Cancer* 82:439–447.

Nagel H, Laskawi R, Wahlers A, Hemmerlein B. 2004. Expression of matrix metalloproteinases MMP-2, MMP-9 and their tissue inhibitors TIMP-1, −2, and −3 in benign and malignant tumours of the salivary gland. *Histopathology* 44:222–231.

Nagler RM, Kerner H, Ben-Eliezer S, et al. 2003. Prognostic role of apoptotic, Bcl-2, c-erbB-2 and p53 tumor markers in salivary gland malignancies. *Oncology* 64:389–398.

Nakano T, Yamamoto H, Hashimoto K, et al. 2013. HER2 and EGFR gene copy number alterations are predominant in high-grade salivary mucoepidermoid carcinoma irrespective of MAML2 fusion status. *Histopathology* 63:378–392.

Nardi V, Sadow PM, Juric D, et al. 2013. Detection of novel actionable genetic changes in salivary duct carcinoma helps direct patient treatment. *Clin Cancer Res* 19:480–490.

Nishimine M, Nakamura M, Kishi M, et al. 2003. Alterations of p14ARF and p16INK4a genes in salivary gland carcinomas. *Oncol Rep* 10:555–560.

Ochal-Choińska AJ, Osuch-Wójcikiewicz E. 2016. Particular aspects in the cytogenetics and molecular biology of salivary gland tumours – Current review of reports. *Contemp Oncol* 20:281–286.

Ohki K, Kumamoto H, Ichinohasama R, et al. 2001. Genetic analysis of DNA microsatellite loci in salivary gland tumours: Comparison with immunohistochemical detection of hMSH2 and p53 proteins. *Int J Oral Maxillofac Surg* 30:538–544.

Okutsu S, Takeda A, Suzuki T, et al. 1993. Expression of ras-P21 and ras gene alteration in pleomorphic adenomas. *J Nihon Univ Sch Dent* 35:200–203.

Ono J, Okada Y. 2018. Study of MYB-NFIB chimeric gene expression, tumor angiogenesis, and proliferation in adenoid cystic carcinoma of salivary gland. *Odontology* 106(3):238–244.

Ortiz R, Melguizo C, Prados J, et al. 2012. New gene therapy strategies for cancer treatment: A review of recent patents. *Recent Pat Anticancer Drug Discov* 7:297–312.

Ouyang L, Shi Z, Zhao S, et al. 2012. Programmed cell death pathways in cancer: A review of apoptosis, autophagy and programmed necrosis. *Cell Prolif* 45:487–498.

Paiva-Fonseca F, De Almeida OP, Ayroza-Rangel AL, Agustin-Vargas P. 2013. Tissue microarray construction for salivary gland tumors study. *Med Oral Patol Oral Cir Bucal* 18:e1–e6.

Papadaki H, Finkelstein SD, Kounelis S, et al. 1996. The role of p53 mutation and protein expression in primary and recurrent adenoid cystic carcinoma. *Hum Pathol* 27:567–572.

Persson M, Andren Y, Mark J, et al. 2009. Recurrent fusion of MYB and NFIB transcription factor genes in carcinomas of the breast and head and neck. *Proc Natl Acad Sci U S A* 106:18740–18744.

Pfeffer MR, Talmi Y, Catane R, et al. 2007. A phase II study of imatinib for advanced adenoid cystic carcinoma of head and neck salivary glands. *Oral Oncol* 43:33–36.

Prabhu S, Kaveri H, Rekha K. 2009. Benign, malignant salivary gland tumors: Comparison of immunohistochemical expression of e-cadherin. *Oral Oncol* 45:594–599.

Pramoonjago P, Baras AS, Moskaluk CA. 2006. Knockdown of Sox4 expression by RNAi induces apoptosis in ACC3 cells. *Oncogene* 25:5626–5639.

Prenen H, Kimpe M, Nuyts S. 2008. Salivary gland carcinomas: Molecular abnormalities as potential therapeutic targets. *Curr Opin Oncol* 20:270–274.

Pusztaszeri MP, Faquin WC 2015. Update in salivary gland cytopathology: Recent molecular advances and diagnostic applications. *Semin Diagn Pathol* 32:264–274.

Rao PH, Roberts D, Zhao YJ, et al. 2008. Deletion of 1p32-p36 is the most frequent genetic change and poor prognostic marker in adenoid cystic carcinoma of the salivary glands. *Clin Cancer Res* 14:5181–5187.

Rosa JC, Felix A, Fonseca I, Soares J. 1997. Immunoexpression of c-erbB-2 and p53 in benign and malignant salivary neoplasms with myoepithelial differentiation. *J Clin Pathol* 50:661–663.

Rugo HS, Herbst RS, Liu G, et al. 2005. Phase I trial of the oral antiangiogenesis agent AG-013736 in patients with advanced solid tumors: Pharmacokinetic and clinical results. *J Clin Oncol* 23:5474–5483.

Saintigny P, Mitani Y, Pytynia KB, et al. 2018. Frequent PTEN loss and differential HER2/PI3K signaling pathway alterations in salivary duct carcinoma: Implications for targeted therapy. *Cancer* 124:3693–3705.

Samples J, Willis M, Klauber-Demore N. 2013. Targeting angiogenesis and the tumor microenvironment. *Surg Oncol Clin N Am* 22:629–639.

Sams RN, Gnepp DR. 2013. P63 expression can be used in differential diagnosis of salivary gland acinic cell and mucoepidermoid carcinomas. *Head Neck Pathol* 7:64–68.

Santana T, Pavel A, Martinek P, et al. 2019. Biomarker immunoprofile and molecular characteristics in salivary duct carcinoma: Clinicopathological and prognostic implications. *Hum Pathol* 93:37–47.

Schache AG, Hall G, Woolgar JA, et al. 2010. Quantitative promoter methylation differentiates carcinoma ex pleomorphic adenoma from pleomorphic salivary adenoma. *Br J Cancer* 103:1846–1851.

Schindler S, Nayar R, Dutra J, Bedrossian CW. 2001. Diagnostic challenges in aspiration cytology of the salivary glands. *Semin Diagn Pathol* 18:124–146.

Schneider S, Kloimstein P, Pammer J, et al. 2014. New diagnostic markers in salivary gland tumors. *Eur Arch Otorhinolaryngol* 271:1999–2007.

Schneider T, Strehl A, Linz C, et al. 2016. Phosphorylated epidermal growth factor receptor expression and KRAS mutation status in salivary gland carcinomas. *Clin Oral Investig* 20:541–551.

Schvartsman G, Pinto NA, Bell D, Ferrarotto R. 2019. Salivary gland tumors: Molecular characterization and therapeutic advances for metastatic disease. *Head Neck* 41:239–247.

Seethala RR, Stenman G 2017. Update from the 4th edition of the World Health Organization classification of head and neck tumours: Tumors of the salivary gland. *Head and Neck Pathol* 11:55–67.

Seethala RR. 2011. Histologic grading and prognostic biomarkers in salivary gland carcinomas. *Adv Anat Pathol* 18:29–45.

Seethala RR. 2017. Salivary gland tumors: Current concepts and controversies. *Surg Pathol Clin* 10:155–176.

Seethala RR, Griffith CC. 2016. Molecular pathology: Predictive, prognostic, and diagnostic markers in salivary gland tumors. *Surg Pathol Clin* 9:339–352.

Sequeiros-Santiago G, Garcia-Carracedo D, Fresno MF, et al. 2009. Oncogene amplification pattern in adenoid cystic carcinoma of the salivary glands. *Oncol Rep* 21:1215–1222.

Shang J, Sheng L, Wang K, et al. 2007. Expression of neural cell adhesion molecule in salivary adenoid cystic carcinoma and its correlation with perineural invasion. *Oncol Rep* 18:1413–1416.

Shao C, Bai W, Junn JC, et al. 2011a. Evaluation of MYB promoter methylation in salivary adenoid cystic carcinoma. *Oral Oncol* 47:251–255.

Shao C, Sun W, Tan M, et al. 2011b. Integrated, genome-wide screening for hypomethylated oncogenes in salivary gland adenoid cystic carcinoma. *Clin Cancer Res* 17:4320–4330.

Shao C, Tan M, Bishop JA, et al. 2012. Suprabasin is hypomethylated and associated with metastasis in salivary adenoid cystic carcinoma. *PLoS One* 7:e48582.

Shay JW, Wright WE. 2005. Senescence and immortalization: Role of telomeres and telomerase. *Carcinogenesis* 26:867–874.

Shieh YS, Hung YJ, Hsieh CB, et al. 2009. Tumor-associated macrophage correlated with angiogenesis and progression of mucoepidermoid carcinoma of salivary glands. *Ann Surg Oncol* 16:751–760.

Shigeishi H, Sugiyama M, Tahara H, et al. 2011. Increased telomerase activity and hTERT expression in human salivary gland carcinomas. *Oncol Lett* 2:845–850.

Shin JA, Li C, Choi ES, et al. 2013. High expression of microRNA127 is involved in cell cycle arrest in MC3 mucoepidermoid carcinoma cells. *Mol Med Rep* 7:708–712.

Shintani S, Mihara M, Nakahara Y, et al. 2000. Infrequent alternations of RB pathway (Rb-p16INK4A-cyclinD1) in adenoid cystic carcinoma of salivary glands. *Anticancer Res* 20:2169–2175.

Sidranski D. 2002. Emerging molecular markers of cancer. *Nat Rev Cancer* 2:210–219

Skalova A, Leivo I. 1996. Cell proliferation in salivary gland tumors. *Gen Diagn Pathol* 142:7–16.

Skalova A, Vanecek T, Sima R, et al. 2010. Mammary analogue secretory carcinoma of salivary glands, containing the ETV6-NTRK3 fusion gene: A hitherto undescribed salivary gland tumor entity. *Am J Surg Pathol* 34:599–608.

Skálová A, Stenman G, Simpson RHW, et al. 2018. The role of molecular testing in the differential diagnosis of salivary gland carcinomas. *Am J Surg Pathol* 42:e11–e27.

Sliwkowski MX, Mellman I. 2013. Antibody therapeutics in cancer. *Science* 341:1192–1198.

Smith SM, Anastasi J, Cohen KS, Godley LA. 2010. The impact of MYC expression in lymphoma biology: Beyond Burkitt lymphoma. *Blood Cells Mol Dis* 45:317–323.

Sowa P, Goroszkiewicz K, Szydelko J, et al. 2018. A review of selected factors of salivary gland tumour formation and malignant transformation. *Biomed Res Int* 2018:2897827.

Sreeja C, Shahela T, Aesha S, Satish MK. 2014. Taxonomy of salivary gland neoplasms. *J Clin Diag* 8:291–293.

Stenman G. 2005. Fusion oncogenes and tumor type specificity-insights from salivary gland tumors. *Semin Cancer Biol* 15:224–235.

Stenman G. 2013. Fusion oncogenes in salivary gland tumors: Molecular and clinical consequences. *Head Neck Pathol* 7(Suppl 1):S12–S19.

Stenner M, Demgensky A, Molls C, et al. 2011. Prognostic value of survivin expression in parotid gland cancer in consideration of different histological subtypes. *Eur J Cancer* 47:1013–1020.

Stenner M, Demgensky A, Molls C, et al. 2012. Prognostic value of proliferating cell nuclear antigen in parotid gland cancer. *Eur Arch Otorhinolaryngol* 269:1225–1232.

Sun J, Luo Y, Tian Z, et al. 2012. Expression of ERBB3 binding protein 1 (EBP1) in salivary adenoid cystic carcinoma and its clinicopathological relevance. *BMC Cancer* 12:499.

Suzuki H, Fujioka Y. 1998. Deletion of the p16 gene and microsatellite instability in carcinoma arising in pleomorphic adenoma of the parotid gland. *Diagn Mol Pathol* 7:224–231.

Talmadge JE, Fidler IJ. 2010. AACR centenial series: The biology of cancer metastasis: Historical perspective. *Cancer Res* 70:5649–5669.

Tang Y, Liang X, Zheng M, et al. 2010. Expression of c-kit and Slug correlates with invasion and metastasis of salivary adenoid cystic carcinoma. *Oral Oncol* 46:311–316.

Taube S, Jacobson J, Lively TG. 2005. Cancer diagnostics: Decision criteria fro marker utilization in the clinic. *Am J Pharmacogenomics* 5:357–364.

Thakor AS, Gambhir SS. 2013. Nanooncology: The future of cancer diagnosis and therapy. *CA Cancer J Clin* 63:395–418.

Todd R, Donoff R, Wong D. 2000. The chromosome: Cytogenetic analysis and its clinical application. *J Oral Maxillofac Surg* 58:1036–1041.

Todd R, Munger K 2003. Oncogenes. In: Dn C (ed.), *Nature Encyclopedia of the Human Genome*. London, Nature Publishing Group.

Todd R, Wong D. 1999. Epidermal growth factor receptor (EGFR) biology and human oral cancer. *Hist Histopath* 14:491–500.

Theocharis S, Gribilas G, Giaginis C, et al. 2015. Angiogenesis in salivary gland tumors: From clinical significance to treatment. *Expert Opin Ther Targets* 19:807–819.

Turgut B, Ozdemir O, Erselcan T. 2006. Evaluation of the p53 tumor suppressor gene mutation in normal rat salivary gland tissue after radioiodine application: An experimental study. *Adv Ther* 23:456–468.

Turk AT, Wenig BM. 2014. Pitfalls in the biopsy diagnosis of intraoral minor salivary gland neoplasms: Diagnostic considerations and recommended approach. *Adv Anat Pathol* 21:1–11.

Tyagi R, Dey P. 2015. Diagnostic problems of salivary gland tumors. *Diagn Cytopathol* 43:495–509.

Vander Poorten V, Bradley PJ, Takes RP, et al. 2012. Diagnosis and management of parotid carcinoma with a special focus on recent advances in molecular biology. *Head Neck* 34:429–440.

Vattemi E, Graiff C, Sava T, et al. 2008. Systemic therapies for recurrent and/or metastatic salivary gland cancers. *Expert Rev Anticancer Ther* 8:393–402.

Vekony H, Roser K, Loning T, et al. 2008. Deregulated expression of p16INK4a and p53 pathway members in benign and malignant myoepithelial tumours of the salivary glands. *Histopathology* 53:658–666.

Verdone L, Caserta M, Di Mauro E. 2005. Role of histone acetylation in the control of gene expression. *Biochem Cell Biol* 83:344–353.

Vermeulen K, Van Bockstaele DR, Berneman ZN. 2003. The cell cycle: A review of regulation, deregulation and therapeutic targets in cancer. *Cell Prolif* 36:131–149.

Vidal L, Tsao MS, Pond GR, et al. 2009. Fluorescence in situ hybridization gene amplification analysis of EGFR and HER2 in patients with malignant salivary gland tumors treated with lapatinib. *Head Neck* 31:1006–1012.

Vidal MT, De Oliveira Araujo IB, Gurgel CA, et al. 2013. Density of mast cells and microvessels in minor salivary gland tumors. *Tumour Biol* 34:309–316.

Vila L, Liu H, Al-Quran SZ, et al. 2009. Identification of c-kit gene mutations in primary adenoid cystic carcinoma of the salivary gland. *Mod Pathol* 22:1296–1302.

Vogelstein B, Kinzler K. 1992. p53 function and dysfunction. *Cell* 70:523–526.

Vogelstein B, Kinzler K. 1998. *The Genetic Basis of Human Cancer*. New York, McGraw-Hill.

Wang L, Sun M, Jiang Y, et al. 2006. Nerve growth factor and tyrosine kinase A in human salivary adenoid cystic carcinoma: Expression patterns and effects on in vitro invasive behavior. *J Oral Maxillofac Surg* 64:636–641.

Wang WM, Zhao ZL, Zhang WF, et al. 2015. Role of hypoxia-inducible factor-1α and CD146 in epidermal growth factor receptor-mediated angiogenesis in salivary gland adenoid cystic carcinoma. *Mol Med Rep* 12:3432–3438.

Wang X, Luo Y, Li M, et al. 2017. Management of salivary gland carcinomas – A review. *Oncotarget* 8:3946–3956.

Watson IR, Takahashi K, Futreal PA, Chin L. 2013. Emerging patterns of somatic mutations in cancer. *Nat Rev Genet* 14:703–718.

Weber A, Langhanki L, Schutz A, et al. 2002. Expression profiles of p53, p63, and p73 in benign salivary gland tumors. *Virchows Arch* 441:428–436.

Williams MD, Chakravarti N, Kies MS, et al. 2006. Implications of methylation patterns of cancer genes in salivary gland tumors. *Clin Cancer Res* 12:7353–7358.

Willis AL, Sabeh F, Li XY, Weiss SJ. 2013. Extracellular matrix determinants and the regulation of cancer cell invasion stratagems. *J Microsc* 251:250–260.

Wong SJ, Karrison T, Hayes DN, et al. 2016. Phase II trial of dasatinib for recurrent or metastatic c-KIT expressing adenoid cystic carcinoma and for nonadenoid cystic malignant salivary tumors. *Ann Oncol* 27:318–323.

Wysocki PT, Izumchenko E, Meir J, et al. 2016 Adenoid cystic carcinoma: Emerging role of translocations and gene fusions. *Oncotarget* 7:66239–66254.

Xie S, Yu X, Li Y, et al. 2018. Upregulation of lncRNA ADAMTS9-AS2 promotes salivary adenoid cystic carcinoma metastasis via PI3K/Akt and MEK/Erk signaling. *Mol Ther* 26:2766–2778.

Xu L, Li S, Stohr BA. 2013. The role of telomere biology in cancer. *Annu Rev Pathol* 8:49–78.

Xu W, Liu L, Lu H, et al. 2019. Dysregulated long non coding RNAs in pleomorphic adenoma tissues of pleomorphic adenoma gene 1 transgenic mice. *Mol Med Rep* 19:4735–4742.

Yamamoto Y, Virmani AK, Wistuba II, et al. 1996. Loss of heterozygosity and microsatellite alterations in p53 and RB genes in adenoid cystic carcinoma of the salivary glands. *Hum Pathol* 27:1204–1210.

Yang X, Zhang P, Ma Q, et al. 2012. EMMPRIN contributes to the in vitro invasion of human salivary adenoid cystic carcinoma cells. *Oncol Rep* 27:1123–1127.

Yang X, Zhang P, Ma Q, et al. 2012. EMMPRIN silencing inhibits proliferation and perineural invasion of human salivary adenoid cystic carcinoma cells in vitro and in vivo;. *Cancer Biol Ther* 13:85–91.

Yin HF, Okad N, Takagi M. 2000. Apoptosis and apoptotic-related factors in mucoepidermoid carcinoma of the oral minor salivary glands. *Pathol Int* 50:603–609.

Yin LX, Ha PK. 2016. Genetic alterations in salivary gland cancers. *Cancer* 122:1822–1831.

Yoo J, Robinson RA. 2000. ras gene mutations in salivary gland tumors. *Arch Pathol Lab Med* 124:836–839.

Yoshizawa JM, Schafer CA, Schafer JJ, et al. 2013. Salivary biomarkers: Toward future clinical and diagnostic utilities. *Clin Microbiol Rev* 26:781–791.

Yue J, Liu X, Zhuo S, Zhang W. 2017. N-RAS expression in patients with salivary adenoid cystic carcinoma: Association with clinicopathologic features and prognosis. *Oral Surg Oral Med Oral Pathol Oral Radiol* 123:242–248.

Zarbo RJ. 2002. Salivary gland neoplasia: A review for the practicing pathologist. *Mod Pathol* 15:298–323.

Zboray K, Mohrherr J, Stiedl P, et al. 2018. AKT3 drives adenoid cystic carcinoma development in salivary glands. *Cancer Med* 7:445–453.

Zhang CY, Mao L, Li L, et al. 2007. Promoter methylation as a common mechanism for inactivating E-cadherin in human salivary gland adenoid cystic carcinoma. *Cancer* 110:87–95.

Zhang X, Cairns M, Rose B, et al. 2009a. Alterations in miRNA processing and expression in pleomorphic adenomas of the salivary gland. *Int J Cancer* 124:2855–2863.

Zhang X, Wang Y, Yamamoto G, Tachikawa T. 2009b. Expression of matrix metalloproteinases MMP-2, MMP-9 and their tissue inhibitors TIMP-1 and TIMP-2 in the epithelium and stroma of salivary gland pleomorphic adenomas. *Histopathology* 55:250–260.

Zhao D, Yang K, Tang X F, et al. 2013. Expression of integrin-linked kinase in adenoid cystic carcinoma of salivary glands correlates with epithelial-mesenchymal transition markers and tumor progression. *Med Oncol* 30:619.

Chapter 10
Tumors of the Parotid Gland

Outline

Introduction
Etiology and Epidemiology
Diagnosis
Surgical Management
  Benign Tumors
    Pleomorphic Adenoma (PA)
  Warthin Tumor
  Malignant Tumors
    Principles of Management of Parotid Carcinoma
Summary
Case Presentation – *How Did This All Start?*
References

Introduction

This chapter will discuss the diagnosis and management of parotid tumors arising from epithelial cells, i.e. salivary derived parotid tumors. Non-epithelial tumors will be discussed in Chapter 15. Although the commonest tumor is the benign pleomorphic adenoma (PA) there is currently much controversy in the literature about the surgical management of this tumor, regarding the place of extra-capsular dissection versus traditional parotidectomy and this will be discussed at length in this chapter and Chapter 19. Changing approaches to neck dissection and adjuvant radiotherapy in malignant parotid tumors will also be highlighted. Wherever possible, recent references will encompass prospective trials, systematic reviews, meta-analysis, and large series based on population data bases, e.g. SEER and NCDB, to improve the scientific evidence base for the recommendations given.

Etiology and Epidemiology

The etiology of salivary gland tumors is largely unknown. There is an increase in salivary tumors from exposure to radiation documented in survivors from Hiroshima and Nagasaki (Saku et al. 1997). In children exposed to therapeutic radiation for treatment of leukemias and lymphomas, there is an increased incidence of secondary salivary cancers. These are most commonly mucoepidermoid carcinomas and the parotid is the most frequently affected salivary gland (Miyatima et al. 2007; Védrine et al. 2006). Second, primary salivary cancers can also occur following chemotherapy alone or with a combination of radiation and chemotherapy. A systematic review showed that 14/58 (24%) of cases of second primary salivary cancers had childhood cancers treated with chemotherapy alone. Interestingly, the latent interval between initial treatment and development of the salivary cancer was much longer (27.2 years) for children treated with only radiation therapy (Verma et al. 2011).

Adults exposed to radiation can also develop salivary cancers, most commonly mucoepidermoid carcinoma. In one study, 18 patients of 3025 cases of salivary gland tumors had received prior radiation therapy. The median age at which cases were irradiated was 22 years (range 5–74 years), the median age of developing their salivary tumor was 54 years (range 21–79 years), with median interval between the radiation and diagnosis of the salivary tumor of 21 years (range 4–64 years) (Beal et al. 2003). (See section "Case Presentation – *How Did this All Start?*" at the end of chapter).

Salivary Gland Pathology: Diagnosis and Management, Third Edition. Edited by Eric R. Carlson and Robert A. Ord.
© 2022 John Wiley & Sons, Inc. Published 2022 by John Wiley & Sons, Inc.
Companion website: www.wiley.com/go/carlson/salivary

An increase in poorly differentiated carcinoma of the parotid that may be associated with Epstein-Barr Virus (EBV) is reported in Inuit people. This association with EBV has also been reported in pediatric patients (Venkateswaran et al. 2000). In lymphoepithelial carcinoma of the parotid, there is a racial predilection with high incidence in Asians (particularly Chinese) and Inuit people. An association with Epstein-Barr Virus (EBV) is common and has treatment implications (Anantharajan et al. 2013). Rarely, these poorly differentiated carcinomas of the parotid gland may represent nuclear protein of the testis (NUT) carcinomas (Agaimy et al. 2018).

Advances in molecular biology have allowed the identification of gene rearrangements and biomarkers in many salivary tumors. These may not only be useful for diagnosis and prognosis but may also be used in novel targeted therapy. Examples are ETV6-NTRK3 fusion gene in secretory carcinoma, chromosomal rearrangements of the gene encoding nuclear protein of the testis (NUT) at 15q14 in the NUT midline carcinoma, EWSR1-ATF1 fusion in hyalinizing clear cell carcinoma, t(11;19)(q21;p13)MECT1-MAML2 translocation for mucoepidermoid carcinoma, and HER2/neu gene amplification in high-grade salivary duct carcinomas. A systematic review of the prognostic value of CRTC1-MAML2 translocations in mucoepidermoid carcinoma found that patients with this translocation had better disease free survival (DFS) and overall survival (OS). However, the authors emphasize that the level of evidence is not as high once important limitations were found in the published studies (Pérez-de-Olivera et al. 2019).

It is thought that Warthin tumors arise from salivary duct remnants enclaved in lymph nodes during embryologic development and that irritation from tobacco smoke may cause these ducts to proliferate (Lamelas et al. 1987). There appears to be a link to heavy smoking and bilateral Warthin's tumors (Klussman et al. 2006). A recent study has linked obesity combined with increased BMI, and also comorbidities associated with metabolic syndrome to patients with Warthin tumor (Kadletz et al. 2019).

At present, data do not show any connection between cell phone use and increased risk of parotid tumors (Lonn et al. 2006). In one systematic review and meta-analysis, cell phone use did show greater odds, i.e. 1.28, to develop a salivary gland tumor. However, only three studies were included in the meta-analysis and they were retrospective in nature (de Siqueira et al. 2017).

There is a reported increase in other solid tumors, particularly breast cancer in conjunction with salivary malignancies (In der Maur et al. 2005). Overall, most salivary tumors show a predilection for females and there may be a link to estrogen.

Salivary gland tumors are rare, 1.5–2 per 100 000 in the United States, and they comprise approximately 3% of head and neck malignancies. The incidence of major salivary gland cancer may be rising. A SEER data study showed an increase from 10.4 per 1 000 000 in 1973 to 16 per 1 000 000 in 2009, an annual percentage change of 0.99. This study also found an increase in small parotid tumors and an increase in tumors with regional and distant disease (Del Signor and Megwalu 2017). In a SEER analysis of 2545 cases of squamous cell carcinoma of the parotid from 1973 to 2009, there was an increase in incidence over the three decades of 1.9% annually, $p < 0.05$ (Pfisterer et al. 2014).

Eighty percent of all salivary tumors are located in the parotid gland and of these tumors approximately 80% will be benign. The "rule of 80s" also states that 80% of parotid tumors are located in the superficial lobe and that 80% of these will be pleomorphic adenomas (PAs). There are publications that suggest a rise in incidence of Warthin tumor in the parotid gland, with more females, at a younger age and a higher incidence of multiple tumors (Franzen et al. 2018).

There may also be geographic variations in the demographics of parotid tumors with perhaps a lower involvement of the parotid in Chinese populations (62.7 and 65.4%). (Gao et al. 2017; Shen et al. 2018). In most series from China, the incidence of adenoid cystic carcinoma (ACC) is higher than that seen in Europe/United States. Some tumors such as polymorphous adenocarcinoma are comparatively rare in the Far East. Mucoepidermoid is the most common malignancy seen in the West; however, in large series from Brazil, ACC is found to be the commonest (58.3%) (Vascocelos et al. 2016). Polymorphous adenocarcinoma is comparatively much commoner in black patients in most Western series. As stated above, salivary tumors are more commonly seen in females and this is particularly true for polymorphous adenocarcinoma and epimyoepithelial carcinomas. It is not known why some salivary tumors have a predilection for certain salivary glands, e.g. acinic cell carcinoma in the parotid and canalicular adenoma and polymorphous adenocarcinoma in the minor glands of the oral cavity. Canalicular adenoma comprises <1% of salivary tumors yet it is the third commonest tumor in the oral cavity. In one systematic review of 430 cases, 66.3% were found in the upper lip (Peraza et al. 2017). This chapter will discuss the epithelial derived salivary tumors of the parotid.

Diagnosis

The diagnosis of a tumor of the parotid gland will be dependent upon the history, clinical examination, imaging, and fine needle aspiration biopsy (FNAB). In most cases, the history will be of a painless slow-growing lump that the patient had been aware of for some months or even years, and that was noticed initially when shaving, washing, or applying makeup. Occasionally, the patient will report a rapidly growing mass but this is not always a malignancy, as a long-standing benign retromandibular tumor that can no longer be accommodated in this space may have "popped out" and become prominent. Pain in a parotid mass is usually an ominous sign and can be an indication of adenoid cystic carcinoma. A history of facial nerve weakness, fixity or ulceration of the skin, or a mass in the neck are also signs of malignancy.

Clinical examination will begin with the cervical nodes and palpation of the parotid. The facial nerve and muscles of facial expression are tested and an intraoral examination of the soft palate and lateral pharynx is done to exclude deep lobe tumors extending into the parapharyngeal space. Parotid tumors will present as smooth sometimes lobulated, firm or hard nontender masses in the superficial lobe. Most are discrete and mobile. Fixation to the skin, ulceration, and deep muscle fixation are signs of malignancy. Facial nerve palsy and associated hard lymph nodes are also signs of parotid cancer. However, only 2.6–22% of parotid cancers will have VII nerve palsy (Ord 1995). Overall, 30% of malignancies are diagnosed on clinical features with palpable cervical nodes, facial nerve palsy, deep fixation, and rapid enlargement being significant signs (Wong 2001) (Figure 10.1). The majority of cancers histologically will present clinically as benign tumors.

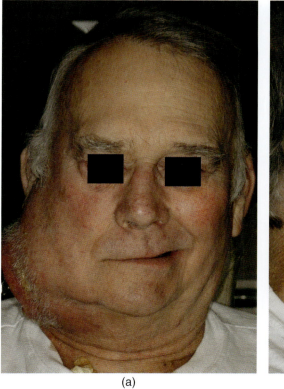
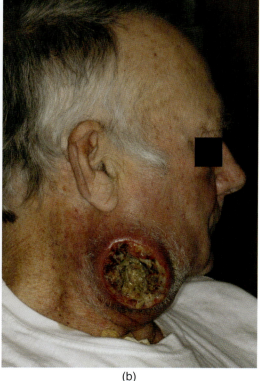

(a)   (b)

Figure 10.1. (a) A 67-year-old gentleman with a rapidly growing right parotid mass. Clinical examination shows facial nerve palsy and hard nodes palpable at levels II and III. (b) Side view shows necrotic ulceration through skin biopsy diagnosed a poorly differentiated carcinoma of the parotid.

The differential diagnosis of parotid tumor includes lesions arising outside the parotid as well as intraparotid masses. Skin lesions such as sebaceous or dermoid cysts are usually distinguished by their superficial origin in the overlying skin. Neoplasms of the masseter and masseteric hypertrophy will become fixed and more prominent on clenching the jaws. Condylar masses usually move with jaw opening and jaw lesions are usually bony hard to palpation. Intraparotid masses that mimic parotid tumors include enlarged parotid nodes and as these may be metastatic, clinical examination of the parotid mass should always include the ear and the scalp for skin cancers. Parotid cysts may be difficult to distinguish from common parotid tumors such as PAs and low-grade mucoepidermoid carcinoma that can present as fluctuant cysts. Tumors arising in the parotid tail may be mistaken for submandibular or neck masses (Figure 10.2) while those arising in the accessory gland may be thought to arise in the cheek itself (Figure 10.3).

In imaging the parotid, technetium scans may confirm a diagnosis of Warthin tumor or oncocytoma but are largely of historical interest. The same is true for sialography, which is no longer used for tumor diagnosis but is useful in diseases of the ductal system. Ultrasound (US) can distinguish cystic from solid masses and may be helpful to guide FNAB. As a diagnostic tool, it has a 72% sensitivity and 86% specificity for detecting malignant tumors (Schick et al. 1998). In the assessment of benign disease and pleomorphic adenomas, sensitivities of 80% and specificity of 86% with an accuracy of 84% are reported (Bialek et al. 2003; Bozzato et al. 2007). Although the use of shear wave elastography can differentiate malignant from benign tumors by its measurement of stiffness, it was not found to significantly improve the predictive power of the US blurred margin classifier (sensitivity 79% and specificity 97%) (Herman et al. 2017). A recent meta-analysis has shown sonoelstography to have limited value in distinguishing benign from malignant parotid tumors (Zhang et al. 2019).

However, CT scanning and MR are the imaging modalities of choice if the clinician feels the information gained is worth the financial cost. Little is added to the diagnosis when imaging tumors in the superficial lobes; however, imaging deep lobe tumors, particularly those with parapharyngeal extension, gives the surgeon useful information. Recent papers have claimed that high-resolution MR using a surface coil may allow imaging of the facial nerve and its relationship to the tumor (Takahashi et al. 2005). Other methods of predicting facial nerve position have been to use anatomic lines drawn on the images, such as the facial nerve line which connects the lateral surface of the posterior belly of the digastric muscle with the lateral surface of the cortical bone of the ascending ramus of the mandible and has been assessed as 88% accurate in determining the location of the tumor in relation to the nerve (Ariyoshi and Shimahara 1998). Another proposed guideline is the Utrecht line connecting the most dorsal point visible of C1 or C2 vertebra to the retromandibular vein (RMV) (de Ru et al. 2002). Magnetic resonance imaging may be helpful in distinguishing benign PAs from malignant tumors, by post-contrast enhancement, a higher T2 signal and lack of invasion (Figure 10.3). The use of diffusion weighted MRI may further improve the ability to distinguish benign from malignant tumors according to two systematic reviews (Liang et al. 2018; Munhoz et al. 2019). In the 2018 systematic review and meta-analysis of MR imaging techniques for parotid tumors, the data showed that MR combined with diffusion weighted imaging or dynamic contrast enhanced showed higher accuracy in diagnosis than conventional MR alone. Pooled analysis of combination treatment showed a sensitivity of 76% and specificity of 80% (Liang et al. 2018). However, Fee and Tran (2003) suggest that neither MR nor ultrasound is accurate enough to be routinely used in the workup of parotid masses and that careful history and examination are sufficient for most cases. This conclusion was echoed by de Ru et al. (2007), who concluded that MRI and palpation are almost equally accurate for assessing tumor location and both are superior to ultrasound. They recommend the use of FNAB as an accurate method of assessing whether a tumor is malignant, and MR only for tumors in the deep lobe or malignant tumors. PET scan and fused PET/CT images have so far not been shown to reliably differentiate between benign and malignant parotid tumors (Rubello et al. 2005), or benign, malignant, and metastatic parotid tumors (Kendi et al. 2016). In examining only malignant salivary tumors for staging and restaging, PET-CT was found to show no significant difference in accuracy between conventional imaging but was more specific, 73 vs. 43% (Sharma et al. 2013).

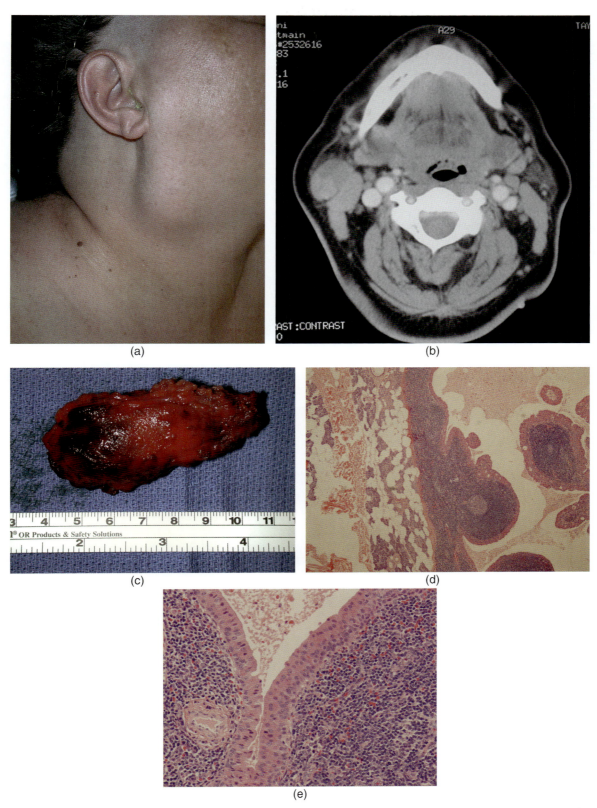

Figure 10.2. (a) A woman with a Warthin tumor in the parotid tail presenting as a neck mass. (b) CT scan confirms the mass is in the parotid tail. (c) Surgical specimen following partial parotidectomy of parotid tail with tumor (see also Figure 10.12). (d and e) Low- and high-power microscopic views of the specimen that identified a Warthin tumor.

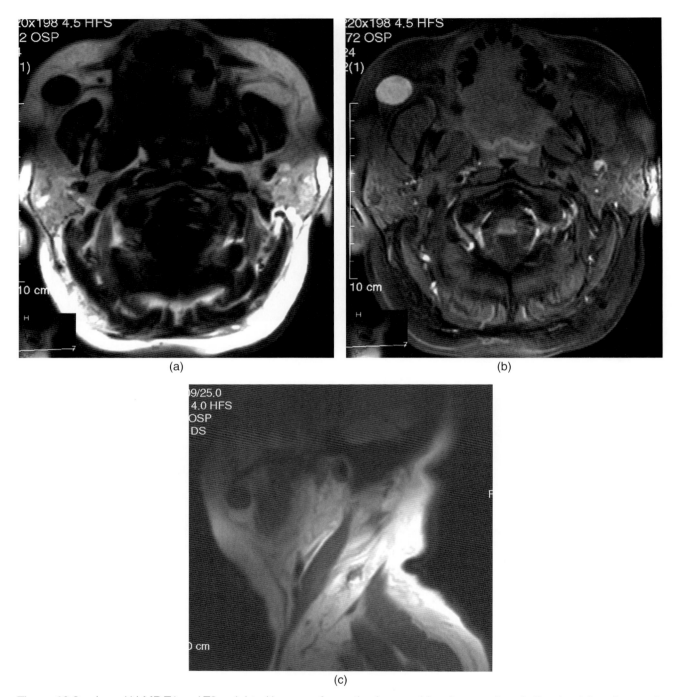

Figure 10.3. (a and b) MR T1 and T2 weighted images of a cystic pleomorphic adenoma deep in the cheek is a diagnostic challenge as to whether this is a minor salivary gland tumor or an accessory parotid tumor. (c) Clinically, this lesion appears to be inferior to the parotid duct as seen in the sagittal view, which would make an accessory lobe tumor unlikely.

FNAB may be utilized to give a preoperative cytologic diagnosis. Open biopsy is contraindicated as it will cause spillage and seeding of benign PAs and lead to increased recurrence (Figure 10.4). Although FNAB will not usually change the proposed treatment plan of parotidectomy, a malignant diagnosis may allow better pre-surgical counseling for possible facial nerve sacrifice. In

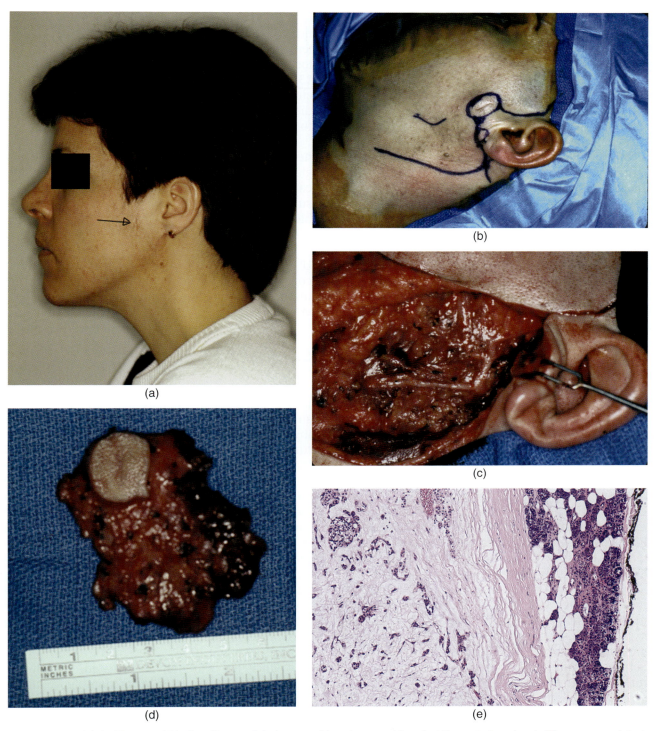

Figure 10.4. (a) A 45-year-old lady with parotid pleomorphic adenoma biopsied through the cheek. The arrow points to the biopsy scar. (b) Surgical incision marked out and includes a skin paddle 1 cm around the biopsy scar. (c) Following superficial parotidectomy with complete nerve dissection. (d) Surgical specimen of parotid with overlying skin. The patient is disease free 10+ years post-surgery. (e) Histopathology confirms the diagnosis of pleomorphic adenoma. Note the marked pseudocapsule of collagen.

addition, when extra-capsular dissection (ECD) or limited superficial parotidectomy is contemplated ("Benign Tumors" and "Pleomorphic Adenoma (PA)"), it is best to have confirmation of the benign nature of the tumor (O'Brien 2003). There is still controversy whether FNAB is mandatory as part of the diagnostic workup for a presumed parotid tumor. Although Schroder et al. (2000) report a sensitivity of 93.1%, specificity of 99.2%, and accuracy of 98.2%, other papers have shown lower figures, sensitivity 81.5% and specificity 97.5% (Longuet et al. 2001).

Zbären et al. (2001) recommended FNAB as a valuable adjunct to preoperative diagnosis, reporting 86% accuracy, 64% sensitivity, and 95% specificity. However, in a study of 6249 participant responses from the data base of the College of American Pathologists Inter-laboratory Comparison Program in Non-Gynecologic Cytology, the sensitivity and specificity for interpreting salivary tumors as benign or malignant were 73 and 91% respectively. Benign cases with the commonest false positive rates were monomorphic adenoma (53%) and intraparotid lymph node (36%). Malignant salivary gland tumors with the highest false negative rate were acinic cell carcinoma (49%), low-grade mucoepidermoid carcinoma (43%), and adenoid cystic carcinoma (33%). It was felt that the data confirmed the difficulty inherent in FNAB of salivary glands (Hughes et al. 2005). A paper from the Memorial Sloane Kettering Hospital concluded that a FNAB biopsy result positive for a malignant or neoplastic process is generally predictive of the final histologic diagnosis, whereas the predictive value of a negative FNAB is low (Cohen et al. 2004). In a study of 996 cases, sensitivity, specificity, and accuracy for malignancy were 82.3, 98.7, and 95.9%, respectively. However, in only 34% of cases did the diagnosis give the correct grade of the cancer (Suzuki et al. 2019). Combining FNAB with ultrasound guidance can improve accuracy and diagnostic yield especially in difficult tumors such as carcinoma ex pleomorphic adenoma where sampling error is a problem. In the diagnosis of pleomorphic adenomas with ultrasound-guided FNAB, sensitivities of 97% and specificity of 98% were published (Carrilo et al. 2009).

An alternative to fine needle biopsy is the ultrasound-guided core needle biopsy, which allows evaluation of tumor architecture as well as cytology. A 2019 systematic review (Kim and Kim 2018) showed a sensitivity of 0.94 and a specificity of 0.98. There were seven hematomas, one temporary facial nerve paralysis caused by the local anesthetic, and zero tumor seeding in the 1315 procedures performed. The authors concluded that core needle biopsy was an excellent diagnostic tool in terms of accuracy, technical performance, and safety.

In a comparative study of 228 US-guided core needle biopsies vs. 371 FNAC of major salivary gland tumors, the core needle biopsy gave significantly higher sensitivity and greater accuracy of sub-typing. The improved results for core needle biopsy were more marked in cases of malignancy (Song et al. 2015). Very similar results were found in another study of 155 US-guided FNAB vs. 257 US-guided core biopsy. The authors suggest that core needle biopsy could emerge as the diagnostic method of choice for a salivary gland mass (Eom et al. 2015).

Surgical Management

The basic surgical procedure for superficial lobe tumors is the superficial parotidectomy in which the superficial lobe of the parotid is removed, preserving the facial nerve unless it is directly infiltrated by tumor. The author's usual incision is the modified Blair or "lazy S." The skin flap is elevated in a plane through the subcutaneous fat superficial to the parotid capsule (Figure 10.5). Recently, the use of a face lift incision has been advocated to improve esthetic results of the scar (Honig 2005; Meningaud et al. 2006). These authors have also combined face lift incisions with a separate SMAS (superficial musculo-aponeurosis) dissection to eliminate hollowing and reduce Frey syndrome. Concerns regarding access to anteriorly sited tumors when using a face lift approach for parotidectomy do not appear to be borne out in anatomic studies (Nouraei et al. 2006), (Figures 10.6 and 10.7).

Once the skin flap is elevated, the sternocleidomastoid muscle (SCM) is identified with the overlying greater auricular nerve whose posterior branch to the earlobe may be preserved if it does not compromise tumor resection (Figure 10.5e). This will retain sensation in the ear lobe skin (Grosheva et al. 2017). The anterior border of the SCM is dissected free of the posterior parotid gland, which is retracted anteriorly. Deeper dissection at the superior end of the SCM will allow

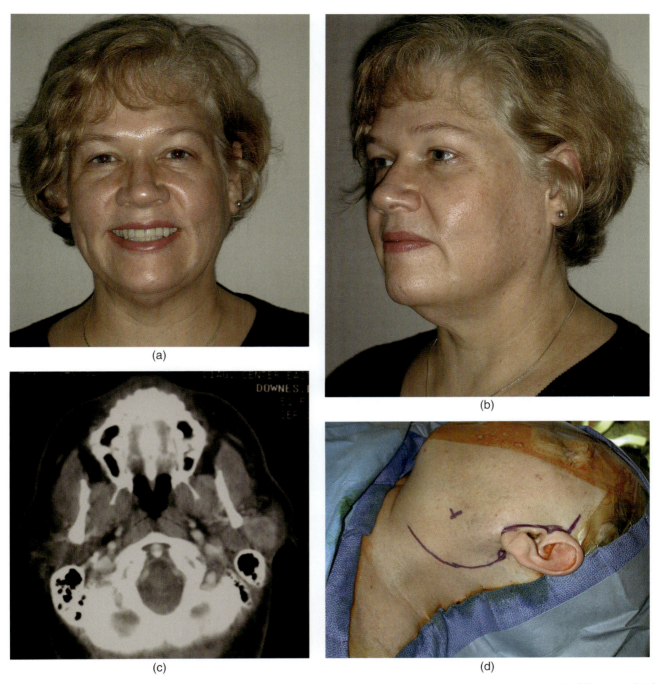

Figure 10.5. (a and b) Patient with pleomorphic adenoma of the left parotid gland preoperatively. (c) CT scan of left parotid showing superficial lobe tumor. (d) Modified Blair incision. (e) Skin flap raised, the instrument indicated the sensory branch of the greater auricular nerve to the ear, which was preserved in this case. (f) The parotidectomy has been commenced from inferiorly and the superficial lobe is being retracted superiorly. The arrow indicates the deep surface of the tumor which was adjacent to the nerve bifurcation and has no normal parotid tissue covering the tumor capsule. (g) Surgical specimen, the tumor is seen superiorly with no good surrounding "cuff" of tissue. (h) The surgical site postparotidectomy with complete dissection of the facial nerve. (i) A free abdominal fat graft is placed to reduce "hollowing" which was a concern of the patient. (j and k) Appearance of patient six month post surgery.

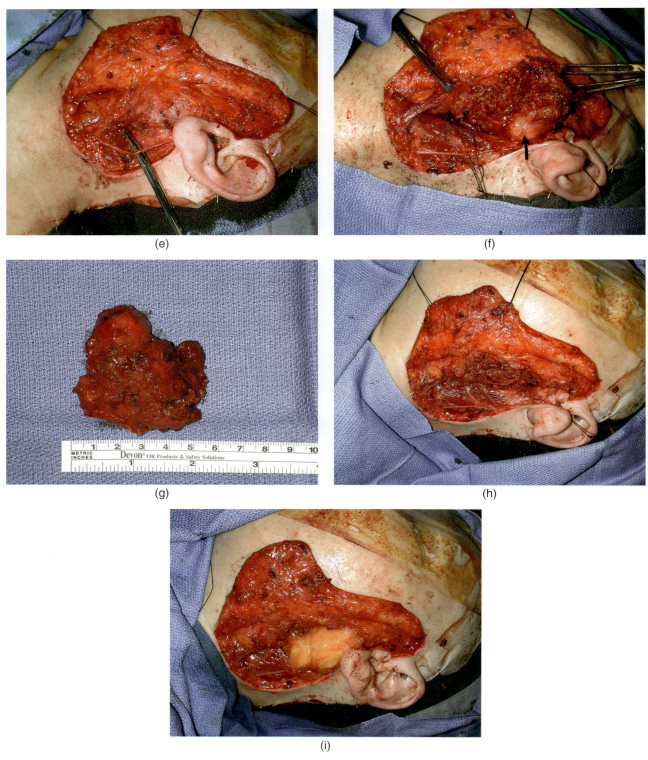

Figure 10.5. (*Continued*).

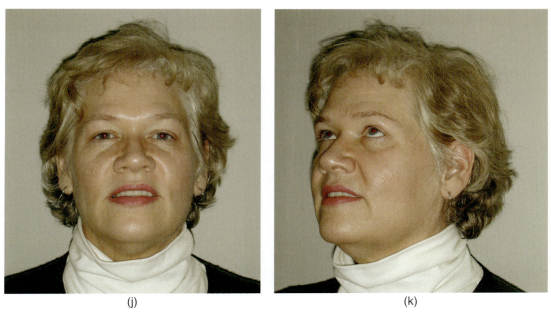

Figure 10.5. (*Continued*).

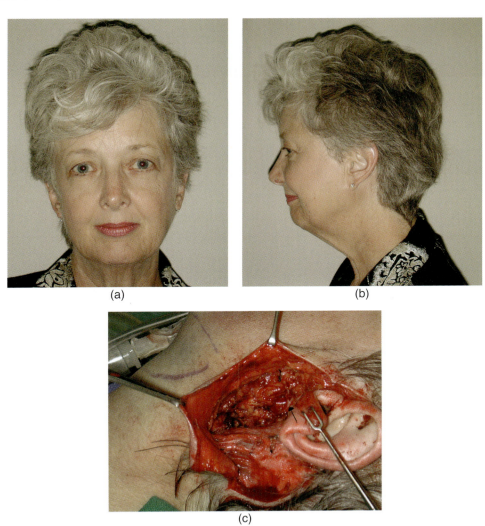

Figure 10.6. (a and b) Post surgery facial views of patient with left parotid pleomorphic adenoma. Patient requests bilateral face lift at the same time as parotidectomy. (c) Surgical access through face lift incision running into occipital hair line. Arrow shows facial nerve trunk being dissected. (d and e) Six months postoperative notice absence of neck incision. Source: Esthetic portions of this case undertaken by Dr. A Pazoki DDS MD.

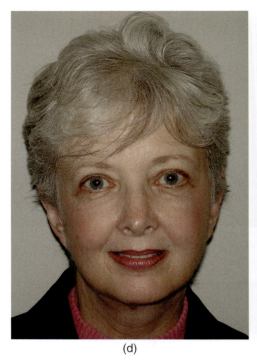
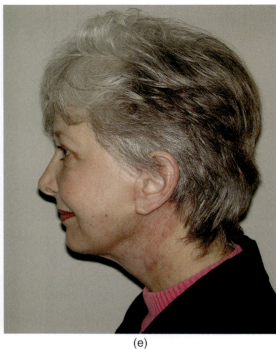

(d) (e)

Figure 10.6. (*Continued*).

identification of the posterior belly of the digastric muscle. The facial nerve trunk lies 4 mm superior to the digastric and at the same depth and this muscle is an important landmark (Figure 10.8). Next, attention is turned to the preauricular region with sharp and blunt dissection down the cartilage of the external auditory meatus to the bony portion of the meatus. A strip of parotid tissue remains which separates the cervical from the preauricular dissection and this tissue is carefully dissected away to the depth of the digastric muscle. Some troublesome bleeding must be controlled with bipolar diathermy under direct vision superficial to where the facial nerve will be identified. The facial nerve trunk can be confirmed with a nerve stimulator and the nerve branches are dissected out peripherally to mobilize and remove the superficial parotid. It is important to keep the dissection superficial to the nerve. The author uses a fine‐mosquitos on top of the nerve spreading the tines to stretch the overlying glandular salivary tissues. Bipolar forceps are used to nibble carefully through the stretched salivary tissue and mobilize the superficial lobe safely.

Intraoperative facial nerve monitoring has been advocated to prevent postoperative facial nerve weakness. A recent systematic review and meta‐analysis have shown the risk of immediate postoperative weakness to be reduced but the long‐term outcome shows no significant difference (Sood et al. 2015). It is usually best to dissect either the frontal or mandibular branches first depending on the site of the tumor and then proceed stepwise inferiorly or superiorly dissecting the branches in order while staying superficial to the nerves.

If the tumor directly overlies the facial nerve trunk, making it impossible to access safely, then the peripheral branches can be identified and followed proximally as a retrograde parotidectomy although the author finds this is more tedious. The mandibular branch of the facial nerve where it crosses the anterior facial vein or the buccal branch with its close relationship to the parotid duct (Pogrel et al. 1996) can be identified initially. Despite a 66% incidence of weakness one‐week post parotidectomy, normal facial nerve function was present in 99% of 136 retrograde parotidectomies in one series (O'Regan et al. 2007). In a recent systematic review and meta‐analysis, the retrograde approach was found to be safe with no significant difference in facial nerve palsy rates compared to the standard antegrade approach. The

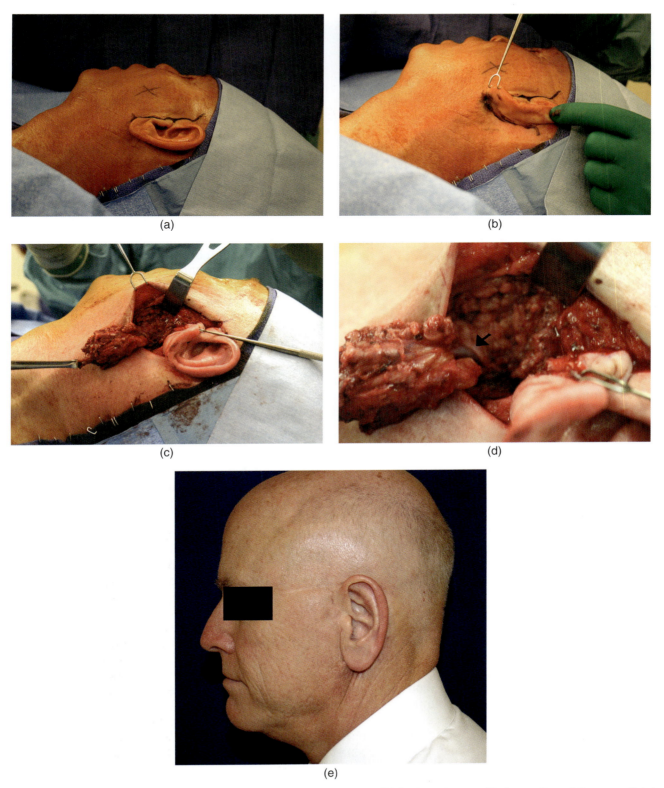

Figure 10.7. (a) Omega incision preauricular limb used to access a PA in the retromandibular portion of the superficial lobe of the parotid. (b) Postauricular limb of the omega incision runs in the postauricular sulcus. (c) Partial parotidectomy of the retromandibular portion of the superficial lobe is almost completed. (d) Arrow points to the cervical-mandibular trunk of the facial nerve as it crosses the retromandibular vein superficially. The rest of the branches of the facial nerve did not require dissection. (e) Three months postoperatively, there is no visible scar.

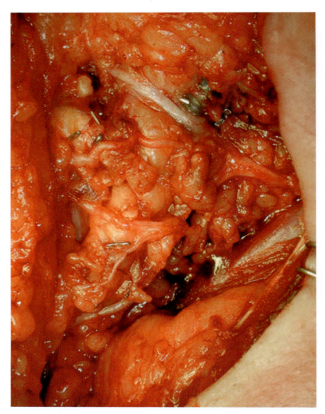

Figure 10.8. Facial nerve trunk 4 mm superior to and at the same depth as the upper border of the posterior belly of the digastric muscle.

authors found the procedure to have a shorter operating time and to require less dissection of healthy tissue (Stankovic et al. 2018).

In tumors of the deep lobe, it is usually necessary to undertake a total parotidectomy. The superficial parotidectomy is performed preserving the facial nerve and dissecting the superficial lobe from superiorly so that it remains attached to the deep lobe inferiorly and at the tail. Most deep lobe tumors will be retromandibular and lie inferior to the trunk of the nerve. The space inferiorly is larger, and by gentle retraction and dissection of the nerve trunk and its branches it can be mobilized off the tumor. Then, with blunt dissection around the tumor, the deep lobe in‐continuity with the superficial lobe can usually be delivered into the neck. It is important to remember that deep lobe tumors are not defined by their position within the parotid gland but by their relationship to the facial nerve. A tumor may clinically look to be in the superficial lobe but be located on the masseter muscle deep to the branches of the facial nerve (Figure 10.9).

In larger tumors, the neoplasm may be impacted between the mandible and the mastoid with no means of mobilizing it without either dislocating the mandible forward or a sub‐sigmoid or "C" osteotomy to give more space. As contemporary surgery has evolved, more emphasis has been placed on reducing morbidity. Deep lobe tumors may be removed without removing the superficial lobe but leaving it attached anteriorly and then replacing it after excising the deep lobe tumor (Coleela et al. 2007). This technique preserves facial contour and 84% of glandular function compared to the contralateral parotid.

In those tumors with parapharyngeal extension, blind finger enucleation may lead to capsular rupture or cause brisk hemorrhage. In order to visualize and safely remove these tumors, an osteotomy of the mandible with or without lip split is utilized (Kolokythas et al. 2007) (Figures 10.10 and 10.11).

The accessory parotid gland (APG) is closely related to the Stensen duct as it curves deep to the anterior border of the masseter muscle. It is present in 21–65% of patients (Frommer 1977; Toh et al. 1993) and tumors in this gland, which are rare, will present as a cheek mass anterior to the main parotid, and may be thought erroneously to be arising in the buccal minor salivary glands. It is important to differentiate between these two as an intraoral approach may be hazardous for accessory lobe tumors due to the vicinity of buccal branches of the facial nerve and a higher propensity for malignant neoplasm in the accessory gland (Yang et al. 2011). An endoscopically assisted transoral approach has been suggested for these tumors, but these are case reports (Woo 2016; Mani et al. 2019).

In one recent review of 152 cases of accessory parotid gland tumors, 30% were found to be malignant (Newberry et al. 2014). A review of 130 patients presenting with a mass in the APG showed 29 (22.4%) to have non‐neoplastic lesions, (vascular malformations, sialadenitis, or cysts). Thirty one of the hundred and one patients with tumors had malignancies (30.7%) (Ma et al. 2018). A review of 65 cases in the Japanese literature showed 44.6% malignant, commonest being MECA, and 55.4% benign, most commonly PA (Iguchi et al. 2013). In another small series, the malignancy rate was 38.5% with MECA most

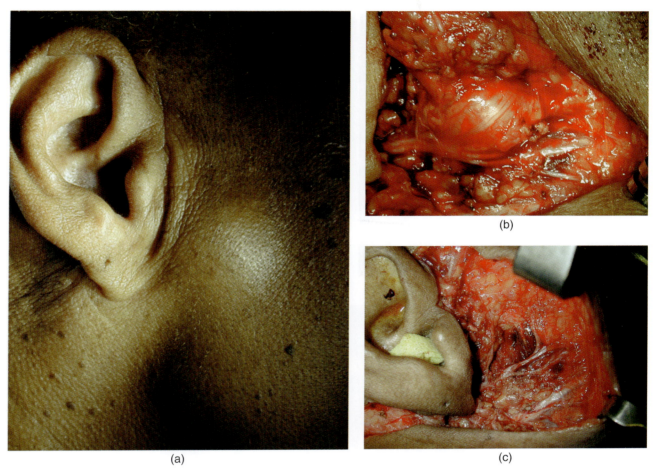

Figure 10.9. (a) A 67-year-old African-American lady with a preauricular swelling, clinically diagnosed as a superficial lobe tumor. (b) The intraoperative view shows the superficial parotidectomy is completed and the superficial lobe is retracted superiorly. The tumor lies deep to the upper branches (buccal and temporal) of the facial nerve. The cervical-mandibular trunk is passing inferior to the tumor. (c) The facial nerve trunk has been mobilized off the tumor, which was lying on the masseter muscle deeply. The masseter can be seen beneath the buccal and temporal branch. Source: This patient was treated under the care of Dr. Andrew Salama DDS, MD. Case by permission of Dr. Salama.

common. The commonest benign tumor was PA (Luskic et al. 2019). In a review of 43 malignancies in the accessory parotid, the commonest cancer was mucoepidermoid carcinoma. Temporary facial paralysis was seen postoperatively in 11 (25.6%) and this was permanent in 3 (7%). Five-year disease specific survival (DSS) was 86% and 10-year DSS 66%. Tumor stage, N stage, neck dissection, and tumor grade were significantly associated with disease-related death but only tumor grade was an independent risk factor (Han et al. 2018).

It is the author's practice to use an extended parotidectomy approach tracing the buccal nerves distally to protect them (Figure 10.12). The commonest pattern seen for the facial nerve is two buccal branches superior to the duct and one inferior, lying at 1 cm distance on average (Tsai et al. 2019). A series of 13 cases of APG benign tumors removed endoscopically through a tragal approach without complications has been published (Zhang et al. 2015).

There is currently a controversy between surgeons regarding superficial parotidectomy or extracapsular dissection. This important topic will be discussed in the section "Pleomorphic Adenoma" as well as in Chapter 19.

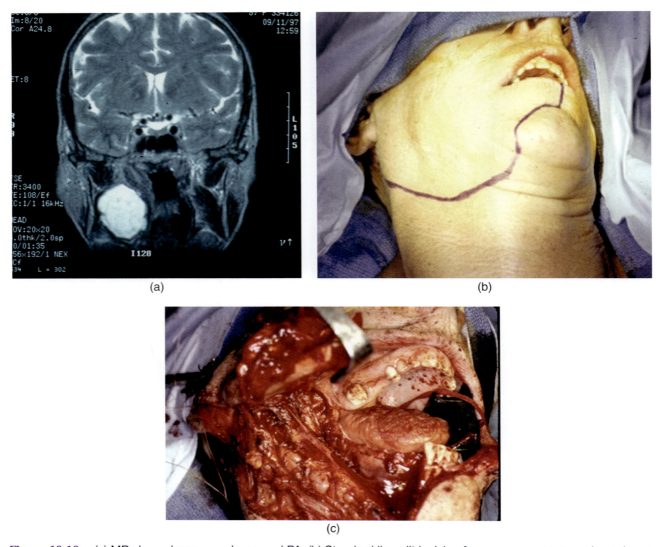

Figure 10.10. (a) MR shows large parapharyngeal PA. (b) Standard lip split incision for an access parasymphyseal mandibulotomy. (c) Mandible is retracted out of the field and the PA is dissected preserving the overlying lingual nerve.

BENIGN TUMORS

Pleomorphic Adenoma (PA)

The PA is the commonest benign salivary gland tumor and the commonest salivary tumor overall, with 80% found in the parotid gland. PA is comparatively rare in young children, and is less frequent in the parotid (25/41 cases, 61%) (Dombrowski et al. 2019), and 63% (Xu et al. 2017) It is slow-growing and can reach giant proportions if neglected, and there is a 2–4% malignant change. PA will recur if the tumor is inadequately removed. Although PAs have a pseudocapsule of compressed fibrous tissue, the buds and pseudopodia from the tumor involve the capsule so that simple enucleation will leave tumor remnants and lead to multifocal recurrence. The concept of whether the capsule is incomplete and whether pseudopodia of tumor involve the parotid tissue is currently being questioned and with it the need for complete superficial parotidectomy. Although parotidectomy is supposed to remove PAs with a cuff or margin of normal tissue to prevent recurrence, the tumor's proximity to the facial nerve frequently means that the dissection at some points leaves no tissue around the capsule. Donovan and Conley's landmark publication in 1984 emphasized that proximity of the tumor to the facial nerve meant that

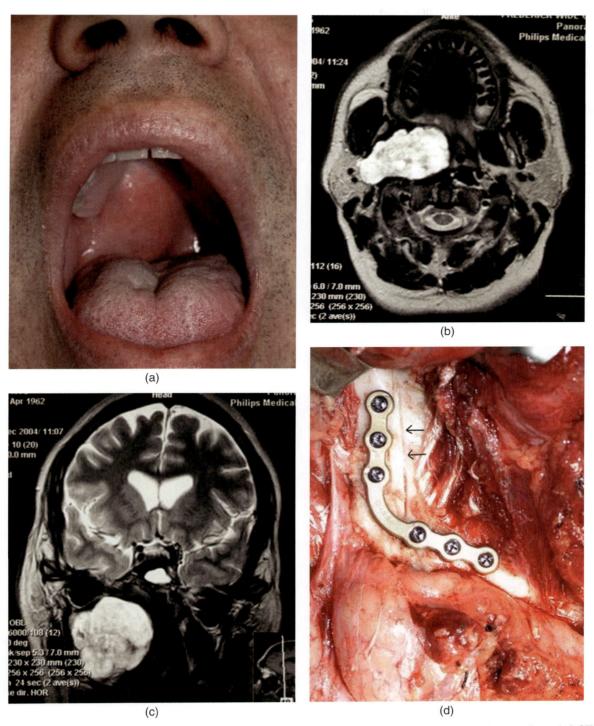

Figure 10.11. (a) Deep lobe parotid tumor with parapharyngeal extension presenting as a palatal mass. (b and c) CT axial and coronal scans show the tumor in the lateral pharyngeal space. (d) The mandible is accessed via a cervical incision from mastoid to chin without lip split. Sub-sigmoid osteotomy cut marked with saw through buccal cortex only (arrows) and plate has been applied prior to completing the osteotomy. (e) Osteotomy marked with a saw through the buccal cortex (long arrow) anterior to the mental nerve (short arrow). Two miniplates applied prior to completing the osteotomy. (f) The plates are removed and the double osteotomy is completed and the osteotomized hemimandible retracted upward and rotated to expose the lateral pharyngeal space and the tumor is being delivered under direct vision. (g) The final specimen which was PA seen in relation to the mandible. (h) The post-resection tumor bed. The plates are reapplied to reconstruct the original position and occlusion for the mandible.

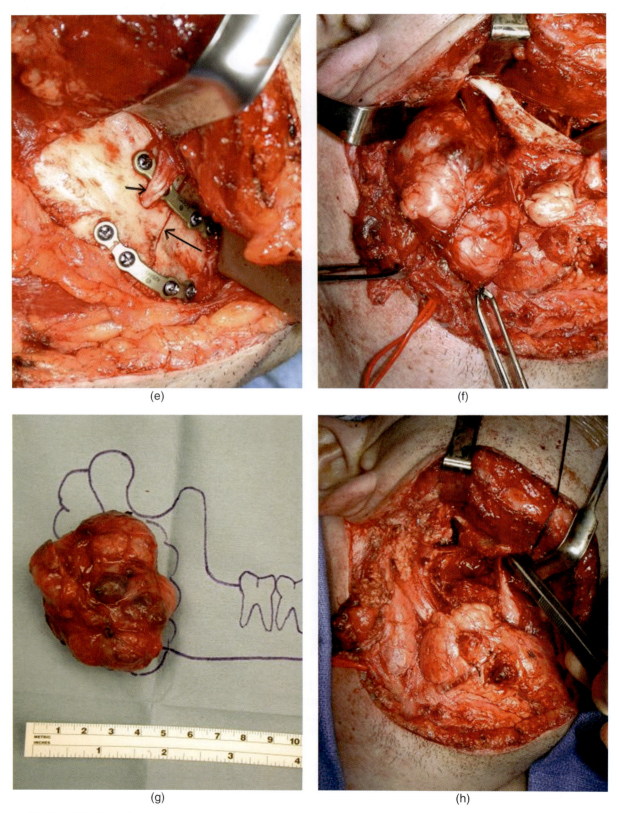

Figure 10.11. (*Continued*).

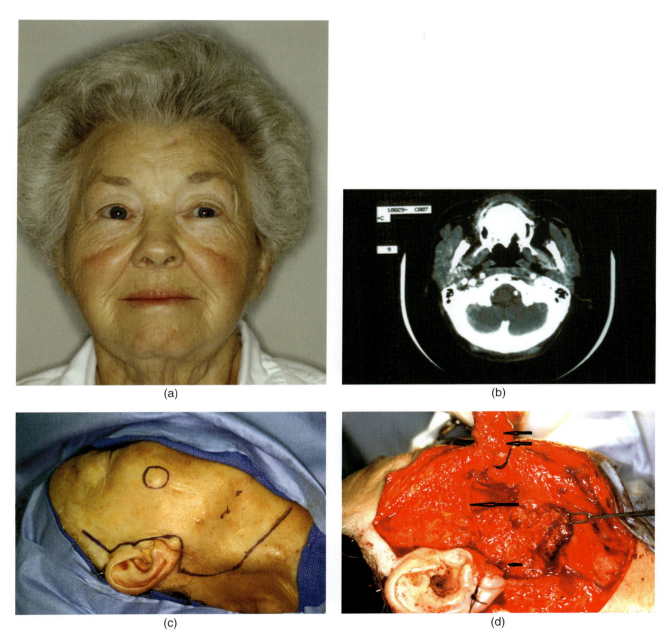

Figure 10.12. (a) Female patient with fullness and mass in anterior right cheek. (b) Axial CT shows a mass in the accessory parotid gland. (c) Proposed extended Blair incision to allow access anteriorly. (d) Intraoperative view shows facial nerve trunk (small arrow), and by dissecting the facial nerve branches anteriorly a strip of superficial parotid has been elevated along with the accessory parotid gland and tumor (indicated by the double arrow). The buccal branches are preserved and the long single arrow shows the superior buccal branch.

limited enucleation or capsular dissection was involved in 60% of their "parotidectomies" (Donovan and Conley 1984). In a recent histologic analysis of the capsular form in PAs, 81% showed capsular exposure following parotidectomy or submandibular gland excision (Webb and Eveson 2001) (Figure 10.13). This paper also showed 57% bosselations, 33% enveloping of the capsule, with 42% microinvasion and 12% "tumor buds" in the capsule; and large >25 mm

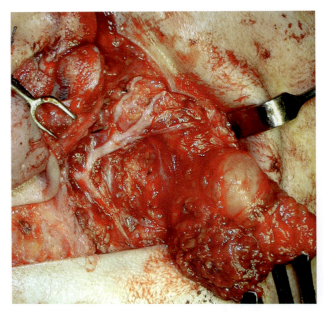

Figure 10.13. The superficial parotidectomy is completed and the superficial lobe is retracted anteriorly and inferiorly. The PA is seen projecting from the deep surface of the superficial lobe with only a thin transparent capsule around its deep surface. The upper and lower trunks of the facial nerve have been spread widely apart by the slowly growing mass and were intimately associated with the PA. There is a concave cavity where the tumor was lying directly on the underlying masseter.

hypocellular tumors had thinner capsules possibly easier to rupture at surgery. This article suggested that a minimum of 1 mm of normal tissue around PA was required as a margin. However, in an article reviewing 475 PAs of the superficial lobe of the parotid, 380 treated by extra-capsular dissection and 95 by superficial parotidectomy, there was no difference in recurrence rate or permanent facial nerve palsy (McGurk et al. 1996). These surgeons postulated that tumor buds or microinvasion into the capsule had little significance and that extra-capsular dissection could be done safely. Witt in a later paper confirmed that capsular exposure occurred in virtually all types of parotid surgery, and could find no difference in recurrence, capsular rupture, tumor–facial nerve interface, and permanent facial palsy between total parotidectomy, superficial parotidectomy, and extra-capsular dissection. However, he recommended against minimum margin resection in extra-capsular dissection (Witt 2002). Further evidence for extra-capsular dissection is provided by a series of 83 cases in which the overall recurrence rate was 6%, but 17.6% when tumor itself was at the margins; however, cases with margins of < 1 mm had a recurrence of only 1.8% (Ghosh et al. 2003). They also reported that microscopic invasion of the capsule had no influence on recurrence, suggesting that a fraction of a millimeter of normal tissue was an adequate margin and that only tumors that actually involved the margin were at risk for recurrence. These authors recommend that preservation of vital structures is a more important consideration than preserving a cuff of normal tissue.

In contrast, Piekarski et al. (2004) found a recurrence rate of 8.2% and an unacceptable rate of complications with extra-capsular dissection (ECD) and did not recommend the technique as too "technically demanding." In a separate publication with 213 patients who were operated for pleomorphic adenoma of the parotid, five of nine primary tumors (56%), which recurred, were found to have pseudopodia extending outside the capsule on histologic review. This was statistically higher than the examined cases that did not recur (8%) and the authors concluded that pseudopodia extending outside the capsule were a significant risk for recurrence (Henriksson et al. 1998). A further cautionary note is raised by the histologic analysis of (Zbären and Stauffer 2007) in which 160 of 218 (73%) of PAs were found to have adverse capsular characteristics, 33% with an incomplete capsule and 13% with satellite nodules. These were most frequently seen in the stroma-rich myxoid subtype. Similar findings with stroma-rich PAs showing 71% of focal absence of a capsule and 33% of satellite nodules have been reported with recommendations against local dissection (Stennert et al. 2004).

It does not appear that extra-capsular dissection is just a "euphemism for enucleation" as some have claimed as recurrence rates are comparable to standard parotidectomy and most papers show lower morbidity. The exact margin required for complete removal of PA remains controversial. A criticism of extra-capsular dissection has been that even if this technique is suitable for a presumed benign PA, what should the surgeon do if the final histopathologic diagnosis turns out to be malignant? In a review of 662 clinically benign parotid tumors, 503 treated by extra-capsular dissection and 159 by superficial parotidectomy, 5% were malignant and there was no difference in 5- or 10-year survival or recurrence rates between the malignant tumors in the two surgical groups, although morbidity was significantly lower in the extra-capsular dissection group (McGurk et al. 2003).

The current evidence is not conclusive but two large meta-analyses published recently comparing ECD to superficial parotidectomy for benign tumors have both concluded that ECD is a viable treatment option. In 2012, Albergotti et al. performed a meta-analysis on nine studies (1882 patients), and found no significant difference between the ECD and parotidectomy groups in terms of recurrence. There was a significantly lower transient facial nerve paresis but not for permanent palsy, and less Frey's syndrome in the ECD cohort. In 2014, Foresta et al. reviewed 1152 articles and 123 studies were included in their meta-analysis. Their conclusions were very similar to the previous analysis with parotidectomy having a higher recurrence rate, incidence of facial nerve paralysis and Frey syndrome. Their conclusion was that ECD was a good surgical treatment for benign parotid tumors < 4 cm in the superficial lobe with no facial nerve involvement.

Despite these studies, it should be noted that Witt and Rejto in a 38-year Ovid Medline search (1970–2008) with statistical analysis demonstrated the complete opposite results. These authors concluded that ECD had a significantly higher recurrence rate and permanent facial nerve palsy than parotidectomy. These findings were echoed in a study of 849 parotidectomies, 55.8% treated with superficial parotidectomy and 44.2% with ECD. In this paper, there were significantly higher rates of facial palsy, positive margins and recurrence for the ECD cohort (Kadletz et al. 2017). The latest systematic review published concluded that ECD shows a trend for reduced risk of complications but not sufficient to establish that ECD is more beneficial than partial superficial parotidectomy (Lin et al. 2019). The current evidence base indicates that ECD has a place in the surgical management of smaller benign superficial lobe tumors of the parotid; however, it is not a procedure for the inexperienced parotid surgeon.

A superficial lobe parotid tumor clinically benign and diagnosed as a PA on FNAB may also be treated with a limited superficial parotidectomy (without complete dissection of the facial nerve), or removal of the entire parotid lobe, and may not require a complete superficial parotidectomy for cure (O'Brien 2003). This is probably most commonly undertaken for tumors in the parotid tail. In 1999, a series of 59 partial parotidectomies with selective nerve dissection for benign and low-grade malignant tumors reported a zero incidence of permanent facial nerve paralysis or paresis and zero recurrence (Witt 1999). In a recent review, Zbären et al. (2013) concluded that formal parotidectomy is not mandatory, and that ECD in the hands of a novice/occasional parotid surgeon may result in higher recurrence. These authors recommend partial superficial parotidectomy as removing a better cuff than ECD to minimize recurrence but less healthy tissue than formal parotidectomy, thus reducing complications (Zbären et al. 2013) (Figure 10.14).

Deep lobe PAs are usually larger and frequently will have less surrounding parotid tissue, especially deeply where they lie against the prevertebral muscles of the neck. Also, the overlying facial nerve will be stretched over their surface often with no intervening glandular tissue. The dissection of the nerve at this point will be capsular at best (see Figure 10.9). However, the inability to obtain a surrounding cuff of parotid does not seem to lead to increased recurrence. Harney et al. (2003) found that the capsules of deep lobe tumors were significantly thicker and that there was less extra-capsular extension of tumor in the deep lobe tumors (58% vs. 79%), which may explain this phenomenon. There are numerous factors that have been postulated as increasing the incidence of recurrence for PA. Rupture of the tumor during its removal is frequently quoted as a major cause. If the capsule of the tumor is ruptured during surgery, then recurrence is not inevitable and perhaps liberal irrigation with sterile water followed by normal saline may be tumoricidal (Webb and Eveson 2001). However, Ghosh et al. (2003) reported that intraoperative capsular rupture does not influence recurrence. In an earlier published study of 213 PA of the parotid, only 2 of 28 cases that ruptured during surgical removal recurred (7.1%), which was not significantly different to the 4.1% recurrence rate for the tumors that had no rupture (Henriksson et al. 1998).

Demographically, numerous authors have noted that PA recurrence is more frequent in younger patients (Abu-Ghanem et al. 2016; Espinosa et al. 2018; Kantas et al. 2018). In the series reported by Aro et al. (2019), a median age of 33.5 years for recurrent PA was found, with 87% occurring in the parotid.

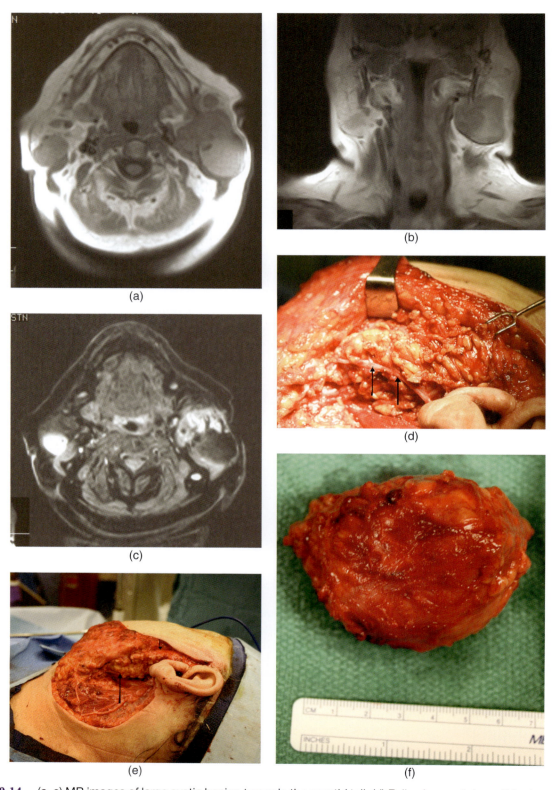

Figure 10.14. (a–c) MR images of large cystic benign tumor in the parotid tail. (d) Following partial parotidectomy, the two arrows point to the dissected cervical-mandibular branch of the facial nerve. The parotid tail tumor has been resected inferior to this nerve branch. The upper branches of the facial nerve have not been dissected in this case. (e) The long arrow points to the resected parotid tail region while the shorter arrow points to the remaining superficial parotid lobe preserved intact. (f) Surgical specimen.

The type of initial surgery is an extremely important cofactor. Both treatment by enucleation and initial surgery with positive margins have been shown to increase the rate of recurrence (Witt and Rejto 2009; Aro et al. 2019). In one series, recurrence following enucleation was 88.9% vs. 4% after superficial parotidectomy and 0% after total parotidectomy (Causevic Vucak and Masic 2014). A recurrence rate of 78.6% following enucleation versus 6% post-superficial parotidectomy with a 49 times risk of recurrence in patients with positive margins (p = 0.001) was reported by Espinosa et al. (2018). It is also important to recognize that initial recurrence is frequently followed by further multiple recurrences in 18–30% of cases (Leonetti et al. 2005; Zbären et al. 2005a; Andreasen et al. 2016; Aro et al. 2019). Additionally, in all series, there was an increase in multifocal disease in up to 73% of cases (Zbären et al. 2005a) and the rate of malignant change was between 3.3 and 9%.

It is difficult to judge the true rate of recurrence of PA from the literature, as long follow-up is necessary. Reoccurrence is seen after at least 10 years following parotid surgery in 16% of cases (range 6.1–11.8 years) (Douville and Bradford 2013). Finally, there has been work to show that hHTH1 may be upregulated in patients who develop recurrent PA (Xu et al. 2018).

As recurrent PA is frequently multinodular and multifocal (Figures 10.15 and 10.16), it requires a more radical en bloc surgery with excision of the previous scar, muscle, overlying skin, and facial nerve if they are involved. Maxwell et al. (2004) in a retrospective study of 35 patients treated with surgery alone found a locoregional control of 77% with a malignant transformation of 5.7%. In a separate study of 42 cases of multinodular recurrence (6 with prior radiation), there were 2 patients with malignant transformation who died of distant metastases. A total of 12 patients had subtotal parotidectomy, 25 total parotidectomy, 5 subtotal petrosectomy, and 14 facial nerve resection. A total of 7 patients of 36 who were followed developed further recurrences (19.4%), all of whom had only undergone subtotal parotidectomy (Leonetti et al. 2005). In a further series of 33 patients 73% with multifocal disease, 9% with malignant transformation, treated surgically; 6 (18%) recurred at an average of 9 years, and 23% of patients with initial enucleation and 14% with initial superficial parotidectomy had permanent partial facial nerve injury (Zbären et al. 2005a). Because of the

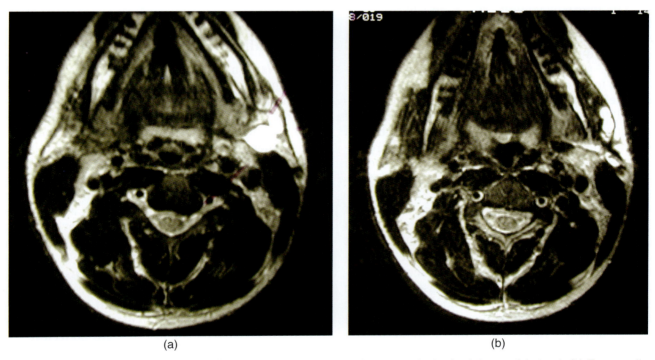

(a) (b)

Figure 10.15. (a) Two large nodules of recurrent pleomorphic adenoma exist in the left parotid gland. (b) Two smaller nodules are seen in the parotid tail.

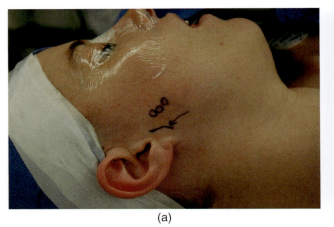 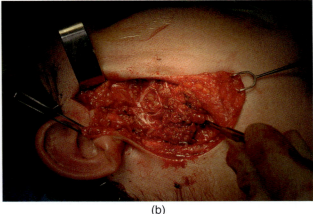

Figure 10.16. (a) A 20-year-old lady who previously had a "cyst" enucleated now presents with multinodular recurrence of pleomorphic adenoma in the superficial parotid. The surgical marking pen delineated three palpable nodules and arrow points to the 1.5 cm incision in front of the earlobe used for the original surgery. (b) Surgery consists of parotidectomy with excision of the previous skin incision. The superficial lobe is being retracted inferiorly. The pickups point to one of the tumor nodules.

scarring and multifocal nature of recurrent PA, the incidence of facial nerve palsy is high at 8.3% (Causevic Vucak and Masic 2014) to 9% (Abu-Ghanem et al. 2016). When the facial nerve cannot be identified, only one-third are preserved, and even when it is identified, only two-thirds are preserved intact according to a Japanese study (Kuriyama et al. 2019). The Danish National Study showed that the risk of facial nerve palsy increased significantly with the number of surgeries recurrences. An OR of 1.86–2.19 was found after the second-fourth surgeries. Overall 63% of patients reported no facial dysfunction (Nøhr et al. 2016).

Renehan et al. (1996) reviewed 144 cases of recurrent PA and suggested a role for radiation in multinodular cases. One paper of 34 cases of recurrent PA with radiation therapy post-gross resection shows a 20-year actuarial control rate of 94% (Chen et al. 2006). Another study of 21 cases, 81% with positive margins and 19% close margins (4 cases were recurrent PA), had a 90% locoregional control at a median follow-up of 92 months. In this cohort, 52% had grade 1 and 19% grade 2 toxicities (Patel et al. 2014). There is one recent systematic review of 8 studies with 366 cases. Only two studies showed a benefit in reduction in recurrence for postoperative radiation therapy (PORT) although four others did show a trend toward lower rates of recurrence. The authors concluded that the evidence suggested adjuvant radiation therapy reduced recurrent rates in recurrent PA without significant adverse effect. They recommended careful use of postoperative radiation therapy (PORT) in patients at high risk of further recurrence, but emphasized the need for further research with well-designed prospective trials (McLoughlin et al. 2019).

WARTHIN TUMOR

The Warthin tumor is the second commonest benign tumor of the parotid. Initially found primarily in males, the incidence has increased in females from 21% in 1952–1962 to 39% in 1983–1992. A smoking history is found in 88% of men and 89% of women (Yoo et al. 1994). As discussed at the beginning of this chapter, it is likely that these tumors arise from salivary gland inclusions trapped in the lymph nodes during development. Because the parotid glands are encapsulated at a later stage than the other major glands, after the development of the lymphoid tissues, lymph tissue is found in the salivary parenchyma and lymph nodes are intraglandular only in the parotid (Goldenberg et al. 2000). In a study of nine cases of parotid Hodgkin lymphoma, eight were in parotid nodes and only one in the parenchyma. Intranodal acinar and ductal salivary inclusions were noticed in six out of eight cases (four out of five in nodular lymphocyte-predominant Hodgkin lymphoma and two out of three classical Hodgkin lymphoma). These inclusions showed proliferation which ranged from lymphoepithelial lesions to Warthin-like (oncocytic) histologically. The authors postulated that entrapment of these proliferating salivary inclusions could mimic Warthin tumor arising in the lymphoma (Agaimy et al. 2015). Case reports of Warthin tumor occurring in conjunction with Hodgkin lymphoma in the parotid gland (Di Napoli et al. 2015) and in cervical nodes are reported (Jun and Ming 2018). It can be postulated that the lymphoma or tobacco use stimulates the salivary inclusions inside the node to grow and form a Warthin tumor.

A combination of FNAB cytology and MRI characteristics may be sufficient to definitively define the Warthin tumor and prevent unnecessary surgery (Espinosa et al. 2018). However, Warthin tumor can cause problems in the diagnosis of head and neck and other cancers as its standard uptake value (SUV) can be very high on PET/CT. It can mimic both metastatic and multiple primary cancers (Rassekh et al. 2014). A similar problem can occur with extra-parotid Warthin tumor in cervical nodes, in patients being worked up for head and neck squamous carcinoma. On PET scan, it is impossible to differentiate these benign lesions from metastatic nodes (Schwartz et al. 2009; Mistry et al. 2015).

If Warthin tumor is diagnosed when small and asymptomatic, it may not require treatment in an old or infirm patient. Warthin's tumors have a tendency to occur in the parotid tail where the majority of parotid lymph nodes occur so partial parotidectomy is often all that is required if the tumor needs to be removed for cosmetic reasons (Figure 10.2).

There is a 17% incidence of multiple ipsilateral or bilateral tumors in Warthin tumor (Klussman et al. 2006). Eight percent of these tumors occur in extra-parotid cervical lymph nodes and may be found at the time of parotidectomy or serendipitously in neck dissection specimens. In an attempt to classify multiple salivary tumors, Seiffert and Donath (1996) concluded that the most common multiple tumors with identical histology were Warthin tumors followed by pleomorphic adenomas. The most common bilateral tumors are oncocytomas, acinic cell carcinomas, and basal cell adenomas. In the case of multiple tumors with different histologies, both Warthin tumor and pleomorphic adenoma can be found in combination with other adenomas and carcinomas (Seiffert and Donath 1996). In a review of 758 patients having parotidectomy, 93 (13%) were found to have multiple tumors. In cases of multiple tumors, 55 (59%) were unilateral, and 13/38 of the bilateral tumors (34%) were diagnosed synchronously. Warthin tumors (65%) were the commonest histologic type (Franzen et al. 2017). Warthin tumor in combination with pleomorphic adenoma is a rare combination (Lefor and Ord 1993) (Figure 10.17).

MALIGNANT TUMORS

Principles of Management of Parotid Carcinoma

There is no universally agreed method for managing parotid cancer; however, prognosis and management are related to two variables: the histologic classification/grade of the tumor and the tumor staging. Essentially, salivary tumors may be divided into low-grade (e.g. low-grade mucoepidermoid carcinoma, acinic cell carcinoma, epimyoepithelial carcinoma) and high-grade lesions (e.g. poorly differentiated carcinoma, high-grade mucoepidermoid carcinoma, salivary duct carcinoma). In reviewing 2465 patients with carcinoma of parotid and submandibular glands, Wahlberg et al. (2002) found a 10-year survival of 88% for acinic cell carcinoma, 80% for mucoepidermoid carcinoma (MEC), and 74% for adenoid cystic carcinoma (ACC) but only 55% for adenocarcinoma unspecified and 44% for undifferentiated carcinoma. It should be noted that five-year survival figures for ACC will give an artificially high value as late local recurrence and distant metastasis may continue over a 20+ year period. Harbo et al. (2002) also found acinic cell carcinoma to have the best one-year survival, but in their Cox hazard regression analysis found T stage, N stage, M stage, and histologic differentiation to be significant in predicting prognosis and recommended the use of both staging and histologic diagnosis to assess prognosis. In other published series, significant factors include extraglandular extension, aggressive histology, and nodal disease (Bhattacharyya and Fried 2005); histologic grade, T stage, N stage, and facial nerve dysfunction (Lima et al. 2005); and N stage and perineural involvement (Hocwald et al. 2001).

The only other predictor of adverse prognosis reported in several series was advancing age (Kirkbridge et al. 2001; Bhattacharyya and Fried 2005; Lima et al. 2005).

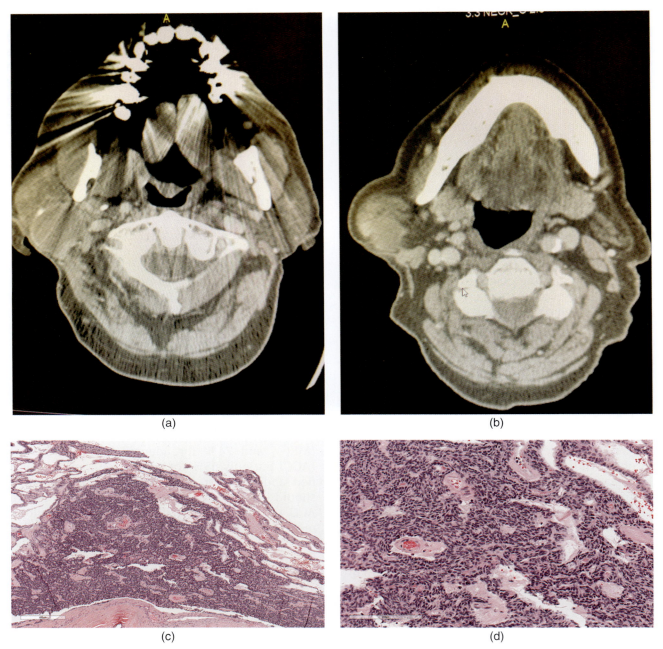

Figure 10.17. (a) Axial CT shows large hypodense mass in the retromandibular portion of the right parotid gland. This lesion appears cystic and could represent a cyst or cystic neoplasm. Note a small area of calcification in the capsule. (b) Axial CT more inferiorly at the level of the parotid tail. The mass at this level is smaller and appears more solid. Note a contrast-enhancing mass superficial to the mass, which could represent a lymph node. (c) Low-power H + E stain shows pleomorphic adenoma consisting of a mixture of epithelial and myoepithelial cells in different patterns, including in this view prominent cyst formation. (d) High power shows extensive spindling of the myoepithelial cells in this view. (e) High power of pleomorphic adenoma with myoepithelial cells stained brown with actin immunohistochemical cytoplasmic stain. The unstained epithelial cells are lining the lumen as noted by the blue arrows. (f) High power of pleomorphic adenoma with myoepithelial cells highlighted by p63 immunohistochemical brown nuclear stain. The arrow points to the unstained epithelial cells lining the lumen. (g) Low power of the Warthin tumor at the parotid tail. The thin capsule separating the tumor from the parotid parenchyma and fibrofatty stroma is best seen on the left. (h) The high power view of the Warthin tumor shows the oncocytic epithelial component and the lymphoid stroma-including prominent germinal centers (center of the picture). The epithelial component is characterized by inner/lining the lumen, columnar cells, and outer cuboidal cells. The courtesy is for Figure 10.17(c-h). Source: By courtesy of Dr. John Papadimitriou, Professor of Pathology, University of Maryland.

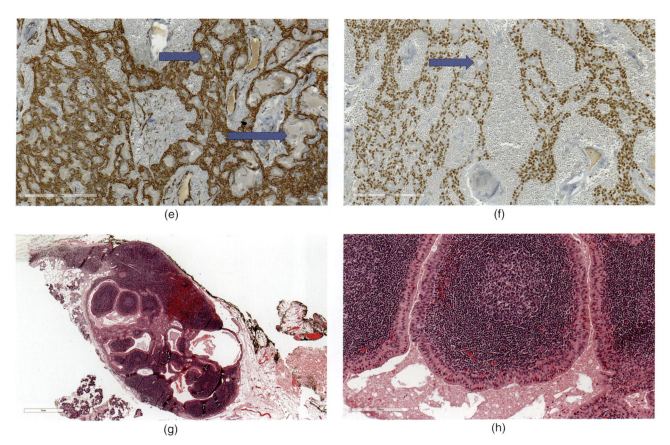

Figure 10.17. (Continued).

The reported survival related to stage varies between authors, which may reflect differences in therapy as well as different patterns of histopathology. Luukkaa et al. (2005) found 5-year survival in Stage I-IV 78, 25, 21, and 23% respectively while (Lima et al. 2005) found 10-year disease-specific survival Stage I-IV 97, 81, 56, and 20%.

In considering management, Kaplan and Johns (1986) divide parotid cancers into four groups to recommend treatment. Group I T1–2 low-grade tumors are treated by parotidectomy with preservation of the facial nerve (Figures 10.18 and 10.19). Group II T1–2 high-grade tumors are treated with parotidectomy plus first echelon nodes removal and postoperative radiation therapy (RT) (Figure 10.20). Group III T3 tumors and any positive nodes and recurrent tumor not in Group IV are treated with radical parotidectomy with sacrifice of the facial nerve, if necessary, and radical neck dissection plus RT. Group IV includes T4 and tumors with significant local extension, and are treated by radical parotidectomy plus skin, muscle and bone as indicated with radical neck dissection and postoperative RT (see Figure 15.16).

Controversy exists in the exact indications for RT and adjuvant therapy, neck dissection, and facial nerve sacrifice in the management of parotid cancer. There is some overlap between these topics. Most recent papers do show that RT is indicated for advanced parotid carcinoma and confers a survival benefit (Bhattacharyya and Fried 2005), or longer disease-free survival (Hocwald et al. 2001). An NCDB study of 4068 patients with locally advanced cancers of major salivary glands showed the five-year OS was 56% in the PORT cohort and 50.6% in surgery alone, which was significant. Female gender was also associated with better OS (Safedieh et al. 2017). An earlier study had shown 10-year local control for T3–4 tumors to be 84% with surgery + PORT as opposed to 18% for surgery alone. Significant benefit for the PORT cohort was also seen in patients with close and positive margins,

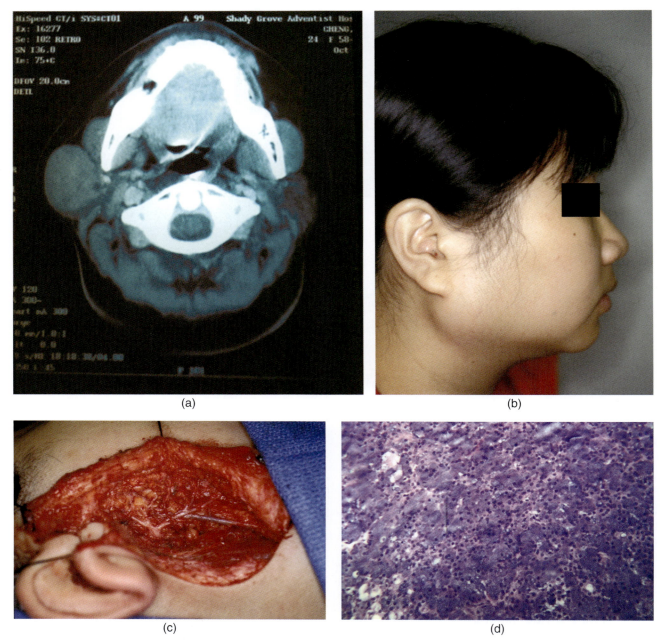

Figure 10.18. (a) CT scan of large superficial lobe tumor in 22-year-old lady. (b) Clinical appearance, the tumor has no signs of malignancy. (c) Complete parotidectomy the facial nerve was not involved. (d) Histopathology acinic cell carcinoma. Patient alive and well 8+ years.

PNI and bone invasion. In cases of positive cervical nodes, PORT improved regional control to 86% vs. 62% in the surgery alone cohort (Terhaard et al. 2005). However, although there is a consensus of agreement regarding the role of radiation in Stage III–IV disease, there is a recent move toward suggesting RT for earlier stage disease. Zbären et al. (2006) retrospectively analyzed T1–2 carcinomas with and without postoperative RT and found local recurrence rates of 3 and 33% respectively and actuarial and disease-free survival of 93% and 92% with and 83% and 70% without RT. In an earlier publication from the same unit, RT was suggested not just for high-grade tumors but also for

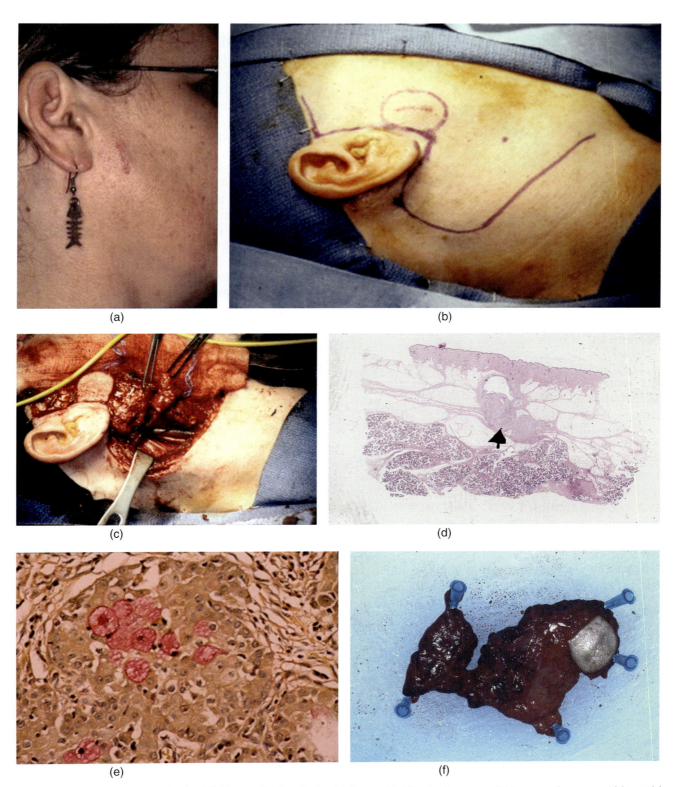

Figure 10.19. (a) Patient who had "skin-cyst" biopsied, which was histologically a parotid low-grade mucoepidermoid carcinoma. Note preauricular biopsy scar. (b) Operative slide shows Blair incision incorporating 1 cm around the biopsy. (c) The level II nodes (first echelon nodes) will be taken in continuity in this case. (d) Histologic slide shows focus of mucoepidermoid carcinoma (arrow) in the biopsy scar between the skin and parotid showing the importance of excising "seeded skin." (e) Mucicarmine stain confirms intracellular mucous. (f) Surgical specimen. (g) Patient is alive and disease free 20 years post-surgery.

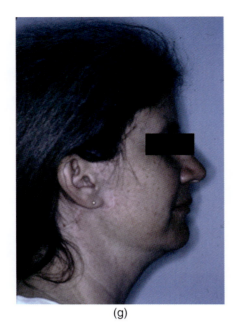

Figure 10.19. (*Continued*).

low-grade T2–4 (Zbären et al. 2003). So, perhaps RT is indicated for earlier stage disease than was previously recommended. The role of elective neck irradiation in the N0 neck will be discussed in the section on neck dissection below.

Regarding fast neutron therapy in the management of advanced salivary cancer with gross residual disease, one study showed a six-year local-regional control of 59%, which became 100% in patients with no evidence of gross residual disease (Douglas et al. 2003). An updated study (2019) of 545 patients treated with neutron RT for salivary cancer, 56% in the parotid gland and 47% ACC, showed 6- and 10-year locoregional controls of 84 and 79% while 6- and 10-year OS was 72 and 62%. Only 3.4% of cases were diagnosed with osteoradionecrosis (Timoshchuk et al. 2019).

Benefits of chemotherapy have not been clearly demonstrated for parotid cancer. A recent critical literature review found very little evidence to support the addition of chemotherapy to radiation in salivary gland cancer (Cerda et al. 2014). In a NCDB study of 2210 cases, there was no advantage in survival outcome between PORT and chemoradiation. Indeed, overall survival was inferior with chemoradiation on multivariable analysis and propensity score-matched analysis compared to radiation alone (Amini et al. 2016). However, high-grade salivary duct cancer SDC which is HER-2 positive may be treated with trastuzumab as targeted therapy, like ductal carcinoma of the breast. Although most papers are case reports, in one series of 13 patients, 8 adjuvant and 5 palliative treatments with metastatic disease, there was a 62% response rate for adjuvant patients with 5/8 disease free at two years. All five of the metastatic patients responded, with a median duration of response of 18 months and one patient had no evidence of disease 52 months following treatment (Limaye et al. 2013). Dual HER-2 inhibition with a combination of trastuzumab and pertuzumab has also been recently reported (Park et al. 2018). High-grade SDC is an aggressive, high-grade tumor with a poor prognosis. In a comprehensive and in-depth review of the literature, Schmitt et al. (2017) report a weighted average of local recurrence of 20%, regional failure of 20%, and distant metastases of 47%. Five-year OS ranged from 12 to 55%, and the weighted average of five-year DFS and OS across studies was 46.6 and 35%. The literature on targeted therapy including HER2/neu is detailed in this paper for interested readers (Schmitt et al. 2017). A case presentation using Herceptin in a HER2/neu positive parotid cancer is detailed in Chapter 14.

Regarding the indications for neck dissection, a National Cancer Database (NCDB) study of 22 652 patients with parotid cancer examined predictors of nodal disease and OS. The commonest tumor types were MECA 31%, acinic cell carcinoma 18%, adenocarcinoma 14%, and adenoid cystic carcinoma (ACC) 9%. The overall incidence for positive nodes was 24.4% (occult nodes were found in 10.2%) but depended on the histologic type of tumor. As would be expected, five-year OS was 79% in N0 cases vs. 40% in N+ cases and 88% for low-grade vs. 69% for high-grade tumors. Adenocarcinoma had the highest mortality for N+ cases and salivary duct carcinoma had the highest cN+ and occult nodes (Xiao et al. 2016). Although lymph node dissection (with PORT, see above) is now recommended for patients with positive nodes, advanced TNM stage, and high-grade tumors, there is an increasing interest in the N0 neck. The relatively high occult regional metastasis rates of 22–45% (Zbären et al. 2003; Stennert et al. 2003) led these authors to recommend an elective neck dissection in the N0 neck for parotid cancer (Figure 10.21). A scoring system based upon points for T stage and histologic type/grade has been proposed. cN0 parotid tumors with a score of

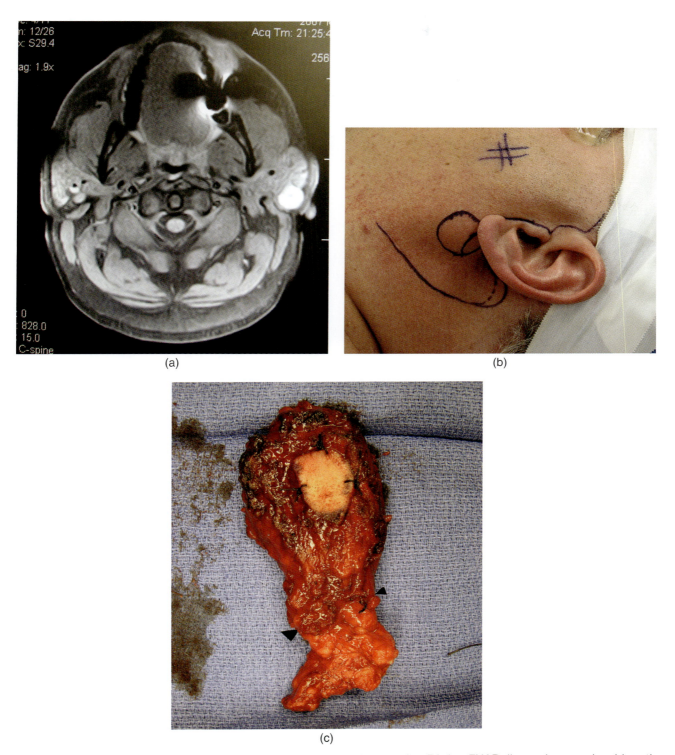

Figure 10.20. (a) MR of parotid tumor which radiologically was diagnosed as PA, but FNAB diagnosis was adenoid cystic carcinoma. (b) In view of cytologic diagnosis proposed, treatment includes resection of overlying skin, which clinically was possibly tethered and level II cervical nodes. (c) Surgical specimen shows parotid with skin. The arrows show where level II nodes and fat are in continuity with the parotid tail. Final diagnosis was cellular PA with the FNAB diagnosis being a false positive.

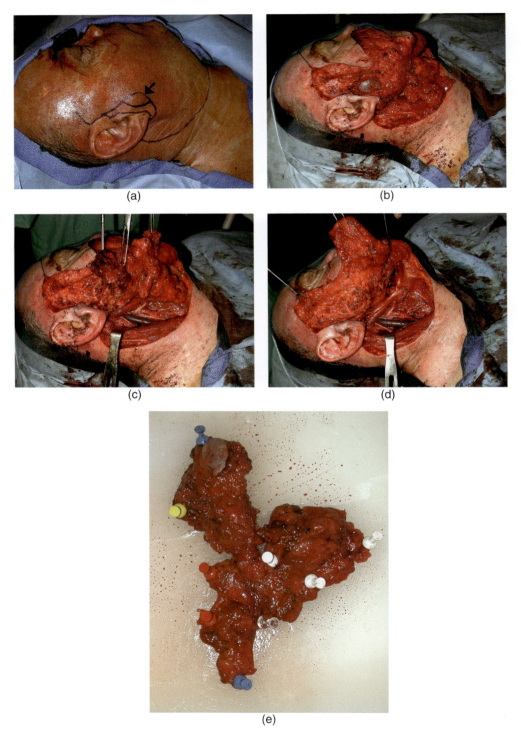

Figure 10.21. (a) High-grade parotid malignancy with skin fixity and N0 neck. Incision modified to include skin excision (arrow), and cervical incision extended to allow supraomohyoid neck dissection. (b) The skin flaps developed with the skin overlying the tumor left on the parotid gland. (c) The selective neck dissection is complete with the specimen in continuity with the parotid gland. The facial nerve trunk has been exposed and the superficial parotidectomy is being performed. (d) The surgical site following parotidectomy and selective neck dissection. (e) The surgical specimen with the parotid superiorly and level I nodes pinned out with white pins.

4 have a 24% risk of occult nodes and for the submandibular gland a score of 3 gives a 33% risk (Terhaard et al. 2005). A systematic review of 19 studies and 2703 patients found 83% were cN0. Patients with END showed a 23% incidence of occult nodal metastases. Regional recurrence occurred in only 5% of cases, which was interpreted as being due to the efficiency of END or RT to the neck (Valstar et al. 2010). Elective selective, neck dissection for high-grade tumors and > T2 low-grade tumors should encompass levels I–III and upper V (Teymoortash and Werner 2002). In comparing elective neck dissection for the N0 neck against observation, Zbären et al. (2005b) found an actuarial and disease-free survival of 80 and 86% for the elective neck dissection patients versus 83 and 69% for the observation group in a retrospective study.

Squamous cell carcinoma of the parotid gland is a rare high-grade tumor with a high propensity for lymph node metastasis. In a SEER population based study (1973–2009), 2545 cases were identified, 79.8% males and 92.9% Caucasians. Five-year OS was 54%, and the significant prognostic factors for poor survival were black race, age > 75 years, higher stage and tumor T3 or >. Elective neck dissection in N0 cases showed a significant increase in DSS 78.3% vs. 51.1%, p < 0.0001. Patients who did not have an END had a > 3 times hazard of death irrespective of whether they received adjuvant radiation therapy (Pfisterer et al. 2014).

An alternative management of the N0 neck in parotid cancers is elective neck irradiation (ENI). A systematic review of 20 studies and practice in the United Kingdom concluded that ENI is a reasonable alternative to END in high-grade tumors or T3/4 disease. The ENI should encompass levels I–III (Ng-Cheng-Hin et al. 2018). In an earlier study of 251 patients, 131 patients treated with ENI to the neck had 0 regional failure whereas the 120 patients without ENI had 26% regional failure (Chen et al. 2007). A similar trial with 59 cases of high-grade cN0 salivary cancers reported 41 having END and 18 ENI. There was a 44% of occult positive neck disease in the END cohort, and 4 (10%) relapsed. There was 0 relapse in the ENI group. The authors concluded that planned END conferred no benefit over ENI if PORT was already planned. Two patients developed fistulas and one osteoradionecrosis (Herman et al. 2013).

Regarding the facial nerve, Spiro and Spiro (2003) recommend preservation unless the nerve is adherent to/embedded in the tumor. They feel that close margins to the nerve can be treated successfully by RT. This view is supported by the work of Carinci et al. (2001) who found that sacrifice of the nerve was not always able to improve survival rate. In a series of 107 patients with parotid cancer, 91 had normal nerve function preoperatively and facial nerve preservation was possible in 79 patients. The 5-year disease-free rate and 5- and 10-year survival rates were 65, 83, and 54% respectively in the preserved nerve cohort and 56, 62, and 42% respectively in the patients with nerve sacrifice. The authors felt that preservation of the facial nerve by careful dissection gave favorable oncologic results (Guntinas-Lichius et al. 2004). A disease-free survival of 69, 37, and 13% in patients with normal, partially and completely impaired facial nerve function preoperatively despite the use of facial nerve sacrifice and postoperative RT indicates what a poor prognosis invasion of the nerve confers (Terhaard et al. 2006). This poor prognosis of patients with facial nerve involvement is confirmed in a study of 129 patients with primary parotid cancers. The results show that 64% of patients with both facial palsy and PNI recurred, 43% with palsy but no PNI recurred, 27% with only PNI and 16% only in patients with neither parameter (Terakedis et al. 2017). The United Kingdom National Multidisciplinary Guidelines for managing salivary tumors recommend that every attempt should be made to preserve the facial nerve if its function is normal preoperatively (Sood et al. 2016).

In specific histologic tumor types, variable results for different treatments have been reported. Mucoepidermoid carcinoma (MECA) is the commonest salivary malignancy and most cases are fortunately of low or intermediate grade. Grade is most commonly based on the ratio of squamous cells to mucous cells in the tumor. A series of 89 cases of MECA at the Mayo clinic, 69 T1–2, 85 N0, and 83 low/intermediate grade, were treated by parotidectomy with "appropriate" neck dissection and only 7 had RT. Kaplan–Meier estimated cancer-specific survival rates at 5, 15, and 25 years were 98.9, 97.4, and 97.4% respectively (Boahene et al. 2004). Using a point grading system for histopathologic features in a series of 234 mucoepidermoid carcinomas of the major salivary glands, cystic component < 20%, 4 or more mitotic figures per 10 high-power fields, neural involvement, necrosis and anaplasia were found to have prognostic significance for parotid MECA (Goode et al. 1998). Intermediate-grade MECA tends to behave more like low-grade MECA while high-grade MECA behaves aggressively with local recurrence, regional and distant metastases in most cases. A recent NCDB survey of 4431 cases of MECA of the parotid gland reported a one-year survival of 92.9% and a five-year OS of 75.2%. Decreased survival was associated with patient age and comorbidities, high-grade MECA, advanced TNM stage, and positive margins. Improved survival was seen in female patients. Intermediate grade was not associated with decreased survival except in patients with tumors T2 or > and/or N2 or > (Rajasekaran et al. 2018).

Other low-grade tumors such as acinic cell carcinoma, epimyoepithelial carcinoma, and low-grade adenocarcinoma all can be treated in a similar manner to low-grade MECA. Acinic cell carcinoma has a propensity for the parotid gland and rivals MECA as the most common tumor in some series. In another recent NCDB survey of 2362 cases of acinic cell carcinoma, 61.3% were female and 75.8% of tumors were < 3 cm in size. High-grade histology was very rare (5.1%) and regional disease was only seen in 8.2% of cases. The five-year OS was 88.6%. Multivariable analysis showed that significant prognostic factors included age > 70 years, high grade, T size > 3 cm and advanced T stage, and pN2 + .Interestingly, histologic grade was a stronger predictor of OS than either T or N stage (Scherl et al. 2018).

A newly described tumor, the mammary analogue secretory carcinoma (MASC) was only defined in 2010. It also behaves mostly as a low-grade tumor. It is defined by its ETV6-NTRK3 fusion gene. In a series of 31 cases, median age was 49 years, 55% were male and 58% of cases arose in the parotid. Only one case had a nodal metastasis; 4/31(12.9%) had neck dissections and 48% had adjuvant radiation therapy. The 5- and 10-year OS was 95% and DFS 89% (Boon et al. 2018). On the other hand, results for high-grade tumors such as primary squamous carcinoma of the parotid are poor. In one published series two thirds were treated with radical surgery and RT and one third with RT alone but five-year actuarial survival and disease-free survival was 31 and 33% respectively (Lee et al. 2001). A 2014 study of 2545 cases of primary squamous cell carcinoma of the parotid, however, showed a five-year DSS survival of 54.4%. Poor prognostic factors included black race, age > 75 years, T3 or greater and high stage (Pfisterer et al. 2014). Infiltrating ductal carcinoma has a particularly poor prognosis. A SEER data review of 252 cases showed significantly better OS for patients treated with PORT for T3–4, N1 and stage 3 disease (Lv et al. 2019).

Malignant change in PA is most commonly seen as carcinoma ex-pleomorphic adenoma and prognosis will depend on the histologic type of malignancy and whether the malignancy has spread outside the capsule. In carcinoma ex-pleomorphic adenoma, the use of postoperative RT improved five-year local control from 49 to 75% and improved survival in patients without cervical metastasis (Chen et al. 2007). Two other forms of malignant PA occur, which are both rare: the "true" malignant mixed tumor or carcinosarcoma where malignant change is seen in both the epithelial and myoepithelial component of the PA and the benign metastasizing PA, which as its name suggests retains a benign histologic appearance despite the presence of metastases. In a recent systematic review, only 80 cases of benign metastasizing pleomorphic adenoma were found between 1942 and 2016. The mean age was 49.5 years and the mean time from PA to metastasis was 14.9 years (range 0–51 years). The commonest sites for metastasis were bone, 36.6%; lung, 33.8%; and cervical nodes, 20.1% (see Figure 11.12) (Knight and Ratnasingham 2015).

It is hard to interpret adenoid cystic carcinoma survival figures in some series as ACC is very slow-growing and 5-year survival is less meaningful in this neoplasm as survival continues to fall on 20-year follow-up. Thus, in series with short follow-up, ACC will erroneously be thought to have a good prognosis. Typical long-term survival figures are 84.3% 2 year, 75.9% 5 year, 50.49% 10 year, and 20.11% after 20 years (Issing et al. 2002). The type of histologic appearance, solid versus cylindrical, and the presence of perineural invasion are important prognostic factors. Even with documented lung metastases, patients can live 5 + years, the average survival between the appearance of lung metastases and death being 32.3 months in one series (van der Waal et al. 2002). Current NCCN guidelines recommend that adjuvant RT should be considered for all ACC (including early stage). A NCDB analysis of 1784 patients with ACC of the major salivary glands (72.4% had parotidectomy) confirmed that PORT was associated with better survival even for early stage disease (pT1–2 N0) (Lee et al. 2017).

The histologic grade of the tumor must be considered as well as TNM staging when interpreting survival results in reported series. Every parotid cancer will be unique and the decision for what is the correct surgery will be made on an individual basis for each patient.

Summary

- Around 80% of parotid tumors are benign, most commonly pleomorphic adenomas.
- Less than one-third of malignant tumors will have obvious clinical signs of malignancy, e.g. facial nerve palsy, ulceration, fixation, or lymphadenopathy.
- Routine use of CT or MR imaging does not appear justified and should be used selectively for malignant neoplasms and deep lobe tumors.
- Preoperative open biopsy is contraindicated and FNAB is still the modality of choice for preoperative histologic diagnosis. Core needle biopsy has been shown to be more accurate in malignant cases.
- Although superficial parotidectomy remains the basic surgical procedure, there is currently much debate regarding the roles of partial parotidectomy and extra-capsular dissection in the management of PA. The role of the capsule and the acceptable margin for PA remains undefined.
- Recurrent PA will frequently require en bloc resection due to its infiltrative and multinodular nature. Cure in this situation is probably achieved in approximately two-thirds of cases.
- Management of malignant parotid tumors will depend on both the histologic diagnosis and the staging of the tumor
- Radiation therapy may be helpful in earlier stage disease and lower grade tumors than previously advocated.
- Selective neck dissection for the N0 neck or elective neck irradiation may be justified in early stage disease given the high reported rate of occult nodes.
- The facial nerve should be preserved in parotid cancer unless it is directly infiltrated by tumor.

Case Presentation – *How Did This All Start?*

A 69-year-old white man was referred by his dentist with a mass in the floor of his mouth in October 2015. The patient had been asymptomatic and the mass was noted incidentally by his general dentist one month prior to referral. He was referred to his local oral and maxillofacial surgeon who performed a biopsy of the floor of mouth that showed a low-grade mucoepidermoid carcinoma. The mass was described in the referring surgeon's letter as indurated, and lateral to Wharton duct in the left sublingual gland.

Interestingly, he had numerous risk factors for salivary gland cancer, which included a previous ipsilateral parotid cancer gland for which he was given postoperative radiation therapy in 1984 and then a lymphoma in 2007 treated with chemotherapy (Chapter 10).

Past Medical History
Hypertension treated with Terazosin, Losartan, and Amlodipine.

Hypercholesterolemia treated with Atorvastatin

He had been diagnosed with aortic valve sclerosis and had a murmur.

Diabetes mellitus treated with Metformin.

In 1984, he was diagnosed with thyroid cancer and underwent thyroidectomy, followed by radioactive iodine therapy. He is currently on thyroxine.

In 1984, he was diagnosed with left parotid cancer, type unknown, and underwent parotidectomy with postoperative radiation therapy.

In 2007, he underwent inguinal node biopsy, which was positive for lymphoma treated with chemotherapy.

He has seasonal allergies

Social History
He is a nonsmoker and drinks alcohol only occasionally.

Examination
He had no obvious facial nerve palsy, and no palpable nodes. Intraorally, he had a 3.5 cm × 1.5 cm submucosal mass in the sublingual gland. The mobile mass was separate from

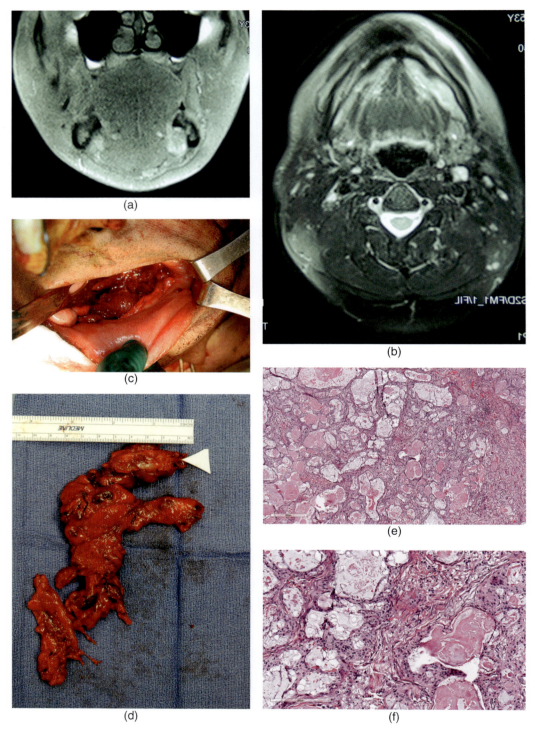

Figure 10.22. (a) Coronal MRI view shows mass in left sublingual gland adjacent to the medial mandible. (b) Axial MRI view shows that lingual cortex of the mandible is intact. The mass in the sublingual gland extends posteriorly to the submandibular gland. (c) Intraoperative view post-resection. The mandible stripped of periosteum is visible in the foreground and the anterior belly of the digastric muscle is seen bulging into the mouth. (d) The gross specimen is placed on a blue surgical towel. The white paper triangle indicates the sublingual gland that is attached to the submandibular gland and neck dissection. (e) Low-power view shows low-grade mucoepidermoid carcinoma, roughly equivalent components of mucous/goblet cells with cyst formation and epidermoid/squamous cells. (f) High-power view of previous slide. Source: Figures 10.22 (e-f) courtesy of Dr. John Papadimitriou, Professor of pathology, University of Maryland.

the mandible. The mass was palpable from the anterior floor of mouth to posterior to the mylohyoid muscle where it appeared to involve the submandibular gland.

Diagnosis

T2 N0 low-grade mucoepidermoid carcinoma of the left sublingual gland.

MRI imaging confirmed a left sublingual gland tumor (Figure 10.22a and b).

The patient underwent surgery on 7 November 2015. In view of the probable extension of the tumor to the submandibular gland, he underwent an in-continuity resection comprising resection of the sublingual gland with the mylohyoid muscle, submandibular gland, and a supraomohyoid neck dissection (Figure 10.22c and d).

The final pathology report showed a 2.6 cm low-grade mucoepidermoid carcinoma with calcifications, limited to the sublingual gland. Margins were negative and 0/12 lymph nodes were involved (Figure 10.22e and f).

Postoperatively, the patient did well. He had a slight facial nerve weakness initially, which resolved within one month. He was followed regularly until June 2018, two years and seven months post his surgery. He was then lost to follow-up.

TAKE-HOME POINTS

1. It is rare for a patient to have two separate major salivary gland cancers and the etiology of his parotid carcinoma and histologic type is unknown. The fact that his facial nerve was intact argues against high-grade or late T stage for his initial primary parotid cancer. Nonetheless, he developed a second primary salivary gland cancer in the sublingual gland 31 years post his parotid cancer. In his medical history, there are three possible risk factors for him developing a further salivary cancer: the radiation to his parotid gland, the radioactive iodine, and his subsequent lymphoma treated with chemotherapy. In this chapter, both chemotherapy and radiation were discussed as etiologic factors for the development of MECA in children treated for leukemia/lymphoma. Certainly, this can also be seen in adults and MECA as a second cancer in adults following radiation, chemotherapy, and hemopoietic stem cell transplant have been described. The radiation to the parotid bed would have encompassed the neck (which would explain the low lymph node yield, usually 22–26 for SOHND). The area of the sublingual gland would also have been in the radiation field. Radioactive iodine is also avidly taken up by salivary gland tissue (see Chapter 16). Radiation is associated with the late development of second primary salivary cancer after many years. However, the chemotherapy given for the lymphoma 11 years previously could also be the major factor. It is impossible to know which of these factors or combination of these factors was responsible but his is a fascinating case.

References

Abu-Ghanem Y, Mizrachi A, Popovtzer A, et al. 2016. Recurrent pleomorphic adenoma of the parotid gland: Institutional experience and review of the literature. *J Surg Oncol* 114(6):714–718

Agaimy A, Wild V, Märkl, et al. 2015. Intraparotid classical and nodular lymphocyte-predominant Hodgkin lymphoma: Pattern analysis with emphasis on associated lymphadenoma-like proliferations. *Am J Surg Pathol* 39(9):1206–1212

Agaimy A, Fonseca I, Martins C et al. 2018. NUT carcinoma of the salivary glands: Clinicopathologic and molecular analysis of 3 cases and a survey of NUT expression in salivary gland carcinomas. *Am J Surg Pathol* 42(7):877–884.

Albergotti WG, Nguyen SA, Zenk J, Gillespie MB 2012 Extracapsular dissection for benign parotid tumors: A meta-analysis. *Laryngoscope* 122(9):1954–1960

Amini A, Waxweiller TV, Bower JV, et al. 2016. Association of adjuvant chemoradiotherapy vs radiotherapy alone with survival in patients with resected major salivary gland carcinoma: Data from the National Cancer data base. *JAMA Otolaryngol Head Neck* 142(1):1100–1110

Anantharajan N, Ravindranathan N, Rajadurai P. 2013. Lymphoepithelial carcinoma of the parotid gland, a very unusual tumor: A case report and review. *Ear Nose Throat J* 92(9):E7–E9.

Andreasen S, Therkildsen MH, Bjørndal, HP. 2016.Pleomorphic adenoma of the parotid gland 1985-2010: A Danish nationwide study of incidence, recurrence rate, and malignant transformation. *Head Neck* 38(Suppl 1):E1364–E1369.

Ariyoshi Y, Shimahara M. 1998. Determining whether a parotid tumor is in the superficial or deep lobe using magnetic resonance imaging. *J Oral Maxillofac Surg* 56:23–27.

Aro K, Valle J, Tarkanen J, et al. (2019). Repeatedly recurring pleomorphic adenoma; a therapeutic challenge. *Acta Otorhinolaryngol Ital.* 39(3):156–161.

Beal KP, Singh B, Kraus D et al. 2003. Radiation -induced salivary gland tumors: A report of 18 cases and a review of the literature. *Cancer J* 9(6):467–471.

Bhattacharyya N, Fried MP. 2005. Determinants of survival in parotid gland carcinoma: A population-based study. *Am J Otolaryngol* 26(1):39–44.

Bialek EJ, Jabukowski W, Karpinska G. 2003. Role of ultrasonography in diagnosis and differentiation of pleomorphic adenomas. *Arch Otolaryngol Head Neck Surg* 129:929–933

Boahene DK, Olsen KD, Lewis JE et al. 2004. Mucoepidermoid carcinoma of the parotid gland: The Mayo clinic experience. *Arch Otolaryngol Head Neck Surg* 130(7):849–856.

Boon E, Valstar MH, van der Graaf WTA, et al. 2018. Clinicopathological characteristics and outcome of 31 patients with ETV6-NTK3 fusion gene confirmed (mammary analogue secretory carcinoma of salivary glands). *Oral Oncol* 82:29–33.

Bozzato A, Zenk J, Greess H et al. 2007. Potential of ultrasound diagnosis of parotid tumors: Analysis of qualitative and quantitative *Parameters* 137:642–646.

Carinci F, Farina A, Pelucchi S et al. 2001. Parotid gland carcinoma: Surgical strategy based on local risk factors. *J Craniofac Surg* 12(5):434–437.

Carrilo JF, Ramirez R, Flores L et al. 2009. Diagnostic accuracy of fine needle aspiration biopsy in preoperative diagnosis of patients with parotid gland masses. *J Surg Oncol* 100:133–138.

Causevic Vucak M, Masic T. 2014. The incidence of recurrent parotid pleomorphic adenoma of the parotid gland in relation to the choice of surgical procedure. *Med Glas (Zenica)* 11(1):66–71.

Cerda T, Sun XS, Vignot S, et al. 2014. A rationale for chemoradiation (vs radiotherapy) in salivary gland cancers? On behalf of the REFCOR (French rare head and neck cancer network). *Crit Rev Oncol Hematol* 91(2):142–158.

Chen AM, Garcia J, Bucci MK, et al. 2006. Recurrent pleomorphic adenoma of the parotid gland: Long term outcome of patients treated with radiation therapy. *Int J Radiol Biol Phys* 66(4):1031–1035.

Chen AM, Garcia J, Bucci MK, et al. 2007. The role of postoperative radiation therapy in carcinoma ex pleomorphic adenoma of the parotid gland. *Int J Radiat Oncol Biol Phys* 67(1):138–143.

Chen AM, Garcia J, Lee NY et al. 2007. Patterns of nodal relapse after surgery and postoperative radiation therapy for carcinomas of the major and minor salivary glands: What is the role of elective neck irradiation. *Int J Radiat Oncol Biol Phys* 67(4):988–984.

Cohen EG, Patel SG, Lin O et al. 2004. Fine needle aspiration biopsy of salivary gland lesions in a selected patient population. *Arch Otolaryngol Head Neck Surg* 130(6):773–778.

Coleela C, Giudice A, Rambali PF Cuccurullo V. 2007. Parotid function after selective deep lobe parotidectomy. *Brit J Oral Maxillofacial Surg* 45:108–111.

Del Signor AG, Megwalu UC 2017. The rising incidence of major salivary cancer in the United States. *Ear Nose Throat J.* 96(3:E13–E16.

Di Napoli A, Mallel G, Bartolazzi A, et al. 2015. Nodular lymphocyte-predominant Hodgkin lymphoma in a Warthin tumor of the parotid gland: A case report and a literature review. *Int J Surg Pathol* 23(5):419–423

Dombrowski ND, Walter NE, Irace AL et al. 2019. Pleomorphic adenoma of the head and neck in children: Presentation and management. *Laryngoscope.* 129(110;2603–2609.

Donovan DT, Conley JJ. 1984.Capsular significance in parotid surgery: Reality and myth of lateral lobectomy. *Laryngoscope* 94(3):324–329

Douglas JG, Koh WJ, Austin-Seymour M, Laramore GE. 2003. Treatment of salivary gland neoplasms with fast neutron radiotherapy. *Arch Otolaryngol Head Neck Surg* 129:944–8.

Douville NJ, Bradford CR. 2013. Comparison of ultrasound -guided Core biopsy versus fine-needle aspiration biopsy in the evaluation of salivary lesions. *Head Neck* 35(11):1657–1661

Eom H-J, Lee JH, Ko M-S et al. 2015. Comparison of fine-needle aspiration and core needle biopsy under ultrasonic guidance for detecting malignancy and for the tissue-specific diagnosis of salivary gland tumors. *AJNR Am J Neuroradiol* 36(6):1188–1193

Espinosa CA, Fernández-Valle Á, Lequerica-Fernández P et al. 2018. Clinicopathologic and surgical study of pleomorphic adenoma of the parotid gland: An analysis of risk factors for recurrence and facial nerve dysfunction. *J Oral Maxillofac Surg* 76(2):347–354

Fee WE Jr, Tran LE. 2003. Evaluation of a patient with a parotid tumor. *Arch Otolaryngol Head Neck Surg* 129:937–938.

Foresta E, Torrini A, Di Nardo F, et al. 2014 Pleomorphic adenoma and benign parotid tumors: Extracapsular dissection vs superficial parotidectomy – Review of literature and meta-analysis *Oral Surg Oral Med Oral Pathol Oral Radiol* 117(6): 663–676

Franzen AM, Coordes A, Franzen CK, Guenzel G. 2017 Are multiple tumors of the parotid gland uncommon or under estimated? *Anticancer Res* 37(9):5263–5267

Franzen AM, Franzen KC, Guenzel T et al. 2018.Increased incidence of Warthin tumours of the parotid gland: A 42-year evaluation. *Eur Arch Ortorhinolaryngol* 275(10):2593–2598

Frommer J. 1977 The human accessory parotid gland: Its incidence, nature and significance. *Oral Surg* 138:671–676

Gao M, Hao Y, Huang MX et al. 2017. Salivary gland tumors in a northern Chinese population: A 50-year retrospective study of 7,190 cases. *Int J Oral and Maxillofac Surg* 46(3):343–349

Ghosh S, Panarese A, Bull PD, Lee JA. 2003. Marginally excised parotid pleomorphic adenomas: Risk factors for recurrence and management. A 12.5-year mean follow up study of histologically marginal excisions. *Clin Otolaryngol* 28:262–266.

Goldenberg D, Flax-Goldenberg R, Joachims HZ, Peled N. 2000. Misplaced parotid glands: Bilateral agenesis of parotid glands associated with bilateral accessory parotid tissue. *J Laryngol Otol* 114:883–885

Goode RK, Auclair PL, Ellis GL. 1998. Mucoepidermoid carcinoma of the major salivary glands: Clinical and histopathologic analysis of 234 cases with evaluation of grading criteria. *Cancer* 82(7):1217–1224.

Grosheva M, Shablis S, Volk GF et al. 2017. Sensation loss after superficial parotidectomy: A prospective controlled multicenter trial. *Head Neck* 39(3):520–526

Guntinas-Lichius O, Klussman JP, Schroeder U et al. 2004. Primary parotid malignant surgery in patients with normal preoperative facial nerve function: Outcome and long-term postoperative facial nerve function. *Laryngoscope* 114(5):949–956.

Han XB, Zhang X, Gao Y et al., 2018. Management and prognosis of cancers in the accessory parotid gland. *J Int Med Res* 46(12):4930–4933

Harbo G, Bungaard T Pedersen D, et al. 2002. Prognostic indicators for malignant tumors of the parotid gland. *Clin Otolaryngol Allied Sci* 27(6):512–516.

Harney MS, Murphy C, Hone S et al. 2003. A histological comparison of deep and superficial lobe pleomorphic adenomas of the parotid gland. *Head Neck* 25(8)649–653.

Henriksson G, Westrin KM, Carlsoo B, Silversward C. 1998. Recurrent primary pleomorphic adenomas of salivary gland origin: Intrasurgical rupture, histopathologic features, and pseudopodia. *Cancer* 82(4):617–620.

Herman MP, Werning JW, Morris CG et al. 2013. Elective neck management. For high-grade salivary gland carcinoma. *Am J Otolaryngol* 34(3):205–208

Herman J, Sedláčková Z, Vachutka J, et al. 2017. Differential diagnosis of parotid gland tumors: Role of shear wave elastography *Biomed Res* 2017:9234672

Hocwald E, Korkmaz H, Yoo GH et al. 2001. Prognostic factors in major salivary gland cancer. *Laryngoscope* 111(8):1434–1439.

Honig JF. 2005. Omega incision face lift approach and SMAS rotation advancement in parotidectomy for the prevention of contour deficiency and conspicuous scars affecting the neck. *Int J Oral Maxillofac Surg* 34(6):612–618.

Hughes JH, Volk EE Wilbur DC. 2005. Pitfalls in salivary gland fine-needle aspiration cytology: Lessons from the College of American Pathologists Interlaboratory Comparison Program in nongynecologic cytology. *Arch Pathol Lab Med* 129(1):26–31.

Iguchi H, Wada T, Yamamoto H et al. 2013.Clinical features of accessory parotid gland tumors. *Nihon Jibiinkoka Gakkai Kaiho* 116(12):1300–1307

In der Maur CD, Klokman WJ, van Leeuwen FE et al. 2005. Increased risk of breast cancer development after diagnosis of salivary gland cancer. *European Journal of Cancer* 41(9):1311–1315.

Issing PR, Hemmanouil I, Wilkens L et al. 2002. Long term results in adenoid cystic carcinoma. (article in German) *Laryngorhinootologie* 81(2):98–105.

Jun L Ming Z 2018. Classical Hodgkin lymphoma arising from heterotopic Warthin's tumor in the cervical lymph node: A case report. *Oncol Lett* 16(1):619–622

Kadletz L Grasi S, Grasi MC et al. 2017. Extracapsular dissection versus superficial parotidectomy in benign parotid gland tumors: The Vienna medical school experience. *Head Neck* 39(2):356–360

Kadletz L, Grasi S, Perisandis C et al., 2019. Rising incidence of Warthin's tumors may be linked to obesity: A single-institutional experience. *Eur Arch Otorhinolaryngol* 276(4):1191–1196

Kantas A, Ho MWS, Mücke T. 2018. Current thinking about the management of recurrent pleomorphic adenoma of the parotid: A structured review. *Brit J Oral Maxillofac Surg* 56(4):243–248

Kaplan MJ, Johns ME. 1986. Salivary gland cancer. *Clin Oncology* 5:525–547.

Kendi ATK, Magliocca KR, Corey A, et al. 2016. Is there a role for PET/CT parameters to characterize benign,8malignant and metastatic parotid tumors? *AJR Am J Roentgenol* 207(3):635–640

Kim HJ, Kim JS 2018. Ultrasound-guided core needle biopsy in salivary glands: A meta-analysis. *Laryngoscope* 128(1):118–125

Kirkbridge P, Liu FF, O'Sullivan B et al. 2001. Outcome of curative management of malignant tumors of the parotid gland. *J Otolaryngol* 30(5):271–279.

Klussman PJ, Wittekindt C, Preuss FS et al. 2006. High risk for bilateral Warthin's tumors in heavy smokers-review of 185 cases. *Acta Otolaryngol* 126(11):1213–1217.

Knight J, Ratnasingham K 2015. Metastasising pleomorphic adenoma: Systematic review *Int. J Surg.* 19:137–145

Kolokythas A, Fernandes RP, Ord RA. 2007. A non-lip-splitting-double mandibular osteotomy technique for resection of tumors in the parapharyngeal and pterygomandibular spaces. *J Oral Maxillofac Surg* 65(3):66–69.

Kuriyama T, Kawata R, Higashino M, et al. 2019. Recurrent benign pleomorphic adenoma of the parotid gland: Facial nerve identification and risk factors for facial nerve paralysis at re-operation. *Auris Nasus Larynx* 46(5):779–784

Lamelas J, Terry JH, Alfonso AE. 1987. Warthin's tumor: Multicentricity and increasing incidence in women. *Am J Surg* 154:347–351.

Lee S, Kim GE, Parks CS et al. 2001. Primary squamous cell carcinoma of the parotid gland. *Am J Otolaryngol* 22(6):400–406.

Lee A, Babak G, Osborn VW et al. 2017. Patterns of care and survival of adjuvant radiation for major salivary adenoid cystic carcinoma. *Laryngoscope* 127(9):2057–2062

Lefor A, Ord RA 1993. Multiple synchronous bilateral Warthin's tumors of the parotid glands with pleomorphic adenoma. Case report and review of the literature. *Oral Surg Oral Med Oral Pathol* 76(3):319–324

Leonetti JP, Marzo SJ, Petrzelli GJ, Herr B. 2005. Recurrent pleomorphic adenoma of the parotid gland. *Otolaryngol Head Neck Surg* 133(3):319–322.

Liang YY, Xu F, Guo Y et al. 2018. Diagnostic accuracy of magnetic resonance imaging techniques for parotid tumors, a systematic review and meta-analysis. *Clin Imaging* 52:36–43

Lima RA, Tavares MR, Dias FL et al. 2005. Clinical prognostic factors in malignant parotid gland tumors. *Otolaryngol Head Neck Surg* 133: 702–708.

Limaye SA, Posner MR, Krane JK, et al. 2013. Trastuzumab for the treatment of salivary duct carcinoma. *Oncologist* 18(3):294–300

Lin YQ, Wang Y, Ou YM et al. 2019. Extracapsular dissection versus partial superficial parotidectomy for the treatment of benign parotid tumors. *Int J Oral Maxillofac Surg.* 48(7):895–901

Longuet M, Nallet E, Guedon C, et al. 2001. Diagnostic value of needle biopsy and frozen section histological examination in the surgery of primary parotid tumors. *Rev Laryngolo Otol Rhinol* 122(1):51–55.

Lonn S, Alholm A, Christensen HC et al. 2006. Mobile phone use and risk of parotid gland tumor. *Am J Epidemiol* 164(7):637–643.

Luskic I, Mamic M, Suton P. 2019. Management of accessory parotid gland tumors: 32-year experience from a single institution and review of the literature. *Int J Oral Maxillofac Surg.* 48(9):1145–1152

Luukkaa H, Klemi P, Leivo I et al. 2005. Salivary gland cancer in Finland 1991-96. *Acta Otolaryngol* 125(2):207–214.

Lv T, Wang Y, Wang X. 2019.Subgroups of parotid gland infiltrating ductal carcinoma benefit from postoperative radiotherapy: A population-based study. *Future Oncol* 15(8):885–895

Ma H, Jin S, Du S, et al. 2018. Pathology and management of masses in the accessory parotid gland region: 24-year experience at a single institution. *J Craniomaxillofac Surg* 46(2):183–189

Mani S, Mathew J, Thomas R, Michael RC 2019. Feasibility of transoral approach to accessory parotid tumors. *Cureus* 11(2):e4003.

Maxwell EL, Hall FT, Freeman JL. 2004. Recurrent pleomorphic adenoma of the parotid gland. *J Otolaryngol* 33(3)181–184.

McGurk M, Renehan A, Gleave EN, Hancock BD. 1996. Clinical significance of the tumor capsule in the treatment of parotid pleomorphic adenomas. *Br J Surg* 83(12):1747–1749.

McGurk M, Thomas BL, Renehan AG. 2003. Extracapsular dissection for clinically benign parotid lumps: Reduced morbidity without oncological compromise. *Br J Cancer* 89(9):1610–1613.

McLoughlin L, Gillanders SL. Smith S, Young O. 2019. The role of adjuvant radiotherapy in management of recurrent pleomorphic adenoma of the parotid gland: A systematic review *Eur Arch Otorhinolaryngol* 276(20:283–295

Meningaud JP, Bertolus C, Bertrand JC. 2006. Parotidectomy: assessment of a surgical technique including facelift incision and SMAS advancement. *J Craniomaxillofac Surg* 34(10):34–37.

Mistry SG, Gouldesbrough D, Bem C. 2015.Multifocal extraparotid tumors mimicking metastatic squamous cell carcinoma of the upper neck. *J Laryngol Otol* 129(5):513–516

Miyatima Y, Ogama A, Kuno K et al. 2007. Mucoepidermoid carcinoma of the parotid gland as a secondary malignancy developed ten years after chemotherapy for childhood acute lymphoblastic leukemia. *Rinsho Ketsueki* 48(6):491–494)

Munhoz L, Ramos EADA, Im DC et al. 2019. Application of diffusion -weighted magnetic resonance imaging in the diagnosis of salivary diseases: A systematic review *Oral Surg, Oral Med Oral Pathol. Oral Radiol.* 128(3):280–310

Newberry TR, Kaufman CR, Miller FR. 2014. Review of accessory parotid tumors: Pathologic incidence and surgical management. *Am J Otolaryngol* 35(1):48–52

Ng-Cheng-Hin B, Glaholm J Awad Z, Gujral DM. 2018. Elective management of the neck in parotid tumours. *Clin Oncol (R Coll Radiol)* 309120;764–772

Nøhr A, Andreasen S, Thirkildsen MH, Homøe P. 2016. Stationary facial nerve paresis after surgery for recurrent parotid pleomorphic adenoma: A follow up study of 219 cases in Denmark in the period 1985-2012. *Eur Arch Otorhinolaryngol* 273(10):3313–3319

Nouraei SA, Al-Yaghchi C, Ahmed J et al. 2006. An anatomical comparison of Blair and facelift incisions for parotid surgery. *Clin Otolaryngol* 31(6):531–534.

O'Brien CJ. 2003. Current management of benign parotid tumors-the role of limited superficial parotidectomy. *Head Neck* 25:946–952.

Ord RA. 1995. Surgical management of parotid tumors. *Oral and Maxillofac Surg Clin of North America* 7(3):529–564.

O'Regan BO, Bharadwaj G, Bhopal S, Cook V. 2007. Facial nerve morbidity after retrograde nerve dissection in parotid surgery for benign disease: A 10-year prospective observational study of 136 cases. *Brit J Oral Maxillofac Surg* 45(2):101–107.

Park JG, Ma TM, Rooper L, et al. 2018. Exceptional responses to pertuzumab, trastuzumab, and docetaxel in human epidermal growth factor receptor-2 high expressing salivary duct carcinomas. *Head Neck* 40(12):E100–E106

Patel S, Mourad w F, Wang C et al. 2014.Postoperative radiation therapy for parotid pleomorphic adenoma with close or positive margins: Treatment outcomes and toxicities. *Anticancer Res* 34(8):4247–4251

Peraza AJ, Wright J, Gómez R. 2017. Canalicular adenoma: A systematic review. *J Craniomaxillofac Surg* 45(10):1745–1758.

Pérez-de-Olivera ME, Wagner VP, Araújo ALD, et al. 2019. Prognostic value of CRTC1-MAML2 translocation in salivary mucoepidermoid carcinoma: Systematic review and meta-analysis. *J Oral Pathol Med* 49(5):386–394.

Pfisterer MJ, Vazquez A, Mady LJ, et al. 2014 Squamous cell carcinoma of the parotid gland: A population based study of 2,545 cases. *Am J Otolaryngol*

Piekarski J, Nejc D Szymczak W et al. 2004. Results of extracapsular dissection of pleomorphic adenoma of the parotid gland. *J Oral Maxillofac Surg* 62(10):1198–1202.

Pogrel MA, Schmidt B, Ammar A. 1996. The relationship of the buccal branch of the facial nerve to the parotid duct. *J Oral Maxillofac Surg* 54(1):71–73.

Rajasekaran K, Stubbs V, Chen J, et al. 2018. Mucoepidermoid carcinoma of the parotid: a national cancer database study. *Am J Otolaryngol* 39(3):321–326.

Rassekh CH, Cost JL, Hogg JP et al. 2014. Positron emission tomography in Warthin's tumor mimicking malignancy impacts the evaluation of head and neck patients. *Am J Otolaryngol.* 36(2):259–263.

Renehan A, Gleave EN, McGurk M. 1996. An analysis of the treatment of 114 patients with recurrent pleomorphic adenoma of the parotid gland. *Am J Surg* 172:710–714.

de Ru JA, Van Bentham PPG, Hordijk GJ. 2002. The location of parotid gland tumors in relation to the facial nerve on magnetic resonance images and computed tomography scans. *J Oral Maxillofac Surg* 60:992–996.

de Ru JA, Maartens SVL, Van Bentham PPG et al. 2007 Do magnetic resonance imaging and ultrasound add anything to the preoperative workup of parotid tumors? *J Oral Maxillofac Surg* 65:945–952.

Rubello D, Nanni C, Castellucci et al. 2005. Does 18 FDG PET/CT play a role in the differential diagnosis of parotid masses. *Panminerva Med* 47(3)187–189.

Safedieh J, Givi B, Osborn V et al. 2017. Impact of adjuvant radiotherapy for malignant salivary tumors *Otolaryngol Head Neck Surg.* 157(6):988–994.

Saku T, Hayashi, Y., Takahara, O. et al. 1997. Salivary tumors among atom bomb survivors, 1950–1987. *Cancer* 79(8):1465–1475.

Scherl C, Kato M G, Erkul E et al. 2018. Outcomes and prognostic factors for parotid acinic cell carcinoma: A National Cancer Database study of 2362 cases. *Oral Oncol* 82:53–60.

Schick S, Steiner, E Gahleitner A et al. 1998. Differentiation of benign and malignant tumors of the parotid gland: Value of pulsed Doppler and lor Doppler sonography. *Eur Radiol* 8:1462–1467.

Schmitt NC, Kang H, Shama A. 2017 Salivary duct carcinoma: An aggressive salivary gland malignancy with opportunities for targeted therapy. *Oral Oncol* 74:40–48.

Schroder U, Eckel HE, Rasche V et al. 2000. Value of fine needle puncture cytology in neoplasms of the parotid gland. *HNO* 48(6):421–429.

Schwartz U, Hurlimann S, Soyka JD et al. 2009. FDG-positive Warthin's tumors in cervical lymph nodes mimicking metastases in tongue cancer staging with PET/CT. *Otolaryngol Head Neck Surg* 140(1):134–135.

Seiffert G, Donath K. 1996. Multiple tumors of the salivary glands-terminology and nomenclature *Eur J Cancer B Oral Oncol* 32B(1):3–7.

Sharma P, Jain TK, Singh H, et al. 2013. Utility of (18)F-FDG PET-CT in staging and restaging of patients with malignant salivary gland tumors: A single-institutional experience. *Nuc Med Commun* 34(3):211–219.

Shen SY, Wang WH, Liang R et al. 2018. Clinicopathologic analysis of 2,,736vsalivary gland cases over a 11-year period in Southwest China. *Acta Otolaryngol* 138(8):746–749.

de Siqueira EC, de Souza FTA, Gomez RS et al. 2017 Does cell phone use increase the chances of parotid gland tumor development? A systematic review and meta-analysis. *J Oral Pathol* 46(7);480–483.

Song IH, Song JS, Sung CO et al. 2015. Accuracy of core needle biopsy versus fine needle aspiration cytology for diagnosing salivary gland tumors. *J Pathol Transl Med* 49(2):136–143.

Sood AJ, Houlton JJ, Nguyen SA, Gillespie MB 2015.Facial nerve monitoring during parotidectomy: A systematic review and meta-analysis. *Otolaryngol Head Neck Surg* 152(4):631–637.

Sood S, McGurk M, Vaz F. 2016. Management of salivary gland tumors: United Kingdom National Multidisciplinary Guidelines. *J Laryngol Otol* 130(S2):S142–S149.

Spiro JD, Spiro RH. 2003. Cancer of the parotid gland: role of seventh nerve preservation. *World J Surg* 27(7):863–867.

Stankovic P, Wittlinger J, Timmesfeld N et al. 2018. Antero- vs. retrograde nerve dissection in parotidectomy: A systematic review and meta-analysis. *Eur Arch Otorhinolaryngol* 275(6):1623–1630.

Stennert E, Kisner D, Jungehuelsing M et al. 2003. High incidence of lymph node metastasis in major salivary gland cancer. *Arch Otolaryngol Head Neck Surg* 129(7):720–723.

Stennert E, Wittekindt C, Klussman JP, Guntinas-Lichas O. 2004. New aspects in parotid surgery. *Otolaryngol Pol* 58(1):109–114.

Suzuki M, Kawata R, Hiashino M et al. 2019. Values of fine-needle aspiration cytology of parotid gland tumors: A review of 996 cases at a single institution. *Head Neck* 41(2):358–365.

Takahashi N, Okamoto K, Ohkubo M, Kawana M. 2005. High-resolution magnetic resonance of the extracranial facial nerve and parotid duct: Demonstration of the branches of the intraparotid facial nerve and its relation to parotid tumors by MRI with a surface coil. *Clin Radiology* 60(3)349–354.

Terakedis BE, Hunt JP, Buchman LO et al. 2017. The prognostic significance of facial nerve involvement in carcinomas of the parotid gland. *Am J Clin Oncol* 40(3):323–328.

Terhaard CHJ, Lubsen H, Rasch CRN et al. 2005. The role of radiotherapy in the treatment of malignant salivary gland tumors. *Int J Radiat Oncol Biol Phys* 61(1):103–111.

Terhaard C, Lubsen H, Tan B et al. 2006. Facial nerve function in carcinoma of the parotid gland. *Eur J Cancer* 42(16):2744–2750.

Teymoortash A, Werner JA. 2002. Value of neck dissection in patients with cancer of the parotid gland and a clinical no neck. *Onkologie* 25(2):122–126.

Timoshchuk M-A, Dekker P, Hippe DS et al. 2019. The efficacy of neutron radiation therapy in treating salivary malignancies. *Oral Oncol* 88:51–57.

Toh H, Kodama J, Fukuda J, et al. 1993. Incidence and histology of human accessory parotid glands. *Anat Rec* 236:586–590.

Tsai CH, Ting CC, Wu SY et al. 2019. Clinical significance of buccal branches of the facial nerve and their relationship with the emergence of Stensen's duct: An anatomic study on adult Taiwanese cadavers *J Craniomaxillofac Surg.* 47(11):1809–1818.

Valstar MH, van den Brekel MWM, Smeele LE. 2010. Iterpretation of treatment outcome in the clinically node-negative neck in primary parotid carcinoma: A systematic review of the literature. *Head Neck* 32(10):1402–1411.

Vascocelos AC, Nör F, Meurer L, et al., 2016. Clinicopathological analysis of salivary gland tumors over a 15-year period. *Braz Oral Res* 30:S1806.

Védrine PO, Coffinet L, Terman S, et al. 2006. Mucoepidermoid carcinoma of salivary glands in the pediatric age group: 18 cases including 11 second malignant neoplasms. *Head Neck* 28(9):827–833.

Venkateswaran L, Gan YJ, Sixbey JW et al. 2000. Epstein-Barr virus infection in salivary gland tumors in children and young adults. *Cancer* 89(2):463–466.

Verma J, Teh BS Paulino AC. 2011. Characteristics and outcome of radiation and chemotherapy-related mucoepidermoid carcinoma of the salivary glands. *Pediatr Blood Cancer* 57(7):1137–1141.

van der Waal JE, Becking AG, Snow GB, van der Waal I. 2002. Distant metastases of adenoid cystic carcinoma of the salivary glands and the value of diagnostic examinations during follow up. *Head Neck* 24(8):779–783.

Wahlberg P, Anderson H, Bjorklund A, et al. 2002. Carcinoma of the parotid and submandibular glands – a study of survival in 2,465 patients. *Oral Oncol* 38(7):706–713.

Webb AJ, Eveson JW. 2001. Pleomorphic adenomas of the major salivary glands: A study of the capsular form in relation to surgical management. *Clin Otolaryngol* 26:134–142.

Witt RL. 1999. Facial nerve function after partial superficial parotidectomy: An 11 year review 1987–1997. *Otolaryngol Head Neck Surg* 121(3):210–213.

Witt RL. 2002. The significance of the margin in parotid surgery for pleomorphic adenoma. *Laryngoscope* 112(12):2141–2154.

Witt RL, Rejto L. 2009. Pleomorphic adenoma: Extra-capsular dissection versus partial superficial parotidectomy with facial nerve dissection. *Del Med J* 81(3):119–25.

Wong DS. 2001. Signs and symptoms of malignant parotid tumors: An objective assessment. *J R Coll Surg Edinb* 46(2):91–95.

Woo SH. 2016. Endoscope -assisted transoral accessory parotid mass excision. *Head Neck* 38(1):E7–E12.

Xiao CC, Zhan KY, White-Gilbertson SJ, Day TA. 2016. Predictors of nodal metastasis in parotid malignancies: A national cancer database study of 22,653 patients *Otolaryngol Head Neck Surg* 154(1):121–130.

Xu B, Aneja A Ghossein R et al. 2017 Salivary gland epithelial neoplasms in pediatric populations a single institution experience with a focus on the histologic spectrum and clinical outcome. *Hum Pathol* 67:37–44.

Xu J, Yang Z-Y, Chen X, Liu X. 2018) HHTM1 induces the metastasis and recurrence of the parotid adenoma by repairing DNA damage. *Eur Rev Med Pharmacol Sci* 22(13):4363–4370.

Yang X, Ji T, Wang L et al. 2011. Clinical management of masses arising from the accessory parotid gland. *Oral Surg Oral Med Oral Pathol* 112:290–297.

Yoo GH, Eisle DW, Askin FB, et al. 1994. Warthin's tumor: A 40 year experience at the Johns Hopkins Hospital. *Laryngoscope* 104(7):799–803.

Zbären P, Stauffer E. 2007. Pleomorphic adenoma of the parotid gland: Histopathologic analysis of the capsular characteristics of 218 tumors. *Head Neck* 29:751–757.

Zbären P, Schar C, Hotz MA et al. 2001. Value of fine-needle aspiration cytology of parotid gland masses. *Laryngoscope* 111:789.

Zbären P, Schupbach J, Nuyens M et al. 2003. Carcinoma of the parotid gland. *Am J Surg* 186(1):57–62.

Zbären P, Tschumi I, Nuyens M, Stauffer E. 2005a Recurrent pleomorphic adenoma of the parotid. *Am J Surg* 189(2):203–207.

Zbären P, Schupbach J Nuyens M Stauffer E. 2005b. Elective neck dissection versus observation in primary parotid cancer. *Otolaryngol Head Neck Surg* 132(3):387–391.

Zbären P, Nuyens M, Caversaccio M et al. 2006. Postoperative radiation for T1 and T2 primary parotid carcinoma: Is it useful? *Otolaryngol Head Neck Surg* 135(1):140–143.

Zbären P, Vander Poorten V, Witt RL, et al. 2013. Pleomorphic adenoma of the parotid: Formal parotidectomy or limited surgery? *Am J Surg* 205(1):109–118.

Zhang D-m, Wang Y-y, Liang Q-x, et al. 2015. Endoscopic assisted resection of benign tumors of the accessory parotid gland. *J Oral Maxillofac Surg* 73(8):1499–1504.

Zhang YF, Li H, Wang XM, Cai YF. 2019. Sonoelastography for differential diagnosis between malignant and benign parotid lesions: A meta-analysis *Eur Radiol* 29(20):725–735.

Chapter 11
Tumors of the Submandibular and Sublingual Glands

Outline

Introduction
Epidemiology and Etiology
Diagnosis
    Submandibular Gland Tumors
    Sublingual Gland Tumors
Management
    Submandibular Gland Tumors
    Sublingual Gland Tumors
Summary
Case Presentation – *But I Took the Road Less Traveled*
References

Introduction

This chapter discusses the diagnosis and management of epithelial derived tumors of the submandibular and sublingual glands. These tumors are much less common than tumors of the parotid gland, although larger series of cases from which to apply evidence-based medicine treatment protocols are beginning to be published. Current approaches, primarily surgical, are highlighted. The diversity of histologic types, paucity of cases, and lack of long-term follow-up result in many of these cases being treated empirically, based on oncologic principles derived from other tumors and sites in the head and neck region. It should also be noted that the recent large series, utilizing national data bases, are not without inherent flaws. The 2015 study of 2626 submandibular tumors was accumulated between the years 1973 and 2011, a period of almost 40 years (Lee et al. 2015). During this period, there have been a number of reclassifications and definitions of "new" tumor entities, e.g. polymorphous low-grade adenocarcinoma was first recognized during this period and recently changed to polymorphous adenocarcinoma. Other examples of new entities are the mammary analogue secretory carcinoma (MASC) and the hyalinizing clear cell carcinoma. It is clear, that over time salivary tumors are not a homogenous group. Recent papers have shown a remarkable heterogenous and diverse set of genetic markers on tumors that may be useful in targeted therapy. Currently, salivary duct carcinoma appears to be the tumor with most promise for this type of therapeutic approach (Saintigny et al. 2018).

Epidemiology and Etiology

The etiology of tumors of the submandibular and sublingual glands is the same as discussed in relation to salivary gland tumors of the parotid gland (see Chapter 10). At a molecular level in a study that examined PCNA, Ki-67, and p53 in pleomorphic adenomas (PAs), mucoepidermoid carcinomas (MECAs), and adenoid cystic carcinoma (ACC), PCNA, Ki-67, and p53 expression for PA and ACC in the submandibular gland was similar to that reported for tumors of the parotid gland and minor salivary glands. However, there was a higher expression of these markers in MECA of the submandibular gland (Alves et al. 2004). This may indicate that MECA of the submandibular gland is potentially more aggressive. For many of the common tumor types, ACC and MECA, there appears to be a higher rate of both regional and distant metastases from both sublingual and submandibular sites compared to the parotid gland.

Approximately 10–15% of all salivary gland tumors will occur in the submandibular gland, and only 0.5–1% in the sublingual gland, such that sublingual tumors are very rare. These tumors are particularly uncommon in young patients. In a series of 763 patients under the age of 30 years with malignant salivary tumors of the major glands, 11.5% were located in the submandibular gland and only 0.4% were located in the sublingual gland. In looking at children younger than 19 years, 27 of 88 submandibular cancers were in pediatric patients, and 0 of 3 were located in the sublingual gland (Rutt et al. 2011). In the submandibular gland, approximately 50% of these tumors are said to be benign. Different series vary in their percentages of benign tumors, from 657 of 1235 tumors (53%) benign (Auclair et al. 1991), 55% benign (Oudidi et al. 2006) which included non-epidermoid cancers, to 39.2% benign (Rapidis et al. 2004).

Pleomorphic adenoma is the commonest benign tumor in the submandibular gland while ACC predominates for malignant tumors. In examining malignant tumors, Bhattacharyya (2004) analyzed 370 cases from the Surveillance, Epidemiology and End Results (SEER) data base, finding ACC in 42.2% and MECA in 22.2% of cases, while Rapidis et al. (2004) in a literature review of 356 cases showed ACC in 45.3%, adenocarcinoma in 14.3%, MECA in 12.9%, and carcinoma ex-pleomorphic adenoma in 11.2% and Auclair et al. (1991) found ACC in 24% and MECA in 19% of 578 cases. ACC was the commonest malignancy (36%) in a series of 2626 submandibular gland cancers. This is the largest series of malignant submandibular gland tumors published at the current time (Lee et al. 2015). In a series of 85 cases, 24% were malignant, and 55% of these malignant tumors were ACCs (Mizrachi et al. 2017). Similar results have been reported with 30% malignancy and 56% ACC (Aro et al. 2018). Although sublingual gland tumors are rare, they are important to recognize as they have an extremely high rate of malignancy. In a review of approximately 4000 patients with salivary tumors collected over a 55-year period, only 18 (0.5%) had sublingual gland tumors all of which were malignant (Spiro 1995). There are very few other large series of sublingual gland tumors in the literature; Yu et al. (2007) reported 30 cases collected over a 50-year period all of which were malignant. Yamazaki et al. reviewed the literature in 1987 and found 83 cases of sublingual gland tumors of which 72 (87%) were malignant. A Danish series of 29 cases showed 96.6% to be malignant (Andreasen et al. 2016). In the author's personal series, of 1013 salivary gland tumors treated between 1990 and 2014, 25 (2.5%) were sublingual gland tumors and all tumors were malignant. Twenty-one of these 25 tumors were epithelial in nature (Table 11.1). Among the other four were three lymphomas and one sarcoma (see Chapter 15 for details). The largest series of malignant sublingual gland tumors was published is 210 (Lee et al. 2016). Adenoid cystic carcinoma appears to be the commonest histologic type "followed by MECA." Published series show ACC 50%, MECA 28% (Spiro 1995), ACC 56.7% (Yu et al. 2007) and ACC 66%, MECA 33% (Perez et al. 2005). Zdanowski et al. (2012) found 66.7% of their sublingual gland tumors were adenoid cystic carcinomas but also commented that 83.3% of their series presented late with stage III or IV disease. In one small series from Japan, 61.5% of malignancies in the sublingual gland were adenoid cystic carcinoma (Kojima et al. 2020).

Diagnosis

SUBMANDIBULAR GLAND TUMORS

Most submandibular gland tumors present with a slow-growing, painless mass inferior to the mandible (Figure 11.1). In a series of 87 submandibular gland carcinomas, 94% presented with a palpable mass and 39% with pain (Kaszuba et al. 2007). As tumors of the gland are rare and inflammatory swelling secondary to sialolithiasis is seen more often, diagnosis may be delayed and patients can present with late disease. In one series, 50% of all referred patients with submandibular gland tumors had already had their submandibular gland removed on the presumption that the involved process was benign (Camilleri et al. 1998). The average tumor size in 370 cases of cancer of the submandibular gland was 2.9 cm (Bhattacharyya 2004). Inflammatory disease, however, is often painful and usually characterized by exacerbations and resolutions of the swelling in relation to eating. In a series of 258 submandibular gland excisions, 119 (46%) had sialolithiasis, 88 (34%) sialadenitis, and 51 (20%) tumors (Preuss et al. 2007).

Table 11.1. Sublingual gland tumors 1990–2020 (Experience of Drs. Carlson and Ord).

Patient	Age	Race	Gender	Pathology	Stage
1	45	B	M	Int. MECA	IV
2	85	W	F	PLGA	I
3	57	W	F	Int. MECA	I
4	46	W	M	Adeno Ca NOS	IV
5	69	W	M	Comedo Adeno Ca	X
6	67	W	F	ACC	II
7	47	B	F	HG MECA	IV
8	54	A	M	LG MECA	I
9	68	W	F	ACC	I
10	70	W	F	LG MECA	III
11	70	B	F	ACC	II
12	58	W	M	LG MECA	I
13	47	W	F	Int. MECA	II
14	56	B	F	ACC	I
15	48	W	F	Int. MECA	I
16	52	C	M	Low-grade MECA	I
17	73	C	F	Intermediate-grade MECA	I
18	47	C	F	Low-grade MECA	I
19	53	C	F	Low-grade MECA	I
20	72	C	M	Low-grade MECA	I
21	55	B	F	ACC	I

Key: B = Black, W = White, A = Asian. M = Male, F = Female, MECA = Mucoepidermoid carcinoma. ACC = Adenoid cystic carcinoma, Adeno Ca = Adenocarcinoma, PLGA = Polymorphous low-grade adenocarcinoma according to 3rd edition of the World Health Organization of Head and Neck Tumors. LG = Low-grade, Int = Intermediate-grade, HG = High-grade, NOS = Not otherwise specified.

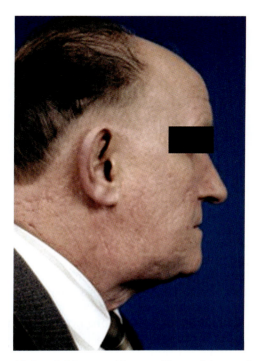

Figure 11.1. A 64-year-old man with a painless submandibular mass.

Examination usually reveals a smooth, firm to hard mass in the submandibular triangle that is most commonly discrete and mobile. Fixation of the mass to the skin or underlying mylohyoid muscle is a sign of malignancy with advanced extra-capsular infiltration (Figure 11.2). Neural involvement of the mandibular branch of the facial nerve with ipsilateral lower lip palsy, the lingual nerve with ipsilateral anesthesia or paresthesia of the tongue or the hypoglossal nerve with ipsilateral palsy of the tongue muscles are also signs of cancer. Associated hard cervical nodes due to regional metastasis may also be present in malignant tumors. However, it may be more difficult to clinically assess whether a submandibular gland tumor is benign or malignant compared to a parotid tumor, as clinical judgment for these tumors has been said to be unreliable (Lee et al. 2013).

The differential diagnosis of a solitary mass in the submandibular triangle with no overt signs of malignancy will include lymphadenopathy, plunging ranula, vascular malformation, and

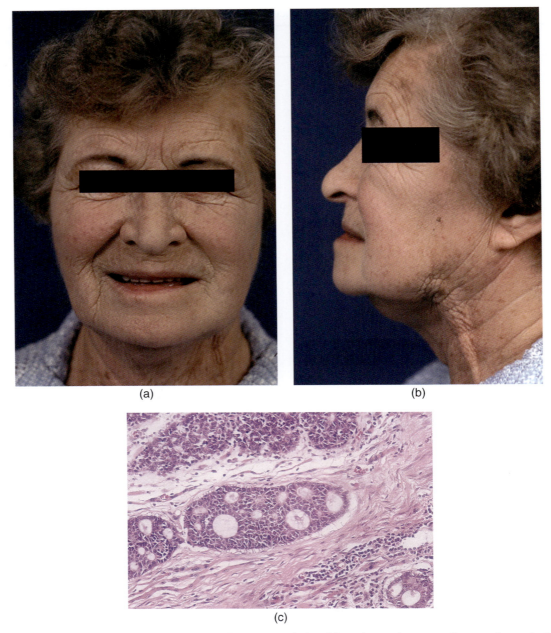

Figure 11.2. (a) Elderly lady with a hard-submandibular mass (adenoid cystic carcinoma on fine needle aspiration biopsy) who presented with a palsy of the marginal mandibular branch of the facial nerve. (b) Lateral facial view shows skin fixation and tethering. (c) Histopathology of adenoid cystic carcinoma of submandibular gland.

branchial cysts. It may be difficult to differentiate a lymph node from the enlarged gland on clinical examination alone. If the mass is bimanually palpable from within the floor of mouth, it is more likely to be a submandibular gland mass, and if it can be "rolled" over the lower border of the mandible on palpation it is a lymph node.

The plunging ranula is usually soft-cystic in consistency but can become firm if chronically encysted. Vascular lesions are also soft, may "pit" on firm pressure or have thrills and murmurs. Branchial cysts lie more posterior and are partially beneath the anterior border of the sternocleidomastoid muscle.

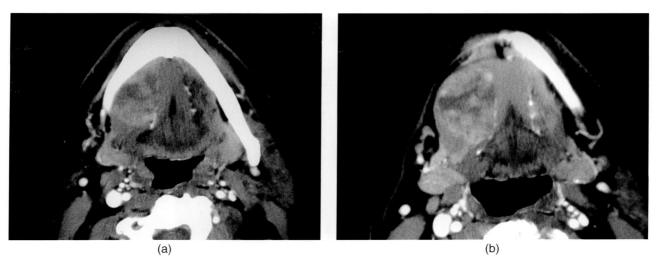

Figure 11.3. (a and b) CT scans showing submandibular mass with differing regions of radiolucency and opacity. Histopathology showed pleomorphic adenoma.

Imaging techniques to delineate submandibular gland lesions include ultrasound, CT, and MR. As the submandibular gland is superficial in the neck, high-resolution ultrasound can distinguish intraglandular from extraglandular masses and can differentiate benign tumors from those that are malignant (Alyas et al. 2005). CT scanning may be useful in detecting early cortical erosion of the mandible and identifying cervical nodes in malignant cases (Figure 11.3). In a study to identify whether a submandibular mass was intraglandular or extraglandular, the accuracy of contrast-enhanced CT was 87%, of CT sialography was 85%, and of MR was 91% (Chikui et al. 2004). These authors did not find displacement of the facial vein and its relationship to the mass a helpful guide. The use of MRI with apparent diffusion coefficient (ADC) can predict malignancy in a submandibular tumor with an accuracy of 84%, a sensitivity of 88%, and specificity of 81% (Razek 2019).

Open biopsy of the submandibular gland mass is contraindicated for similar reasons that were discussed in relation to the parotid gland (see Chapter 10). Fine needle aspiration biopsy (FNAB) is the method of choice for these tumors, one literature review finding an overall accuracy of greater than 80% in skilled hands, which is comparable with the accuracy of frozen section (Pogrel 1995). A further review of submandibular swellings of all types including sialadenitis assessed preoperatively using FNAB cytology/core biopsies showed an accuracy of 88% with sensitivity of 71.4% and specificity of 94.4% (Taylor et al. 2011). Not all authors have found such high success with FNAB: 9/12 patients with class III cytology turned out to be malignant in one study. The authors concluded that FNAC proved useful but has its limitations, and advised that wide margins should always be obtained with submandibular tumors even when clinical exam and cytology indicates no malignancy (Atula et al. 2017). The United Kingdom National Guidelines for salivary gland tumors recommend US-guided FNAC in all salivary gland tumors and cytology to be reported by an expert histopathologist (Sood et al. 2016).

We have used ultrasound-guided FNAB for difficult cases with success. In one case of a 6 mm MECA identified on MR, we were able to obtain a FNAB positive for MECA (Figure 11.4). Ultrasound-guided core needle biopsy has also been used in the submandibular gland (Bahn et al. 2011). As discussed in Chapter 10, recent studies have supported the use of core needle biopsy over FNAB for salivary gland tumors. A 2015 study of 412 cases (101 in the submandibular gland) showed core needle biopsy (CNB) to be significantly more accurate for diagnosis of malignant tumors (Eom et al. 2015). A meta-analysis in 2018 showed a sensitivity of 0.94 and specificity of 0.98 for CNB in salivary glands (Kim and Kim 2018).

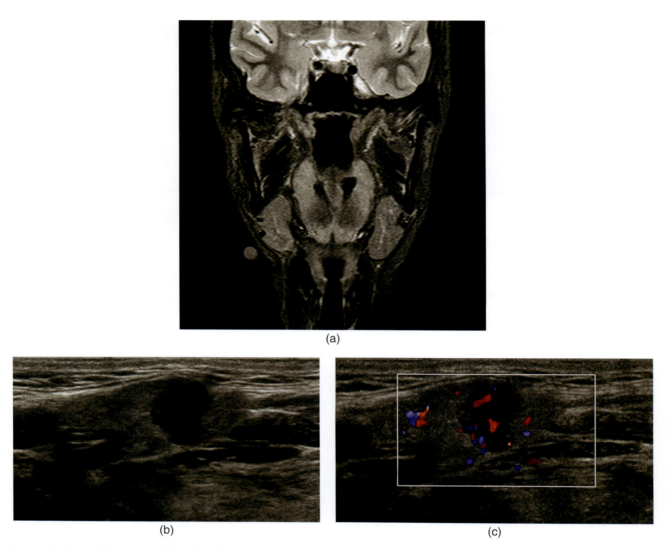

Figure 11.4. (a) T2 coronal MR with skin marker overlying the palpable nodule. Image shows a hypodense 6 mm mass in the inferior of the right submandibular gland. (b) High-resolution ultrasound (c) and color Doppler ultrasound confirm the mass. An ultrasound-guided biopsy was performed that showed epithelial cells consistent with mucoepidermoid carcinoma. The patient underwent a supraomohyoid neck dissection that confirmed a 6 mm focus of MECA within the submandibular gland.

SUBLINGUAL GLAND TUMORS

Tumors of the sublingual gland present as a mass in the floor of mouth that is usually painless and slow-growing. They may be large enough to impair tongue movement with speech difficulty or to prevent wearing a lower denture (Figure 11.5). Occasionally, they may cause obstruction of Wharton duct either due to pressure or malignant infiltration and present with a submandibular swelling. Virtually 100% of these tumors are malignant and involvement of the lingual nerve or hypoglossal nerve with ipsilateral anesthesia or weakness of the tongue may be seen. Examination by palpation reveals a firm to hard mass which may be tender and fixed to the lingual periosteum. Infiltration of the tongue muscles with slurring of speech or dysphagia can occur.

The only other sublingual gland entity on the differential diagnosis is a ranula which can resemble a cystic tumor. Clinically, a prominent sublingual gland may be seen when a mass (e.g. in the submandibular gland, a lateral dermoid cyst, or a

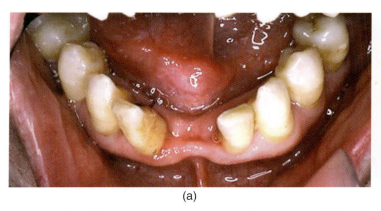 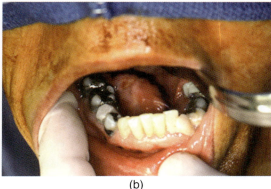

Figure 11.5. (a) Adenocarcinoma of right sublingual gland. (b) Polymorphous low-grade adenocarcinoma of the sublingual gland. Source: Re-published with permission from Blanchaert et al. (1998) DOI-https://doi.org/10.1016/S0901-5027(98)80307-X.

thyroglossal cyst) pushes the sublingual gland superiorly from below the mylohyoid muscle. Although this can be confusing clinically, subsequent imaging will reveal the true cause.

Imaging is usually by CT or MR. CT scans will be more accurate for early cortical bone invasion (Figure 11.6). In MR imaging, T1 weighted signal intensity of carcinomas in and near the sublingual gland is lower than that of the gland whereas T2 weighted signal intensity of carcinomas exceeds that of the gland (Sumi et al. 1999).

In the sublingual gland, histologic diagnosis is usually accomplished by incisional biopsy through the overlying oral mucosa. In deeply seated lesions, FNAB may be useful. Some studies caution that FNAC is less accurate for diagnosis of sublingual gland tumors (Andreasen et al. 2016).

Management

SUBMANDIBULAR GLAND TUMORS

As in all salivary gland tumors, surgery is the primary modality of treatment. When the diagnosis is established preoperatively as benign PA by FNAB, then an extra-capsular excision of the submandibular gland is indicated (Figures 11.7 and 11.8). Pleomorphic adenoma should be treated in the same manner as for the parotid gland (see Chapter 10). There is some evidence that the capsule of PAs in the submandibular gland is thinner than in the parotid (Webb and Eveson 2001) and it is important to maintain a margin of normal tissue around the tumor. If the entire gland and tumor is not removed, but the PA merely enucleated, there is a higher risk of recurrence (Laskawi et al. 1995). In this dissection, it is easy to maintain a little extra fat and connective tissue over areas where the PA may approach the surface of the gland (Figure 11.9). In a series of 15 PAs of the submandibular gland, 20% were in the surface of the gland (Laskawi et al. 1995) (Figure 11.10). However, the submandibular gland PA has a low recurrence rate, 0% in 72 cases followed for a mean of 82 months. A histopathological study of these 72 cases found all of the tumors were encased by a complete and intact capsule. Pseudopodia were seen in only 15.3% and satellite nodules in 4.2%, with a stroma rich/myxoid appearance in 25% and cellular in 20.8%.

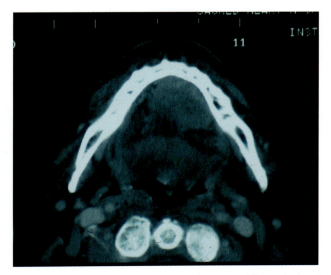

Figure 11.6. CT scan of large malignant sublingual gland tumor.

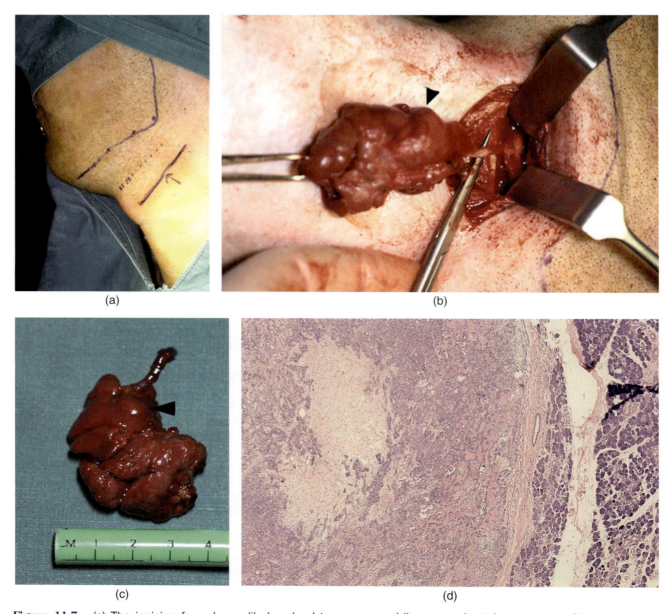

Figure 11.7. (a) The incision for submandibular gland tumor removal lies approximately one to two fingers breadths below the lower border of the mandible and is placed in a natural skin crease. (b) The submandibular gland is separated from its duct, which is indicated by the sharp scissors. The arrow points to the tumor in the hilum. (c) Surgical specimen with arrow indicating PA. (d) Histopathology shows pleomorphic adenoma of submandibular gland.

However, a complete rim of healthy intact tissue around the tumor and its capsule was only seen in 31.9% of cases. The authors concluded that due to the consistent presence of an intact capsule and low incidence of adverse histopathologic features, an excellent oncologic result could be obtained despite capsular exposure (Mantsopoulos et al. 2018).

The marginal mandibular branch of the facial nerve lies between the platysma superficially and the capsule of the submandibular gland (superficial layer of the deep cervical fascia) deeply and can be preserved either by identifying it and dissecting it along its course and retracting it superiorly or by ligating and cutting the anterior facial vein inferior to the nerve and using traction on the

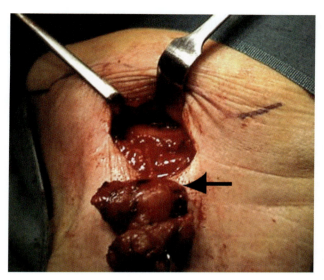

Figure 11.8. Another case of submandibular pleomorphic adenoma dissected to the duct. The larger tumor at the hilum is indicated by the arrow.

tied distal end of the vessel to retract the nerve out of the field (the Hayes Martin maneuver). In one systematic review of 28 studies (1861 halves), at least one branch of the marginal mandibular nerve ran below the inferior border of the mandible (Marcuzzo et al. 2019). The incidence of transient palsy of the marginal mandibular branch of the facial nerve was 7% in excising benign tumors and 21% in excising malignant tumors, with only one case (<1%) of permanent palsy in one series (Preuss et al. 2007). The facial artery is sacrificed if it passes through the gland itself, but if it lies superficial, then its numerous small branches including the submental branch can be clipped and the main vessel preserved.

An alternative approach for pleomorphic adenoma of the submandibular gland is a gland sparing resection as a minimally invasive surgery similar to the use of extra-capsular dissection in the parotid (see Chapter 10). In a prospective study of 20 patients with pleomorphic adenoma of the submandibular gland treated by local excision of the tumor only, with limited negative margins, the submandibular gland and its function were preserved in all cases (Roh and Park 2008). Although the authors reported no recurrence, their median follow-up was only 36 months, which may not be long enough to be confident that the patients are truly cured. However, a more recent randomized prospective trial reports 40 patients with benign submandibular tumors allocated 20 to gland excision and 20 to gland preservation. There was no recurrence in either cohort with follow-up 38 months to 5 years. The authors found less nerve injury to the lingual and mandibular branch of the facial nerve, less hollowing with better facial contour and preservation of salivary function. The authors recommended the gland preserving technique as the first choice for benign submandibular gland tumors (Min et al. 2013). Further evidence for this minimally invasive approach comes from a series of 31 patients, 11 treated with partial sialoadenectomy. Again, there was no recurrence (follow-up 41–82 months) and better salivary function, with improved facial contour (Ge et al. 2016).

Another technique that has been suggested to minimize scar and reduce nerve injury has been removal of the submandibular gland with a pleomorphic adenoma from an intraoral approach. One study reports 12 cases and found only short-term morbidity with temporary lingual nerve paresis and limitation of tongue movement. One patient out of twelve recurred, with a follow-up range of 20 months to 10 years (Hong and Yang 2008).

In recurrent PA, the disease will frequently be multinodular as in the parotid and, as 45% of these cases involve the subcutaneous tissue under the previous operative scar, excision of the scar with a margin of the surrounding skin is recommended as part of the en bloc excision (Laskawi et al. 1995).

Where a definite diagnosis of benign tumor is not established preoperatively or when a low-grade malignant tumor is diagnosed, an en bloc resection of level I is safest. If the final histologic diagnosis is benign no important structures have to be sacrificed, only the gland and tumor plus fat with lymph nodes. If the tumor is a low-grade malignancy, then no further surgery is indicated. In the case of a high-grade tumor, a selective or radical neck dissection can be completed at the same time (Figure 11.11).

In undertaking the level I dissection, the cervical skin flap is lifted in a subplatysmal plane and the marginal mandibular branch of the facial nerve is preserved. The anterior belly of the digastric muscle is identified and its fascia dissected free. The fascia is dissected off the mylohyoid muscle, freeing the fat and nodes from the digastric, mylohyoid, and inferior border of the mandible. The posterior edge of the mylohyoid muscle is retracted to identify the lingual nerve. This nerve is preserved if it is uninvolved, by cutting its branch to

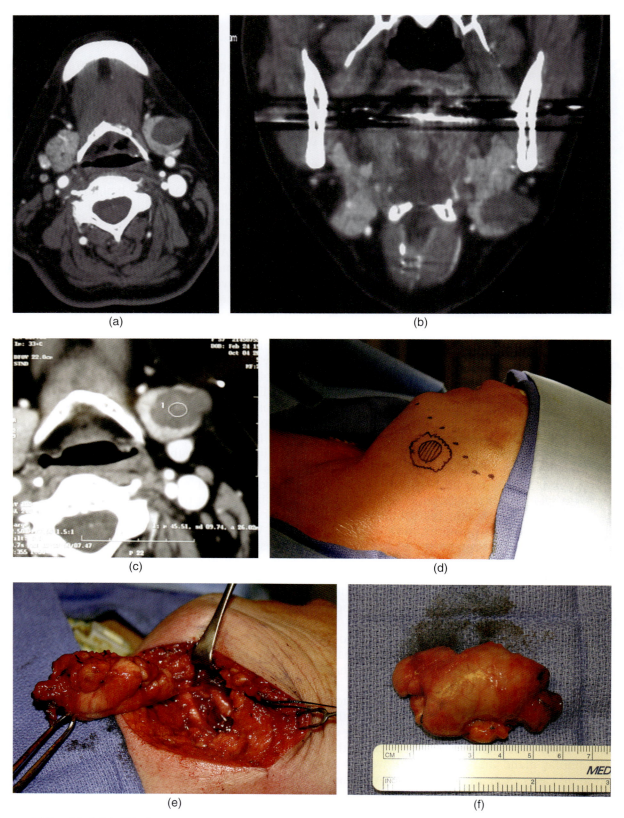

Figure 11.9. (a) Axial CT shows tumor projecting beyond the gland surface. (b) Coronal CT confirms the surface involvement. (c) High-power axial CT scan shows the tumor marked with a circle. (d) Operative picture showing the tumor marked by palpation. (e) Intraoperative view of extra-capsular dissection preserving soft tissue over the tumor surface. (f) Surgical specimen.

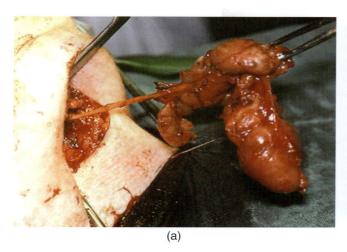 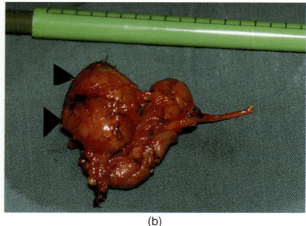

Figure 11.10. (a) Submandibular gland attached only by its duct. The pleomorphic adenoma is large and hangs beneath the gland attached only by the enveloping fascia of the capsule. (b) Surgical specimen with arrows pointing to the large PA which has no real attachment to the gland.

the gland and allowing the nerve to retract superiorly. The Wharton duct is sectioned and the proximal end of the facial vein and artery tied off or dissected free as indicated to release the specimen. In low-grade N0 tumors, a neck dissection is usually not indicated but the excision can be extended to encompass lymph node levels II and III as a standard supraomohyoid neck dissection. The Dutch Oncology Group has proposed a scoring system based upon T stage and histologic type/grade. This appears to show that submandibular gland tumors with less risk factors than similar tumors in the parotid have a higher rate of occult nodes. N0 parotid tumors with a score of 4 have a 24% risk of occult nodes and for the submandibular gland a lesser score of 3 gives a 33% risk (Terhaard et al. 2005). Perhaps the clinician should have a lower threshold for elective neck dissection for the submandibular gland. If lymph nodes are clinically involved, then a type I modified radical neck dissection is required.

In high-grade tumors or advanced low-grade tumors with extra-capsular infiltration and involvement of the skin, muscle or mandible extended resections with resection of these structures will be necessary to obtain clear margins. These resections will be dictated by the size and extent of the tumor. In N0 cases, selective neck dissection levels I–III or I–IV will be used and modified radical neck dissections for clinically positive necks. In one series, the five-year overall survival (OS) and disease free survival (DFS) rates were 76.9 and 67.3% respectively.

Fixed mass, positive neck nodes, and positive margin status were relevant predictors of OS and disease specific survival (DSS). Node stage was the relevant predictor for disease outcome (Liu et al. 2018).

In the case of ACC, widespread infiltrative growth beyond the palpable tumor makes obtaining clear margins challenging. The propensity for perineural invasion with ACC will necessitate sacrifice of involved nerves, e.g. lingual, hypoglossal, and facial, tracing the nerves proximally using frozen section guidance to determine clearance. Unfortunately, "skip" metastases can occur along the nerve and a negative frozen section is no guarantee of success. In a systematic review of ACC, the incidence of perineural invasion ranged from 29.4 to 62.5% and was associated with local recurrence (Dantas et al. 2015). A case presentation of disseminated spread of adenoid cystic carcinoma by perineural spread along large cranial nerves is presented at the end of this chapter. ACC is more prone to metastasize hematogenously than through lymphatics such that a selective neck dissection is usually sufficient.

Robotic surgery has also been reported in the surgery of submandibular gland tumors. In a report of utilizing a robotic approach through a trans-hairline incision for 25 submandibular resections, which included benign and malignant tumors, no positive margins were seen and no tumor recurrence reported (Yang 2018).

Postoperative radiation therapy is administered for high-grade tumors, positive margins,

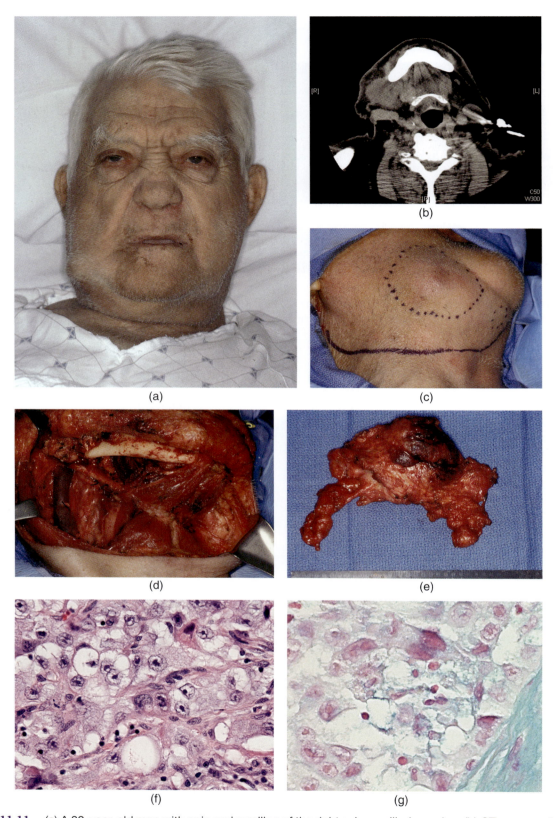

Figure 11.11. (a) A 82-year-old man with pain and swelling of the right submandibular region. (b) CT scan confirms a right submandibular gland mass diagnosed as malignant on fine needle aspiration biopsy. (c) Intraoperative view showing neck dissection incision marked on the skin. (d) Level I excision combined with a selective neck dissection in view of high-grade cytology. (e) Operative specimen. (f) Hematoxylin and eosin stain shows mucous cells and mitotic figures. (g) Alcian Blue stain confirms a diagnosis of high-grade mucoepidermoid carcinoma. (h) One-year postoperative view of the patient. He died three years postoperatively with distant metastases of the lung.

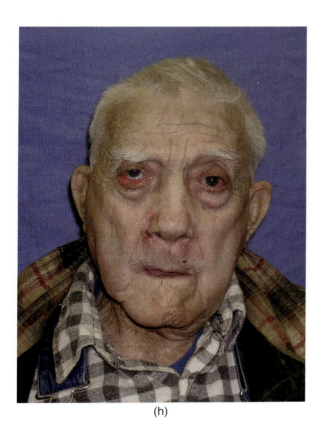

(h)

Figure 11.11. (Continued).

positive nodes, and perineural spread if re-resection is not possible. Chemotherapy has not been shown to improve survival in salivary gland cancer.

Prognosis will depend on the histologic grade and the stage of the tumor. The largest series reported of 2626 cases from the SEER database found an OS and DSS at 5 and 10 years of 54 and 67%, and 40 and 60% respectively. Multivariate Cox regression analysis revealed that the independent predictors for OS and DSS were age, tumor grade, and TNM stage for negative predictors and female sex, and surgical resection for positive survival benefit. A larger than 3 cm tumor size had a significantly worse prognosis and radiation therapy's effect on survival depended on tumor size and histologic type (Lee et al. 2015). Some authors (Anderson et al. 1991) have found a crude 10-year survival of 50% with 10% local recurrence and 39% of cases having metastasized at the time of diagnosis. In the series reported by Rapidis et al. (2004), 8 of 14 patients died during follow-up with a survival rate of 38.5%, but 11 of 14 of these patients presented with stage III or IV disease. Bhattacharyya (2004) analyzed 370 cases of submandibular gland cancer from the SEER data base, and reported a 59.7% five-year survival; however, this figure is high as 42.2% of his cases were ACC with a mean survival of 99 months. In the same series, the patients with squamous cell carcinoma had a mean survival of 52 months. Younger age, low-grade histology, and the use of radiation therapy were factors in improving survival. Weber et al. (1990) found a 69% five-year survival, with extra-capsular infiltration and lymph node metastases indicating a poor prognosis. Stages TI-TIVA had a case-specific five-year survival of 88% compared to 55% for T4B, and five-year survival of 86% for negative nodes compared to 30% for positive nodes.

More recent papers have confirmed the propensity of submandibular gland tumors to have a higher failure rate from distant metastases (Figure 11.12). In a Brazilian study of 255 major salivary carcinomas, the percentage of distant metastasis seen was 42% for the submandibular gland, 20%

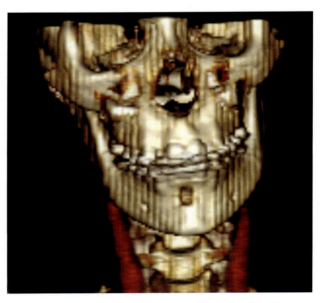

Figure 11.12. Three-dimensional CT scan of a 15-year-old Caucasian girl who had a pleomorphic adenoma of the submandibular gland removed four years earlier when she was 11 years old. She presented with an oval radiolucent lesion in the mandibular symphysis thought to be a cyst. This was removed and histologically was benign PA. The final diagnosis was benign metastasizing pleomorphic adenoma.

for the parotid gland, and 17% for the sublingual gland (Mariano et al. 2011). Again, this may be due to the high percentage of adenoid cystic carcinomas found at this site. However, in an interesting study which compared parotid and submandibular adenoid cystic carcinomas and their propensity for earlier systemic dissemination, the authors found more abundant tumor-associated blood vessels in the submandibular gland microenvironment. This study postulates a true site difference in the behavior of adenoid cystic carcinomas (Shin et al. 2014).

Actuarial five-year locoregional control, distant metastasis-free survival, disease-free and overall survival rates were 69.7, 65.8, 52.8, and 56.8% respectively for carcinomas in the submandibular gland (Roh et al. 2008). In multivariate analysis, T category and histological grading were prognostic for disease-free survival and T category and resection margins for locoregional control. Around 33.9% of this series initially had or developed distant metastases. Another series showed actuarial five-year locoregional control, distant metastasis-free survival, and disease-free survival of 80.5, 86.1, and 71.85% respectively (Mallik et al. 2010). In this study, overall stage grouping, perineural invasion, and radiotherapy dose were significant predictors of locoregional control. In addition, overall stage grouping and T stage affected disease-free survival, with a nonsignificant trend for worse outcomes with extra-glandular involvement. A further series of 50 patients showed 70% were T1–2 and 30% were node positive. High-grade lesions were identified in 64% of cases. OS, DSS, and RFS at 5 years were 66.4, 57.1 and 76.6%, and at 10 years 72.1, 69.1 and 62.4%. pT status, pN status, and perineural involvement (PNI) significantly affected prognosis (Lombardi et al. 2018).

Most published series have found a survival benefit conferred by radiation therapy with 75% of patients receiving adjuvant radiation in one study (Camilleri et al. 1998). Storey et al. (2001) reported actuarial locoregional control of 88% at 5 and 10 years; however, the corresponding disease-free survival rates were 60 and 53% due to 36% of patients with locoregional control developing distant metastases. Nonetheless, the median survival time for patients with locoregional control was 183 months compared to 19 months for those patients without locoregional control. In a similar study of adjuvant radiation therapy, cancer-specific survival was 79 and 57% at 5 and 10 years, with local control of 85 and 74% respectively. Twenty percent of their patients (all ACC) developed distant metastases (Sykes et al. 1999). A retrospective study of 87 patients compared two cohorts of patients." "One cohort received initial enucleation of the gland (subcapsular dissection) with no evidence of residual primary or nodal disease followed by postoperative radiation therapy. The second cohort had evidence of gross residual primary or nodal disease, grossly positive margins or piecemeal removal following initial treatment who underwent further definitive surgical resection followed by postoperative radiation therapy. This study found no difference in locoregional control, disease specific survival or overall survival (Kaszuba et al. 2007). This suggests patients without evidence of gross residual disease post-enucleation might be satisfactorily treated with radiation therapy without further surgery. The United Kingdom National Guidelines for salivary gland tumors recommend radiotherapy for all malignant submandibular tumors except in cases of small low-grade tumors that have been completely excised (Sood et al. 2016).

In a series of 22 patients with ACC of the submandibular gland, disease-free survival at 5 years of 57% and at 10 years of 41% and overall survival of 70 and 37% respectively were found (Cohen et al. 2004). These authors concluded that early diagnosis, wide surgical intervention, and postoperative radiotherapy were associated with a favorable prognosis while not surprisingly large tumor size, positive surgical margins, perineural invasion, and local recurrence were negative prognostic factors.

In comparing submandibular gland cancers to parotid cancer, a worse overall prognosis was associated with submandibular gland tumors (Hocwald et al. 2001). In addition, the likelihood of developing distant metastasis is greater in the submandibular gland than the parotid (Schwenter et al. 2006); however, this may be due to the higher percentage of ACC. In one large series of 370 cases, only 12 (2.9%) presented with distant metastases, but 24.9% were found to have positive regional nodes (Bhattacharyya 2004). Interestingly, in this retrospective review extraglandular extension and nodal positivity did not affect survival. Another study found that mortality from submandibular cancer was mostly due to distant metastases and that the main predictors for this were positive nodes N2 or > and high tumor grade (Yamada et al. 2018). Goode et al. (1998) in a study of 234 cases of MECA of the major salivary glands stated that MECAs with equal histopathologic grade had a better prognosis when their tumors were in the parotid gland rather than in the submandibular gland. This finding was confirmed in a Swedish study of 2465 major salivary gland tumors (Wahlberg et al. 2002). High-grade MECA is also more common in the submandibular gland, with 32 of 82 cases (39%) occurring in this gland (Bhattacharyya 2004). A study from Eastern China of 376 cases of mucoepidermoid carcinoma found that the highest rates of cervical node metastases were found in the submandibular gland (Liu et al. 2014).

SUBLINGUAL GLAND TUMORS

Virtually all sublingual gland tumors will be malignant and, as for all salivary tumors, primary surgery is the treatment of choice. Prognosis will be determined by the histologic grade and the stage of the tumor.

In the very rare benign tumor or with small low-grade carcinomas, a transoral wide local resection may be successfully performed (Blanchaert et al. 1998). This will be easier to undertake in edentulous patients and Wharton duct will require a sialodochoplasty procedure (Figure 11.13). In most cases, due to grade, tumor size, the presence of teeth, and involvement of mandibular periosteum/bone, a wider access will be required. In dealing with adenoid cystic carcinomas, extension to surrounding structures, particularly the mandibular bone and the lingual nerve, will be greater than clinically appreciated. Preoperative imaging with MR will be essential (Figure 11.14). If the periosteum is uninvolved and can be safely peeled from the lingual bone, a standard "pull-through" approach or a lip split with mandibulotomy can be used (Figure 11.15). The result of the lip split/mandibulotomy was functionally better than the pull-through approach in a comparative study (Devine et al. 2001). As both of these methods of access involve entering the neck, a supraomohyoid neck dissection is usually carried out in the N0 neck even for low-grade tumors (Figure 11.16). Both lingual and hypoglossal nerves can be involved by these tumors at an early stage, particularly with the ACC (Figure 11.17). Sacrifice of the nerve with

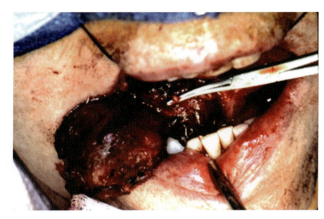

Figure 11.13. Delivering sublingual gland with low-grade (polymorphous adenocarcinoma) malignant tumor via an intraoral wide local excision. Source: Re-published with permission from Blanchaert et al. (1998) DOI-https://doi.org/10.1016/S0901-5027(98)80307-X.

proximal tracing and frozen section guidance as described for the submandibular tumors may be needed. Due to local infiltration of the lingual nerve, submandibular duct, and the oral portion of the submandibular gland, the submandibular gland and neck dissection are usually removed in continuity. A case presentation of disseminated perineural spread of adenoid cystic carcinoma is presented at the end of this chapter.

In tumors fixed to periosteum or where minimal cortical erosion is present, an oblique marginal mandibular resection angling the cut to take a greater height of the lingual plate will be utilized (Figure 11.18). The marginal mandibular resection can be performed with the pull-through or mandibulotomy approach, but is most commonly performed intraorally. Where the medullary bone is invaded, a segmental mandibular resection with a composite en bloc resection of the floor of mouth is safest and will provide excellent access (Figure 11.19). In these larger soft tissue resections, a thin pliable flap such as the radial forearm flap probably gives the best results in maintaining tongue mobility. Where the mandible has been resected, a fibular flap (Rinaldo et al. 2004) or deep circumflex iliac artery (DCIA) flap is appropriate.

Most malignant tumors of the sublingual gland are adenoid cystic carcinomas which have a low incidence of lymph node metastasis (10% in Sun et al. 2010 study), but selective neck dissection

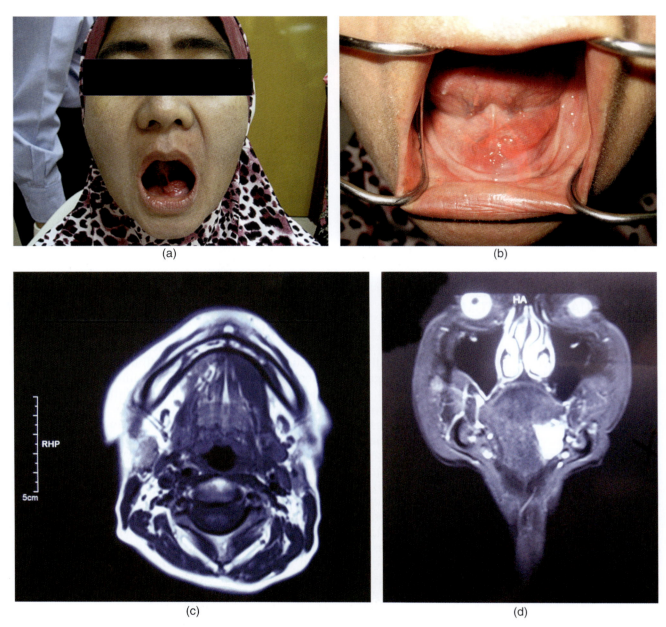

Figure 11.14. (a and b) A 48-year-old Asian female with ACC of left sublingual gland. Clinically, it appears to be in the floor of mouth well away from the mandible. (c and d) Axial MR demonstrates the mass in the left sublingual gland approximates the mandible. Coronal MR shows deep invasion of the tongue musculature with presumed involvement of the lingual and possibly hypoglossal cranial nerves. Source: Photographs by permission of Dr. N Ravindranathan. Director of the Pantai Jerudong Specialist Center Brunei.

is recommended. When positive nodes are present, type I modified radical neck dissection is required. ACC of the sublingual gland has a higher percentage of regional metastasis (24.7%) than any major other major salivary gland site (International Head and Neck Scientific Group 2017). Adjuvant radiation therapy is indicated for positive nodes, perineural invasion, extra-capsular nodal spread, positive margins, and high-grade histology. In one small series, the overall nodal involvement was 57%, with 33% for T1–2 and 75% for T3–4. All patients received post-operative radiation therapy (PORT) (Huang et al. 2016).

Tumors of the Submandibular and Sublingual Glands **361**

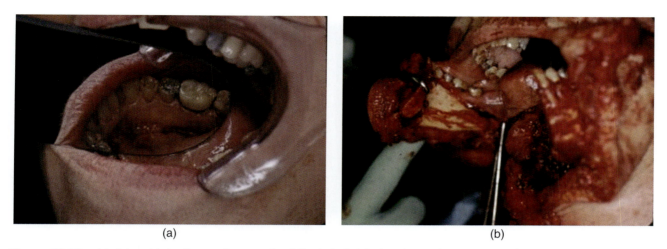

Figure 11.15. (a) Adenoid cystic carcinoma of sublingual gland closely approximated to the mandible (seen via an intraoral mirror photograph). (b) Following lip split and mandibulotomy, the periosteum is found to be uninvolved and is stripped from the mandible which is preserved.

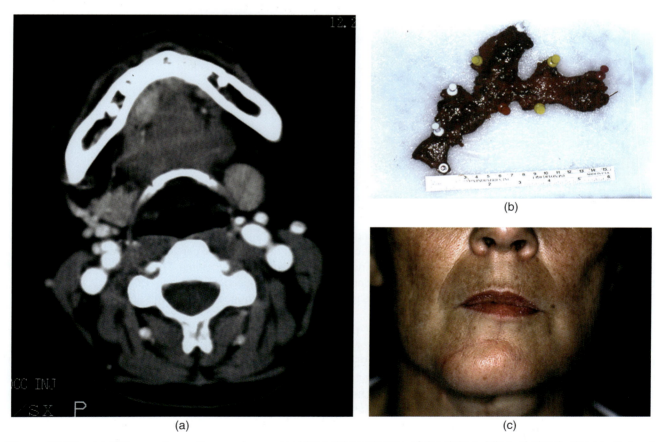

Figure 11.16. (a) CT scan shows low-grade mucoepidermoid carcinoma of the right sublingual gland, close to but not involving the mandible. (b) This tumor was accessed via a lip split incision and mandibulotomy. Bilateral supraomohyoid neck dissections were undertaken as can be seen in the surgical specimen. (c) Cosmetic result of lip split incision. Patient is alive and tumor-free 13 years postoperatively.

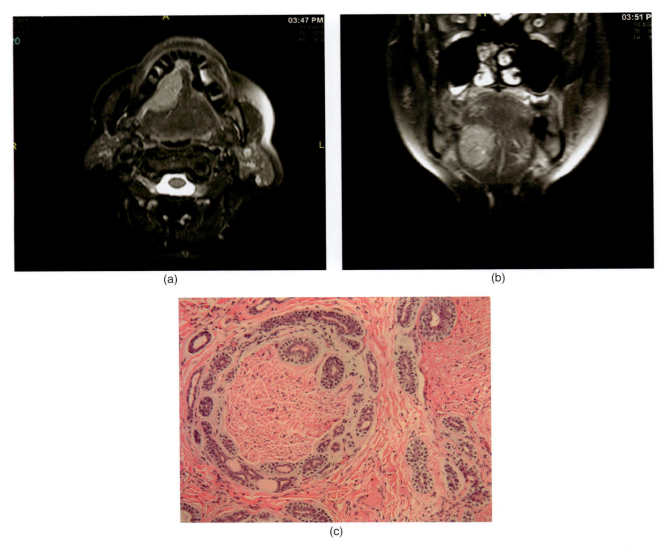

Figure 11.17. (a and b) MR imaging shows mass in right sublingual gland in a 70-year-old female with two-year history of floor of mouth pain. Biopsy showed basal cell adenocarcinoma but adenoid cystic carcinoma was suspected clinically. (c) Final histopathology shows infiltration of the lingual nerve by adenoid cystic carcinoma. The lingual nerve was removed to the skull base and the submandibular gland in continuity with the sublingual gland. Source: Dr. John C. Papadimitriou, Professor of Pathology, Department Pathology University of Maryland. Reproduced with permission of Dr. Papadimitriou.

Prognosis for these tumors is difficult to assess as the literature is mostly composed of case reports and small series. Spiro (1995) reported only 3 of 18 patients (16.6%) dying of their tumor with a median follow-up of 74 months. However, Yu et al. (2007) reported distant metastases and local recurrence as the main cause of death with local recurrence rates of 30% and distant metastases of 26.7%. In this series, 56.7% of tumors were stage III. In a study of 38 sublingual gland cancers, 28.9% had T3–4 tumors and 15.8% had pN+. The local recurrence rate at five years was 18.4% and the distant metastatic rate was 23.7%. Patient age, N stage, and limited tongue mobility were independent predictors of locoregional recurrence and mortality (Liu et al. 2017). A SEER data base study of 210 cases found five-year OS and DSS of 69 and 83% respectively. Multivariate analysis showed that female gender and surgical resection correlated with increased survival, while increased age and stage had a negative effect on survival. Radiation

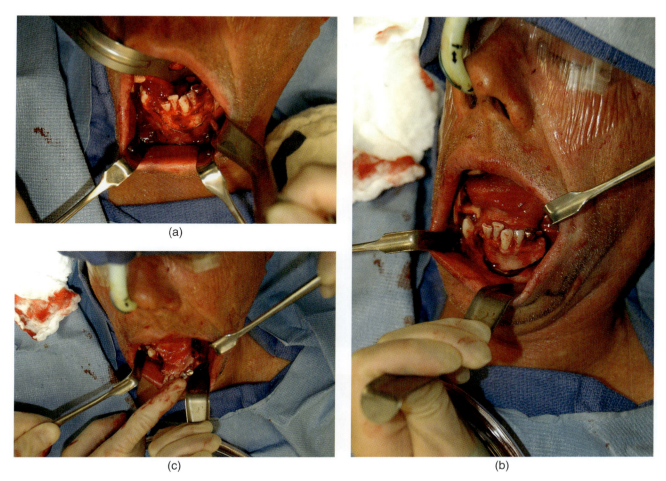

Figure 11.18. (a) Intraoperative view of a 53-year-old man with a mass of the left anterior floor of the mouth stuck to the lingual periosteum behind the left canine and lateral incisors. Biopsy shows intermediate-grade MECA. The mental nerve is preserved on the left side and the marginal resection is marked with a Bovie on the buccal bone. (b) Bone cut has been completed on the buccal side the cut is angled inferiorly to the lower border on the lingual side. (c) The marginal resection is mobilized anteriorly. The right and left Wharton papillae are seen close to the midline mucosal cut. In this case staged T1N0, both left and right Wharton duct were transplanted to the posterior floor of mouth and the submandibular glands preserved. The patient is alive without disease 16 years post-surgery.

therapy in those patients with ACC was correlated with increase in survival (Lee et al. 2016). Other authors have found DSS to be determined by stage and less by histopathology (Andreasen et al. 2016).

Most malignant sublingual gland tumors are ACC and distant metastasis may be 33% for these tumors (Andreasen et al. 2016). When incidence of ACC metastasis to the lung is examined, the sublingual gland has the highest risk of all salivary sites. Other risk factors identified are tumor size >2.5 cm and PNI (Seok et al. 2019). In examining all sites of ACC in the head and neck, the sublingual gland has the worst OS. But PORT to >60 Gy gave a better prognosis (Takebayashi et al. 2018).

It is reasonable to conclude that although 5-year survival from submandibular and sublingual gland cancer is reasonable, the high percentage of ACC found in these glands leads to continuing decrease in survival at 10 years and beyond due to late local recurrence and distant metastases.

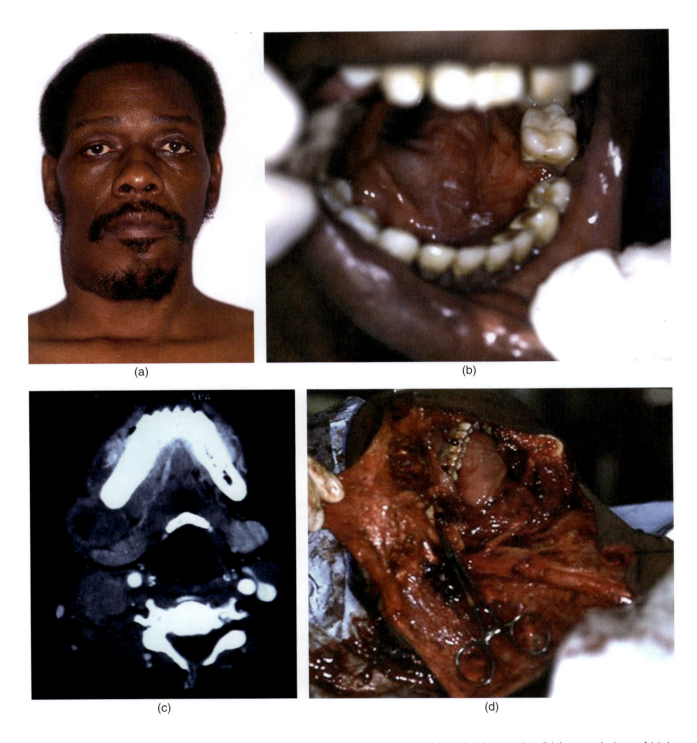

Figure 11.19. (a) A 46-year-old African-American man with right cervical lymphadenopathy. (b) Intraoral view of high-grade mucoepidermoid carcinoma fixed to the right mandible. (c) CT scan confirms a large necrotic node. (d) An intraoperative view of a modified radical neck dissection and hemi-mandibulectomy with lip split was performed. (e) Postoperative panoramic film showing a reconstruction plate. (f) Post-chemoradiation, patient has developed a mediastinal metastasis that is eroding through the manubrium sterni. Scar on right chest is from the pectoralis major flap. Patient died within weeks from lung metastases. Source: Republished with permission from Ord (2000).

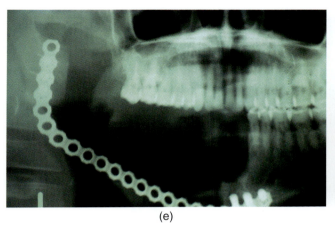
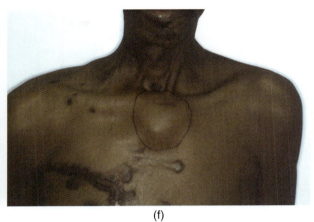

(e) (f)

Figure 11.19. (Continued).

Summary

- Submandibular gland tumors comprise only 10% of salivary tumors.
- Most submandibular swellings are inflammatory in etiology.
- Approximately 50% of submandibular tumors will be malignant.
- Open biopsy should not be used for submandibular gland tumors. FNAB is the preoperative diagnostic method of choice.
- Sublingual gland tumors comprise <1% of salivary tumors.
- Ninety percent of sublingual gland tumors are malignant.
- ACCs followed by MECA are the commonest cancers in both the submandibular and sublingual glands.
- Submandibular gland and sublingual gland malignancies appear to have a worse prognosis than similar malignancies in the parotid gland.
- Distant metastasis is more common from the sublingual and submandibular gland than the parotid gland.
- Surgical management is based on both histologic diagnosis and stage for malignancies in the submandibular and sublingual glands

Case Presentation – *But I Took the Road Less Traveled*

A 70-year-white male was seen in November 2007 with a two- to three-month history of swelling of the left palate which he thought was decreasing in size. Biopsy had shown an adenoid cystic carcinoma.

Past Medical History
Hypertension for which he took Lisinopril.
Hypercholesterolemia for which he was taking Zocor.
Osteoarthritis for which he was taking Lodine.
He had a tonsillectomy as a young boy.
He was allergic to Sulfa drugs and Allopurinol.

Social History
He had a 30-pack year history of cigarettes but had quit 10 years ago. He drank two beers each day.

Examination
He had no palpable lymph nodes in the neck. Intraorally, there was a firm, submucosal mass 1.5 × 2 cm in the area of the palatine foramen (Figure 11.20a).

Diagnosis
T1 ACC left palate.
The diagnosis and possible treatment plans were discussed at length with the patient and he was seen in a week with his CT (Figure 11.20b and c) and MR scans (Figure 11.20d–f) of the head and neck. The scans showed involvement of the floor of sinus and nose. The tumor did not extend high superiorly and the pterygoid plates were grossly uninvolved. The resection was planned to be through the left canine socket at a high Le Fort I level. The patient decided he wished for reconstruction with a flap

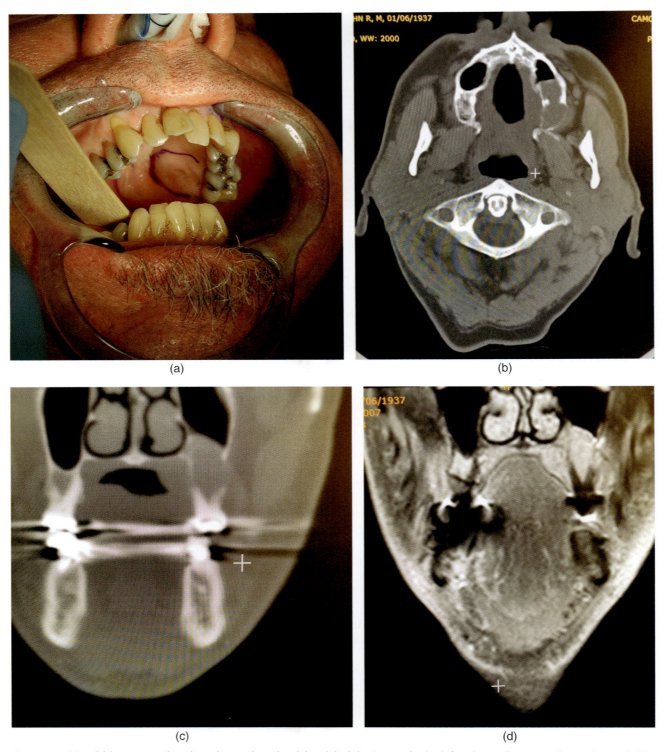

Figure 11.20. (a) Intraoperative view shows the raised, hard, indolent mass in the left palate adjacent to the molar teeth. The surgical marking pen has delineated the palpable margins. The central ulceration is from the preoperative biopsy. Note that the tumor is situated over the greater palatine foramen. (b) Axial CT bone window shows thinning and erosion of the bone of the posterior maxilla to the pterygoid plates and invasion of the maxillary sinus. (c) Coronal CT bone window confirms perforation of the buccal sinus wall, hard plate, and lateral wall of the nasal cavity. (d) Coronal MRI shows extension of the adenoid cystic carcinoma to the midline of the palate and destruction of the alveolar bone around the roots of the maxillary molar.

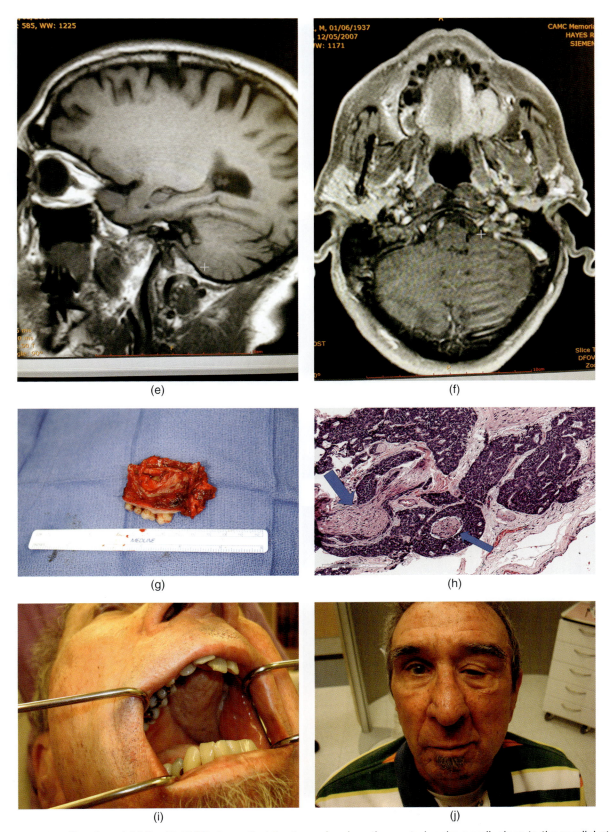

Figure 11.20. (*Continued*) (e) Sagittal MRI shows that the tumor involves the posterior sinus wall, close to the medial pterygoid muscle. (f) Axial MRI shows enhancement along the course of the greater palatine nerve. (g) The resection specimen following partial maxillectomy. Note the pterygoid plates and pterygoid muscles have been removed posteriorly with the maxilla to try and encompass the greater palatine nerve, which was traced cephalad. (h) Adenoid cystic carcinoma cribriform type with extensive perineural invasion indicated by the two blue arrows. The nerve is large and most likely represents the greater palatine nerve. Source: By courtesy of Dr. John Papadimitriou, Professor of pathology, University of Maryland. (i) Postoperative view showing the well-healed radial forearm flap reconstruction of the left palate. (j) Patient presents with left ptosis.

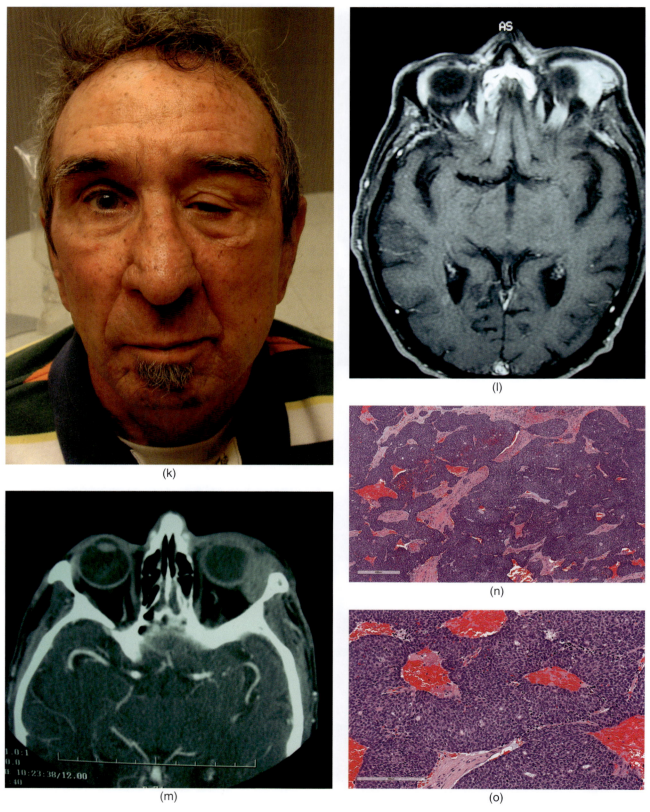

Figure 11.20. (*Continued*) (k) In this closer frontal view, the mass in the left lacrimal gland is better appreciated. (l) Axial MR shows an enhancing mass in the left lacrimal gland. (m) Axial MR shows the globe displaced medially by the lacrimal gland tumor. (n) Left lacrimal gland biopsy shows adenoid cystic carcinoma mostly solid type. Source: By courtesy of Dr. John Papadimitriou, Professor of pathology, University of Maryland. (o) High power view of solid adenoid cystic carcinoma in the lacrimal gland. Source: By courtesy of Dr. John Papadimitriou, Professor of pathology, University of Maryland.

rather than an obturator and he was planned for a radial forearm flap. As this would involve entering the neck to find vessels, it was also planned to undertake an elective supraomohyoid neck dissection.

Surgery was carried out on 3 January 2008, and a posterior maxillectomy was performed (Figure 11.20g). Final pathology was reported as showing a moderately differentiated adenoid cystic carcinoma (ACC), 2.3 cm maximum diameter. The tumor was staged pT2 N0. The sinus was involved, and 0/16 lymph nodes contained metastases. Margins were reported as negative. He had extensive perineural and lymphatic invasion, and tumor was seen in lymphatic spaces at the anterior margin (Figure 11.20h).

The head and neck tumor board recommended radiation therapy. He completed his radiation on 9 April 2008, and was seen on 4 June 2008, when he was doing well apart from some muffled hearing, which was thought to be due either to edema and fluid in the middle ear post-radiation or due to disruption of the tensor veli palatini muscle from his maxillectomy (Figure 11.20i). He was given an appointment with his otologist. The patient was next seen in our clinic on 8 October 2008. His history had evolved since he had been seen at our clinic. In July 2008, he had developed ptosis, thought initially to be from a Horner's syndrome. He was referred to an oculoplastic surgeon who told him that he had an orbital tumor and had arranged a biopsy in a week's time. On examination, he had a hard mass in his lacrimal gland compressing his globe and causing a marked ptosis (Figure 11.20j and k). This was confirmed on his MRI (Figure 11.20m and n). We liaised with the oculoplastic surgeon expressing our concern that this was related to his maxillary ACC.

Biopsy consisted of removal of the lacrimal gland and confirmed an ACC solid-type (Figure 11.20n and o). He was represented to the head and neck tumor board where the recommendation was for a sub-cranial exenteration of the orbit. The patient wished to explore the possibility of further radiation therapy, perhaps proton or neutron therapy. He was seen by his radiotherapist on 31 October 2008 for consultation and at that time a re-staging PET/CT scan showed concerning uptake at T5-T6 vertebrae, suggestive of metastases. Core needle biopsy in West Virginia showed metastatic ACC in the thoracic vertebrae on 19 November 2008. At this point, the patient decided against further radical surgery in the orbit. He completed 3850 Gy radiation to his thoracic spine on 31 December 2008 and 45 Gy of IMRT radiation to the left orbit and base of skull on 8 January 2009. He was not seen again for follow-up in Maryland and presumably succumbed to distant metastases.

TAKE-HOME POINTS

1. As stated in this chapter, adenoid cystic carcinoma (ACC) is the commonest malignant salivary gland tumor found in the sublingual and submandibular glands. It was emphasized that any of the major nerves adjacent to the tumor that were involved should be traced proximally and sacrificed, due to the propensity of this tumor to show perineural involvement (PNI). As can be seen from this case, perineural involvement can allow the tumor to disseminate widely and recur at a distance. Technically, even though the recurrence in this case was in the lacrimal gland, a separate organ, this would be classed as a local recurrence. The spread can be insidious as in this case, but pain is usually a sign of PNI. In speculating how this tumor traveled from the left palate to the ipsilateral lacrimal gland, the most obvious route is via the greater palatine nerve. The ACC would accompany the greater palatine nerve to the sphenopalatine ganglion at the apex of the pterygopalatine fossa, and leave the ganglion via its ganglionic nerves to the maxillary branch of the trigeminal nerve. Then, traveling along the zygomatic branch of the maxillary nerve, it could reach the lacrimal nerve via the communicating branch of the zygomatic nerve. There are alternative routes of course. The ACC could have started in the lesser palatine nerve to the sphenopalatine ganglion. Another route from the sphenopalatine ganglion would be proximal along the maxillary nerve to the trigeminal ganglion in Meckel's cave and then along the ophthalmic branch of the trigeminal nerve to the lacrimal nerve. However, the case illustrates how an ACC in the palate can potentially spread to the orbit, skull base, or brain. Unfortunately, even tracing the nerve proximally and sectioning it in an area which is negative for ACC on frozen section cannot guarantee success as ACC can have "skip" lesions which extend beyond a portion of apparently uninvolved nerve

2. Although ACC is usually thought of as being a slow-growing tumor that can take up to 20 years to result in death of the patient, in this case in 12 months the tumor spread to the lacrimal gland and bony vertebrae. The solid type of ACC is said to have the worse prognosis and the orbital recurrence was classified as solid-type.
3. Finally, ACC does not usually metastasize via the lymphatic system but usually via the blood stream. The lung is the commonest site but, as in this case, the bones may be affected.

References

Alves FA, Pires FR, DeAlemeda OP et al. 2004. PCNA, Ki-67 and p53 expression in submandibular salivary gland tumors. *Int. J Oral Maxillofac Surg* 33(6):593–597.

Alyas F, Lewis K, Williams M et al. 2005. Diseases of the submandibular gland as demonstrated using high resolution ultrasound. *Br J Radiol* 78(928):362–369.

Anderson LJ, Thrkildsen MH, Ockelman HH et al. 1991. Malignant epithelial tumors in the minor salivary glands, the submandibular gland and the sublingual gland. *Cancer* 68:2431–2437.

Andreasen S, Bjørndal K. Agander TK et al. 2016. Tumors of the sublingual gland: A national clinicopathological study of 29 cases. *Eur J Otorhinolaryngol* 273(11):3847–3856.

Aro K, Tarkkanen J, Saat R et al. 2018. Submandibular gland cancer: Specific features and treatment considerations. *Head Neck* 40(1):154–162.

Atula T, Panigrahi J, Tarkknen J. et al. 2017. Preoperative evaluation and surgical planning of submandibular tumors. *Head Neck* 39(6):1071–1077.

Auclair PL, Ellis GL, Gnepp DR et al. 1991. Salivary gland neoplasms: general considerations. In: Ellis GL, Auclair PL, Gnepp DR (eds), *Surgical Pathology of the Salivary Glands*. Philadelphia, WB Saunders, pp. 144–145.

Bahn YE, Lee SK, Sun YK, Kim SP. 2011. Sonographic appearance of mucosa-associated lymphoid tissue lymphoma of the submandibular gland confirmed with sonographically guided core needle biopsy. *J Clin Ultrasound* 39(4):228–232.

Bhattacharyya N. 2004. Survival and prognosis for cancer of the submandibular gland. *J Oral Maxillofac Surg* 62(4):427–430.

Blanchaert RH, Ord RA, Kumar D. 1998. Polymorphous low-grade adenocarcinoma of the sublingual gland. *Int J Oral Maxillofac Surg* 27:115–117.

Camilleri IG, Malata CM, McLean NR, Kelly CG. 1998. Malignant tumors of the submandibular salivary gland: A 15 year review. *Br J Plast Surg* 51(3):181–185.

Chikui T, Shimizu M, Goto TK et al. 2004. Interpretation of the origin of a submandibular mass by CT and MR imaging *Oral Surg Oral Med Oral Pathol Radiol Endod* 98(6):721–729.

Cohen AN, Damrose EJ, Huang RY et al. 2004. Adenoid cystic carcinoma of the submandibular gland: A 35 year review *Otolaryngol Head Neck Surg* 131(6):994–1000.

Dantas AN, Freitas de Moraais E, de Paiva Macedo R A., et al. 2015.) Clinicopathological characteristics and perineural invasion in adenoid cystic carcinoma: A systematic review. *Braz J Otorhinolaryngol* 81(3):329–325.

Devine JC, Rogers SN, McNally D et al. 2001. A comparison of aesthetic, functional and patient subjective outcomes following lip-split mandibulotomy and mandibular lingual releasing access procedures. *Int J Oral Maxillofac Surg* 30(3):199–204.

Eom H-J, Lee JH, Ko M-S et al. 2015. Comparison pf fine-needle aspiration and core needle biopsy under ultrasonographic guidance for detecting malignancy and for tissue-specific diagnosis of salivary gland tumors. *AJNR Am J Neuroradiol* 36(6):1188–1193.

Ge N, Peng X, Zhang L et al. 2016.Partial sialoadenectomy for the treatment of benign tumors in the submandibular gland. *Int J Oral Maxillofac Surg* 46(6):750–755.

Goode RK, Auclair PL, Ellis GL. 1998. Mucoepidermoid carcinoma of the major salivary glands: Clinical and histopathologic analysis of 234 cases with evaluation of grading criteria. *Cancer* 82(7):1217–1224.

Hocwald E, Korkmaz H, Yoo GH et al. 2001. Prognostic factors in major salivary gland cancer. *Laryngoscope* 111(8):1434–1439.

Hong KH, Yang YS. 2008 Intraoral approach for the treatment of submandibular salivary gland mixed tumors. *Oral Oncol* 44(5):491–495.

Huang T-T, Chou Y-F, Wen Y-H, Chen P-R. 2016. Resected tumors of the sublingual gland:15 years' experience *Br J Oral Maxillofac Surg* 54(6):625–628.

International Head and Neck Scientific Group 2017. Cervical lymph node metastasis in adenoidcystic carcinoma of the major salivary glands. *J Laryngol Otol* 131(2):96–105N.

Kaszuba SM, Zafero ME, Rosenthal DI et al. 2007. Effects of initial treatment on disease outcome for patients with submandibular gland carcinoma. *Arch Otolaryngol Head Neck Surg* 133(6):546–550.

Kim HJ, Kim JS. 2018. Ultrasound-guided core needle biopsy in salivary glands: A meta-analysis. *Laryngoscope* 128(1):118–125.

Kojima T, Hori R, Tanaka S et al. 2020. A retrospective multicenter study of sublingual gland carcinoma in Japan. *Auris Narus Larynx* 47(1):111–115.

Laskawi R, Ellies M, Arglebe C, Schott A. 1995. Surgical management of benign tumors of the submandibular gland: A follow up study. *J Oral Maxillofac Surg* 53(5):506–508.

Lee WH, Tseng TM, Hsu HT, et al. 2013. Salivary gland tumors: A 20-year review of clinical diagnostic accuracy at a single center. *Oncol Lett* 7(2):583–587.

Lee RJ, Tan A P, Tong E L et al. 2015. Epidemiology, prognostic factors and treatment of malignant submandibular gland tumors: A population-based cohort analysis *JAMA Otolaryngol Head Neck Surg* 141(10),905–912.

Lee RJ, Tong EL, Patel R et al. 2016. Malignant sublingual gland tumors: Demographics, prognostic factors, and treatment outcomes. *Oral Surg Oral Med Oral Pathol Oral Radiol* 121(2):180–187.

Liu S, Ow A, Ruan M, et al. 2014.Prognostic factors in primary salivary gland mucoepidermoid carcinoma: An analysis of 376 cases in an eastern Chinese population. *Int J Oral Maxillofac Surg* 43(6):667–673.

Liu Y, Hong L, Qin L et al. 2017. Prognostic factors in malignant sublingual salivary gland tumors. *J Oral Maxillofac Surg* 75(7):1542–1548.

Liu Y, Qin L, Zhuang R-T et al. 2018.Nodal stage: Is it a prognostic factor for submandibular cancer? *J Oral Maxillofac Surg* 76(8):2018.

Lombardi D, Accorona R, Lambert A et al. 2018. Long-term outcomes and prognosis in submandibular gland malignant tumors: A multicenter study. *Laryngoscope* 128(12):2745–2750.

Mallik S, Agarwak J, Gupta T, et al. 2010. Prognostic factors and outcome analysis of submandibular gland cancer: A clinical audit. *J Oral Maxillofac Surg* 68(9):2104–2110.

Mantsopoulos K, Goncalves M, Kock M et al. 2018. Submandibular gland pleomorphic adenoma: Histopathological capsular characteristics and correlation with the surgical outcome. *Ann Diagn Pathol* 34:166–169.

Marcuzzo AV, Suran-Brunell AN, Dal Cin E, et al. 2019. Surgical anatomy of the marginal mandibular nerve: A systematic review and meta-analysis. *Clin Anat* 33, 739–750.

Mariano FV, da Silva SD, Chulan TC, et al. 2011. Clinicopathological factors are predictors of distant metastasis from major salivary gland carcinomas. *Int J Oral Maxillofac Surg* 40(5):504–509.

Min R, Zun Z, Siyi L, et al. 2013. Gland-preserving surgery can effectively preserve gland function without increased recurrence in treatment of benign submandibular tumor. *Br J Oral Maxillofac Surg* 51(7):615–619.

Mizrachi A, Bachar G, Unger Y et al. 2017. Submandibular salivary gland tumors: Clinical course and outcome of a 20-year multicenter study. *Ear Nose Throat* 96(3):E17–E20.

Ord RA. 2000. Salivary gland disease. In: Fonseca R (ed.), *Oral and Maxillofacial Surgery, Volume 5, Surgical Pathology*. Philadelphia, WB Saunders Co., pp. 288–289,

Oudidi A, El-Alami MN, Boulaich M et al. 2006. Primary submandibular gland tumors: Experience based on 68 cases. *Rev Laryngol Otol Rhinol (Bord)* 127(3):187–190.

Perez DE, Pires FR, Fábio de Abreu Alves et al. 2005. Sublingual gland tumors: Clinicopatholgic study of six cases. *Oral Surg Oral Med Oral Pathol Radiol Endod* 100(4):449–453.

Pogrel MA. 1995. The diagnosis and management of tumors of the submandibular and sublingual glands. *Oral Maxillofac Clin N Am* 7(3):565–571.

Preuss SF, Klussmann JP, Wittekindt C et al. 2007. Submandibular gland excision: 15 years of experience *J Oral Maxillofac Surg* 65:953–957.

Rapidis AD, Stavrianos S, Lagogiannis G, Faratzis G. 2004. Tumors of the submandibular gland: Clinicopathologic analysis of 23 patients. *J Oral Maxillofac Surg* 62(10):1203–1208.

Razek AAKA 2019. Prediction of malignancy of submandibular gland tumors with apparent diffusion coefficient *Oral Radiol* 35(1):11–15.

Rinaldo A, Shaha AR, Pellitteri PK et al. 2004. Management of malignant sublingual salivary gland tumors. *Oral Oncol* 40:2–5.

Roh J-L, Park CI. 2008. Gland-preserving surgery for pleomorphic adenoma in the submandibular gland. *Br J Surg.* 95(10):1252–1256.

Roh JL, Choi SH, Lee SW, et al. 2008.Carcinomas arising in the submandibular gland: High propensity for systemic failure. *J Surg Oncol*:97(6):533–537.

Rutt AL, Hawkshaw MJ, Lurie D, Sataloff RT 2011.Salivary gland cancer in patients younger than 30 years. *Ear Nose Throat J* 90(4):174–184.

Saintigny P, Mitani Y, Pytynia KB et al. 2018. Frequent PTEN loss and differential HER2/PI3Ksignalling pathway alterations in salivary duct carcinoma: Implications for targeted therapy. *Cancer* 124(18):36933705.

Schwenter I, Obrist P, Thumfart W, Sprinzi G. 2006. Distant metastasis of parotid tumors *Acta Otolaryngol* 126(4):340–345.

Seok J, Lee DY, Kim WS et al. 2019. Lung metastasis in adenoid cystic carcinoma of the head and neck. *Head Neck* 41(11):3976–3983.

Shin DY, Jang KS, Kim BY, et al. 2014 Comparison of adenoid cystic carcinomas: Focus on systemic metastasis and tumor-associated blood vessels. *J Oral Pathol Med* 43(6):441–447.

Sood S, McGurk M Vaz F. 2016. Management of salivary gland tumors: United Kingdom National Multidisciplinary Guidelines. *J Laryngol Otol* 130(S2):S142–S149.

Spiro RH. 1995. Treating tumors of the sublingual glands, including a useful technique for repair of the floor of mouth after resection. *Am J Surg* 170(5):457–460.

Storey MR, Garden AS, Morrison WH et al. 2001. Postoperative radiotherapy for malignant tumors of the submandibular gland. *Int J Radiat Oncol Phys* 51(4):952–958.

Sumi M, Izumi M, Yonetsu K, Nakamura T. 1999. Sublingual gland: MR features of normal and diseased states. *Am J Roentgenol* 172(3):717–722.

Sun G, Yang X, Tang E, et al. 2010 The treatment of sublingual gland tumors. *Int J Oral Maxfac Surg* 39:863–868.

Sykes AJ Slevin NJ, Birzgalis AR, Gupta NK. 1999. Submandibular gland carcinoma: An audit of local control and survival following adjuvant radiotherapy. *Oral Oncol* 35(2):187–190.

Takebayashi S, Shinohara E, Tamaki H et al. 2018. Adenoid cystic carcinoma of the head and neck: A retrospective multicenter study. *Acta Otolaryngol* 138(1):73–79.

Taylor MJ, Serpell JW, Thompson P. 2011. Preoperative fine needle cytology and imaging facilitates the management of submandibular salivary gland lesions. *ANZ J Surg* 81(1–2):70–74.

Terhaard CHJ, Lubsen H, Rasch CRN et al. 2005. The role of radiotherapy in the treatment of malignant salivary gland tumors. *Int J Radiat Oncol Biol Phys* 61(1):103–111.

Wahlberg P, Anderson H, Bjorklund A, et al. 2002. Carcinoma of the parotid and submandibular glands – A study of survival in 2,465 patients *Oral Oncol* 38(7):706–713.

Webb AJ, Eveson JW. 2001. Pleomorphic adenomas of the major salivary glands: A study of the capsular form in relation to surgical management. *Clin Otolaryngol* 26:134–142.

Weber RS, Byers RM, Petit B et al. 1990. Submandibular gland tumors. *Arch Otolaryngol Head Neck Surg* 116:1055–1060.

Yamada K, Honda K, Tamaki H et al. 2018. Survival in patients with submandibular gland carcinoma-results of a multi-institutional retrospective study. *Auris Nasus Larynx* 45(5):1066–1072.

Yamazaki T, Kotani A, Kawakami T. 1987. Basal cell carcinoma of the sublingual gland. *J Oral Maxillofac Surg* 45:270–273.

Yang T-L 2018. Robotic surgery for submandibular gland resection through a trans-hairline approach: The first human series and comparison with applicable approaches. *Head Neck* 40(4):793–800.

Yu T, Gao GH Wang XY et al. 2007. A retrospective clinicopathologic study of 30 cases of sublingual gland malignant tumors. (in Chinese) *Hua Xi Kou Qiang Yi Xue Za Zhi* 25(1):64–66.

Zdanowski R, Dias FL, Barbosa MM, et al. 2012. Sublingual gland tumors: Clinical, pathologic, and therapeutic analysis of 13 patients treated in a single institution. *Head Neck* 33(4):476–481.

Chapter 12
Tumors of the Minor Salivary Glands

Outline

Introduction
Etiology of Minor Salivary Gland Tumors
Diagnosis of Minor Salivary Gland Tumors
Treatment of Minor Salivary Gland Tumors
    General Principles of Surgery for Minor Salivary Gland Tumors
    Surgical Treatment of Benign Minor Salivary Gland Tumors
        Pleomorphic Adenoma
        Canalicular Adenoma
    Surgical Treatment of Malignant Minor Salivary Gland Tumors
        Mucoepidermoid Carcinoma
            Central Mucoepidermoid Carcinoma
        Adenoid Cystic Carcinoma
        Polymorphous Adenocarcinoma
        Acinic Cell Carcinoma
        Epithelial-Myoepithelial Carcinoma
        Secretory Carcinoma
    Surgical Management of the Neck for Minor Salivary Gland Malignancies
    The Role of Radiation Therapy in the Management of Minor Salivary Gland Malignancies
    The Role of Chemotherapy in the Management of Minor Salivary Gland Malignancies
Summary
Case Presentation – *Two Peas in a Pod*
References

Introduction

The evaluation, diagnosis, and treatment of a patient with a mass occupying the territory of minor salivary gland tissue in the palate, buccal mucosa, and lips represent intellectually stimulating disciplines. This statement is clearly derived from the relative paucity of lesions in these anatomic areas. Salivary gland tumors in general are quite rare, accounting for only 0.2–6.6% of all human tumors (Chidzonga et al. 1995). Both geographic and racial factors may explain the relative paucity of these tumors (Ansari 2007). The average annual incidence of salivary gland tumors per 100 000 population is 4.7 for benign tumors and 0.9 for malignant tumors (Ansari 2007). Both neoplastic and non-neoplastic entities are diagnosed in the salivary glands, including the minor salivary glands, thereby adding to the stimulating nature of the differential diagnosis, microscopic diagnosis, and treatment of minor salivary gland tumors. Data regarding the true incidence of salivary gland tumors in general may be difficult to obtain. This is not only due to the rarity of these tumors, but also to the previous nonroutine nature of reporting of these diagnoses to hospital tumor registries, and the occasional treatment of these lesions in office settings (Melrose 1994). It has been estimated that minor salivary gland tumors account for only 2–5% of all head and neck tumors, with malignant minor salivary gland tumors accounting for only 2–4% of all head and neck cancers (MacIntosh 1995), and 10–15% of all salivary gland cancers (Hay et al. 2019).

In 1985, Regezi et al. reported on 238 minor salivary gland tumors among a total of 72 282 (0.33%) oral biopsy specimens diagnosed over a 19-year period (Regezi et al. 1985). Similarly, Rivera-Bastidas et al. reported 62 minor salivary gland tumors from a total of 9000 oral biopsies (0.7%) during a 24-year period (Rivera-Bastidas et al. 1996). A review of 40 000 head and neck tumors over a 40-year period revealed 196 (0.5%)

Salivary Gland Pathology: Diagnosis and Management, Third Edition. Edited by Eric R. Carlson and Robert A. Ord.
© 2022 John Wiley & Sons, Inc. Published 2022 by John Wiley & Sons, Inc.
Companion website: www.wiley.com/go/carlson/salivary

minor salivary gland tumors. Approximately, 10% of all salivary gland tumors arise in the minor glands (Ord 1994). Of these minor salivary gland tumors, 70% occur in the oral cavity, 25% in the nasal cavity/sinuses/nasopharynx, and 3% occur in the larynx (MacIntosh 1995). Of the oral minor salivary gland tumors, at least 50% have been diagnosed in the palate, per most large series (Eveson and Cawson 1985; Spiro 1986).

In addition to relatively low numbers of minor salivary gland tumor diagnoses, there are controversies regarding the precise microscopic diagnosis of these tumors. In Waldron's review of 426 oral minor salivary gland tumors (Waldron et al. 1988), each of these cases was reviewed by the three authors and complete concurrence of the microscopic diagnoses was reached in 346 cases (81.2%). In 49 cases, there were minor disagreements as to the diagnoses, mainly related to the subclassification of the tumors. Significant disagreement, regarding a benign versus malignant diagnosis of the neoplasm, was noted in 21 cases (5%). Moreover, following the authors' review, their diagnoses were compared to those of the contributing pathologists. There was complete agreement in 374 cases (87.8%). These statistics exemplify the complex nature of intraoral minor salivary gland tumors, thereby questioning the exact incidence of these neoplasms as well as their specific diagnoses.

Minor salivary gland tumors occur in the oral cavity or other sites in the head and neck such as the paranasal sinuses, nasopharynx, nasal cavity, larynx, oropharynx, and trachea, although the oral cavity is the most commonly involved anatomic site (Carlson and Schlieve 2019). These tumors develop not only as benign and malignant entities, but also as a spectrum of cell types within these glands (Carlson 1998). The frequency of benign versus malignant tumors occurring throughout the minor glands in the oral cavity is one feature that distinguishes these tumors from their counterparts in the major glands. One series reported 15% of parotid gland tumors and 37% of submandibular gland tumors to be malignant (Eveson and Cawson 1985). In general terms, published series record that approximately 20–70% of minor salivary gland tumors are malignant (Epker and Henny 1969; Ord 1994) (Table 12.1). It seems that the center that reports the incidence of benign versus malignant minor salivary gland tumors of the oral cavity is the primary bias in these reports. For example, tertiary care referral centers with a cancer initiative may be preferentially referred patients with malignant diagnoses. Spiro's report of his 35-year experience with salivary gland neoplasia at Memorial Sloan Kettering Cancer Center is a case in point. He reported on 2807 patients, 607 of whom had minor salivary gland tumors. The frequency of malignant tumors in this report was 87%. The Armed Forces Institute of Pathology reported 2945 cases of minor salivary gland tumors in 1991. By contrast, 49% of these cases were malignant. Numerous other series have reported similar figures, such that it has become reasonably well accepted that approximately 50% of minor salivary gland tumors of the oral cavity are benign and 50% are malignant.

Etiology of Minor Salivary Gland Tumors

Risk factors for salivary gland tumors have been studied extensively. Carcinoma of the major salivary glands, for example, has identified a relationship with prior radiation therapy and previous skin cancer Spitz et al. 1984). Another study reported 31 patients who had both a newly diagnosed salivary gland tumor and a history of radiation therapy to the head and neck region (Katz and Preston-Martin 1984). Radiation therapy had been administered with a range of 11–66 years prior to the development of the salivary gland tumors. No course of radiation therapy was administered for a malignant condition, but rather for acne, hypertrophied tonsils, keloids, and other benign conditions. As such, it is reasonable to assume that a low dose of radiation therapy was administered. Only three cases of minor salivary gland tumors were identified among these 31 cases, including two adenoid cystic carcinomas and one mucoepidermoid carcinoma. One of the tumors was in the palate and two were in the cheek/retromolar region.

Benign and malignant salivary gland tumors have also been linked to exposure to ionizing radiation related to the atomic bombings in Hiroshima and Nagasaki during World War II. One hundred forty-five salivary gland tumors have been studied in survivors of these bombings (Saku et al. 1997). One hundred nineteen major gland tumors (27 malignant tumors, 82 benign tumors, 10 undetermined tumors) and 26 minor

Table 12.1. Incidence of minor salivary gland tumors.

Authors	Year	Location	# of cases	Histology
AFIP	1991	USA	2945	Benign 51% Malignant 49%
Chau, Radden	1986	Australia	98	Benign 62% Malignant 38%
Chidzonga, Perez, Alvarez	1995	Zimbabwe	282	Benign 80% Malignant 20%
Eveson, Cawson	1985	England	336	Benign 54% Malignant 46%
Isacsson, Shear	1983	Sweden	201	Benign 28% Malignant 72%
Ito, Ito, Vargas et al.	2005	Brazil	113	Benign 37% Malignant 63%
Jabar	2006	Libya	75	Benign 39% Malignant 61%
Lopes, Kowalski, Santos, Almeida	1999	Brazil	196	Benign 35% Malignant 65%
Potdar, Paymaster	1969	India	110	Benign 49% Malignant 51%
Regezi, Lloyd, Zarbo, McClatchey	1985	USA	238	Benign 65% Malignant 35%
Rivera-Bastidas, Ocanto, Acevedo	1996	Venezuela	62	Benign 55% Malignant 45%
Satko, Stanko, Longauerova	2000	Slovakia	31	Benign 48% Malignant 52%
Spiro	1986	USA	607	Benign 13% Malignant 87%
Stuteville, Corley	1967	USA	80	Benign 10% Malignant 90%
Toida, Shimokawa, Makita et al.	2004	Japan	82	Benign 67% Malignant 33%
Waldron, El-Mofty, Gnepp	1988	USA	426	Benign 58% Malignant 42%
Ansari	2007	Iran	18	Benign 11.1% Malignant 88.9%
Dhanuthai, Boonadulyarat, Jaengjongdee, Kuruedee	2009	Thailand	311	Benign 47.3% Malignant 52.7%
Gao, Hao, Huang et al.	2017	China	1787	Benign 38.1% Malignant 61.9%
Liao, Chih-Chao, Ma, Hsu	2020	Taiwan	46	Benign 78.3% Malignant 21.7%

gland tumors (14 malignant tumors, 12 benign tumors) were identified. Among the 41 malignant tumors, the frequency of mucoepidermoid carcinoma was disproportionately high, and among the 94 benign tumors, the frequency of the Warthin tumor was high.

The association between first primary benign and malignant neoplasms of the salivary glands and the subsequent development of breast cancer has also been investigated (Abbey et al. 1984). This study identified a fourfold to fivefold increased risk of a second primary breast cancer following the first salivary gland tumor. Of note is that all primary salivary gland tumors were of the major glands, and three of the four patients described had benign salivary gland tumors. While no association between minor salivary gland neoplasia and breast cancer was established, the study nonetheless attempted to develop a relationship between salivary gland neoplasia and breast cancer. Moreover, the study investigated subsequent breast cancer in patients with a history of salivary gland neoplasia, rather than vice versa. As such, a risk factor for salivary gland tumor development would not be established in patients with breast cancer. In addition, minor salivary gland neoplasia was not represented in this cohort of patients. In the final analysis, there is some evidence to identify risk factors for the development of minor salivary gland tumors, yet not as much evidence as exists for the development of major salivary gland tumors.

Diagnosis of Minor Salivary Gland Tumors

The diagnosis of a minor salivary gland tumor begins with the establishment of a differential diagnosis. This differential diagnosis should be classified categorically and in order of decreasing likelihood (Carlson 1998). The evaluation of a lesion of the palate, lip, or buccal mucosa might suggest inflammatory, neoplastic and non-neoplastic entities. Ultimately, the differential diagnosis is based on the patient's history, physical examination, and the anatomic location of the pathologic entity under scrutiny. In general terms, benign and malignant minor salivary gland tumors present as painless, slowly enlarging intraoral masses. When present, ulceration predicts a malignant diagnosis, although many minor salivary gland malignancies do not create ulceration of the oral mucosa. Pain is an ominous sign and is associated with perineural invasion, typically by adenoid cystic carcinoma. A painful enlargement of the minor salivary glands is malignant until proved otherwise. The presence or absence of pain therefore represents an important element of the patient's history. Special imaging studies may be obtained prior to performing the biopsy, if required at all, or they may be obtained after the establishment of a diagnosis based on incisional biopsy. Experience shows, however, that their purpose is to anatomically delineate the extent of the tumor rather than to assist in the establishment of the diagnosis. The experienced salivary gland surgeon may detect nuances on imaging studies that favor various diagnoses on the differential diagnosis. While fine needle aspiration biopsy is arguably an essential element of the diagnosis of parotid neoplasms, it has no practical role in the diagnosis of minor salivary gland neoplasms. Rather, an incisional biopsy should be routinely performed, for example, when planning treatment of palatal tumors due to the diverse nature of possible histopathologic diagnoses, as well as the diverse nature of surgical treatment plans based on benign vs. malignant diagnoses.

Other minor salivary gland tumor sites, such as the buccal mucosa and upper lip, require greater attention to the differential diagnosis to determine whether incisional or excisional biopsy best serves the needs of the patient. In many instances, the differential diagnosis may strongly support a benign neoplasm such that proceeding directly to excision is the most appropriate therapy. For example, a tumor in the upper lip that is freely moveable and associated with normal overlying mucosa indicates that an excisional biopsy may be performed in most instances due to the high likelihood of a benign tumor. A minor salivary gland tumor of the buccal mucosa, like the palate, has a diverse number of possibilities on the differential diagnosis such that an incisional biopsy should be considered to establish the diagnosis (Table 12.2). There are instances, however, where a freely moveable buccal mucosal tumor may be excised without preceding incisional biopsy, like the upper lip tumor previously described.

Treatment of Minor Salivary Gland Tumors

GENERAL PRINCIPLES OF SURGERY FOR MINOR SALIVARY GLAND TUMORS

The treatment of minor salivary gland tumors is distinctly surgical. The specific type of surgery is a function of the anatomic site of the tumor, the invasion of surrounding structures, and the histopathologic diagnosis, provided an incisional biopsy has been performed. In general terms, a palatal minor salivary gland tumor requires an incisional biopsy to definitively establish the histopathologic

Table 12.2. Incidence of benign and malignant minor salivary gland tumors at commonly observed anatomic sites.

Authors	Year	Palate	Lip	Cheek
AFIP	1991	Benign 53%	Benign 73%	Benign 50%
		Malignant 47%	Malignant 27%	Malignant 50%
Chau, Radden	1986	Benign 67%	Benign 77%	Benign 64%
		Malignant 33%	Malignant 23%	Malignant 36%
Eveson, Cawson	1985	Benign 53%	Benign 73%	Benign 50%
		Malignant 47%	Malignant 27%	Malignant 50%
Isacsson, Shear	1983	Benign 78%	Benign 71%	Benign 89%
		Malignant 22%	Malignant 29%	Malignant 11%
Jabar	2006	Benign 58%	Benign 46%	Benign 46%
		Malignant 42%	Malignant 54%	Malignant 54%
Lopes, Kowalski, Santos, Almeida	1999	Benign 42%	Benign 60%	Benign 0%
		Malignant 58%	Malignant 40%	Malignant 100%
Potdar, Paymaster	1969	Benign 49%	Benign 67%	Benign 78%
		Malignant 51%	Malignant 33%	Malignant 22%
Regezi, Lloyd, Zarbo, McClatchey	1985	Benign 30%	Benign 88%	Benign 43%
		Malignant 70%	Malignant 12%	Malignant 57%
Rivera-Bastidas, Ocanto, Acevedo	1996	Benign 56%	Benign 18%	Benign 50%
		Malignant 44%	Malignant 82%	Malignant 50%
Spiro	1986	Benign 26%	Benign 18%	
		Malignant 84%	Malignant 82%	
Stuteville, Corley	1967	Benign 4%	Benign 33%	Benign 27%
		Malignant 96%	Malignant 67%	Malignant 73%
Toida, Shimokawa, Makita et al.	2004	Benign 69%	Benign 67%	Benign 60%
		Malignant 31%	Malignant 33%	Malignant 40%
Waldron, El-Mofty, Gnepp	1988	Benign 58%	Benign 75%	Benign 54%
		Malignant 42%	Malignant 25%	Malignant 46%
Dhanuthai, Boonadulyarat, Jaengjongdee, Jiruedee	2009	Benign 56%	Benign 87%	Benign 65%
		Malignant 44%	Malignant 13%	Malignant 15%
Gao, Hao, Huang et al.	2017	Benign 45.8%	Benign 50.6%	Benign 31.6%
		Malignant 54.2%	Malignant 49.4%	Malignant 68.4%
Liao, Chih-Chao, Ma, Hsu	2020	Benign 100%		Benign 100%
		Malignant 0%		Malignant 0%

diagnosis prior to the tumor surgery. This biopsy should be performed in the center of the mass to not seed the surrounding normal tissue (Freedman and Jones 1994). The decision as to whether to perform an incisional biopsy of buccal mucosal and lip masses thought to represent minor salivary gland tumors rests on the surgeon's intuition as to the benign vs. malignant nature of the mass. Smooth, freely moveable submucosal masses without fixation to the overlying mucosa are likely benign and may be treated with excisional biopsies without first performing an incisional biopsy due to the high likelihood of a benign process. By contrast, sizeable masses with mucosal fixation in these areas should probably be subjected to incisional biopsy to establish the diagnosis due to the concern for malignant disease. As with tumor surgery for other diagnoses, minor salivary gland tumor surgery requires a preoperative assessment of the anatomic barriers. Physical examination and imaging studies serve to delineate invasion of surrounding anatomic barriers by the tumor. In the palate, for example, it is important to determine whether the palatal bone has been invaded by the tumor. Benign tumors typically do not invade bone, but may "cup it out." In such situations, it is not necessary to resect bone. Malignant tumors of the palate display variable involvement of the palatal

Table 12.3. Management of the anatomic barriers in minor salivary gland tumor surgery.

Histology	Site		
	Palate	Lip	Buccal mucosa
Benign	– Mucosal sacrificing – Periosteal sacrificing – Bone sparing	– Mucosal sparing – Muscle sparing – Skin sparing	– Mucosal sparing – Muscle sparing – Skin sparing
Malignant	– Mucosal sacrificing – Periosteal sacrificing – Bone sacrificing (variable)	– Mucosal sacrificing – Muscle sacrificing – Skin sparing (variable)	– Mucosal sacrificing – Muscle sacrificing – Skin sparing (variable)

bone. Imaging studies, particularly coronal bone windows, must be obtained to assess the involvement of the anatomic barrier of palatal bone. Minor salivary gland tumors of the upper lip and buccal mucosa exhibit different behavior regarding their invasion of the anatomic barrier of the surrounding mucosa. In general terms, it is appropriate to preserve the mucosa surrounding a benign minor salivary gland tumor of these sites, while a malignant tumor surgery in these sites requires sacrifice of the surrounding mucosa (Table 12.3).

Treatment of minor salivary gland tumors is predicated on the histopathologic diagnosis, which largely predicts the biologic behavior of the neoplasm. Descriptive surgical terms may describe the sacrifice of surrounding soft and hard tissues as a matter of convenience (Carlson 1998). For example, surgical management of palatal tumors may be as straightforward as a periosteal sacrificing, bone sparing wide local excision with split thickness dissection of the soft palate. This specific surgical procedure is the main procedure performed for benign palatal tumors and also has a role to play in some low-grade malignancies (Carlson 1998). The bone sparing, periosteally sacrificing wide local excision with full thickness sacrifice of the soft palate is reserved for deeply infiltrative low-grade malignancies of the palate. The most aggressive surgery for palatal minor salivary gland tumors is the maxillectomy, specifically reserved for the highly aggressive minor salivary gland malignancies of the palate.

SURGICAL TREATMENT OF BENIGN MINOR SALIVARY GLAND TUMORS

The treatment of benign tumors of the minor salivary glands centers on the pleomorphic adenoma, with a brief discussion of the surgery for the canalicular adenoma. The three most common minor salivary gland anatomic sites will be considered, including the palate, the lip, and the buccal mucosa.

Pleomorphic Adenoma

The terms pleomorphic adenoma and mixed tumor are equally satisfactory and interchangeable when describing this common minor salivary gland tumor. The designation mixed is based on the tumor's mixtures of neoplastic elements such that each mixed tumor has unique features (Melrose 1994). It has also been pointed out that the designation refers to the tumor showing combined features of epithelioid and connective tissue-like growth (Waldron 1991). There is universal agreement that the pleomorphic adenoma is the most common salivary gland tumor. The Armed Forces Institute of Pathology (AFIP) data of 13749 salivary gland tumors showed 6880 cases of pleomorphic adenoma of which 4359 were in the parotid gland and 1277 were located in minor salivary gland tissue (Auclair et al. 1991). The palate accounted for 711 of these 6880 cases of pleomorphic adenoma (10.3%), and was the second most common site for this tumor in the AFIP data. The 711 cases in the palate represent 56% of cases located in the minor salivary glands. Interestingly, the AFIP data subclassified palatal pleomorphic adenomas into those occurring on the hard palate (118 cases) and those occurring in the soft palate (110 cases). There were 483 cases that were not specified as to location in the palate. The subclassification of specific anatomic location in the palate is of significance when working up these cases and planning surgical treatment for these patients. Those pleomorphic adenomas located primarily in the soft palate require investigation as to involvement of the parapharyngeal space.

Treatment of the palatal pleomorphic adenoma is based on the realization that this tumor does not possess a capsule that would be produced by the tumor. This notwithstanding, the tumor does exhibit a pseudocapsule represented by a loose fibrillar network surrounding the tumor that is produced by the host. In addition, the periosteum on the superior aspect of the tumor does serve as a very competent anatomic barrier such that palatal bone may be preserved in this tumor surgery, even when the bone has been "cupped out" clinically and radiographically. Under such circumstances, the pleomorphic adenoma does not invade bone histologically such that bone resection is not warranted. In fact, it is reasonable to proceed with surgery without obtaining CT scans preoperatively. A periosteally sacrificing wide local excision is performed, observing at least a 5-mm linear margin surrounding the clinically apparent tumor (Figure 12.1). While these tumors are submucosal in nature, the mucosa must be sacrificed with the tumor due to the intimate proximity of the tumor and the overlying mucosa (Yih et al. 2005). The most appropriate linear margin of uninvolved soft tissue included at the periphery of the tumor seems to be a source of controversy (Ord 1994; Pogrel 1994; Carlson 1998). The soft palate musculature is dissected in a split thickness fashion to prevent an oral-nasal communication. A preoperatively fabricated palatal stent protects the exposed bone in the postoperative period until granulation tissue appears on the bone surface of the palate. There is no need to provide reconstruction of this exposed bone surface, as mucosalization ultimately occurs predictably. Negative soft-tissue margins in the specimen predict a curative surgery without recurrence of the tumor (Beckhardt et al. 1995).

As previously stated, the pleomorphic adenoma that develops in the soft palate may be different from the pleomorphic adenoma of the hard palate, in terms of its anatomic progression. Tumors located on the hard palate will grow into the oral cavity in an exophytic fashion (Figure 12.2), while tumors of the soft palate (Figure 12.3) may descend into the parapharyngeal space in an endophytic fashion (Carlson 1998). As such, when considering the surgical treatment for a pleomorphic adenoma of the soft palate, the surgeon should obtain CT scans preoperatively to determine possible involvement of the parapharyngeal space. When dissection of the parapharyngeal space by the tumor is noted, a combined transoral/transcutaneous approach to tumor extirpation is indicated. A mandibular osteotomy for effective dissection of the tumor bed and protection of the great vessels in the neck may be indicated.

Pleomorphic adenomas are known to occur in other minor salivary gland sites, including the lip, buccal mucosa, and tongue. Lip tumors accounted for 297 cases in the AFIP files, of which a majority occurred in the upper lip. Lower lip pleomorphic adenomas are very rare. The buccal mucosa accounted for 126 cases in the AFIP series. The surgery required for removal of pleomorphic adenomas in the lip and buccal mucosa involves an excision of the tumor and associated minor salivary gland tissue. The plane of dissection is "peripseudocapsular" in nature. This ensures an anatomic barrier of fascia surrounding the tumor. These tumor surgeries are curative provided tumor spillage does not occur intraoperatively. Subtherapeutic ablation of these tumors in the form of an enucleation will certainly predispose the patient to persistent disease. Such recurrences were noted to be multifocal in nature as originally described in the major salivary glands (Foote and Frazell 1953).

Malignant pleomorphic adenomas of salivary gland origin are uncommon neoplasms. The broad heading, malignant mixed tumor, includes three different clinical and pathologic entities: *carcinoma ex-pleomorphic adenoma, carcinosarcoma, and metastasizing pleomorphic adenoma*. Carcinoma ex-pleomorphic adenoma, perhaps the most commonly referenced malignant pleomorphic adenoma, is a pleomorphic adenoma in which a second neoplasm develops from the epithelial component that fulfills the criteria for malignancy. These features include invasiveness, destruction of normal tissues, cellular anaplasia, cellular pleomorphism, atypical mitoses, and abnormal architectural patterns (Gnepp and Wenig 1991). The Armed Forces Institute of Pathology data showed 326 cases of carcinoma ex-pleomorphic adenoma which accounted for 2.4% of their 13 749 cases. A significant majority of these tumors were in the parotid gland (64.4%); however, these malignancies occurred in the minor salivary glands, as well. The palate accounted for 36 of 57 cases in the minor glands, with the upper lip (6 cases), tongue (4 cases), and cheek (4 cases) also represented. A review of this tumor shows that preoperative duration of a benign pleomorphic adenoma is the main determining

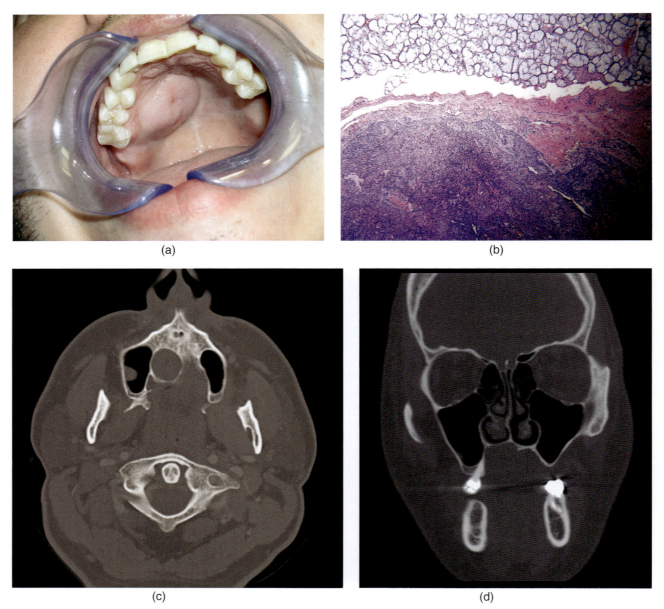

Figure 12.1. The clinical appearance of a pleomorphic adenoma of the palate (a). An incisional biopsy (b) was performed that established the definitive preoperative diagnosis owing to a diverse differential diagnosis containing benign as well as malignant diagnoses. Preoperative CT scans were obtained to precisely define the anatomic extent of the tumor (c, d, and e). The CT scans identify "cupping out" of the bone that need not translate to the performance of a resection. A periosteal sacrificing, bone sparing wide local excision with split thickness sacrifice of the soft palate was therefore performed with a 5–10 mm linear mucosal margins (f). In so doing, the periosteum serves as the superior anatomic barrier on the specimen (g). A periosteal elevator is used judiciously to reflect the specimen inferiorly while effectively negotiating and preserving the periosteum on the superior aspect of the specimen (h). The specimen's mucosal side (i) and periosteal side (j) are noted. The histopathology of the tumor specimen (k) shows the tumor approaching, but well contained within the superiorly located pseudocapsule. The remaining tissue bed (l) is covered with a surgical stent and allowed to heal with tertiary intention. No tissue coverage of the palate is required. The tissue bed is noted at six months postoperatively (m). Effective mucosalization of the exposed bone surface of the hard palate and exposed muscle surface of the soft palate has occurred. No signs of tumor recurrence exist. (b) = hematoxylin and eosin, original magnification × 40. (k) = hematoxylin and eosin, original magnification × 40.

Tumors of the Minor Salivary Glands

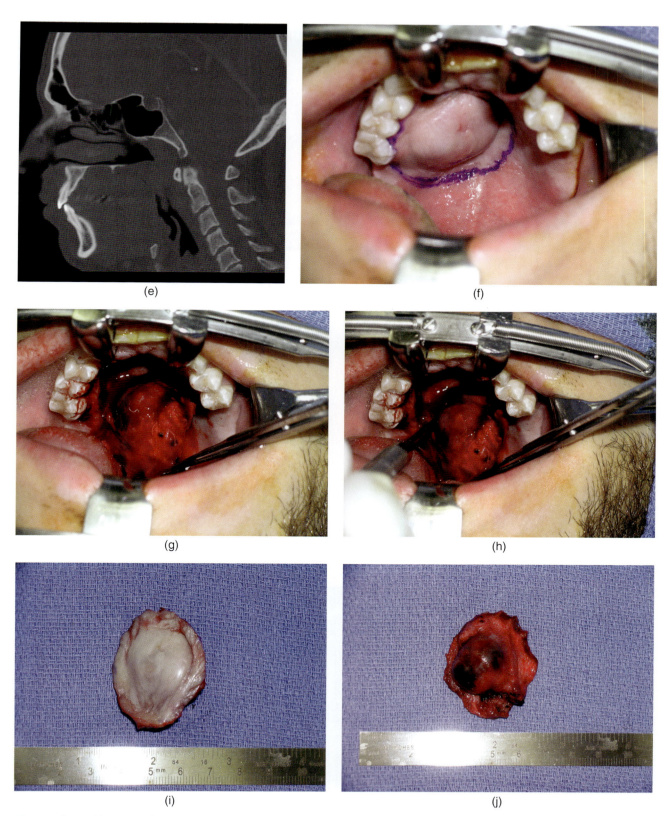

Figure 12.1. *(Continued).*

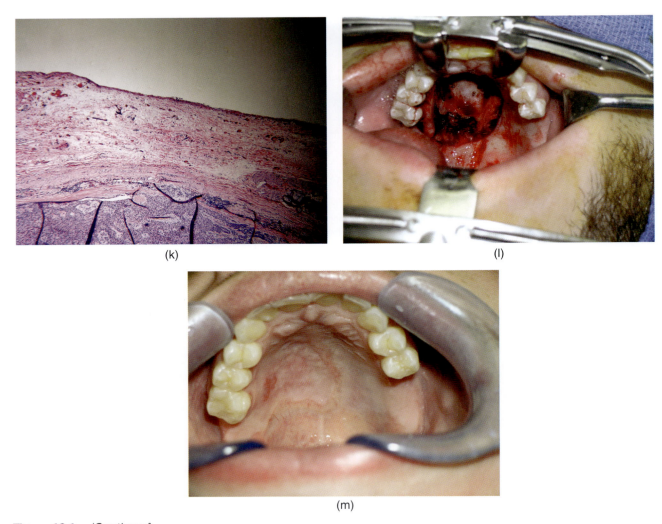

Figure 12.1. (Continued).

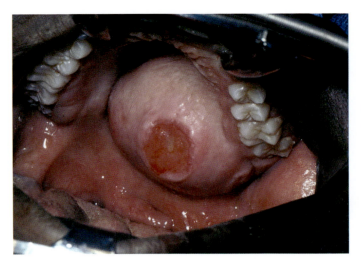

Figure 12.2. A large pleomorphic adenoma that is primarily located over the hard palate. As such, it is permitted to grow in an exophytic fashion, with cupping out of the palatal bone, but no involvement of the parapharyngeal space. Source: Reprinted with permission from: Carlson ER: Salivary Gland Pathology – Clinical Perspectives and Differential Diagnosis, In: The Comprehensive Management of Salivary Gland Pathology, Oral and Maxillofacial Surgery Clinics of North America 7, 361–386, WB Saunders Co., 1995.

Tumors of the Minor Salivary Glands   **383**

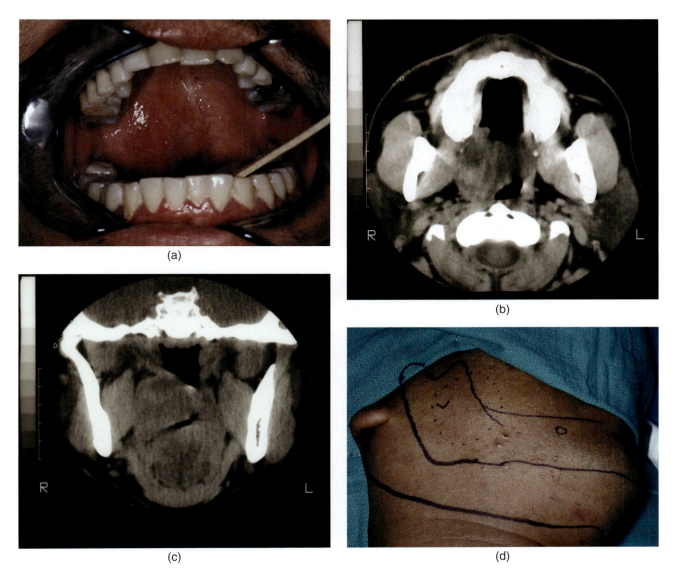

Figure 12.3. The clinical appearance of a pleomorphic adenoma that is located primarily in the soft palate (a). Its chronic growth permitted entry into the parapharyngeal space, as noted on CT scans (b and c). Due to the relative inability to dissect this tumor bed entirely transorally, a decision was made to perform a combined transcutaneous and transoral approach to the tumor ablation with an Attia double osteotomy of the mandible. Wide transcutaneous access was accomplished for this tumor surgery (d). Dissection of the mandible was performed in a subperiosteal fashion, while maintaining as much periosteum and muscle as possible on the lateral surface of the mandible (e). Bone plates were placed on the mandible in preparation for the osteotomy (f). The plates were then removed and an Attia double osteotomy of the mandible was performed that involved a horizontal resection of the mandible superior to the mandibular foramen and a vertical resection of the mandible anterior to the mental foramen. Superior reflection of the mandibular segment was then able to be accomplished (g). Reflection of the medial surface of the medial pterygoid muscle permitted entry into the parapharyngeal space with identification of the tumor (h). With the great vessels of the neck protected, the tumor ablation continued intraorally with development of the tumor dissection surrounding the pseudocapsule (i). The combination of transcutaneous access and transoral access permitted safe delivery of the specimen (j). Histopathology identified a pleomorphic adenoma with tumor present in the pseudocapsule, but with negative margins (k). Following delivery of the specimen, the plates are replaced on the mandible and closure occurred (l). The six-month postoperative view of the palate is noted (m). This surgery provided curative surgery for this patient's tumor. Reprinted with permission from: Carlson ER, Schimmele SR: The Management of Minor Salivary Gland Tumors of the Oral Cavity, In: Surgical Management of Salivary Gland Disease, The Atlas of the Oral and Maxillofacial Surgery Clinics of North America 6, 75–98, WB Saunders Co., 1998.

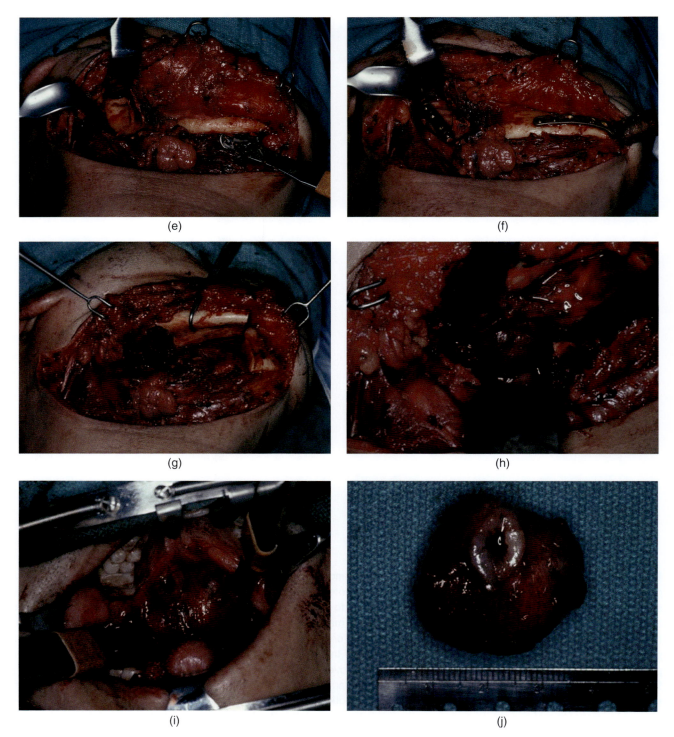

Figure 12.3. (*Continued*).

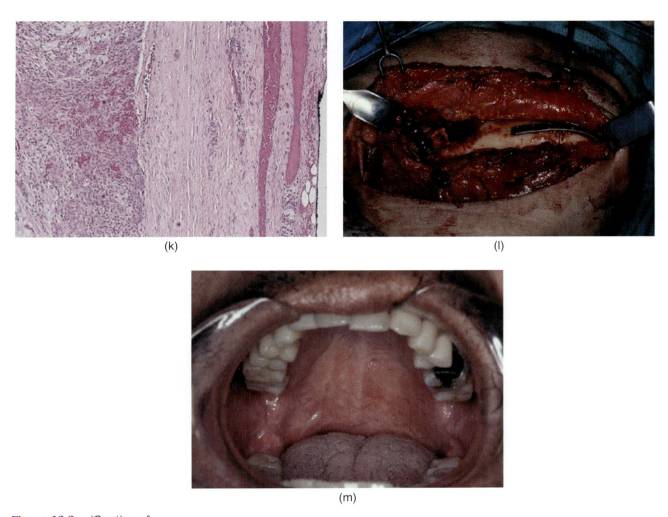

Figure 12.3. (Continued).

factor regarding malignant transformation. Specifically, the incidence of malignancy progressively increases from 1.6% for tumors present for less than 5 years to 9.4% for tumors present for periods longer than 15 years (Gnepp and Wenig 1991). The other predisposing condition for the development of this malignancy is recurrence of a benign pleomorphic adenoma. This fact supports a curative approach to the pleomorphic adenoma from the outset, with abandonment of the subtherapeutic enucleation of these tumors in the parotid gland or minor salivary gland tissues. The prognosis for this malignancy is generally considered dismal, with 71% of patients exhibiting metastatic disease during the course of their disease.

Carcinosarcoma, also known as true malignant pleomorphic adenoma, is a tumor defined by histologic evidence of malignancy in both the epithelial and stromal elements of the tumor. These tumors are rarer than the carcinoma ex-pleomorphic adenoma, accounting for only eight cases in the AFIP registry, and none occurred in the minor salivary glands. Other cases presented in the literature do identify the existence of this diagnosis in the minor salivary glands.

Metastasizing mixed tumor is a histologically benign pleomorphic adenoma, but located in distant sites. The pleomorphic adenomas are known to arise in major as well as minor salivary glands, and the metastatic foci have been identified in the cervical lymph nodes, spine, and liver (Gnepp and Wenig 1991). Data on the interval from removal of the primary tumor to the identification of the first metastasis is 1.5–51 years, with an average of 16.6 years.

Canalicular Adenoma

The canalicular adenoma is a benign tumor that has a significant predilection for the upper lip (Figure 12.4). In the past, this tumor was more commonly referred to as a monomorphic adenoma. Historically, Gardner recommended that the term monomorphic adenoma be used as a nosologic group of epithelial salivary gland tumors that are not pleomorphic adenomas (Gardner and Daley 1983). The canalicular adenoma and basal cell adenoma identify specific forms of monomorphic adenomas (Daley et al. 1984). The canalicular adenoma classically occurs in the upper lip in elderly women (Kratochvil 1991). In fact, canalicular adenomas typically affect an older population compared to pleomorphic adenomas (Ord 1994).

The canalicular adenoma is typically an asymptomatic, slow-growing, and freely moveable mass that uncommonly exceeds 2 cm in widest diameter. They may resemble mucoceles which are uncommonly located in the upper lip. Of the 121 canalicular adenomas in the AFIP files, 89 of them occurred in the upper lip. The second most common site was the buccal mucosa (Auclair et al. 1991). The tumor is encapsulated such that an excision of the tumor in any anatomic site in a pericapsular fashion represents a curative surgery provided tumor spillage does not occur (Figure 12.5). The canalicular adenoma is multifocal in 20% of cases (Ord 1994). If recurrence is believed to have occurred, it might represent a new primary tumor (Melrose 1994).

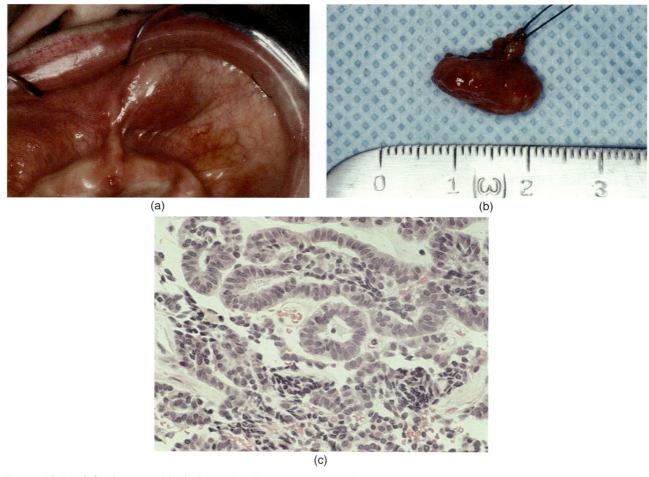

Figure 12.4. A freely moveable, indurated, submucosal mass of the upper lip in an elderly woman, highly suggestive of a canalicular adenoma (a). Based on this assumption, an incisional biopsy is not required. A pericapsular dissection of this mass was performed in association with surrounding minor salivary gland tissue, thereby allowing for delivery of the specimen (b). The histopathology of the specimen confirms the clinical impression of canalicular adenoma (c). Source: Reprinted with permission from: Carlson ER, Schimmele SR: The Management of Minor Salivary Gland Tumors of the Oral Cavity, In: Surgical Management of Salivary Gland Disease, The Atlas of the Oral and Maxillofacial Surgery Clinics of North America 6, 75–98, WB Saunders Co., 1998.

SURGICAL TREATMENT OF MALIGNANT MINOR SALIVARY GLAND TUMORS

The malignant diagnoses in the minor salivary glands are more diverse than their benign counterparts. These malignant diagnoses may be low grade, intermediate grade, or high grade, and many tumors represent histopathologic diagnostic challenges. As with the benign minor salivary gland tumors, surgery represents the hallmark of therapy for malignant minor salivary gland tumors, and the principles of surgery have not changed significantly over the past several decades (Bell et al. 2005). In addition to eradication of the primary malignancy, consideration should be given for neck dissection in very specific circumstances, as well as postoperative radiation therapy in this cohort of patients.

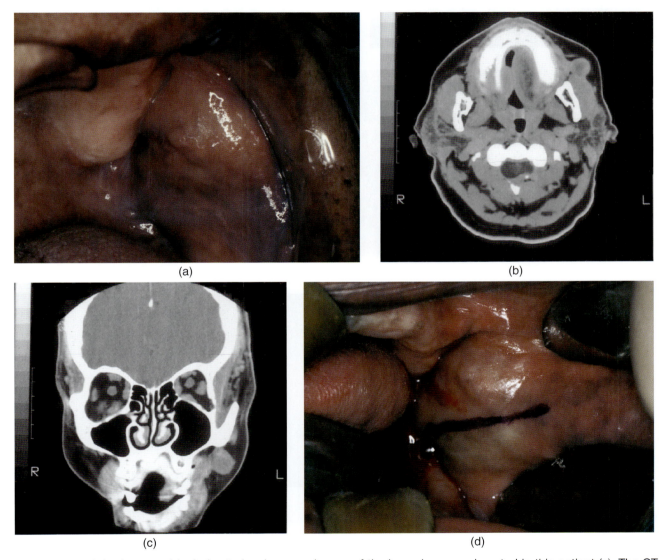

Figure 12.5. A freely moveable, indurated, submucosal mass of the buccal mucosa is noted in this patient (a). The CT scans (b and c) show a well-circumscribed mass of this region. A benign neoplastic process occupies a high position on the differential diagnosis such that a mucosal sparing excision of the mass with transoral access can be performed without first obtaining an incisional biopsy (d). A pericapsular dissection is performed (e), thereby permitting delivery of the specimen (f). Stenson duct was intimately attached to the tumor and therefore sacrificed with the tumor. Histopathology identified canalicular adenoma (g) with an uninvolved capsule (h). The appearance of the site is noted to be well healed at nine months postoperatively (i). Source: Reprinted with permission from: Carlson, ER, Salivary Gland Pathology – Clinical Perspectives and Differential Diagnosis, In: The Comprehensive Management of Salivary Gland Pathology, Oral and Maxillofacial Surgery Clinics of North America 7, 361–386, WB Saunders Co., 1995.

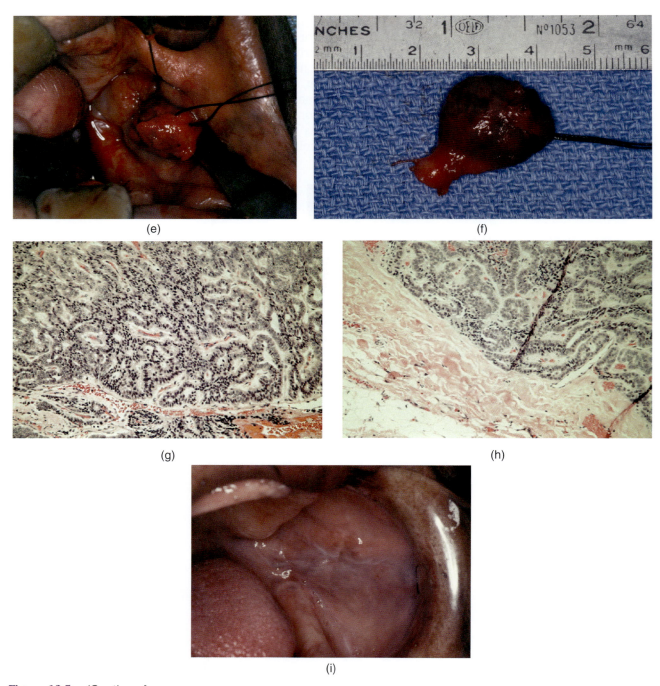

Figure 12.5. (Continued).

Hay et al. (2019) retrospectively reviewed 450 patients with malignant minor salivary gland tumors of which 305 tumors (68%) were found in the oral cavity. Of these 305 tumors, 45% were mucoepidermoid carcinomas and 27% were adenoid cystic carcinomas. While not stratified anatomically as to tissue of origin (oral cavity vs. oropharynx, larynx, trachea, nasal cavity, or paranasal sinuses), 130 patients underwent neck dissection as part of their surgical treatment, 64 patients (49%) with pathologically negative necks and 66 patients with pathologically positive necks. Features predictive of failure for overall survival on univariate analysis were age equal or greater than 60 years, male gender, history of tobacco use, perineural invasion, lympho-vascular invasion, close or positive surgical margins, and stage.

Mimica et al. (2019) retrospectively reviewed 867 salivary gland malignancies, 446 (51.4%) of which were in the minor salivary glands. There were 247 (55.4%) minor salivary gland malignancies in women and 199 (44.6%) minor salivary gland malignancies in men in this study. Although categorization of tumors as originating in the minor vs. the major glands was not performed as a function of survival following surgery, the overall cohort of 867 salivary gland malignancies demonstrated that female gender was a favorable prognostic index in this study. Superior disease-specific survival was observed in female patients. When stratifying results as a function of histologic risk, low- and intermediate-risk cancers faired equally well in men and women, but with regard to the disease-specific survival for high-risk cancers, there was a significant difference between the 5-year disease-specific survival in men (49%) and women (68%) and the 10-year disease-specific survival in men (34%) and women (55%).

Lombardi et al. (2017) have emphasized the primary goal of surgery for malignant minor salivary gland tumors to be the achievement of clear margins as part of radical surgery. Frequently the most common minor salivary gland malignancy, adenoid cystic carcinoma is characterized by its proclivity to exhibit perineural spread with inherently poor long-term survival of patients. In addition, the adenoid cystic carcinoma is frequently diagnosed in late stages, thereby impacting treatment surgical outcomes. The mucoepidermoid carcinoma and polymorphous adenocarcinoma of minor salivary gland origin, by contrast, permit a less aggressive approach to resection and with more favorable outcomes following surgery. The recommendation of a less aggressive approach to resection and more favorable outcomes translates to the observation that these malignancies are capable of perineural invasion but not perineural spread. One notable yet exceptionally rare example of a palatal mucoepidermoid carcinoma with intracranial extension exists in the literature (Dossani et al. 2016).

The concept of dedifferentiation/high-grade transformation (HGT) of salivary gland cancer is well established (Nagao 2013). High-grade transformation is defined as the histologic progression of a low-grade cancer to a high-grade cancer. This process can occur at the time of initial presentation or as part of a recurrence of the cancer. HGT was originally described in relationship to a dedifferentiated chondrosarcoma where low-grade chondrosarcoma was juxtaposed to a histologically different high-grade sarcoma, specifically an anaplastic fibrosarcoma or osteosarcoma (Dahlin and Beabout 1971). Following the first report of HGT of an acinic cell carcinoma (Stanley et al. 1988), this process has been described in relationship to adenoid cystic carcinoma, epithelial-myoepithelial carcinoma, polymorphous adenocarcinoma, myoepithelial carcinoma, mucoepidermoid carcinoma, and hyalinizing clear cell carcinoma (Nagao 2013). The concept of HGT is important to consider when contemplating surgical treatment of salivary gland cancers since these cancers are more aggressive than conventional cancers, associated with a more guarded prognosis, and accompanied by a higher local recurrence rate and cervical lymph node metastases. A wider surgical resection and neck dissection should be considered under these circumstances (Nagao 2013).

Mucoepidermoid Carcinoma

The mucoepidermoid carcinoma is the second most common tumor of the salivary glands overall, the most common salivary gland malignancy overall, and the most common minor salivary gland malignancy (Auclair and Ellis 1991). During the greater than 70 years since its first description, this neoplasm has generated significant debate regarding the possible existence of a benign variant, the optimal number of grades, and the proper treatment for certain minor salivary gland lesions. The term *mucoepidermoid tumor* was first introduced by Stewart, Foote, and Becker in 1945 in their publication of 45 cases (Stewart et al. 1945). In this report, only two grades were utilized, including relatively favorable (benign) and highly unfavorable (malignant) tumors. The authors indicated that the adjective benign was rarely ever applicable in an absolute sense and as used in their report did not imply innocent behavior. The benign adjective did indicate, however, that the authors had not observed metastasis from these tumors. The designation malignant indicated a histologic structure that was associated with the ability to produce regional lymph node and distant metastases. This notwithstanding, the authors explicitly referred to and separated the benign and malignant tumors in their series of 45 cases in this report, of which there were 26 "benign" tumors and 19 "malignant" tumors. In 1953, this grading scheme was modified to include three grades due to the development of metastases related to tumors previously referred to as benign (Foote and Frazell 1953). These investigators accepted all of these tumors as malignant, and clinical and pathologic correlation suggested that separation into low-, intermediate-, and high-grade malignant subgroups might be useful, mainly due to histologically overlapping qualities. The designation of intermediate grade was recognized as behaving more like the low-grade tumors than the high-grade tumors. Interestingly, despite the authors' recognition that all of these tumors were malignant, the designation *mucoepidermoid tumor* persisted throughout their paper. Subsequent studies were undertaken to more objectively determine if a benign variant existed. One such study investigated 23 mucoepidermoid carcinomas with a malignant course, such as evidence of local extension of tumor outside the capsule, local recurrences, histologically verified metastases, or death due to the tumor (Eneroth et al. 1972). Fifteen patients showed local recurrences, 13 showed histologically verified metastases, and 22 patients died of their disease. In 7 of the 23 cases, histology revealed highly or moderately differentiated structures, and in 3 of these cases, the primary tumor as well as the lymph node metastases were highly differentiated. Six of the 23 patients had tumors in the palate with 2 of these patients developing recurrences, 1 with lymph node metastases, and 5 of the patients died due to their disease. The authors concluded by stating that well-differentiated metastases in cases with a malignant course contradicted the existence of a benign variety of mucoepidermoid carcinoma, such that all of these neoplasms should be considered cancers (Eneroth et al. 1972).

Of the 712 mucoepidermoid carcinomas occurring in the minor salivary glands in the AFIP registry, 305 (43%) of these tumors were located in the palate, 93 (13%) in the buccal mucosa, and 58 (8%) in the lip, with 37 specifically designated as the upper lip and 12 specifically designated as the lower lip (Auclair et al. 1991). While the AFIP data is generally recognized as being representative of the incidence of most salivary gland tumors, some authors have identified the mucoepidermoid carcinoma to be more common in minor salivary gland sites than in major salivary gland sites (Plambeck et al. 1996).

Histologic grading of mucoepidermoid carcinomas is an essential exercise from the surgeon's perspective. Histologic grade connotes biologic aggressiveness, prognosis, and provides the surgeon with important information with which to plan surgical treatment (Evans 1984; Brandwein et al. 2001). This notwithstanding, the World Health Organization's fourth edition of classification of head and neck tumors is less dogmatic about grading of the mucoepidermoid carcinoma (Seethala 2017). Mucoepidermoid carcinomas are composed of three cell types: mucous secreting, epidermoid, and intermediate. The intermediate cell is appropriately named because it is likely the progenitor of the two other cells (Batsakis and Luna 1990). Three grading schemes have found general acceptance among pathologists, and differences in biologic behavior could be demonstrated as a function of grade, even though clinical stage has also been considered an important prognosticator. Indeed, Brandwein et al. found that only 5% of low-grade mucoepidermoid carcinomas of the major glands and only 2.5% of low-grade mucoepidermoid carcinomas of the minor glands metastasized to regional lymph nodes or resulted in death. Spiro indicated that survival of patients with minor salivary gland carcinoma is significantly influenced by the clinical stage and the histologic grade, but the applicability of grading to survival was limited to patients with mucoepidermoid carcinoma or adenocarcinoma in their study (Spiro et al. 1991). They determined that staging was important in all patients regardless of the histologic diagnosis.

The mucoepidermoid carcinoma is the most common salivary gland malignancy in children (Auclair et al. 1991; Luna et al. 1991; Ord 1994; Rogerson 1995). Although most of these tumors are noted in the parotid gland, the palate is the second most common site of involvement. Most appear to occur in teenagers, and the majority are low-grade or intermediate-grade histology. Mucoepidermoid carcinoma in children appears to follow a more favorable course with cure rates of 98–100% (Ord 1994).

Surgical treatment of the mucoepidermoid carcinoma of minor salivary gland origin is primarily a function of the anatomic site of the tumor and its histologic grade. Those arising in the palate are not only the most common, but also the most variable in so far as surgical treatment is concerned. It is the histologic grade that is of utmost importance when determining treatment in the palate. Large series show that the low-grade cancer is most common in this anatomic site (Pires et al. 2007). Incisional biopsy is clearly essential to establish the histopathologic diagnosis, as previously described. Computerized tomograms are essential in planning surgical treatment of palatal mucoepidermoid carcinomas as they assess the involvement of the underlying palatal bone. When the palatal bone does not appear to be involved by the cancer, a bone sparing, periosteal sacrificing wide local excision with split thickness sacrifice of the soft palate musculature is the surgical treatment of choice (Figure 12.6). Like the surgery for the palatal pleomorphic adenoma, the periosteum serves as the anatomic barrier on the superior aspect of

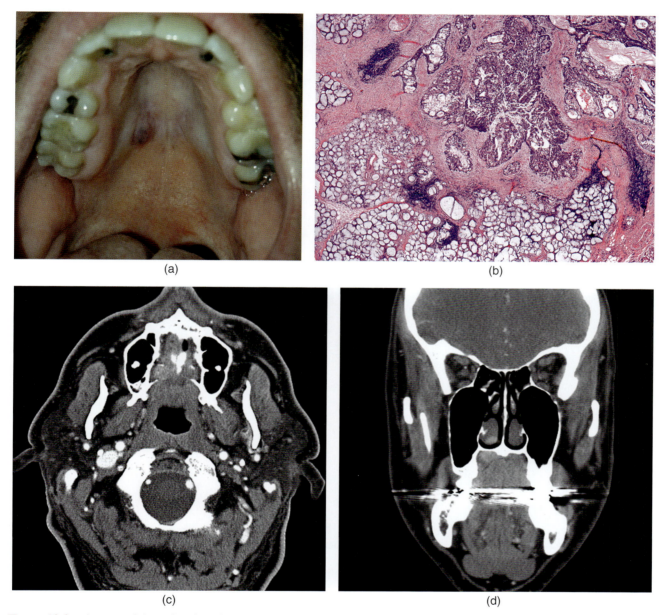

Figure 12.6. A mass of the palate in a 45-year-old man (a). The extensive differential diagnosis, including benign and malignant entities, requires an incisional biopsy for diagnosis prior to performing definitive tumor surgery. The biopsy identifies low-grade mucoepidermoid carcinoma (b). CT scans (c–g) identify no concerning erosion of the palatal bone that would otherwise require a resection of the palate. As such, a periosteal sacrificing, bone sparing wide local excision with split thickness sacrifice of the soft palate is planned with 1 cm mucosal linear margins based on the appearance of the remaining cancer following healing related to the incisional biopsy (h). Like the surgery for pleomorphic adenoma (Figure 12.1), a sharp dissection is performed with a periosteal elevator between the periosteum on the superior aspect of the tumor specimen and the overlying palatal bone. The specimen is delivered (i and j). Histopathology identified low-grade mucoepidermoid carcinoma (k) with negative, but a close margin at the periosteal surface (l). Despite the close nature of this microscopic margin, the palatal bone need not be removed and the patient does not require adjuvant radiation therapy. Mucosalization of the exposed bone and soft palate musculature is noted at 12 months postoperatively (m). This surgery provided curative care for this patient's tumor.

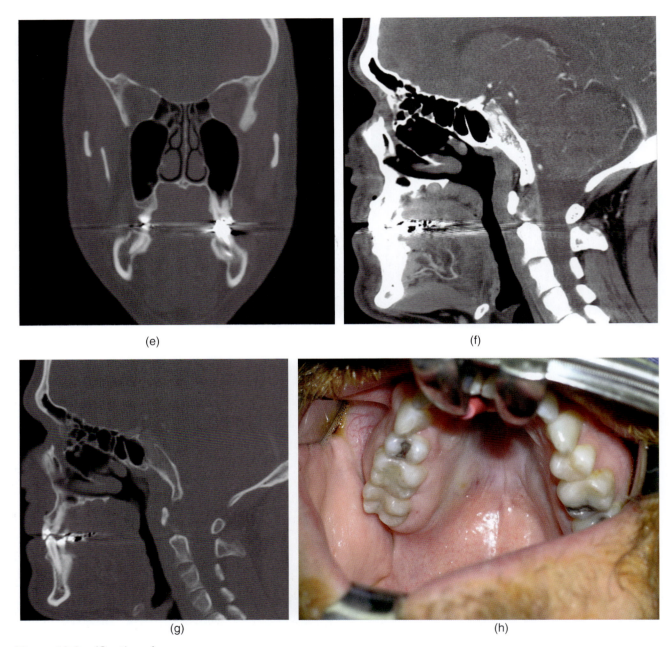

Figure 12.6. (Continued).

the tumor specimen, and tumor-free periosteal frozen and permanent sections should be obtained to confirm this concept. When the periosteum has not been invaded by the cancer and all radial soft tissue margins are free of tumor, this surgery has a high frequency of cure. When the palatal bone is noted to be invaded by tumor on preoperative CT scans, however, its sacrifice is indicated as part of a traditional partial maxillectomy (Figure 12.7). Ord and Salama (2012) reviewed their series of 18 mucoepidermoid carcinomas of the palate, 17 of which were low grade. Sixteen patients underwent soft-tissue excision only of their tumors with periosteum serving as the deep anatomic barrier on the specimen due to the absence of bone erosion on preoperatively obtained CT scans. One patient required bone sacrifice due to intraoperative suspicion for bone erosion, and one patient underwent bone sacrifice due to preoperative CT suspicion for bone erosion. Interestingly, only the patient with CT evidence of bone erosion demonstrated microscopic evidence of bone invasion by the tumor. No local recurrences were identified in these 18 patients with a mean follow-up period of 44 months. The authors concluded that the periosteum represents an effective anatomic barrier margin for palatal mucoepidermoid carcinomas.

The designation of an intermediate mucoepidermoid carcinoma of the palate may change the recommended surgical treatment of the tumor in this, and other anatomic sites, with a more aggressive surgical procedure required for curative intent (Figure 12.8). This is particularly true if the designation of intermediate grade is made by the pathologist based on the worst microscopic pattern observed in the tumor. For example, a mucoepidermoid carcinoma that is predominantly low grade, but that shows a component of intermediate-grade cancer, will likely be designated intermediate

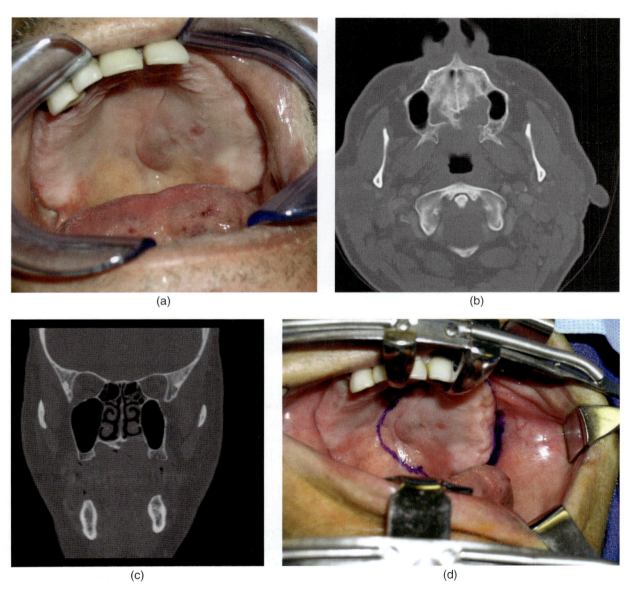

Figure 12.7. A mass of the left palate (a) that demonstrated low-grade mucoepidermoid carcinoma on incisional biopsy. Axial (b) and coronal (c) CT scans demonstrated bone invasion by the tumor such that a partial maxillectomy was planned. One centimeter linear margins in bone and soft tissue were included at the periphery of the resection (d and e). Decalcified histopathologic sections (f – hematoxylin and eosin, original magnification × 140) confirmed the destruction of bone by the tumor. The defect (g) underwent obturation and showed no evidence of disease at two years postoperatively (h).

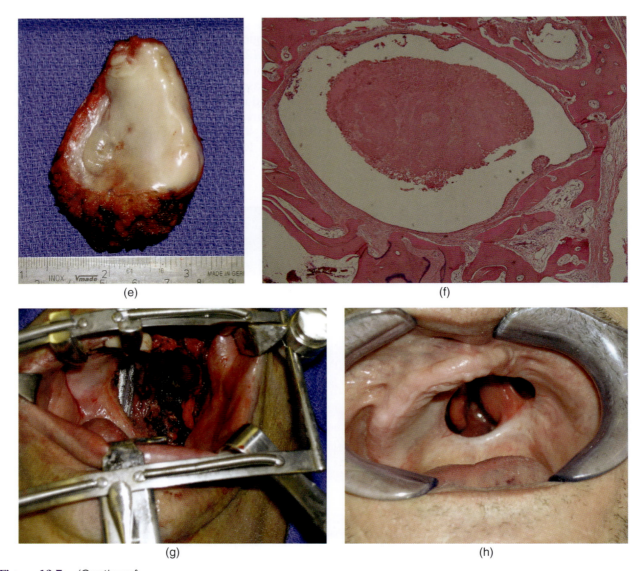

Figure 12.7. (*Continued*).

grade. This notwithstanding, the behavior of such a tumor is likely to be low grade in nature. This scenario is different from a cancer that is designated intermediate grade that shows a predominantly intermediate-grade pattern with intermixed low-grade cancer. The surgeon may wish to offer more aggressive surgical therapy in the form of a partial maxillectomy for the mucoepidermoid carcinoma of the palate that is predominantly intermediate grade on microscopic sections. While rare, a high-grade mucoepidermoid carcinoma of the palate would require a partial maxillectomy, and prophylactic surgical removal of the cervical lymph nodes in the case of an N0 neck, or a therapeutic neck dissection in the case of an N+ neck. Postoperative radiation therapy would also be administered in such circumstances.

Mucoepidermoid carcinoma of the buccal mucosa is the second most common minor salivary gland site affected. In contrast to benign neoplasms of this anatomic site, a mucosal sacrificing tumor surgery is required, with attention to the sacrifice of surrounding submucosal anatomic barriers. The same is true of the lip (Figure 12.9).

Survival of patients with mucoepidermoid carcinomas of the minor salivary glands is clearly related to grade. Five-year survival rates have been estimated at 90% and 15-year survival rates have

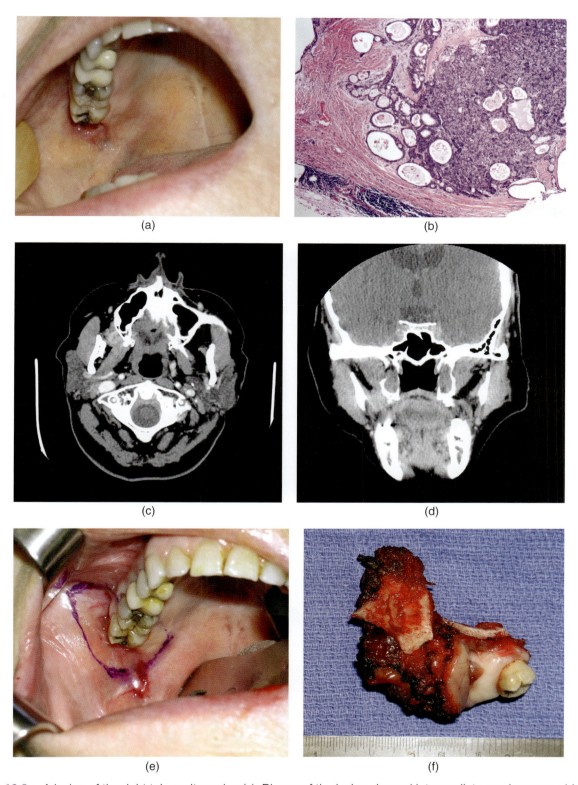

Figure 12.8. A lesion of the right tuberosity region (a). Biopsy of the lesion showed intermediate-grade mucoepidermoid carcinoma (b). Computerized tomograms identified an enhancing mass located lateral to the right tuberosity, and in close proximity to the coronoid process (c and d). Definitive tumor surgery involved a transoral partial maxillectomy and coronoidectomy en bloc (e) which permitted effective removal of the cancer (f). The resultant defect was obturated and allowed to contract significantly over time (g). Soft-tissue reconstruction was accomplished with a buccal fat flap and advancement of the mucosa (h–j). The reconstruction healed well as noted at six years postoperatively (k).

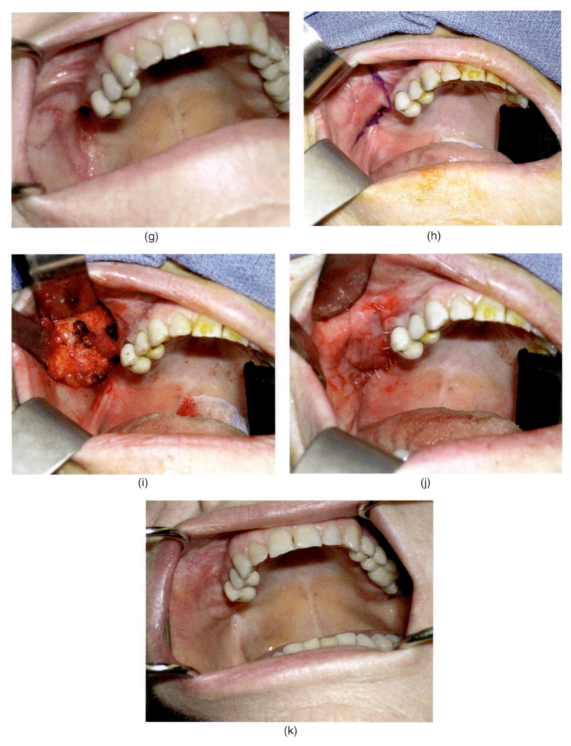

Figure 12.8. (*Continued*).

been estimated at 82% for low-grade mucoepidermoid carcinomas (Ord 1994). In their study of 37 patients with mucoepidermoid carcinoma of the palate, Li et al. (2012) identified an overall survival of 84.4% at 5 and 10 years.

Central Mucoepidermoid Carcinoma

Salivary gland cancers of the jaws most frequently involve direct intraosseous extension of primary malignancies arising from the major or minor salivary glands (Woolgar et al. 2013). Centrally

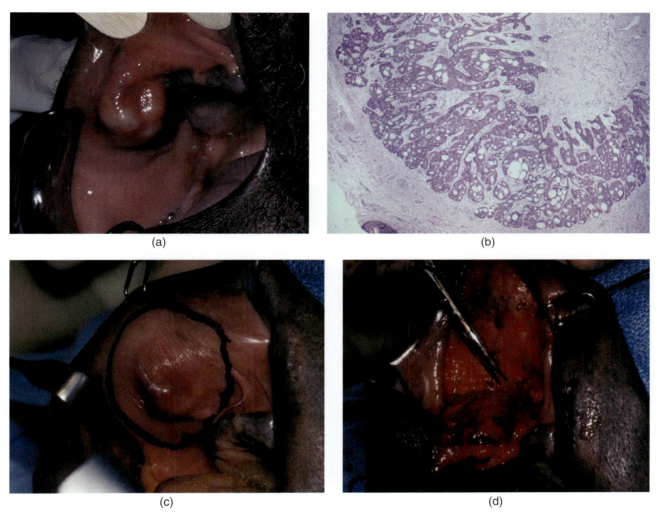

Figure 12.9. An indurated upper lip mass that was fixed to surrounding mucosa (a). Due to the likely but equivocal malignant nature of the mass, incisional biopsy is essential for the establishment of the diagnosis prior to definitive surgical therapy. The histopathology identified intermediate-grade mucoepidermoid carcinoma (b). A wide local excision of the mass with oral mucosal sacrifice was planned (c). A surgical plane was developed between the dermis of the upper lip and the musculature on the deep aspect of the tumor specimen (d). The specimen was delivered and oriented for the pathologist with sutures (e). Final histopathology identified intermediate-grade mucoepidermoid carcinoma with perineural invasion (f). The defect was reconstructed immediately with a full thickness skin graft (g). A prophylactic neck dissection was not performed as part of this cancer surgery due to the low concern for occult neck disease associated with this diagnosis. The patient underwent postoperative radiation therapy and the surgical site was noted to be well healed at one year postoperatively without signs of recurrent disease (h). Source: Reprinted with permission from: Carlson, ER, Salivary Gland Pathology – Clinical Perspectives and Differential Diagnosis, In: The Comprehensive Management of Salivary Gland Pathology, Oral and Maxillofacial Surgery Clinics of North America 7, 361–386, WB Saunders Co., 1995.

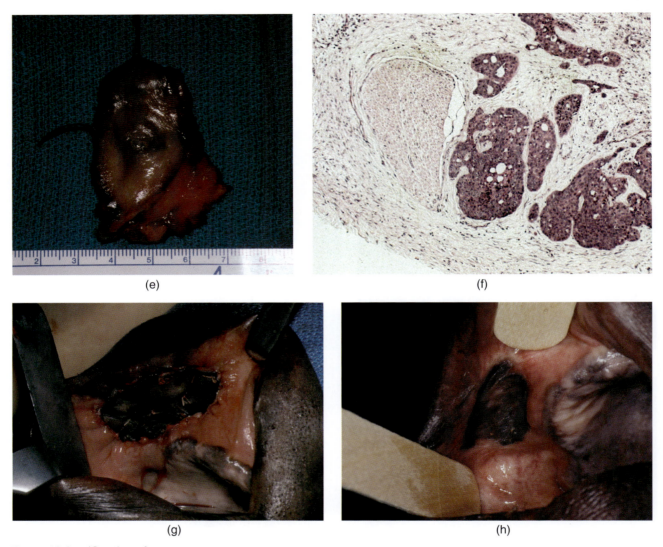

Figure 12.9. *(Continued).*

occurring malignant salivary gland tumors are very rare. While academic understanding and the international literature would primarily point to the identification of mucoepidermoid carcinoma of the jaws in this category of tumor, other malignant salivary gland tumor diagnoses have been identified in the jaws (Li et al. 2008). Adenoid cystic carcinoma seems to be the second most common central salivary gland malignancy of the jaws (Woolgar et al. 2013). Central mucoepidermoid carcinoma is considered an exceedingly rare subgroup, accounting for approximately 2–4% of all cases of mucoepidermoid carcinoma (Chiu et al. 2012). This primary malignancy occurs most frequently in the fourth and fifth decades of life with a male-to-female ratio of 1:1.4 (Zhou et al. 2012). These malignancies are most commonly located in the mandible, and specifically in the molar/ramus region, and a predominantly unilocular or multilocular radiographic character is noted (Zhou et al. 2012) (Figure 12.10a). Most cases are classified as low-grade malignancies. The exact pathogenesis is uncertain; however, several hypotheses have been documented in the literature including ectopic salivary gland tissue resulting from entrapment during embryonic development of minor salivary glands, inclusions of embryonic rests of submandibular or sublingual glands, or seromucinous glands displaced from the maxillary sinus into the maxilla;

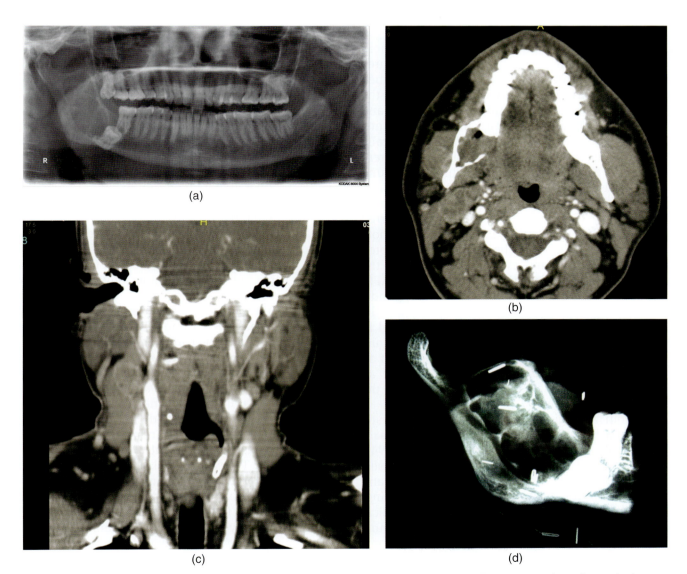

Figure 12.10. A central mucoepidermoid carcinoma of the right mandibular ramus. The panoramic radiograph demonstrates a multilocular radiolucency (a). The patient demonstrated an enlarged right level II lymph node that is also apparent on the MRI study (b and c). The patient underwent a composite resection including a disarticulation resection of the right mandible and type I modified radical neck dissection. The specimen radiograph is noted (d).

development in a submucosal gland with intraosseous extension; and neoplastic transformation of the epithelial lining of odontogenic cysts (Chiu et al. 2012). The latter possibility is most favored as transition of cyst lining to carcinoma is evident in some cases (Zhou et al. 2012; Spoorthi et al. 2013). Preferred treatment is radical resection of the tumor (Figure 12.10). The value of neck dissection for N0 disease is debatable as cervical lymph node metastases seem to occur in fewer than 10% of cases (Chiu et al. 2012; Takano et al. 2012). Patients require therapeutic neck dissections when cervical lymph node metastases are apparent on clinical examination and or on imaging studies (Figure 12.10). A transcutaneous approach for resection of the mandible for central mucoepidermoid carcinoma with a clinically negative neck examination additionally represents justification for elective neck dissection. Distant metastasis is rare but has been reported in the lungs, brain, and clavicle (Chiu et al. 2012; Zhou et al. 2012).

Adenoid Cystic Carcinoma

Like the mucoepidermoid carcinoma, the adenoid cystic carcinoma is a very diverse tumor with three histologic variants. These have been described morphologically, rather than by grade as is the case with the mucoepidermoid carcinoma, and include the tubular, cribriform, and solid variants. The adenoid cystic carcinoma is characteristically slow-growing, with a high propensity for recurrent disease. It is highly infiltrative, exhibits profound neurotropism, and is associated with a dismal long-term survival rate. This malignancy was first described by Theodor Billroth in 1859 and referred to as cylindroma (Tomich 1991). In 1953, Foote and Frazell proposed the currently accepted nomenclature, adenoid cystic carcinoma. Of the 600 cases of adenoid cystic carcinoma in the AFIP files, 312 were noted in the major salivary glands, and 288 were noted in the minor salivary glands. The palate was the most common site affected in the minor salivary glands, followed by the tongue. Adenoid cystic carcinoma accounts for 8.3% of all palatal salivary gland tumors and 17.7% of all malignant palatal salivary gland tumors in the AFIP series (Tomich 1991).

From a surgical perspective, adenoid cystic carcinoma is probably the most challenging salivary gland tumor for the surgeon (Ord 1994). While straightforward to perform in most cases, radical resection is fraught with recurrences and ultimate distant metastases. This notwithstanding, palatal tumors should be managed with radical maxillectomy, observing 1–2 cm linear margins, and with resection of the greater palatine neurovascular bundle to foramen rotundum with frozen section guidance (Figure 12.11). The presence or absence of tumor in association with this nerve should be documented as far superior as possible.

Cervical lymph node metastases are thought to be rare such that prophylactic neck dissection is not required in the patient with an N0 neck associated with a palatal adenoid cystic carcinoma as the incidence of cervical metastases is approximately 10% (Min et al. 2012). Elective neck dissection for N0 disease should be considered due to the proximity to lymphatic vasculature associated with adenoid cystic carcinoma at other sites (Figure 12.12). Min et al. (2012) performed a retrospective study of 616 patients with adenoid cystic carcinoma of the head and neck, 422 patients with involvement of minor salivary gland sites, and 194 patients with tumors located in the major salivary glands. Sixty-two of the 616 patients were confirmed to have cervical lymph node metastases, an incidence of approximately 10%. These authors identified the base of tongue, mobile tongue, and floor of mouth as the most frequent sites of lymph node metastases, with incidences of 19.2, 17.6, and 15.3% respectively. The incidence of cervical lymph node metastases from the 166 patients with adenoid cystic carcinoma of the hard/soft palate was less than 10%.

Postoperative radiation therapy is generally considered advisable for all patients with adenoid cystic carcinoma of the minor salivary glands, regardless of the adequacy of the resection (Ord 1994; Dragovic 1995; Triantafillidou et al. 2006). The prognosis associated with adenoid cystic carcinoma of the minor salivary glands is inferior to that of the major salivary glands (Nascimento et al. 1986; Ampil and Misra 1987). In addition, it has been found that the best prognosis for the adenoid cystic carcinoma is associated with the tubular variant, while the solid variant (Figure 12.13) is associated with the worst prognosis (Perzin et al. 1978). It has also been pointed out that perineural invasion of major nerves and positive margins at surgery, in addition to the solid variant of adenoid cystic carcinoma, are associated with increased treatment failures (Fordice et al. 1999). Typical survival statistics for adenoid cystic carcinoma in general include 60% for 5-year survival, 30% for 10-year survival, and 7% for survival at 20 years (Ord 1994). It has been pointed out that adenoid cystic carcinoma of minor salivary gland sites has a worse prognosis, with a 0% survival at 20 years (Ord 1994). The presence of perineural spread has a significant impact on survival. Five-year survival rates of patients with perineural spread have been found to be 36.9% while 5-year survival rates have been found to be 93.8% in patients without perineural spread (Ord 1994). In their review of 26 cases of adenoid cystic carcinoma of the intraoral minor salivary glands, Luksic et al. (2014) found disease-specific survival rates of 62% at 5 years, 53% at 10 years, and 27% at 15 years for patients with perineural invasion compared with 90% for those patients who did not have invasion at the same follow-up intervals. These authors found that perineural invasion was associated with a higher incidence of distant metastases. The lungs are the most common site of distant metastatic spread of adenoid cystic carcinoma, typically with multiple lobe involvement (Figure 12.14).

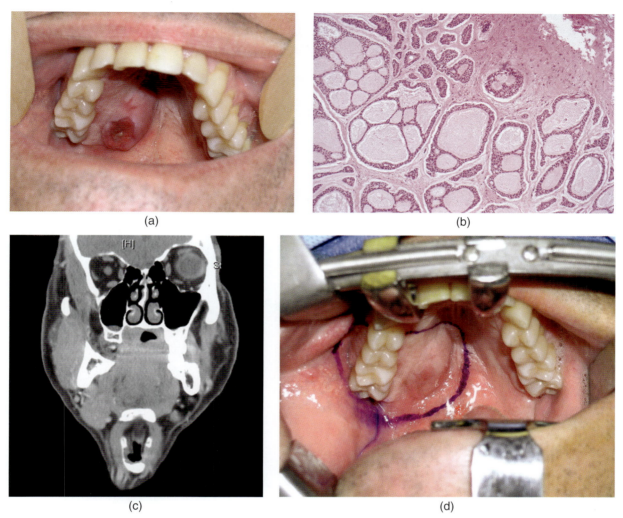

Figure 12.11. A 52-year-old man with a six-month history of a palatal mass (a). Incisional biopsy showed adenoid cystic carcinoma (b). Computerized tomograms identified a soft-tissue mass and minimal invasion of the palatal bone (c). A maxillectomy was planned for this patient observing 1 cm linear margins in bone and soft tissue (d). The bony cuts were created throughout the maxilla and the Smith splitter (e) was utilized to separate the specimen from the remaining facial skeleton (f). The specimen was delivered and inspected from the palatal side (g) and the nasal/sinus side (h) to clinically confirm the efficacy of the resection. Frozen sections were obtained to microscopically examine the soft tissue margins as well as a segment of greater palatine nerve in the superior aspect of the defect. All frozen sections were negative thereby not requiring additional sampling of the nerve or mucosa. Final histopathology identified adenoid cystic carcinoma invading the maxillary bone (i). The patient underwent postoperative radiation therapy and was without evidence of cancer at one year postoperatively (j). This view provides anatomic delineation of the eustachian tube in the defect. He successfully underwent soft-tissue reconstruction with a temporalis muscle flap one year postoperatively and healed uneventfully as noted at four years postoperatively (k). He was doing well until seven years postoperatively, when back pain led to an MRI (l) that identified a compression fracture of T1 with loss of vertebral bone height and osseous retropulsion. A biopsy was performed that identified metastatic adenoid cystic carcinoma of T1. He developed significant progression of disease in his lungs (m), liver (n), and T1 (o) at 12 years postoperatively. He died of his disease shortly thereafter.

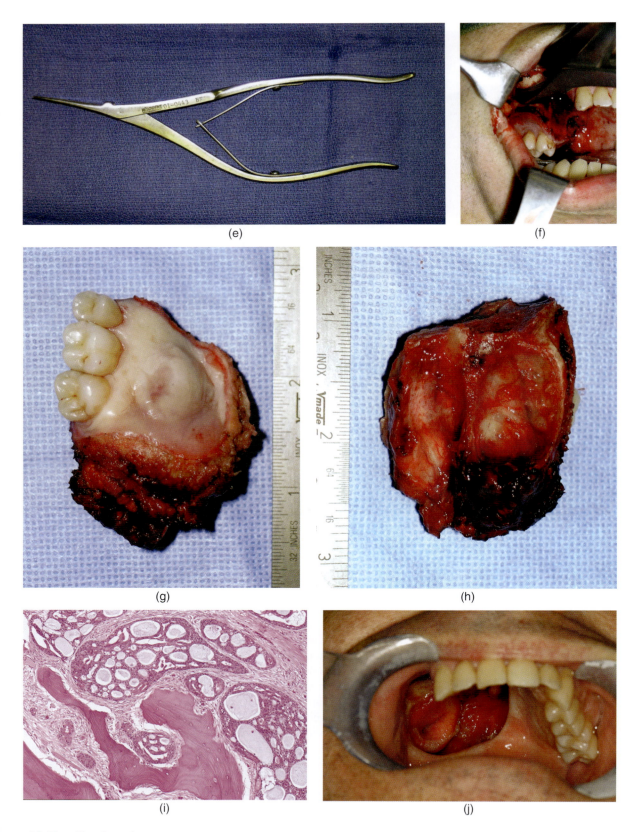

Figure 12.11. (Continued).

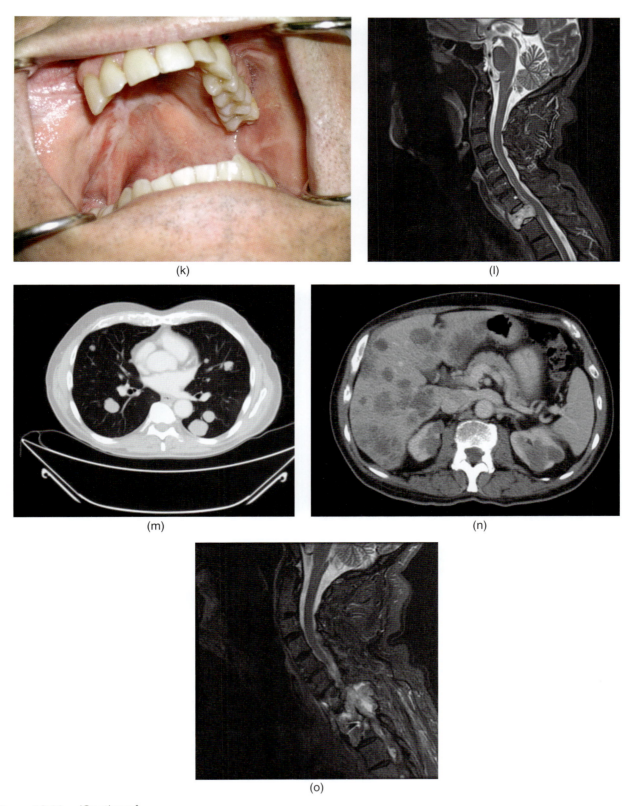

Figure 12.11. (Continued).

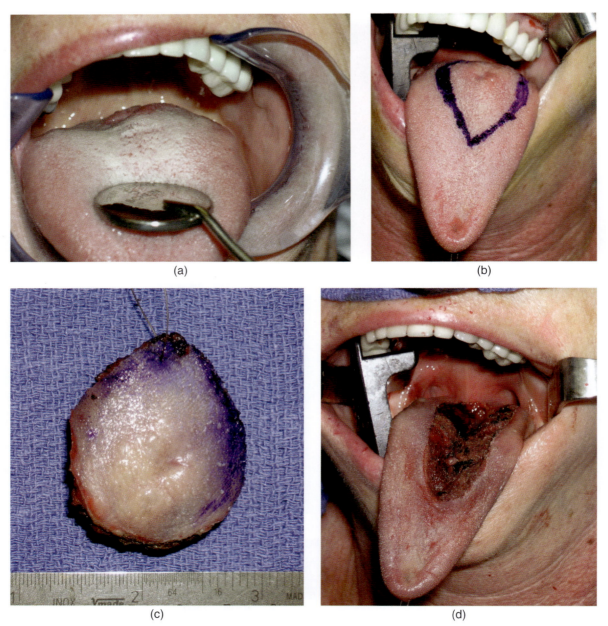

Figure 12.12. A mass of the dorsum of the tongue (a) that demonstrated adenoid cystic carcinoma on incisional biopsy. A wide excision of the dorsum of the tongue, observing one centimeter linear margins (b and c) was performed with primary closure of the tongue defect (d and e). The tongue specimen showed classic cribriform architecture associated with the adenoid cystic carcinoma (f: hematoxylin and eosin, original magnification × 40). Bilateral supraomyohyoid neck dissections were performed (g and h). One lymph node with metastatic adenoid cystic carcinoma was identified (i). The patient underwent postoperative radiation therapy to the tongue and bilateral cervical lymph nodes. She developed a right upper lobe lung metastasis at four years postoperatively (j) that was treated with wedge resection and postoperative radiation therapy. The patient developed a paraspinal soft-tissue metastatic mass at the T6–T7 region at six years postoperatively for which she received radiation therapy. Her tumor was sent for genomic sequencing that demonstrated no Her-2 neu, PD-L1, or EGFR mutations. She received chemotherapy with Alimta, methotrexate, carboplatin, cisplatin, and oxaliplatin. Her nine-year postoperative chest CT showed no evidence of disease (k). The patient demonstrates no evidence of disease at 10 years postoperatively (l, m, and n).

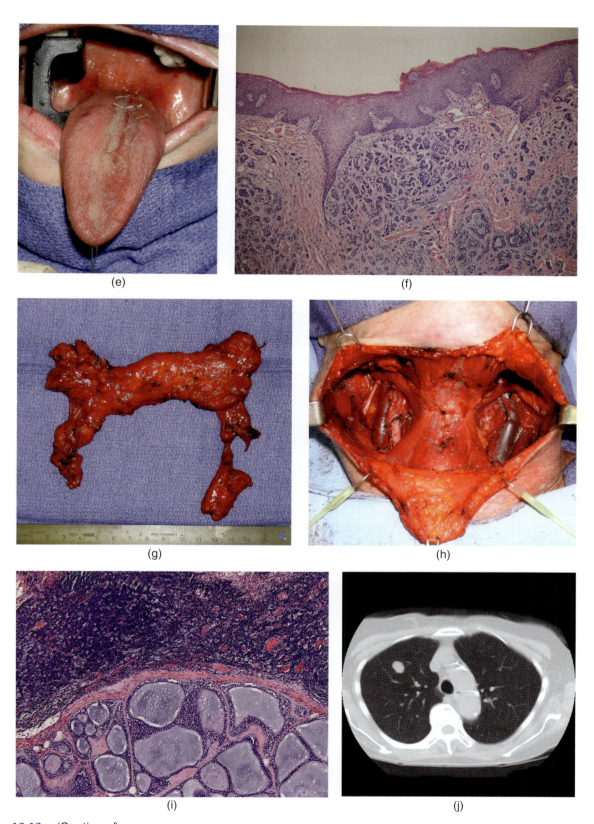

Figure 12.12. (*Continued*)

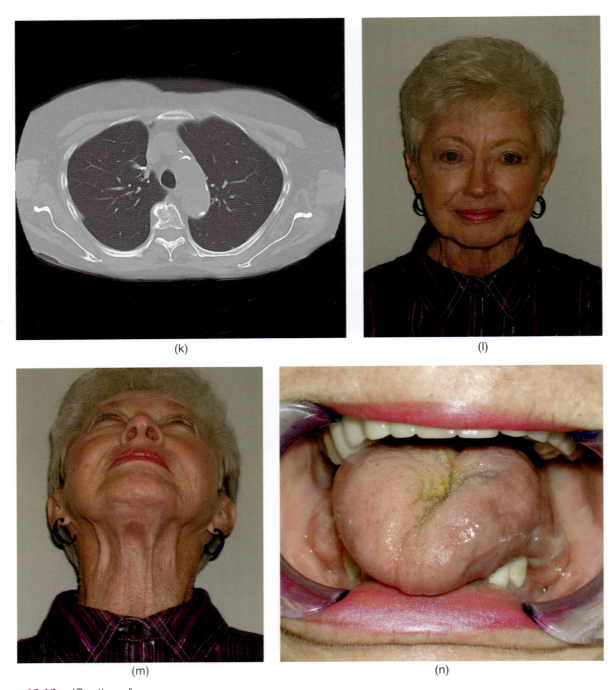

Figure 12.12. (Continued)

Polymorphous Adenocarcinoma

In 1983, two separate investigations reported on low-grade adenocarcinomas of minor salivary glands referred to as terminal duct carcinoma (Batsakis et al. 1983) and lobular carcinoma (Freedman and Lumerman 1983). Terminal duct carcinoma was designated to specify the histogenesis of the tumor which was thought to be the progenitor cell of the terminal duct. Lobular carcinoma was suggested as nomenclature due to the morphology of the tumor resembling lobular carcinoma of the breast. A review of these reports

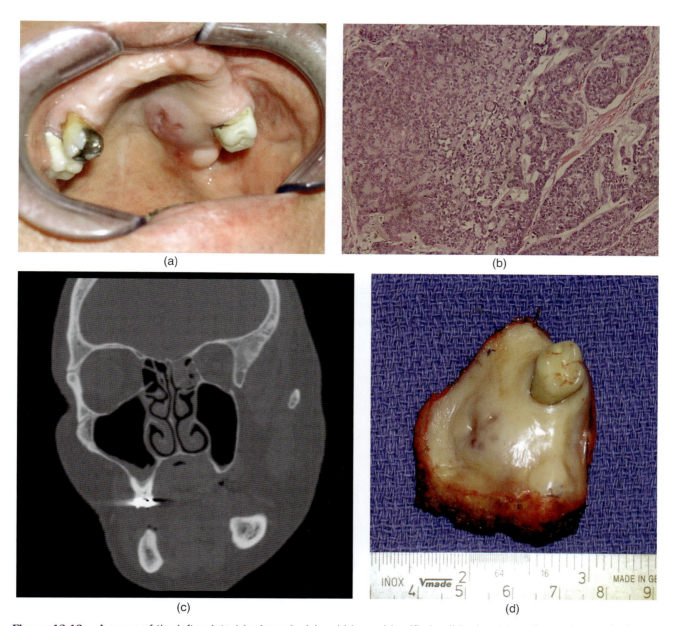

Figure 12.13. A mass of the left palate (a) whose incisional biopsy identified solid adenoid cystic carcinoma (b: hematoxylin and eosin, original magnification × 100). Coronal CT images identified subtle erosion of the palatal bone (c). A partial maxillectomy was performed observing 1 cm linear margins in bone and soft tissue (d).

indicates that the authors were independently describing the same neoplasm (Wenig and Gnepp 1991). Prior to this time, it was thought that these neoplasms were classified as either adenoid cystic carcinoma or adenocarcinoma (Regezi et al. 1991). High-power evaluation of theretofore named polymorphous low-grade adenocarcinoma and adenoid cystic carcinoma permitted the distinction between the two malignancies as adenoid cystic carcinoma showed ductal type structures lined by multiple cells in thickness, while polymorphous low-grade carcinoma showed ductal type structures more commonly lined by single cell layers (Figure 12.15). An Indian filing pattern was also appreciated in polymorphous low-grade adenocarcinoma. The common morphologic features of polymorphous low-grade adenocarcinoma and adenoid cystic carcinoma led researchers to

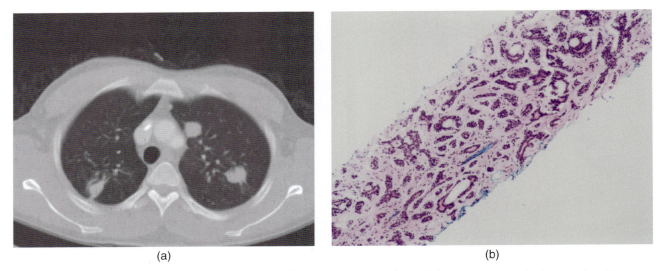

Figure 12.14. A representative axial cut of a chest CT (a) of a patient with multiple pulmonary metastases related to recurrent adenoid cystic carcinoma of the palate. A CT-guided core biopsy of one of the nodules identified metastatic adenoid cystic carcinoma (b: hematoxylin and eosin, original magnification × 40).

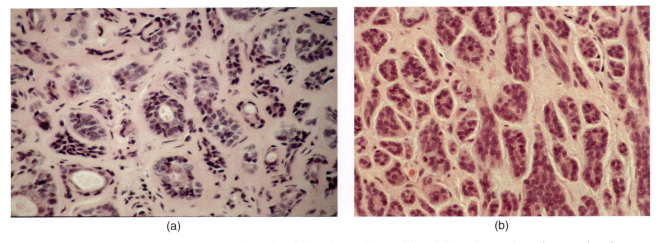

Figure 12.15. Subtle differences between the adenoid cystic carcinoma (a) and the polymorphous low-grade adenocarcinoma (b). The adenoid cystic carcinoma characteristically shows multiple cell layered ductal structures, while the polymorphous low-grade adenocarcinoma shows single cell layered ductal structures. Source: Reprinted with permission from Carlson (1995). (a) and (b) = hematoxylin and eosin, original magnification × 100.

investigate methods of distinguishing these diagnoses (Beltran et al. 2006). In 1984, Evans and Batsakis described 14 cases of a distinctive minor salivary gland neoplasm that they named polymorphous low-grade adenocarcinoma. This term emphasized the features of this neoplasm, including their cytologic uniformity and histologic diversity, variable growth patterns from solid to papillary to cribriform to fascicular, and relative lack of nuclear atypia (Evans and Batsakis 1984). Mitotic figures were infrequent and tumor necrosis was only seen in one case. Perineural invasion was commonly noted in this malignancy. The tumors were distinctly unencapsulated and deeply infiltrative of bone and surrounding soft tissues. Radical surgical procedures were required for tumor control, but no distant metastases were noted. The authors judged from their survey of adenocarcinomas of the major salivary glands that the polymorphous low-grade adenocarcinoma was at least primarily an oral neoplasm. Batsakis and El-Naggar (1991) later subclassified polymorphous low-grade adenocarcinomas into papillary and nonpapillary forms. The papillary form was found to exhibit a more aggressive course with a higher rate of recurrence at the primary site, metastasis to cervical lymph nodes, and distant metastasis (Batsakis and El-Naggar 1991). The AFIP registry identified 75 cases of this neoplasm, and all were in the minor salivary glands (Wenig and Gnepp 1991). Forty-four of these cases were in the palate (58.6%), with the upper lip and buccal mucosa showing 12 cases each. Involvement of other oral minor salivary gland sites has been reported; however, this is quite rare (Kennedy et al. 1987; de Diego et al. 1996).

In 2017, the World Health Organization designated the *polymorphous adenocarcinoma* in its fourth edition, eliminating the term low grade of this tumor's nomenclature due to emerging evidence showing recurrence rates of up to 19% and cases of transformation of high-grade malignancies (Kikuchi et al. 2019; Mimica et al. 2019). Further, at base of tongue sites, a distinctive cribriform architecture was noted in tumors that prompted reclassification of the cribriform adenocarcinoma of minor salivary gland (CAMSG) (Seethala 2017). CAMSG commonly metastasizes to cervical lymph nodes, and often at the time of the patient's presentation (Boyd 2019). Despite significant debate among those contributing to the fourth edition of the classification of salivary gland malignancies, the decision was to maintain CAMSG within the polymorphous adenocarcinoma subheading (Seethala 2017; Carlson and Schlieve 2019).

Since its original description in minor salivary gland sites, cases of polymorphous adenocarcinoma have been reported in all of the major salivary glands such that this tumor cannot be stated to be exclusive to minor salivary gland tissue (Merchant et al. 1996; Barak et al. 1998; Blanchaert et al. 1998; Nagao et al. 2004).

Treatment of polymorphous adenocarcinoma should involve surgery with curative intent. The specific surgical procedure is based on the anatomic site. Surgical removal of these tumors in the palate requires a thorough assessment of the palatal bone with computerized tomograms. Bone involvement by this tumor is not an inherent property of this neoplasm, but rather seems to be a function of chronicity of the tumor. Since these malignancies are not fast-growing, many patients might have long histories of their presence, such that palatal bone infiltration by the tumor occurs over time. In addition, the characteristically deeply infiltrative nature of these tumors into surrounding soft tissues, regardless of the chronicity of the tumor, is such that the soft palate typically requires full thickness sacrifice in most cases. These features are clearly a departure from the treatment of mucoepidermoid carcinoma of the palate where grade has historically represented the main determining factor in planning surgical treatment. Once a biopsy diagnosis of polymorphous adenocarcinoma of the palate has been established, therefore, CT scans should be obtained to examine the quality of the palatal bone. If the bone is unaltered by the tumor, a bone sparing, periosteal sacrificing wide local excision with full thickness sacrifice of the soft palate may be performed (Figure 12.16). Due to the tumor's neurotropism, the greater palatine neurovascular bundle should be sampled for frozen sections superiorly. Since perineural spread is not characteristic of this tumor, it is unlikely to find tumor tracking along the nerve, in contradistinction to adenoid cystic carcinoma of the palate where tumor may be found surrounding this nerve at foramen rotundum. An immediate surgical obturator is fabricated preoperatively for insertion at the time of ablative surgery to permit the patient to begin taking an oral diet on the day of surgery. If the bone is eroded by the tumor, a traditional maxillectomy is necessary, also resulting in a full thickness sacrifice of the soft palate (Figure 12.17). An immediate surgical obturator must also be fabricated preoperatively for insertion at the time of surgery when a maxillectomy is planned for this diagnosis.

The surgical treatment of polymorphous adenocarcinoma of the upper lip or buccal mucosa is similar to that of a mucoepidermoid carcinoma of these regions. The basic approach involves a mucosal sacrificing wide local excision with attention to submucosal anatomic barriers being included on the specimen to ensure tumor free margins (Figure 12.18).

The use of radiation therapy has been assessed in the management of polymorphous adenocarcinoma. In a clinicopathologic study of 164 cases of this malignancy, 17 patients underwent incisional, excisional, or wide local excision followed by radiation therapy (Castle et al. 1999). Adjuvant radiation therapy was not found to affect survival. Their study showed that patients who

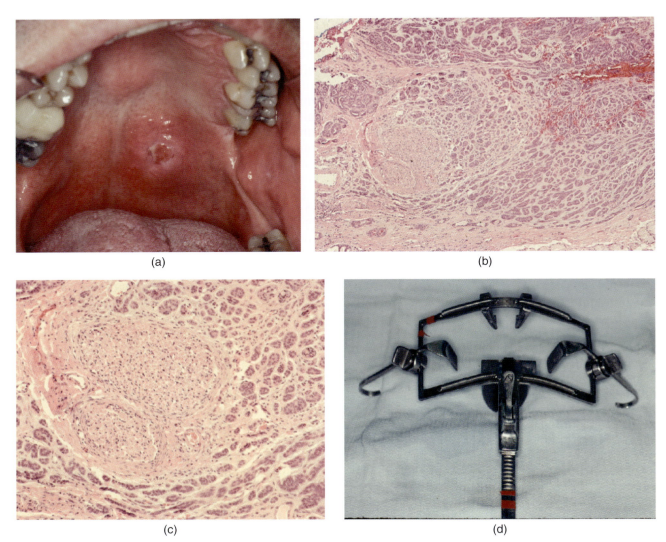

Figure 12.16. A 51-year-old man with a mass of the soft palate that had been reportedly present for only two months (a). Incisional biopsy showed a microscopically cribriform tumor with obvious perineural invasion (b and c). A diagnosis of polymorphous low-grade adenocarcinoma was made. Computerized tomograms did not reveal involvement of the palatal bone such that a periosteal sacrificing, bone sparing wide local excision with full thickness sacrifice of the soft palate was performed. A Dingman mouth gag was utilized to provide acceptable retraction to perform this surgery (d). One centimeter linear margins in mucosa were planned (e). The specimen is delivered (f). Final histopathology ultimately identified a negative periosteal surface, thereby justifying the preservation of palatal bone (g). The greater palatine neurovascular bundle was clamped prior to delivery of the specimen to procure a 1 cm segment of nerve for frozen section analysis (h). The hemostat remained on the nerve stump while the frozen section was being evaluated. If the nerve was positive for cancer, the nerve would be pulled down to procure additional frozen sections to clear the cancer. The defect (i) was addressed with an immediate obturator that had been fabricated preoperatively (j and k). The exposed palatal bone is covered with immature granulation tissue at one month postoperatively (l), which undergoes maturation by three months postoperatively (m). At one-year postoperatively, the patient's defect has demarcated well (n), and a definitive obturator has been fabricated (o). The patient is free of disease at 24 years postoperatively. Source: Reprinted with permission from Carlson (1995).

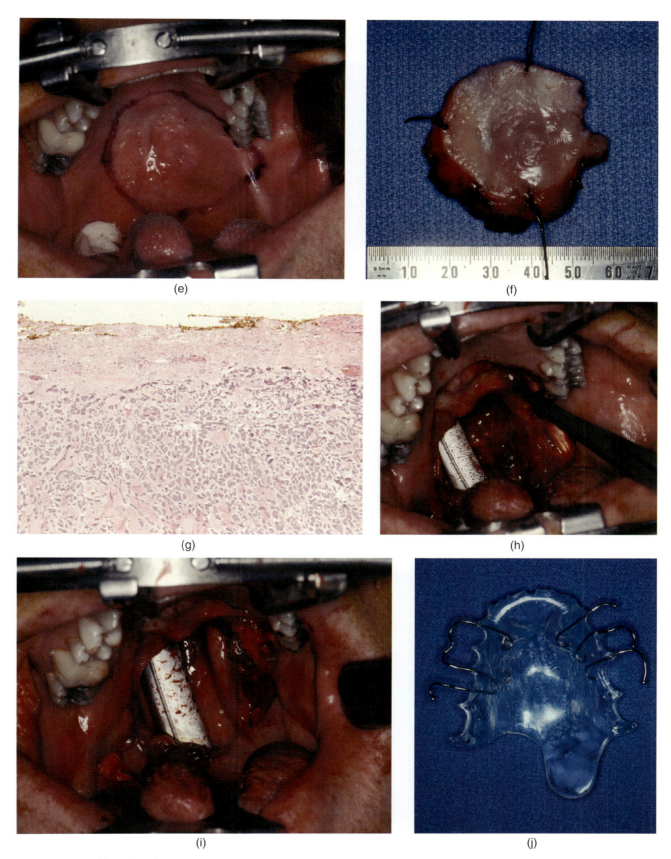

Figure 12.16. (Continued).

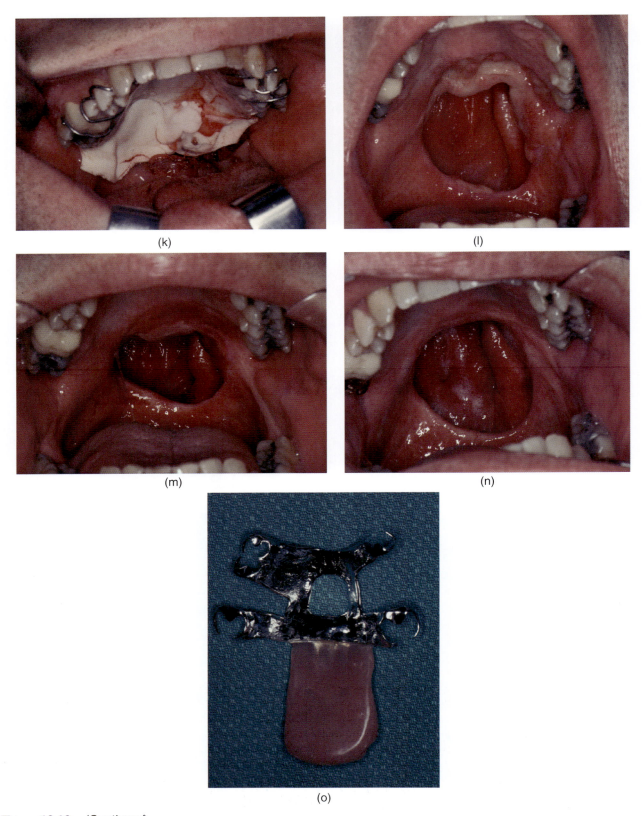

Figure 12.16. (Continued).

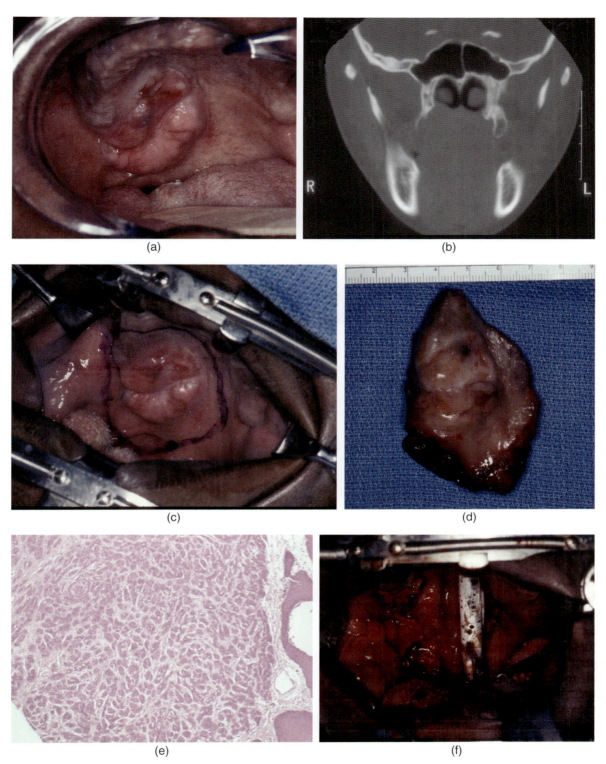

Figure 12.17. A biopsy-proven polymorphous low-grade adenocarcinoma of the palate in a 53-year-old woman that had been present for several years according to the patient (a). Computerized tomograms were obtained that identified destruction of bone by the cancer (b). As such, a maxillectomy was performed, observing 1 cm linear margins in bone and soft tissue (c). The maxillectomy specimen delivered (d). The histopathology confirmed the involvement of the maxillary bone by the tumor (e). The large ablative defect (f) was addressed with an immediate obturator (g). One year postoperatively, the patient showed no signs of recurrent disease (h).

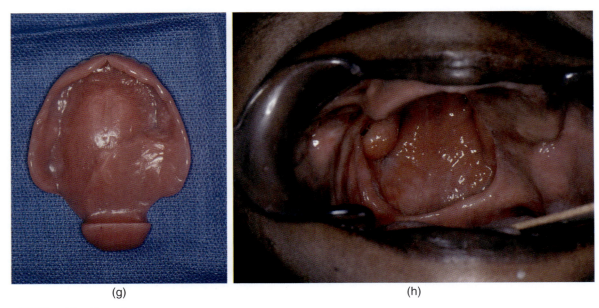

Figure 12.17. (*Continued*).

were treated with radiation therapy were more likely to have evidence of disease at last follow-up when compared with patients who did not have radiation therapy. Furthermore, there was no statistically significant difference in the overall patient outcome based on the type of initial treatment given or for any additional treatment rendered, whether it is additional surgery, radiation therapy, or chemotherapy. Based on this report and others (Crean et al. 1996), the treatment for polymorphous adenocarcinoma of minor salivary glands remains surgical. It has been estimated that approximately 80% of patients survive their disease without evidence of tumor at periods from between several months to 25 years after removal (Wenig and Gnepp 1991). One case has been reported where death occurred from this neoplasm with direct extension to vital structures of the head (Aberle et al. 1985). In addition, while rare, metastasis to cervical lymph nodes (Kumar et al. 2004) and to distant organs (Hannen et al. 2000) has been reported from polymorphous adenocarcinomas originating in the palate. These reports indicate that cervical lymph node involvement should be suspected in patients with papillary cystic change in the tumor, and that periodic chest X-ray examination should be performed postoperatively when this variant of tumor is diagnosed. In addition, while regional and distant metastases are rare related to this tumor, long-term follow-up is recommended due to the possibility for late recurrences (Fife et al. 2013).

Acinic Cell Carcinoma

Acinic cell carcinoma is a very rare malignancy of the minor salivary glands. It has been estimated to represent approximately 2.5–3% of salivary gland tumors in general (Spiro 1986; Guimaraes et al. 1989), and about 4% of minor salivary gland tumors (Castellanos and Lally 1982). Indeed, acinic cell carcinoma is not represented in many studies of minor salivary gland tumors (Isacsson and Shear 1983; Chau and Radden 1986; Jabar 2006), and other studies show only a very limited number of these cases (Toida et al. 2005; Lopes et al. 1999). The acinic cell carcinoma behaves most similarly to the low-grade mucoepidermoid carcinoma (Ord 1994). In fact, like the low-grade mucoepidermoid carcinoma, the acinic cell carcinoma was originally purported to be a benign neoplasm (Ellis and Auclair 1991a). For the first half of the twentieth century, these tumors were thought to be benign. In 1953, Buxton and his group were the first to ascribe a malignant character to many of these tumors (Buxton et al. 1953). These were identified as serous cell adenocarcinomas, after which time Foote and Frazell classified these tumors as acinic cell adenocarcinomas (Foote and Frazell 1953).

The AFIP registry shows 886 acinic cell carcinomas, of which 753 were in the major salivary glands (85%), and 133 (15%) in the minor salivary glands. The most common site of minor salivary gland involvement was the buccal mucosa, accounting for 43 cases (32%), followed by the lip (38 cases = 29%). Tumors in the upper lip were three times more common than tumors in the lower lip. The palate was the only other significant anatomic site to be affected by this tumor, and accounted for 22 cases (17%). A female preponderance was noted, with a mean age of 44 years. In their series of 21 cases of acinic cell carcinoma of minor salivary glands, Omlie and Koutlas (2010)

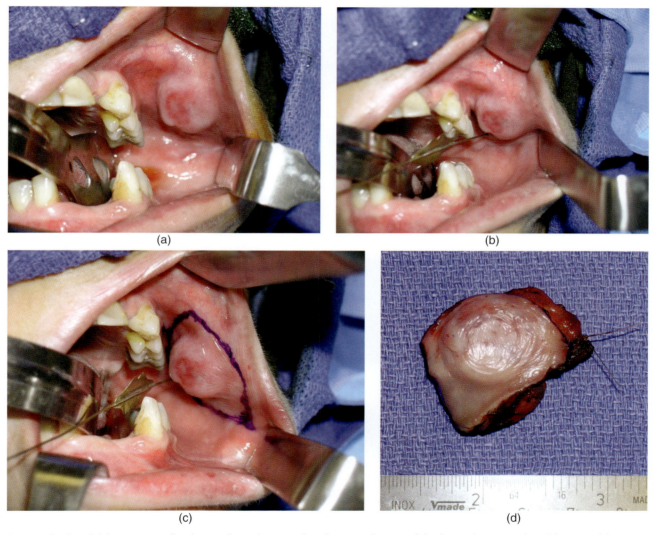

Figure 12.18. A biopsy proved polymorphous low-grade adenocarcinoma of the buccal mucosa in a 53-year-old woman with a five-year history of this mass (a). The characteristically thick tumor blocked immediate visualization of the Stenson duct that was cannulated and was noted to be free from the margin of the tumor (b). A mucosal sacrificing wide local excision with 1 cm linear margins and isolation of the Stenson duct was performed (c). The specimen was delivered without tumor spillage and with a deep anatomic barrier margin of fat within the cheek (d and e). Microscopic analysis of the tumor identified a 3.5 cm thick polymorphous adenocarcinoma (f) with negative margins and perineural invasion (g). The defect was reconstructed with a buccal fat flap (h). There was no need for radiation therapy postoperatively. Acceptable healing is noted without tumor recurrence at 12 months postoperatively (i). (f): hematoxylin and eosin, original magnification × 10. (g): hematoxylin and eosin, original magnification × 40.

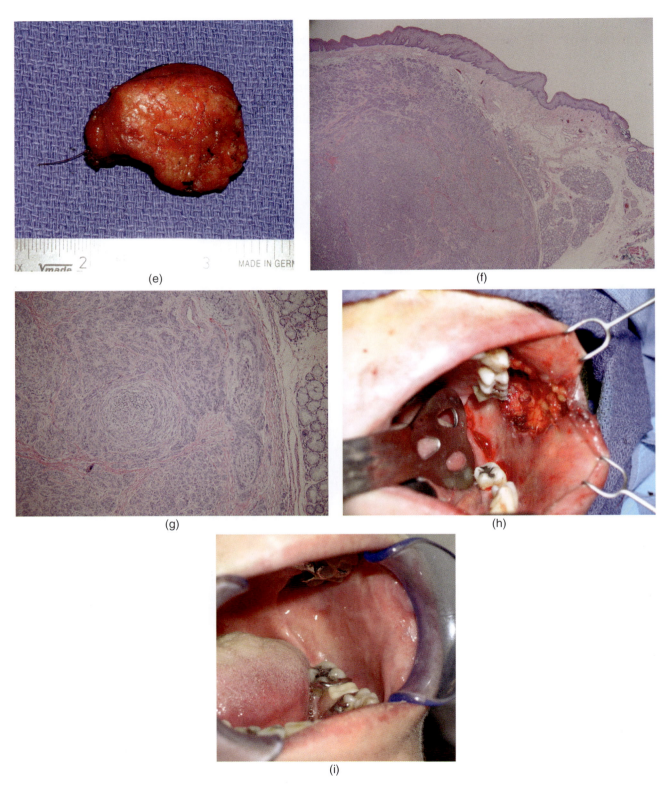

Figure 12.18. (Continued).

identified 7 cases in the buccal mucosa, 6 in the palate, 5 in the upper lip, 1 in the lower lip, and 2 in the retromolar mucosa. Fifteen of the 21 patients were men.

Surgery for acinic cell carcinoma is performed in a similar fashion as that of low-grade mucoepidermoid carcinoma. Tumors of the buccal mucosa and upper lip are treated with mucosal sacrificing wide local excisions, including 1 cm linear margins, with attention to the necessary sacrifice of surrounding anatomic barriers (Figure 12.19). Tumors of the palate can be treated with bone sparing, periosteally sacrificing wide local excisions with split thickness sacrifice of the soft palate. Computerized tomograms may be obtained preoperatively to confirm the lack of bone erosion. Cure is most commonly realized and recurrences and regional and distant metastases are rare when these malignancies are treated with curative intent (Omlie and Koutlas 2010). Cervical lymph node metastases are rare such that prophylactic neck dissections are not recommended. Distant metastatic spread of the acinic cell carcinoma of minor salivary gland origin is also uncommon, although metastases have been identified in the lungs, liver, brain, and bone (Triantafillidou et al. 2010). Five and 10-year survival rates are generally quite favorable, and reported as 82 and 68% respectively (Hickman et al. 1984).

Epithelial-Myoepithelial Carcinoma

The epithelial-myoepithelial carcinoma is very rare, representing approximately 1% of all salivary gland tumors (Angiero et al. 2009). It most commonly occurs in the parotid gland but has been noted in the minor salivary glands. This malignancy has been categorized as an intermediate-grade malignancy according to the AFIP classification (Ellis and Auclair 1991b) although Angiero et al. (2009) have classified this malignancy as primarily low grade. Only 57 cases were identified in their series, with 50 cases diagnosed in the major salivary glands (88%), and 7 cases (12%) in the minor salivary glands (Corio 1991). Of the seven cases in the minor salivary glands, four were located in the palate, one in the tongue, and two cases were not specified as to anatomic location. A mean age of 59 years was noted in these 57 cases. This tumor is known to be highly differentiated, yet it is malignant due to infiltrative and destructive growth patterns, the presence of necrosis, perineural involvement, and metastases (Corio et al. 1982). Corio et al. presented 16 cases of this neoplasm and found 12 cases to involve the parotid gland, 3 cases in the submandibular gland and 1 case in the buccal mucosa (Corio et al. 1982).

Standardized recommendations for surgery for the epithelial-myoepithelial carcinoma are difficult to make due to the rare nature of this malignancy. Nonetheless, evaluation of involved anatomic barriers with physical examination and CT scans generally permits an effective approach to eradication of these malignancies in various minor salivary gland sites (Figure 12.20). In such circumstances, the surgeon respects well-established principles of linear and anatomic barrier margins when operating salivary gland tumors, while also relying on past experiences with other low- and intermediate-grade minor salivary gland malignancies. In so doing, tumor-free margins can be obtained while performing surgery like that for a diagnosis of low- or intermediate-grade mucoepidermoid carcinoma. Recurrences have been reported (Corio 1991), but appropriate surgical management of epithelial-myoepithelial carcinomas of the minor salivary glands should be performed with curative intent. Quantitative survival statistics are not published in the literature.

Secretory Carcinoma

In 2010, Skalova et al. described 16 cases of a new salivary gland cancer that they named mammary analogue secretory carcinoma due to its morphologic, molecular, and immunohistochemical similarities to secretory carcinoma of the breast. The unique molecular characteristic to salivary gland tumors is the fusion of the ETV6 gene on chromosome 12 and the NTRK3 gene on chromosome 15 with translocation t(12;15)(p13;q25), harboring ETV6-NTRK3. In 2017, the World Health Organization changed the name of this cancer to secretory carcinoma. This cancer accounts for approximately 4% of malignant salivary gland tumors (Li et al. 2019). It is generally thought to represent a low-grade cancer that typically presents in middle-aged adults and shows no gender predilection (Mathew et al. 2019). A slow-growing painless mass in the parotid gland is most common for this diagnosis, but cases have also been diagnosed in the minor salivary glands (Boon et al. 2018; Li et al. 2019) (see Chapter 8 case presentation).

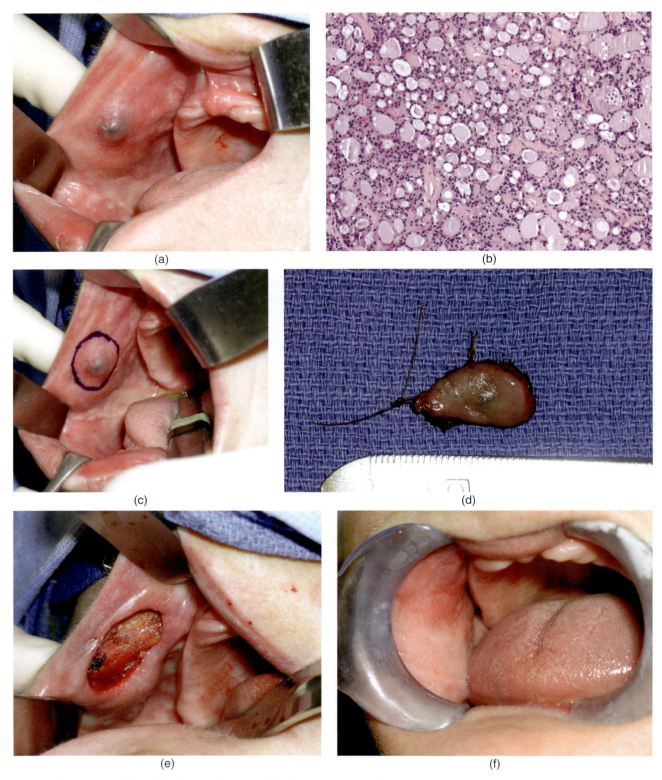

Figure 12.19. An acinic cell adenocarcinoma of the buccal mucosa in a 52-year-old woman (a and b). A mucosal sacrificing wide local excision observing 1 cm linear margins was performed (c). Excision of the specimen (d) occurred without tumor spillage. The defect (e) was reconstructed with mucosal flaps so as to not distort the appearance of the upper lip. Acceptable healing without tumor recurrence is noted at six years postoperatively (f).

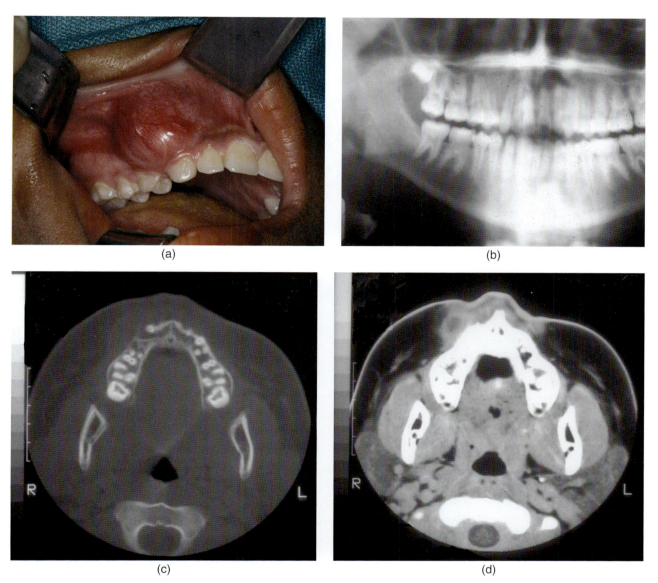

Figure 12.20. A mass of the right maxillary gingiva in a 12-year-old girl (a). Panoramic radiograph demonstrates alteration of the bone between the first premolar and canine teeth with divergence of the roots of these teeth (b). Computerized tomograms demonstrate a soft-tissue mass with involvement of the maxillary bone (c and d). Incisional biopsy showed epithelial-myoepithelial carcinoma (e). A partial maxillectomy observing 1 cm linear margins in bone and soft tissue was performed (f). The specimen was removed without tumor spillage (g and h). Final histopathology showed destruction of bone by the cancer (i). The specimen radiograph demonstrated acceptable bone margins in the specimen (j). The resultant ablative defect of the maxilla (k) was reconstructed with an immediate obturator device (l). The use of the obturator permitted contracture of the defect as noted at one month postoperatively (m). By three months postoperatively, the defect had demarcated significantly (n). An interim obturator was fabricated that allowed for better seal of the defect (o and p). The patient functioned well with a definitive obturator (q) until soft-tissue reconstruction was planned with a buccal fat flap and advancement of the buccal mucosa (r–t). The appearance of the healed flap is noted at one year postoperatively (u).

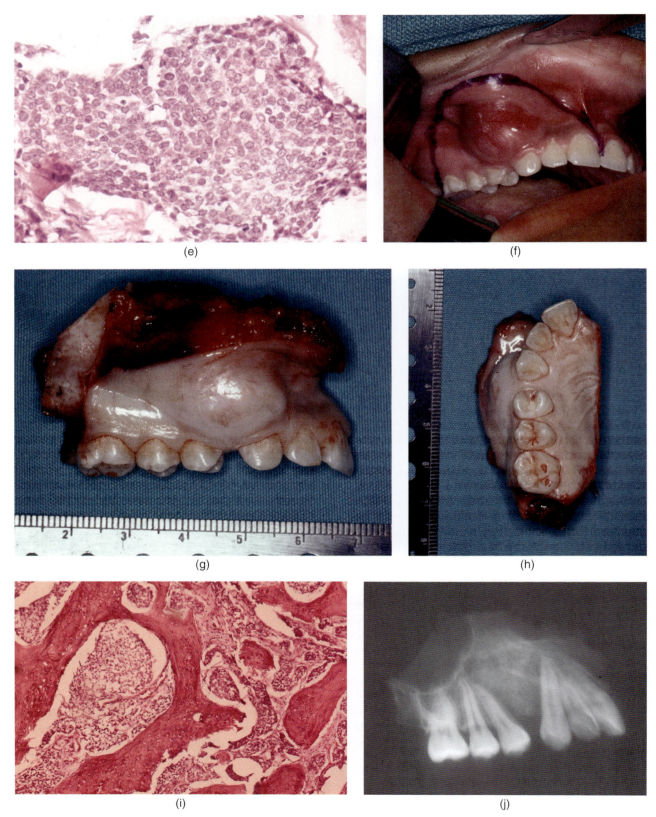

Figure 12.20. (Continued).

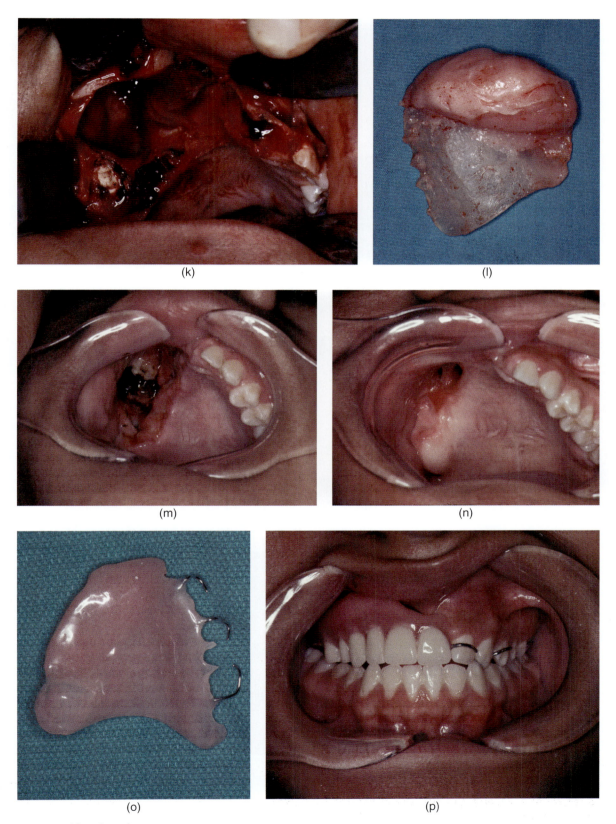

Figure 12.20. (Continued).

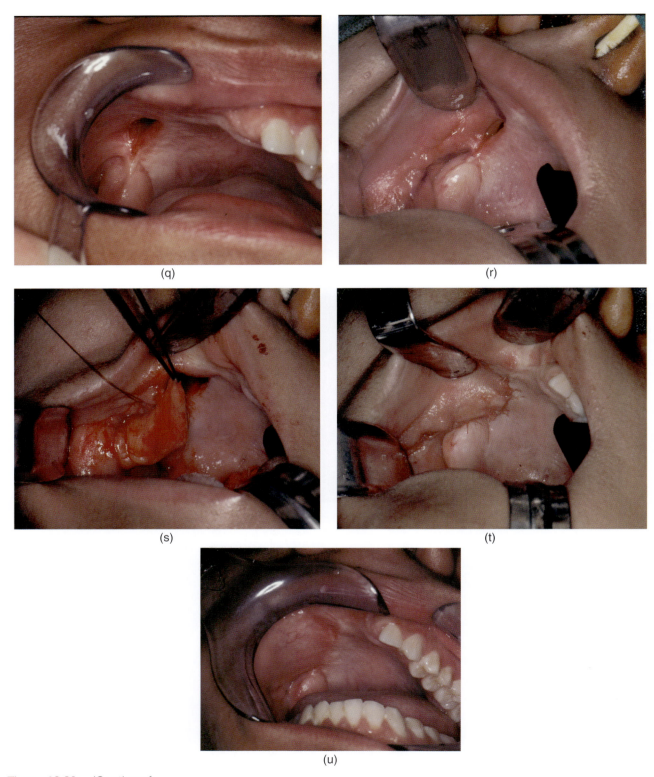

Figure 12.20. (Continued).

Boon et al. (2018) retrospectively studied 31 cases of secretory carcinoma. Eighteen tumors were located in the parotid gland, 12 cases were located in the minor salivary glands, and 1 case was located in the submandibular gland. Of the minor salivary gland sites, five were in the lip, and two tumors were in the palate. Twenty of the cases had been previously diagnosed as acinic cell carcinoma ($n = 16$), polymorphous adenocarcinoma ($n = 3$), and adenocarcinoma, NOS ($n = 1$). All patients underwent surgical resection of their tumors and four patients underwent neck dissection, with one patient demonstrating positive lymph nodes. One patient experienced a local recurrence 50 years postoperatively. None of the patients experienced a regional or distant metastasis.

Li et al. (2019) reported two cases of secretory carcinoma of the palate. The final pathology confirmed the diagnosis of secretory carcinoma with cells staining positive for S-100 and mammaglobin. The authors indicated that the diagnostic sensitivity of mammaglobin and S-100 is approximately 95%. Finally, the authors indicated that the gold standard for diagnosis of secretory carcinoma is detection of the ETV6-NTRK3 fusion transcript by reverse transcription-polymerase chain reaction. This notwithstanding, the immunohistochemistry and characteristic microscopic morphology has become the basis for diagnosis of this salivary gland cancer.

SURGICAL MANAGEMENT OF THE NECK FOR MINOR SALIVARY GLAND MALIGNANCIES

Surgical management of the neck is a controversial and intriguing concept for surgeons managing oral/head and neck malignant disease. At the core of this discipline is an assessment of occult disease in patients with clinically negative necks. To this end, there seems to be a consensus in the literature that occult neck disease is relatively uncommon related to minor salivary gland malignancies compared to squamous cell carcinoma of the oral/head and neck. Moreover, it is also uncommon for patients with minor salivary gland malignancies to present with clinically palpable neck disease related to these tumors. Spiro found 53 patients presenting with cervical metastases among 378 patients (14%) with minor salivary gland malignancies (Spiro et al. 1991). Another 26 patients (7%) developed subsequent cervical metastases for an overall rate of nodal involvement of 21%. Interestingly, nine patients underwent an elective neck dissection, all of whom showed histologically confirmed metastatic disease. The authors do not, however, discuss the incidence of occult and clinically apparent metastases as a function of anatomic site of the primary minor salivary gland malignancy. Sadeghi et al. identified nine patients presenting with cervical metastases related to minor salivary gland malignancies, five of which were present in the tongue base (Sadeghi et al. 1993). Beckhardt et al. found N+ necks in only 3% of their patients with malignant minor salivary gland tumors of the palate, while Chung identified only 2 of 20 patients with malignant salivary gland tumors of the palate presenting with cervical metastases (Chung et al. 1978; Beckhardt et al. 1995). The latter three studies only discussed clinical staging of the neck without comments regarding their histology such that limited information is available regarding the true rate of metastasis to the cervical lymph nodes. In the final analysis, it seems that the incidence of occult neck disease related to a minor salivary gland malignancy of the oral cavity is sufficiently low to negate the need for elective neck dissection. Indications for neck dissection in these patients, therefore, are limited to patients who present with cervical metastases; those patients whose preoperative imaging studies document changes in the cervical lymph nodes consistent with metastatic disease; and those patients with high-grade malignancies, regardless of the clinical and radiographic imaging results.

THE ROLE OF RADIATION THERAPY IN THE MANAGEMENT OF MINOR SALIVARY GLAND MALIGNANCIES

It was once thought that salivary gland malignancies were radioresistant (Dragovic 1995). This previously stated misconception can no longer be considered valid in the twenty-first century. As such, radiation therapy is indicated in the postoperative management of all high-grade malignant minor salivary gland tumors, as well as in patients with positive surgical margins, positive regional lymph nodes, and recurrent tumor (Dragovic 1995). This being the case, it is important to remember that surgery is the primary therapy for minor salivary gland malignancies. Shingaki et al.'s review of the role of radiation therapy in 44 patients with salivary gland cancers, 34 of whom were treated for minor salivary gland cancers, examined the results of surgery vs. surgery and postoperative radiation therapy in these patients (Shingaki et al. 1992). Interestingly, no patients experienced recurrent disease when negative surgical margins were found in the specimen, regardless of whether surgery or surgery and postoperative radiation therapy was performed. All patients with positive surgical margins developed recurrent disease when surgery was the modality of treatment, and 8 of 15 patients (53%) with positive surgical margins developed recurrent disease when their salivary gland cancer was treated with a combination of surgery and postoperative radiation therapy. While not broken down to major vs. minor salivary gland primary sites, these results do point to the significant benefit of obtaining negative margins in the resected specimen. The reader is directed to Chapter 13 for more details regarding the use of radiation therapy in the management of salivary gland tumors.

THE ROLE OF CHEMOTHERAPY IN THE MANAGEMENT OF MINOR SALIVARY GLAND MALIGNANCIES

There are few reports on the benefit of systemic chemotherapy in the management of salivary gland cancers. Chemotherapy is generally reserved for the palliative management of advanced, non-resectable disease where radiation therapy has already been administered. Most patients for whom chemotherapy is considered will have diagnoses of mucoepidermoid carcinoma, adenoid cystic carcinoma, or high-grade adenocarcinoma (Laurie and Licitra 2006). The expression of c-kit in adenoid cystic carcinoma, overexpression of Her-2 in mucoepidermoid carcinoma, overexpression of epithelial growth factor receptor in adenocarcinoma, and androgen receptor positivity in salivary duct carcinoma make the use of imatinib, trastuzumab, cetuximab, and antiandrogen therapy at least theoretically beneficial (Laurie and Licitra 2006). While these agents may be of value in treating difficult cases of minor salivary gland malignancies, there is a need to conduct high-quality clinical trials in patients with these cancers. The reader is directed to Chapter 14 for more details regarding the use of chemotherapy in salivary gland malignancies.

Summary

- Approximately 10% of all salivary gland tumors arise in the minor glands.
- Approximately 1% of head and neck tumors occur within the minor salivary glands, although some authors believe that this figure is somewhat higher.
- Seventy percent of minor salivary gland tumors arise in the oral cavity.
- Fifty percent of oral minor salivary gland tumors are found in the palate.
- Fifty percent of oral minor salivary gland tumors are benign and 50% are malignant.
- Inconclusive evidence exists for cause and effect relationships with minor salivary gland tumors.
- An incisional biopsy is almost always indicated prior to definitive management of a palatal minor salivary gland tumor due to the near equal distribution of benign and malignant diagnoses.
- An excisional biopsy of a buccal mucosal or upper lip minor salivary gland tumor may be acceptable without first obtaining the histopathologic diagnosis provided signs of benign disease exist.
- Benign tumors of the palate, buccal mucosa, and upper lip may be excised without special imaging studies.
- When present, ulceration predicts a malignant diagnosis, although many minor salivary gland malignancies do not create ulceration of the oral mucosa.
- Pain is associated with perineural invasion, most commonly seen with adenoid cystic carcinoma.
- Malignant tumors of the palate should undergo special imaging studies to determine involvement of the palatal bone.
- Malignant tumors of the buccal mucosa and upper lip do not require imaging prior to ablative surgery.
- Surgery represents the primary treatment of minor salivary gland tumors.
- Surgical removal of minor salivary gland tumors requires a scientific approach to the surrounding anatomic barriers.

- High cure rates are anticipated following removal of pleomorphic adenomas and canalicular adenomas of minor salivary gland sites.
- High cure rates are anticipated following removal of low-grade mucoepidermoid carcinomas and polymorphous low-grade adenocarcinomas of minor salivary gland sites.
- Variable cure rates are associated with surgery for intermediate- and high-grade mucoepidermoid carcinomas and adenoid cystic carcinomas of minor salivary glands.

Case Presentation – *Two Peas in a Pod*

A 65-year-old man was referred with an incisional biopsy diagnosis of mucoepidermoid carcinoma of the palate (Figure 12.21a). He reported that the mass had been present for approximately three years and was growing slowly. He experienced mild dysphagia but no odynophagia and had sustained no weight loss over the past three years. There were no signs of additional oral or oropharyngeal pathology noted on physical examination.

Past Medical History
The patient reported a past medical history of hypertension, gastroesophageal reflux disease, chronic obstructive pulmonary disease, celiac disease, and atrial fibrillation. He was taking diltiazem, dabigatran, esomeprazole, hydralazine, and losartan. He reported no known drug allergies.

Imaging
The patient underwent a CT scan of the maxillofacial region that demonstrated the anatomic extent of the mass (Figure 12.21b–e). This CT study also identified serendipitous findings of a 2.4 cm left buccal space mass (Figure 12.21f) and a 3.2 cm mass of the fourth ventricle of the brain with numerous coarse internal calcifications (Figure 12.21g). The patient underwent an MRI of the brain that further defined the fourth ventricle mass that extended out the foramen of Luschka. (Figure 12.21h–j). A presumptive diagnosis of ependymoma was established.

Surgical Intervention
The patient underwent transoral, full thickness resection of his palatal mucoepidermoid carcinoma while observing 1 cm linear margins (Figure 12.21k). The specimen is noted (Figure 12.21l) that required sacrifice of the patient's uvula. Final pathology identified a low-grade mucoepidermoid carcinoma with negative margins (Figure 12.21m and n). The surgical defect is noted (Figure 12.21o). A submucosal excision of the patient's left buccal space mass with intact surrounding anatomic barriers was also performed (Figure 12.21p and q). Final pathology of this mass identified a low-grade epithelial-myoepithelial carcinoma (Figure 12.21r and s). The patient's palatal defect healed uneventfully (Figure 12.21t) and he functions with a definitive obturator with no evidence of disease of either tumor at six years postoperatively. He has had no surgery for his presumed ependymoma of the fourth ventricle, and he remains asymptomatic.

TAKE-HOME POINTS

1. CT imaging of a diagnosed tumor can occasionally result in a serendipitous second diagnosis, and although rarely, a third diagnosis, as occurred in this case.
2. Imaging studies should be critically examined by tumor surgeons for planning ablative surgery while also being part of multidisciplinary tumor conferences to discuss expert interpretations by radiologists for completeness.

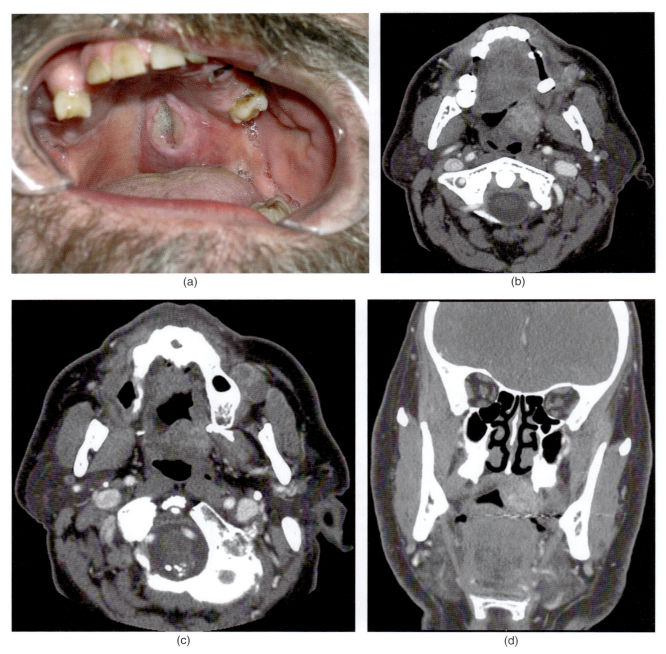

Figure 12.21. A large palatal mass (a) that was diagnosed as mucoepidermoid carcinoma on incisional biopsy. The CT scans of the maxillofacial region demonstrates a 3.7 cm palatal mass that closely approximates the pterygoid musculature and extends across the midline (b–e). This CT study also identified a 2.4 cm left buccal space mass (f) and a 3.2 cm mass of the fourth ventricle of the brain with numerous coarse internal calcifications (g). The patient underwent an MRI of the brain that further defined the fourth ventricle mass that extended out the foramen of Luschka. (h–j). A presumptive diagnosis of ependymoma was established. The palatal mass was widely excised transorally (k). The specimen is noted (l) that required sacrifice of the patient's uvula. Final pathology established a diagnosis of low-grade mucoepidermoid carcinoma on routine stains (m) and mucicarmine stains (n). The surgical defect is noted (o). The patient's left buccal space mass was excised transorally (p) and the tumor's intact pseudocapsule is noted (q). Final pathology of this mass identified low-grade epithelial-myoepithelial carcinoma (r and s). The patient's palatal defect healed uneventfully and was without evidence of disease at five years postoperatively (t). (m) = hematoxylin and eosin, original magnification × 200. (n) = mucicarmine, original magnification × 100. (r) = hematoxylin and eosin, original magnification × 40. (s) = hematoxylin and eosin, original magnification × 400.

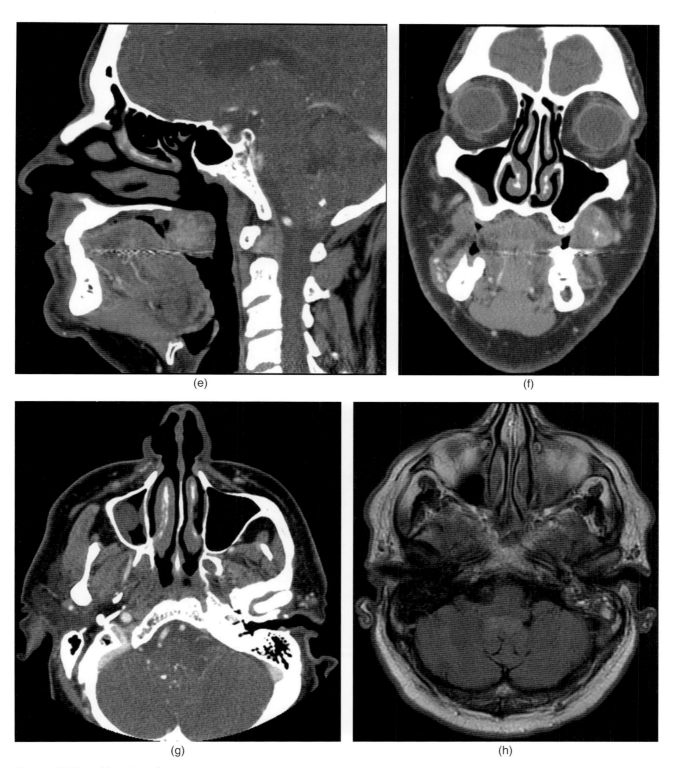

Figure 12.21. (*Continued*).

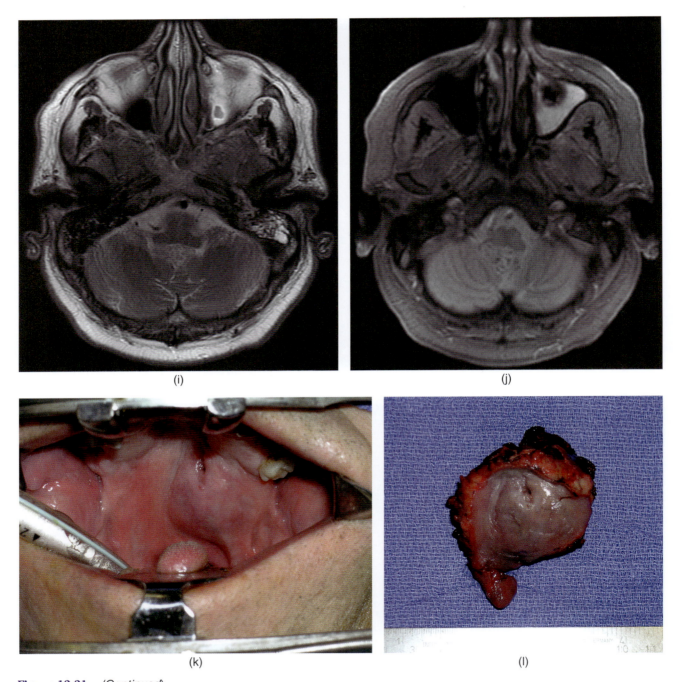

Figure 12.21. (Continued).

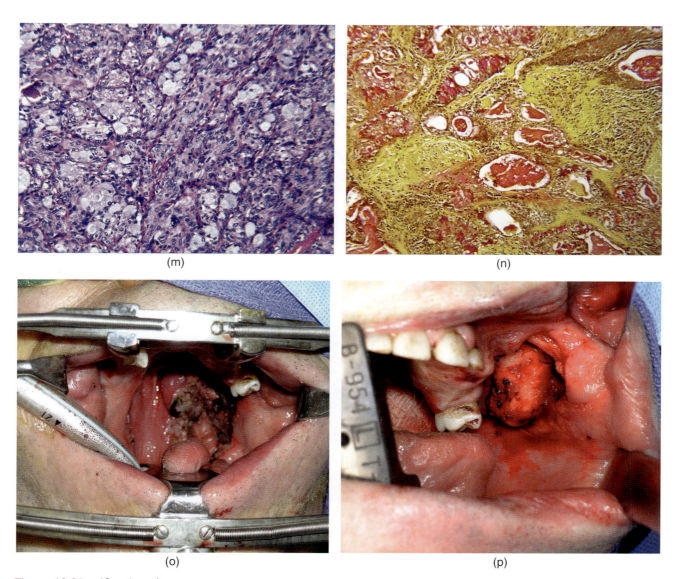

Figure 12.21. (*Continued*).

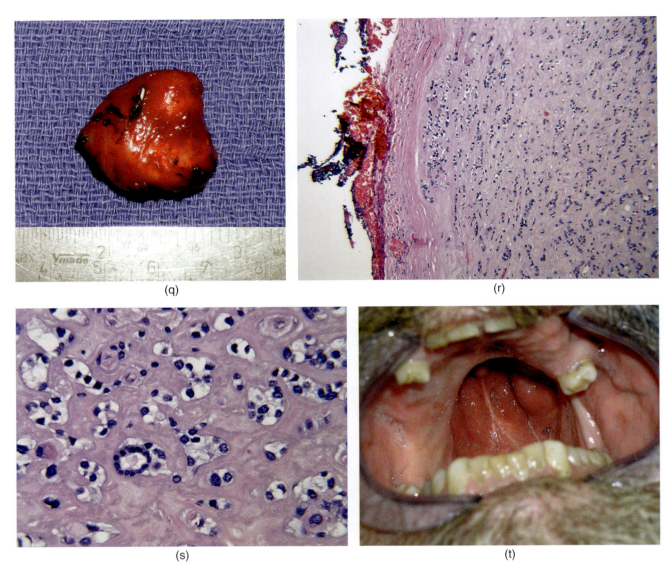

Figure 12.21. (*Continued*).

References

Abbey LM, Schwab BH, Landau GC, Perkins ER. 1984. Incidence of second primary breast cancer among patients with a first primary salivary gland tumor. *Cancer* 54: 1439–1442.

Aberle AM, Abrams AM, Bowe R et al. 1985. Lobular (polymorphous low-grade) carcinoma of minor salivary glands: A clinicopathologic study of 20 cases. *Oral Surg Oral Med Oral Pathol* 60: 387–395.

Ampil FL, Misra RP. 1987. Factors influencing survival of patients with adenoid cystic carcinoma of the salivary glands. *J Oral Maxillofac Surg* 45: 1005–1010.

Angiero F, Sozzi D, Seramondi R, Valenta MG. 2009. Epithelial-myoepithelial carcinoma of the minor salivary glands: Immunohistochemical and morphological features. *Anticancer Res* 29: 4703–4710.

Ansari MH. 2007. Salivary gland tumors in an Iranian population: A retrospective study of 130 cases. *J Oral Maxillofac Surg* 65: 2187–2194.

Auclair PL, Ellis GL. 1991. Mucoepidermoid carcinoma. In: Ellis GL, Auclair PL, Gnepp DR (eds), *Surgical Pathology of the Salivary Glands*. Philadelphia, WB Saunders Co., pp. 269–298.

Auclair PL, Ellis GL, Gnepp DR. 1991. Salivary gland neoplasms: General considerations. In: Ellis GL, Auclair PL, Gnepp DR (eds), *Surgical Pathology of the Salivary Glands*. Philadelphia, WB Saunders Co., pp. 135–164.

Barak AP, Grobbel M, Rabaja DR. 1998. Polymorphous low-grade adenocarcinoma of the parotid gland. *Am J Otolaryngol* 19: 322–324.

Batsakis JG, El-Naggar AK. 1991. Terminal duct adenocarcinomas of salivary tissues. *Ann Otol Rhinol Laryngol* 100: 251–253.

Batsakis JG, Luna MA. 1990. Histopathologic grading of salivary gland neoplasms: I. Mucoepidermoid carcinomas. *Ann Otol Rhinol Laryngol* 99: 835–838.

Batsakis JG, Pinkston GR, Luna MA, et al. 1983. Adenocarcinomas of the oral cavity: A clinicopathologic study of terminal duct carcinomas. *J Laryngol Otol* 97: 825–835.

Beckhardt RN, Weber RS, Zane R et al. 1995. Minor salivary gland tumors of the palate: Clinical and pathologic correlates of outcome. *Laryngoscope* 105: 1155–1160.

Bell RB, Dierks EJ, Homer L, Potter BE. 2005. Management and outcome of patients with malignant salivary gland tumors. *J Oral Maxillofac Surg* 63:917–928.

Beltran D, Faquin WC, Gallagher G, August M. 2006. Selective immunohistochemical comparison of polymorphous low-grade adenocarcinoma and adenoid cystic carcinoma. *J Oral Maxillofac Surg* 64:415–423.

Blanchaert RH, Ord RA, Kumar D. 1998. Polymorphous low-grade adenocarcinoma of the sublingual gland. *Int J Oral Maxillofac Surg* 27:115–117.

Boon, E., Valstar, M.H., van der Graaf, W.T.A., et al. (2018). Clinicopathological characteristics and outcome of 31 patients with ETV6-NTRK3 fusion gene confirmed (mammary analogue) secretory carcinoma of salivary glands. *Oral Oncol* 82:29–33.

Boyd AS. 2019. Cutaneous metastases from a cribriform adenocarcinoma of the minor salivary glands. *Am J Dermatopathol* 42:439–441.

Brandwein MS, Ivanov K, Wallace DI et al. 2001. Mucoepidermoid carcinoma. A clinicopathologic study of 80 patients with special reference to histological grading. *Am J Surg Pathol* 25: 835–845.

Buxton RW, Maxwell JH, French AJ. 1953. Surgical treatment of epithelial tumors of the parotid gland. *Surg Gynecol Obstet* 97:401–416.

Carlson ER. 1995. Salivary gland pathology – Clinical perspectives and differential diagnosis. In: *The Comprehensive Management of Salivary Gland Pathology, Oral and Maxillofacial Surgery Clinics of North America* 7, Philadelphia, WB Saunders Co, 361–386.

Carlson ER. 1998. The management of minor salivary gland tumors of the oral cavity. *Atlas Oral Maxillofac Surg Clin North Am* 6:75–98.

Carlson ER, Schimmele SR. 1998. The management of minor salivary gland tumors of the oral cavity. In: *Surgical Management of Salivary Gland Disease, The Atlas of the Oral and Maxillofacial Surgery Clinics of North America* 6, Philadelphia, WB Saunders Co, 75–98.

Carlson ER, Schlieve T. 2019. Salivary gland malignancies. *Oral Maxillofac Surg Clin North Am* 31:125–144.

Castellanos JL, Lally ET. 1982. Acinic cell tumor of the minor salivary glands. *J Oral Maxillofac Surg* 40:428–431.

Castle JT, Thompson LDR, Frommelt RA et al. 1999. Polymorphous low grade adenocarcinoma. A clinicopathologic study of 164 cases. *Cancer* 86:207–219.

Chau MNY, Radden BG. 1986. Intra-oral salivary gland neoplasms: A retrospective study of 98 cases. *J Oral Pathol* 15:339–342.

Chidzonga MM, Lopez-Perez VM, Portilla-Alvarez AL. 1995. Salivary gland tumours in Zimbabwe: Report of 282 cases. *Int J Oral Maxillofac Surg* 24:292–297.

Chiu GA, Woodwards RT, Benatar B, Hall R. 2012. Mandibular central mucoepidermoid carcinoma with distant metastasis. *Int J Oral Maxillofac Surg* 41:361–363.

Chung CK, Rahman SM, Constable WC. 1978. Malignant salivary gland tumors of the palate. *Arch Otolaryngol* 104:501–504.

Corio RL. 1991. Epithelial-myoepithelial carcinoma. In: Ellis GL, Auclair PL, Gnepp DR (eds), *Surgical Pathology of the Salivary Glands*. Philadelphia, WB Saunders Co., pp. 412–421.

Corio RL, Sciubba JJ, Brannon RB, Batsakis JG. 1982. Epithelial-myoepithelial carcinoma of intercalated duct origin. A clinicopathologic and ultrastructural assessment of sixteen cases. *Oral Surg Oral Med Oral Path* 53:280–287.

Crean SJ, Bryant C, Bennett J, Harris M. 1996. Four cases of polymorphous low-grade adenocarcinoma. *Int J Oral Maxillofac Surg* 25: 40–44.

Dahlin DC, Beabout JW. 1971. Dedifferentiation of low-grade chondrosarcoma. *Cancer* 28:461–466.

Daley TD, Gardner GD, Smout MS. 1984. Canalicular adenoma: Not a basal cell adenoma. *Oral Surg Oral Med Oral Path* 57:181–188.

de Diego JI, Bernaldez R, Prim MP, Hardison D. 1996. Polymorphous low-grade adenocarcinoma of the tongue. *J Laryngol Otol* 10:700–703.

Dossani RH, Akbarian-Tefaghi H, Lemmonnier L, et al. 2016. Mucoepidermoid carcinoma of palatal minor salivary glands with intracranial extension: A case report and literature review. *J Neurol Surg Rep* 77:e156–e159.

Dragovic J. 1995. The role of radiation therapy in the management of salivary gland neoplasms. *Oral Maxillofac Surg Clin North Am* 7:627–632.

Ellis GL, Auclair PL. 1991a. Classification of salivary gland neoplasms. In: Ellis GL, Auclair PL, Gnepp DR (eds), *Surgical Pathology of the Salivary Glands*. Philadelphia, WB Saunders Co., pp. 129–134.

Ellis GL, Auclair PL. 1991b. Acinic cell carcinoma. In: Ellis GL, Auclair PL, Gnepp DR (eds), *Surgical Pathology of the Salivary Glands*. Philadelphia, WB Saunders Co., pp. 299–317.

Eneroth CM, Hjertman L, Moberger G, Soderberg G. 1972. Mucoepidermoid carcinomas of the salivary glands with special reference to the possible existence of a benign variety. *Acta Otolaryngol* 73:68–74.

Epker BN, Henny FA. 1969. Clinical, histopathological and surgical aspects of intraoral minor salivary gland tumors: Review of 90 cases. *J Oral Surg* 27:792–804.

Evans HL. 1984. Mucoepidermoid carcinoma of salivary glands: A study of 69 cases with special attention to histologic grading. *Am J Clin Pathol* 81:696–701.

Evans HL, Batsakis JG. 1984. Polymorphous low-grade adenocarcinoma of minor salivary glands. A study of 14 cases of a distinctive neoplasm. *Cancer* 53:935–942.

Eveson JW, Cawson RA. 1985. Salivary gland tumors. A review of 2410 cases with particular reference to histological types, site, age and sex distribution. *J Pathol* 146:51–58.

Fife TA, Smith B, Sullivan CA. 2013. Polymorphous low-grade adenocarcinoma: A 17 patient case series. *Am J Otolaryngol* 34:445–448.

Foote FW, Frazell EL. 1953. Tumors of the major salivary glands. *Cancer* 6:1065–1133.

Fordice J, Kershaw C, El-Naggar A, Goepfert, H. 1999. Adenoid cystic carcinoma of the head and neck. Predictors of morbidity and mortality. *Arch Otolaryngol Head Neck Surg* 125:149–152.

Freedman PD, Jones AC. 1994. A pathologist's approach to tissue diagnosis. *Oral Maxillofac Surg Clin North Am* 6:357–375.

Freedman PD, Lumerman H. 1983. Lobular carcinoma of intraoral minor salivary glands. *Oral Surg Oral Med Oral Pathol* 56:157–165.

Gao M, Hao Y, Huang MX et al. 2017. Salivary gland tumours in a northern Chinese population: A 50-year retrospective study of 7190 cases. *Int J Oral Maxillofac Surg* 46:343–349.

Gardner DG, Daley TD. 1983. The use of the terms monomorphic adenoma, basal cell adenoma, and canalicular adenoma as applied to salivary gland tumors. *Oral Surg Oral Med Oral Path* 56:608–615.

Gnepp DR, Wenig BM. 1991. Malignant mixed tumors, ch 20. In: Ellis GL, Auclair PL, Gnepp DR (eds), *Surgical Pathology of the Salivary Glands*. Philadelphia, WB Saunders, p. 350.

Guimaraes DS, Amaral AP, Prado LF, Nascimento AG. 1989. Acinic cell carcinoma of salivary glands: 16 cases with clinicopathologic correlation. *J Oral Pathol Med* 18:396–399.

Hannen EJM, Bulten J, Festen J et al. 2000. Polymorphous low grade adenocarcinoma with distant metastases and deletions on chromosome 6q23-qter and 1q23-qter: A case report. *J Clin Pathol* 53:942–945.

Hay AJ, Migliacci J, Zanoni DK, McGill M, Patel S, Ganly I. 2019. Minor salivary gland tumors of the head and neck - Memorial Sloan Kettering experience: Incidence and outcomes by site and histologic type. *Cancer* 125: 3354–3366.

Hickman RE, Cawson RA, Duffy SW. 1984. The prognosis of specific types of salivary gland tumors. *Cancer* 54:1620–1624.

Isacsson G, Shear M. 1983. Intraoral salivary gland tumors: A retrospective study of 201 cases. *J Oral Pathol* 12:57–62.

Ito RA, Ito K. Vargas PA et al. 2005. Salivary gland tumors in a Brazilian population: A retrospective study of 496 cases. *Int J Oral Maxillofac Surg* 34:533–536.

Jabar MA. 2006. Intraoral minor salivary gland tumors: A review of 75 cases in a Libyan population. *Int J Oral Maxillofac Surg* 35:150–154.

Katz AD, Preston-Martin S. 1984. Salivary gland tumors and previous radiotherapy to the head or neck. Report of a clinical series. *Am J Surg* 147:345–348.

Kennedy KS, Healy KM, Taylor RE, Strom CG. 1987. Polymorphous low-grade adenocarcinoma of the tongue. *Laryngoscope* 97:533–536.

Kikuchi K, Nagao T, Ide F, Takizawa S, Sakashita H, Tsujino I, Li THJ, Kusama K. 2019. Palatal polymorphous adenocarcinoma with high-grade transformation: A case report and literature review. *Head Neck Pathol* 13: 131–139.

Kratochvil FJ. 1991. Canalicular adenoma and basal cell adenoma. In: Ellis GL, Auclair PL, Gnepp DR (eds), *Surgical Pathology of the Salivary Glands*. WB Saunders Co., pp. 202–224.

Kumar M, Stivaros N, Barrett AW et al. 2004. Polymorphous low-grade adenocarcinoma – A rare and aggressive entity in adolescence. *Br J Oral Maxillofac Surg* 42:195–199.

Laurie SA, Licitra L. 2006. Systemic therapy in the palliative management of advanced salivary gland cancers. *J Clin Oncol* 24:2673–2678.

Li A, Chen Y, Liu S, et al. 2019. Mammary analogue secretory carcinoma of the minor salivary gland: Report of two cases. *Int J Clin Exp Pathol* 12:4338–4343.

Li Q, Zhang XR, Liu XK et al. 2012. Long-term treatment outcome of minor salivary gland carcinoma of the hard palate. *Oral Oncol* 48:456–462.

Li Y, Li LJ, Huang J et al. 2008. Central malignant salivary gland tumors of the jaw: Retrospective clinical analysis of 22 cases. *J Oral Maxillofac Surg* 66:2247–2253.

Liao WC, Chih-Chao C, Ma H, Hsu CY. 2020. Salivary gland tumors. A clinicopathologic analysis from Taipei veterans general hospital. *Ann Plast Surg* 84, supplement 1, S26–S33.

Lombardi D, McGurk M, Poorten VV, et al. 2017. Surgical treatment of salivary malignant tumors. *Oral Oncol* 65:102–113.

Lopes MA, Kowalski LP, Santos GC, Almeida OP. 1999. A clinicopathologic study of 196 intraoral minor salivary gland tumours. *J Oral Pathol Med* 28:264–267.

Luksic I, Suton P, Macan K, Dinjar K. 2014). Intraoral adenoid cystic carcinoma: Is the presence of perineural invasion associated with the size of the primary tumour, local extension, surgical margins, distant metastases, and outcome? *Br J Oral Maxillofac Surg* 52:214–218.

Luna MA, Batsakis JG, El-Naggar AD. 1991. Salivary gland tumors in children. *An Otol Rhinol Laryngol* 100:869–871.

MacIntosh RB. 1995. Minor salivary gland tumors: Types, incidence and management. *Oral Maxillofac Surg Clin North Am* 7:573–589.

Mathew J, Carvalho M, Chorneyko K, Salama S. 2019. A challenging case of mammary analogue secretory carcinoma: Case study with ultrastructural and cytogenetic correlation. *Case Rep Pathol*; 2019:7468691.

Melrose RJ. 1994. Clinicopathologic features of intraoral salivary gland tumors. *Oral Maxillofac Surg Clin North Am* 6:479–497.

Merchant WJ, Cook MG, Eveson JW. 1996. Polymorphous low-grade adenocarcinoma of parotid gland. *Br J Oral Maxillofac Surg* 34:328–330.

Mimica X, McGill M, Hay A, et al. 2019. Sex disparities in salivary malignancies: Does female sex impact oncological outcome? *Oral Oncol* 94:86–92.

Min R. Siyi L, Wenjun Y et al. 2012. Salivary gland adenoid cystic carcinoma with cervical lymph node metastasis: A preliminary study of 62 cases. *Int J Oral Maxillofac Surg* 41:952–957.

Nagao T. 2013. "Dedifferentiation" and high-grade transformation in salivary gland carcinomas. *Head Neck Pathol* 7:S37–S47.

Nagao T, Gaffey TA, Kay PA et al. 2004. Polymorphous low-grade adenocarcinoma of the major salivary glands: Report of three cases in an unusual location. *Histopathology* 44:164–171.

Nascimento AG, Amaral ALP, Prado LAF et al. 1986. Adenoid cystic carcinoma of salivary glands. A study of 61 cases with clinicopathologic correlation. *Cancer* 57:312–319.

Omlie JE, Koutlas KG. 2010. Acinic cell carcinoma of minor salivary glands: A clinicopathologic study of 21 cases. *J Oral Maxillofac Surg* 68:2053–2057.

Ord RA. 1994. Management of intraoral salivary gland tumors. *Oral Maxillofac Surg Clin North Am* 6:499–522.

Ord RA, Salama AR. 2012. Is it necessary to resect bone for low-grade mucoepidermoid carcinoma of the palate? *Br J Oral Maxillofac Surg* 50:712–714.

Perzin KH, Gullane P, Clairmont AC. 1978. Adenoid cystic carcinomas arising in salivary glands. A correlation of histologic features and clinical course. *Cancer* 42:265–282.

Pires FR, Pringle GA, de Almeida OP, Chen SY. 2007. Intraoral minor salivary gland tumors: A clinicopathological study of 546 cases. *Oral Oncol* 43:463–470.

Plambeck K, Friedrich RE, Schmelzle R. 1996. Mucoepidermoid carcinoma of salivary gland origin: Classification, clinical-pathological correlation, treatment results and long-term follow-up in 55 patients. *J Craniomaxillofac Surg* 24:133–139.

Pogrel MA. 1994. The management of salivary gland tumors of the palate. *J Oral Maxillofac Surg* 52:454–459.

Potdar GG, Paymaster JC. 1969. Tumors of minor salivary glands. *Oral Surg Oral Med Oral Path* 28:310–319.

Regezi JA, Lloyd RV, Zarbo RJ, McClatchey KD. 1985. Minor salivary gland tumors. A histologic and immunohistochemical study. *Cancer* 55:108–115.

Regezi JA, Zarbo RJ, Stewart JCB, Courtney RM. 1991. Polymorphous low-grade adenocarcinoma of minor salivary gland. A comparative histologic and immunohistochemical study. *Oral Surg Oral Med Oral Pathol* 71:469–475.

Rivera-Bastidas H, Ocanto RA, Acevedo AM. 1996. Intraoral minor salivary gland tumors: A retrospective study of 62 cases in a Venezuelan population. *J Oral Pathol Med* 25:1–4.

Rogerson KC. 1995. Salivary gland pathology in children. *Oral Maxillofac Surg Clin North Am* 7:591–598.

Sadeghi A, Tran LM, Mark R et al. 1993. Minor salivary gland tumors of the head and neck: Treatment strategies and prognosis. *Am J Clin Oncol* 16:3–8.

Saku T, Hayashi Y, Takahara O et al. 1997. Salivary gland tumors among atomic bomb survivors, 1950–1987. *Cancer* 79:1465–1475.

Seethala, S. 2017. Update from the 4th edition of the world health organization classification of head and neck tumours: Tumors of the salivary gland. *Head Neck Pathol* 11:55–67.

Shingaki S, Ohtake K, Nomura T, Nakajima T. 1992. The role of radiotherapy in the management of salivary gland carcinomas. *J Craniomaxillofac Surg* 20:220–224.

Skalova A, Vanecek T, Sima R, et al. 2010. Mammary analogue secretory carcinoma of salivary glands, containing the ETV6-NTRK3 fusion gene: A hitherto undescribed salivary gland tumor entity. *Am J Surg Pathol* 34:599–608.

Spiro RH. 1986. Salivary neoplasms: Overview of a 35-year experience with 2,807 patients. *Head & Neck Surg* 8:177–184.

Spiro RH, Thaler HT, Hicks WF et al. 1991. The importance of clinical staging of minor salivary gland carcinoma. *Am J Surg* 162:330–336.

Spitz MR, Tilley BC, Batsakis JG et al. 1984. Risk factors for major salivary gland carcinoma. A case-comparison study. *Cancer* 54:1854–1859.

Spoorthi BR, Rao RS, Rajashekaraiah PB et al. 2013. Predominantly cystic central mucoepidermoid carcinoma developing from a previously diagnosed dentigerous cyst: Case report and review of the literature. *Clinics and Practice* 3:e19.

Stanley RJ, Weiland LH, Olsen KD et al. 1988. Dedifferentiated acinic cell (acinous) carcinoma of the parotid gland. *Otolaryngol Head Neck Surg* 98:155–161.

Stewart FW, Foote FW, Becker WF. 1945. Mucoepidermoid tumors of salivary glands. *Ann Surg* 122:820–844.

Takano M, Kasahara K, Matsui S et al. 2012. A case of mucoepidermoid carcinoma associated with maxillary cyst. *Bull Tokyo Dent Coll* 53:119–125.

Toida M, Shimokawa K, Makita H et al. 2005. Intraoral minor salivary gland tumors: A clinicopathological study of 82 cases. *Int J Oral Maxillofac Surg* 34:528–532.

Tomich CE. 1991. Adenoid cystic carcinoma. In: Ellis GL, Auclair PL, Gnepp DR (eds), *Surgical Pathology of the Salivary Glands* Philadelphia, WB Saunders Co., pp. 333–349.

Triantafillidou K, Dimitrakopoulos J, Iordanidis F, Koufogiannis D. 2006. Management of adenoid cystic carcinoma of minor salivary glands. *J Oral Maxillofac Surg* 64:1114–1120.

Triantafillidou K, Iordanidis F, Psomaderis K et al. 2010. Acinic cell carcinoma of minor salivary glands: A clinical and immunohistochemical study. *J Oral Maxillofac Surg* 68:2489–2496.

Waldron CA. 1991. Mixed tumor (pleomorphic adenoma) and myoepithelioma. In: Ellis GL, Auclair PL, Gnepp DR (eds), *Surgical Pathology of the Salivary Glands*. Philadelphia, WB Saunders Co., pp. 165–186.

Waldron CA, El-Mofty SK, Gnepp DR. 1988. Tumors of the intraoral minor salivary glands: A demographic and histologic study of 426 cases. *Oral Surg Oral Med Oral Path* 66:323–333.

Wenig BM, Gnepp DR. 1991. Polymorphous low-grade adenocarcinoma of minor salivary glands. In: Ellis GL, Auclair PL, Gnepp DR (eds), *Surgical Pathology of the Salivary Glands*. Philadelphia, WB Saunders Co., pp. 390–411.

Woolgar JA, Triantafyllou A, Ferlito A et al. 2013. Intraosseous carcinoma of the jaws – A clinicopathologic review. Part I: Metastatic and salivary-type carcinomas. *Head Neck* 35:895–901.

Yih WY, Kratochvil FJ, Stewart, JCB. 2005. Intraoral minor salivary gland neoplasms: Review of 213 cases. *J Oral Maxillofac Surg* 63:805–810.

Zhou CX, Chen XM, Li TJ. 2012. Central mucoepidermoid carcinoma: A clinicopathologic and immunohistochemical study of 39 Chinese patients. *Am J Surg Pathol* 36:18–26.

Chapter 13
Radiation Therapy for Salivary Gland Malignancies

Joseph R. Kelley, MD, PhD[1] and Max Ofori, MD[2]

[1]Director of Clinical Research, GenesisCare USA of North Carolina
[2]Division of Radiation Oncology, University of Tennessee Medical Center, Knoxville, TN, USA

Outline

Introduction
Low-Risk Salivary Gland Malignancies
Moderate-Risk Salivary Gland Malignancies
High-Risk Salivary Gland Malignancies
Evolution of Radiation Techniques in Salivary Gland
    Malignancies
Complications of Radiation Therapy in Salivary Gland
    Malignancies
  Xerostomia
  Osteoradionecrosis
  Dysphagia
Radiation Technique for Low- and Moderate-Risk
    Salivary Gland Tumors
Radiation Technique for High-Risk Salivary Gland Tumors
  Adenoid Cystic Carcinoma
Advanced Radiation Therapy Techniques
  Proton Therapy
  Neutron Therapy
  Carbon ion Therapy
Summary
References

Introduction

Tumors of the salivary glands represent an uncommon but complex challenge in the field of head and neck cancer. These tumors account for only 3–5% of all head and neck cancers but comprise greater than 37 morphologically distinct neoplasms with variable natural histories, treatment approaches, and clinical outcomes. In the past, these neoplasms were thought to be resistant to radiation therapy. However, improvements in radiation techniques show that salivary gland tumors are highly responsive to radiation therapy. A recent trial showed a 60% improvement in local control of salivary gland tumors after radiation therapy (Terhaard et al. 2005). Other studies confirm this improvement in local control and document a survival advantage for radiation therapy (Pohar et al. 2005; Herman et al. 2013).

Histology is the strongest predictor of clinical outcome in salivary gland tumors. The biology of the malignancy predicts its risk of spread to the nodes and nerves, thus determining the optimal treatment approach. The wide variety of histologic types found in salivary gland tumors gives a wide range of clinical outcomes. This has made it difficult to determine the optimal treatment approach in these rare tumors. Combining patients with different cell types increases numbers of these rare tumors on trial but blurs the risk of disease in patients and obscures the benefits of treatment. It is more useful to segregate salivary gland tumors by their inherent biology. This gives a better indication of the risk of spread, required treatment, and expected outcomes. Adenoid cystic carcinoma displays a unique growth pattern and requires a treatment approach quite distinct from the other histologic types. Even though adenoid cystic carcinoma is the second most common malignancy, it should not be combined with other cell types and

---

Salivary Gland Pathology: Diagnosis and Management, Third Edition. Edited by Eric R. Carlson and Robert A. Ord.
© 2022 John Wiley & Sons, Inc. Published 2022 by John Wiley & Sons, Inc.
Companion website: www.wiley.com/go/carlson/salivary

will be addressed last in this chapter to highlight its different risk of spread and radiation therapy technique. The remaining salivary gland tumors can be divided into three risk groups based on their risk of local recurrence, nodal spread, and survival. This chapter will explore low-, moderate-, and high-risk groupings and discuss the variations in radiation technique required for each cohort.

Low-risk salivary gland tumors include acinic cell carcinoma, pleomorphic adenoma, and well-differentiated mucoepidermoid carcinoma. These tumors have a low rate of local recurrence and an exceedingly low rate of nodal spread. As a result, local excision is often curative and adjuvant radiation is not usually required. Moderate-risk salivary gland tumors include large T3/T4 tumors and smaller mucoepidermoid carcinomas that are moderately differentiated or that contain lympho-vascular space invasion or perineural invasion. Patients in the moderate-risk group carry a low risk of nodal spread but a significant risk for local recurrence. They benefit from adjuvant radiation therapy to the surgical bed and may occasionally require treatment of the regional nodes. High-risk salivary gland tumors include poorly differentiated mucoepidermoid carcinoma, adenocarcinoma, salivary duct carcinoma, undifferentiated carcinoma, and the rare squamous cell carcinoma that is not the result of a cutaneous lesion spread to the parotid gland. These high-risk patients frequently develop local recurrence and have a significant risk of occult spread to regional lymph nodes. Some studies have found that up to 50% of high-risk patients are node positive at time of neck dissection (Regis De Brito Santos et al. 2001). As a result, the best treatment for high-risk salivary gland tumors is resection followed by adjuvant radiation to the surgical bed and ipsilateral lymph nodes. A description of these three risk groups of salivary gland tumors is noted in Figure 13.1. A treatment algorithm based on these three risk groups of salivary gland tumors is noted in Figure 13.2 and is discussed throughout this chapter.

Radiation technique has improved just as our understanding of salivary gland tumor biology has increased. Classic radiation techniques used a large simple field to ensure coverage of the region at risk, limiting the dose to the tumor while creating toxicity to a large area. Intensity-modulated radiation therapy (IMRT) spares uninvolved normal tissue, allowing dose escalation to the tumor and at-risk nodes and is now the standard of care. Advances in proton therapy and other heavy particle therapy may further protect normal tissues of the head and neck and enhance the therapeutic ratio of radiation therapy. This chapter will examine radiation techniques as they relate to salivary gland tumors and discuss the excellent outcomes seen with radiation therapy for salivary gland malignancies.

Low-Risk Salivary Gland Malignancies

Pleomorphic adenomas; acinic cell carcinoma; and small, well-differentiated mucoepidermoid carcinoma

Low-risk salivary gland tumors	Moderate-risk tumors	High-risk tumors
Well Differentiated Mucoepidermoid Carcinoma	Well Differentiated Mucoepidermoid Carcinoma With Adverse Features*	Poorly Differentiated Mucoepidermoid Carcinoma
Acinic Cell Carcinoma	Moderately Differentiated Mucoepidermoid Carcinoma	Undifferentiated Carcinoma Adenocarcinoma
Pleomorphic Adenoma		Salivary Duct Carcinoma Squamous Cell Carcinoma
	Carcinoma Ex-Pleomorphic Adenoma	
	*Adverse features with Moderate Risk Lympho-Vascular Space Invasion Perineural Invasion, T3/T4 Tumor Margin Close <5 mm, Margin Positive	Adverse High-Risk Features Facial Nerve Involvement Clinical Node Positive Unresectable Disease

Figure 13.1. Salivary gland tumors are divided into three risk groups based on histology, tumor size, and margin status.

Treatment low-risk	Treatment moderate-risk	Treatment high-risk
Resection and Observation	Adjuvant Radiation Target Tumor Bed Radiation Dose 50-60Gy	Adjuvant Radiation Target Tumor Bed Radiation Dose 60-70Gy
	Consider Cervical Irradiation Levels I-III Radiation Dose 50-54Gy	Cervical Node Irradiation Levels I-V Radiation Dose 50-54Gy

Figure 13.2. A basic treatment algorithm for patients with salivary gland tumors based on risk grouping. Low-risk tumors can often be observed after resection with negative margins. Moderate-risk tumors benefit from adjuvant radiation to the operative bed even after resection with negative margin. Patients with moderate-risk tumors may benefit from radiation to the ipsilateral cervical lymph nodes if they have a high T-Stage (T3/T4) or multiple adverse features. Patients with high-risk salivary gland tumors require radiation therapy to the resection bed and regional lymph nodes.

comprise a low-risk category of salivary gland tumors (Figure 13.1). These tumors have a low rate of local recurrence and low rates of nodal involvement. They are often cured by surgical resection and do not normally require adjuvant radiation therapy.

Pleomorphic adenoma is the most common benign salivary gland tumor. These tumors normally develop in the parotid gland but may arise in submandibular, sublingual, or minor salivary glands. The preferred treatment for pleomorphic adenomas is surgical resection with cranial nerve preservation. Local control remains excellent at around 95% and adjuvant radiation is not commonly required (O'Brien 2003; Mendenhall et al. 2008). Postoperative radiation is recommended in the small subset of patients with positive margins or multifocal recurrences. Ravasz reported local control in 77 of 78 patients (99%) when tumor spillage or positive margins were treated with conventional radiation to a dose of 60–75 Gy (Ravasz et al. 1990). Radiation can also be effective in the setting of recurrence pleomorphic adenoma. Chen et al. (2006b) reported on 34 patients at the University of California San Francisco with recurrent pleomorphic adenomas treated to a low median dose of 50Gy (range 45–60Gy) and still saw excellent results with local control in 94% of patients. Thus, surgery is the mainstay of treatment for pleomorphic adenoma, but adjuvant radiation improves outcomes in patients with positive margins or in patients who develop multinodular recurrence.

Acinic cell carcinoma is a slowly growing, low-grade lesion that is most common in the parotid but can affect any salivary gland. Patients treated with definitive resection show excellent outcomes with five-year local control and overall survival of 90%. A review from Memorial Sloan Kettering found that lympho-vascular space invasion and perineural invasion both predicted a decrease in disease-free survival. High-grade tumors, node involvement, extra-capsular invasion, and positive margins decreased both disease-free survival and overall survival (Gomez et al. 2009). Cho et al. (2016) examined 179 low-grade salivary gland cancer cases where risk factors for recurrence and the role of postoperative radiation therapy were analyzed. Low-grade tumors have good outcomes with recurrence-free survival and overall survival of 89.6 and 96.6% at 10 years, respectively. Postoperative radiation was beneficial in patients with advanced T stage, perineural invasion, lympho-vascular invasion, or extraparenchymal extension. Consistent with other studies of head and neck squamous cell carcinoma, the presence of regional nodal involvement and positive margins carried the worst prognosis.

Liu et al. (2017) reviewed a retrospective cohort study of patients with acinic cell carcinoma of the parotid gland to estimate five-year survival rates. They found that age was a predictor of outcome with patients older than 60 years, showing decreased survival. Patients with a fixed mass at clinical presentation, high-grade tumor, perineural invasion, or lympho-vascular space invasion also had lower survival. Again, positive margin or nodal involvement reduced overall survival and disease-free survival. A retrospective review from the National Cancer Database of 2362 cases looked at the prognostic factors associated with acinic cell carcinoma (Scherl et al. 2018). Overall patients with acinic cell showed good outcomes with a five-year overall survival of 88%. The study found that age over 70 years, advanced T stage (>3 cm), and high-grade tumors define an aggressive subgroup. The strongest predictor of survival was histologic grade, which was a stronger predictor of survival than T and N classifications.

Not all acinic cell carcinomas are indolent, however. A study performed by Chintakuntlawar et al. (2016) looked at 48 cases using archived pathology material from Mayo Clinic Rochester. They identified high-grade transformation based on an infiltrative growth pattern, anaplasia, prominent nucleoli, and brisk mitotic activity. Patients with high-grade transformation showed poor prognosis with decreased relapse-free survival and overall survival with hazard ratios of 10.4 and 9.3 respectively. Involvement of the base of skull also makes acinic cell carcinoma a more serious malignancy. Breen et al. (2012) found a 10-year overall survival of 80% for all patients with acinic cell carcinoma. However, some patients with recurrence along the base of skull showed a very poor prognosis with a two-year overall survival of only 50%. These patients often suffered recurrences many years after initial therapy that demonstrates the need for long-term follow-up for these patients, including those patients with low risk for recurrent disease.

A report from the University of Michigan identified a subgroup of patients with acinic cell carcinoma with an increased rate of distant metastasis (Ali et al. 2020). In a retrospective review of cases between 2000 and 2017, patients with T4, high-grade tumors with gross perineural invasion showed high rates of distant failure within the lungs with two-year disease-free survival of only 20%. These high-risk acinic cell carcinoma patients may benefit from adjuvant systemic therapy and would clearly need frequent surveillance imaging of the chest.

In summary, low-risk salivary gland tumors represent a local threat. With adequate surgical resection, these tumors show low rates of local recurrence or nodal spread and no adjuvant radiation therapy is required. Terhaard et al. (2005) showed a local control rate as high as 95% at five years in low-risk patients treated with surgery alone. Another trial (Armstrong et al. 1992) found only two patients with occult nodal disease out of 53 neck dissections. As a result, low-risk salivary gland tumors have an excellent prognosis with overall survival at 5 years of 97% and 10-year survival of 94% (Patel et al. 2014).

Moderate-Risk Salivary Gland Malignancies

Moderate-risk salivary gland tumors include mucoepidermoid carcinoma with moderate differentiation or low-grade tumors that contain either lympho-vascular space invasion or perineural invasion (Figure 13.1). Larger tumors and tumors with bone involvement (T3 or T4) also fall within the moderate-risk group. Patients with positive margins or "close margins" can also be placed in the moderate-risk group. These moderate-risk salivary gland tumors have a significant risk of local recurrence and benefit from adjuvant radiation therapy to the postoperative tumor bed.

Surgery is the primary treatment for salivary gland tumors. Patients with gross residual disease should be considered for re-resection at a high-volume center. If additional surgery is not possible, then patients benefit from radiation therapy targeting the region of gross residual disease to 70 Gy. A clear dose response has been seen in these patients. Salivary gland tumors with microscopically positive margins should also be evaluated for additional surgery. If not completely resected, then microscopic residual disease is recommended to a radiation dose of 60–66 Gy. Patients with close resection margins (<5 mm) also have increased rates of local recurrence. As a result, close margin is an adverse risk factor that can place a patient in the moderate-risk category. One study (Terhaard et al. 2005) found 55% recurrence in close margin patients with surgery alone but control in 95% of patients after adjuvant radiation.

The biology of the salivary gland tumor predicts its rate of local recurrence and hence benefit from radiation therapy. Salivary gland tumors that demonstrate lympho-vascular space invasion or perineural invasion have a higher tendency for microscopic spread. As a result, these two characteristics are adverse features that may cause a tumor to fall within the moderate-risk category. In a large study of more than 500 patients (Terhaard et al. 2005), 10-year tumor control in salivary gland tumors with perineural invasion was only 60% after surgery alone but increased to 88% with adjuvant radiation. The size of a tumor also indicates the risk of subclinical disease and the benefit for adjuvant radiation therapy. A review of patients at UCSF (Chen et al. 2006a) showed that T1/T2 salivary gland tumors showed good local control at

10 years with 81% controlled by surgery alone. However, T3 or T4 tumors had a higher recurrence rate with a local control at 10 years of only 39%. Bone invasion also significantly increases the recurrence risk following surgery. The Dutch Head and Neck Oncology Cooperative Group found local control of only 54% with surgery alone in the presence of bone invasion with adjuvant radiation improving outcome to a local control of 86% (Terhaard et al. 2005). As a result, most authors place T3 and T4 tumors in a moderate-risk group that requires adjuvant radiation.

Location of the salivary gland tumor is a matter of debate in its risk for tumor recurrence and hence benefits from radiation. Some authors recommend adjuvant radiation for all submandibular gland tumors and for all salivary gland tumors involving the minor glands. However, the location of a salivary gland tumor may not be as significant a predictor for risk of recurrence as was once thought. A SEER review of 2667 patients with minor salivary gland tumors showed that biology of the tumor was most predictive of risk (Lloyd et al. 2010). A predictive index was identified based on male sex, T3/T4 tumors, and pharyngeal site of tumor but the most predictive factor was high-risk histology. Minor salivary gland tumors with only one of these factors showed node involvement in only 2% of patients. Patients with three of these risk factors showed 41% node positivity and patients with all four risk factors developed nodal disease in 70% of cases.

Researchers in the Netherlands have carefully examined risk factors associated with salivary gland tumors and developed a simple predictive treatment algorithm (Al-Mamgani et al. 2012). Patients with incomplete or close resection margins, perineural invasion, and T3–4 tumors are treated with adjuvant radiation. The risk of nodal recurrence is assigned based on points given for T stage, histology, and location of tumor. Patients with a low score (T1 acinic cell carcinoma of the parotid gland) show recurrence rates after surgery alone of less than 5%. Salivary gland tumors with a moderate score (T2 mucoepidermoid carcinoma of the oral cavity or parotid) carry a 12–33% risk or nodal recurrence and benefit from adjuvant radiation to the resection bed along with cervical node levels I–III. Patients with four or five risk factors show high recurrence rates of 50–60% and require comprehensive radiation to the tumor bed and neck nodes. In a trial of 186 patients, no patient developed a local recurrence following the Dutch treatment guidelines and the cause-specific survival was an impressive 80% (Al-Mamgani et al. 2012).

A study examining primary salivary gland tumors treated with surgical resection and adjuvant radiation to 60–66 Gy reported that histologic grade was predictive of recurrence on multivariate analysis (Szewczyk et al. 2018). Another study of 62 patients with moderate to poorly differentiated mucoepidermoid carcinoma found good outcomes after adjuvant radiation (Akbaba et al. 2019). They determined local regional control of 89 and 84% at three years and five years respectively. Treatment was well tolerated in this study with grade 3 acute toxicity reported in only 15% of patients.

The largest study reported thus far for salivary gland tumors examined 8242 patients within the National Cancer Database (NCDB) (Bakst et al. 2017). All patients were treated with definitive resection and then outcomes were followed between observation and adjuvant radiation. Low-risk patients did not benefit from postoperative radiation. High-risk patients defined as positive margin or extra-capsular extension showed a survival benefit from radiation with a hazard ratio of 0.76. Intermediate-risk patients did not show a statistical improvement in survival after radiation but the study was limited by the inclusion of a large number of patients with adenoid cystic carcinoma who require long-term follow-up to see a survival improvement and by the fact that the NCDB does not report perineural invasion. A large study based on SEER review looked at 2170 patients with salivary gland tumors and found a survival benefit for adjuvant radiation (Mahmood et al. 2011). This report listed high T stage (T3/T4), high-grade, and nodal involvement as risk factors that increased the benefit of radiation therapy.

In summary, moderate-risk salivary gland malignancies include well-differentiated tumors with adverse features such as lympho-vascular space invasion, perineural invasion. Tumors with close (<5mm) or positive margins are included as are patients with advanced T stage (T3/T4). Moderately differentiated mucoepidermoid carcinoma and carcinoma ex-pleomorphic adenoma also fall within the moderate-risk category. All of these patients have increased risk of local recurrence and benefit from adjuvant radiation to the resection bed with some patients benefitting from elective nodal irradiation (Figure 13.3).

Elective Nodal Irradiation (ENI) is delivered to Cervical Levels IB, II, and III
Consider ENI to Cervical Levels IA, IV, or V based on anatomic location of tumor
Elective Nodal Irradiation Dose is 2Gy × 25 Fractions to 50Gy

Always Treat ENI	Adenocarcinoma
	Squamous Cell Carcinoma
	Mucoepidermoid Carcinoma Grade 3
	Salivary Duct Carcinoma
	Undifferentiated Carcinoma
Consider Treat ENI	Carcinoma Ex-Pleomorphic Adenoma
	Mucoepidermoid Carcinoma G2 with 1 Adverse Feature
	Acinic Cell Carcinoma G3 or with 2 Adverse Features
	Adenoid Cystic Carcinoma with T3/T4 or Other Adverse Features
	Adverse Features: T3/T4 Stage, Tumor > 3 cm
	Skin Invasion
	Lymphovascular Space Invasion
	Perineural Invasion
	Extra-Glandular Extension
	Facial Nerve Invasion/Paralysis

Figure 13.3. Elective nodal irradiation should always be delivered to cervical levels IB-III with consideration of levels IB, IV and V based on the anatomic extent of tumor. High risk tumors should always receive radiation to a dose of 50Gy to the at-risk nodal stations. Moderate risk tumors benefit from radiation therapy when presenting with advanced T-Stage, facial nerve invasion or other high risk features.

High-Risk Salivary Gland Malignancies

Patients with salivary gland tumors are placed in the high-risk group based on histology, involvement of the facial nerve, bulky clinically positive neck disease, or unresectable disease. High-risk salivary gland tumors include aggressive histologic types such as adenocarcinoma, undifferentiated carcinoma, high-grade mucoepidermoid carcinoma, salivary duct carcinoma, and squamous cell carcinoma (Figure 13.1). These tumors frequently develop microscopic invasion beyond the salivary gland and unfortunately tend to spread to the regional nodes even at an early stage. Patients with these histologic types demonstrate frequent local recurrence even after optimal surgical resection and commonly show occult nodal disease in the setting of a clinically and radiographically negative neck.

Many reports have found frequent involvement of the cervical nodes in patients with high-risk histologic types. Classic studies at Memorial Sloan-Kettering showed occult nodal disease in 18% of adenocarcinomas, in 14% of high-grade mucoepidermoid carcinomas, and in as many as 41% of squamous cell carcinomas (Armstrong et al. 1992). Lau et al. (2014) reported on patients with clinically negative necks treated between 1999 and 2013 with elective node dissection and found 35% node positivity in adenocarcinoma and poorly differentiated mucoepidermoid carcinoma with cervical neck levels II and III most frequently involved. Other studies of high-risk patients demonstrate node involvement at time of neck dissection in more than 50% of cases (Regis De Brito Santos et al. 2001; Stennert et al. 2003). Salivary gland tumors with both high-risk histology and T3 or T4 stage are found to be node positive in 76% of neck dissections. Despite these high rates of nodal spread in high-risk patients, salivary gland tumors remain almost exclusively a unilateral disease. Rates of involvement on the contralateral cervical nodes are extremely rare. A review of 251 salivary gland tumors found no instances of contralateral neck failures (Chen et al. 2007) and another study from MSK found that treatment for the opposite neck was unnecessary (Harrison et al. 1990). As a result, patients with high-risk tumors are commonly treated by surgical resection of the primary tumor along with an ipsilateral neck dissection followed by adjuvant radiation (Figure 13.2).

Treatment of the clinically negative neck in high-risk patients has become controversial. Despite neck dissection, high-risk patients continue to develop recurrences. An older review of patients at MSK showed that resection alone yielded a local control of only 17% in high-risk patients (Armstrong et al. 1990). Adjuvant radiation to the tumor bed and ipsilateral neck decreases local recurrence and increases survival in high-risk salivary gland tumors, and some authors now suggest that radiation alone can control clinically negative occult nodal disease in these patients. A review of patients at the University of California San Francisco (Chen et al. 2007) showed that adjuvant radiation controlled high-risk salivary gland tumors without the need for neck dissection. This group of high-risk histologies showed perineural invasion in 74% of patients and had a 56% rate of margin positivity. In these patients, elective nodal irradiation in place of neck dissection showed no nodal failures in more than 250 treated patients and gave a five-year survival rate of 81%. Herman et al. (2013) examined elective node dissection compared with elective nodal irradiation at the University of Florida. In their study, all patients underwent resection of the primary tumor followed by postoperative radiation. Clinically, N0 patients treated with elective node dissection showed a 10% recurrence in the neck at five years while no neck recurrences developing in the group treated with elective neck irradiation (ENI). The resulting cause-specific survival in patients with neck dissection was 84% compared with 94% in the ENI group, leading the authors to conclude that high-risk patients do not benefit from a planned neck dissection.

There may be controversy over the optimal treatment of clinically node negative patients, but patients with bulky or unresectable salivary gland tumors clearly benefit from comprehensive neck dissection and then require adjuvant radiation. A review from UCSF (Chen et al. 2007) examined this treatment approach in high-risk patients. Salivary gland tumor patients who were medically inoperable, who refused surgery or those who were deemed inoperable due to the location and extensiveness of the primary tumor were treated with definitive radiation. A clear dose response was seen in these high-risk patients. Those treated with radiation to a total dose of less than 66Gy had a local control at 5 and 10 years of 53 and 40% respectively. If, however, unresectable salivary gland tumors were treated with modern radiation technique to more than 66Gy, then the resulting local control at 5 years was 92% and control at 10 years remained high at 81%.

Surgery and adjuvant radiation therefore benefit high-risk salivary gland tumors and this approach is also favored when the facial nerve is invaded by parotid tumors. Involvement of the facial nerve remains one of the worst prognostic factors in salivary gland tumors. A review of patients at Johns Hopkins treated by surgery and adjuvant radiation showed an overall local control at 10 years of 90% with an overall survival at 5 years of 74% (North et al. 1990). However, if patients presented with facial nerve paresis, then control was poor with local control in only 50% and a dismal five-year survival rate at less than 10%. As a result, patients presenting with facial nerve palsy are recommended for en bloc resection with sacrifice of the facial nerve followed by high dose adjuvant radiation.

The outcomes for patients with high-risk salivary gland tumors are increasing. The abovementioned studies show that these tumors are sensitive to radiation and that, with optimal surgical care and carefully delivered radiotherapy local control even in high-risk patients is good. Unfortunately, these patients still suffer from distant metastatic disease and the overall survival has not kept pace with local control. A recent report of 54 patients with salivary duct carcinoma treated patients with resection and adjuvant radiation to 60Gy (Johnston et al. 2016). Local control at five years was 70% despite the frequent observation of close or positive margins. Unfortunately, metastatic disease developed in more than 50% of patients and the overall survival at five years was only 43%. This argues for concurrent chemotherapy along with radiation or adjuvant chemotherapy in high-risk patients. This combined chemoradiation approach is a standard of care in other head and neck cancers and is the clear trend in treatment for lung and GI malignancies.

A small retrospective review of high-risk salivary gland cancer patients did not show a benefit to chemoradiation over adjuvant radiation therapy alone. Despite higher risk features, patients treated with concurrent chemoradiation had a local-regional control rate of 80% but there was not a statistically significant improvement in progression-free survival (Mifsud et al. 2016). The RTOG 1008 trial is examining concurrent chemotherapy in high-risk salivary gland malignancies. Patients with high-grade mucoepidermoid, adenocarcinoma, salivary duct carcinoma, and high-grade adenoid cystic carcinoma are being randomized to surgery followed by IMRT to 60–66Gy in a control arm and IMRT with concurrent weekly cisplatin in the experimental arm. The results of this trial are anticipated to show a further benefit in local control and hopefully will translate into a survival benefit for high-risk salivary gland patients.

Evolution of Radiation Techniques in Salivary Gland Malignancies

An understanding of radiation techniques requires a brief introduction to target terminology in radiation oncology. All radiation planning is performed on a CT scan that allows for radiation dose calculation based on tissue density. Surgery is the primary treatment for salivary gland malignancies and all visible and palpable tumor tissue is ideally resected prior to radiation therapy. If the patient is medically unresectable or if surgically unresectable, gross residual disease must be treated with radiation therapy, then the gross tumor volume or GTV is contoured during radiation planning and treated to a dose of 70Gy.

After resection of gross tumor, radiation oncology then defines a clinical treatment volume (CTV) within the resection bed. This CTV region accounts for the preoperative tumor location and may extend for 1–2 cm beyond the GTV to account for microscopic residual disease. The CTV is then expanded by 3–5 mm to account for patient setup error and defined as the planning target volume (PTV). Radiation dose is delivered to the PTV.

Early radiation techniques for salivary gland tumors were crude and had poor outcomes. Initially, a combination of photons and electron beam therapy was used to try to cover salivary gland targets but had limited protection of the surrounding normal structures (Figure 13.4). Three-dimensional conformal radiation therapy (3D-CRT) was then developed using radiation portals with different angles and energies of photon radiation to cover the area of risk while attempting to protect normal tissue (Figure 13.5). 3D-CRT has now been replaced by intensity-modulated radiation therapy (IMRT) and volumetric modulated arch therapy (VMAT) as

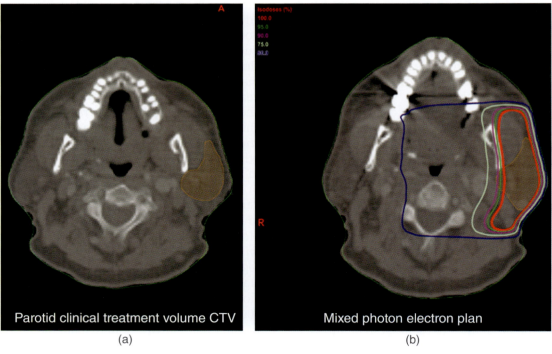

Figure 13.4. Axial images of a patient with an intermediate grade mucoepidermoid carcinoma of the left parotid gland are shown in panel A. The parotid gland is contoured as a clinical treatment volume (CTV) and shown in orange. Panel B shows a mixed beam of photon and electron energy to treat salivary gland tumors. Here the Clinical Target Volume (CTV) is shown in orange. Electron radiation delivers its dose to a superficial zone of tissue. Photon radiation beams penetrate further into the patient to treat the deep tissues. A combined photon–electron radiation plan targets the CTV while providing some protection to the contralateral oropharynx which receives 50% of the dose and to contralateral parotid gland that receives a low exit dose of radiation. The radiation prescription dose is shown in red. The 95% isodose line is shown in dark green. The 90% isodose line is shown in purple. The 75% isodose line is shown in light green. The 50% isodose line is shown in blue.

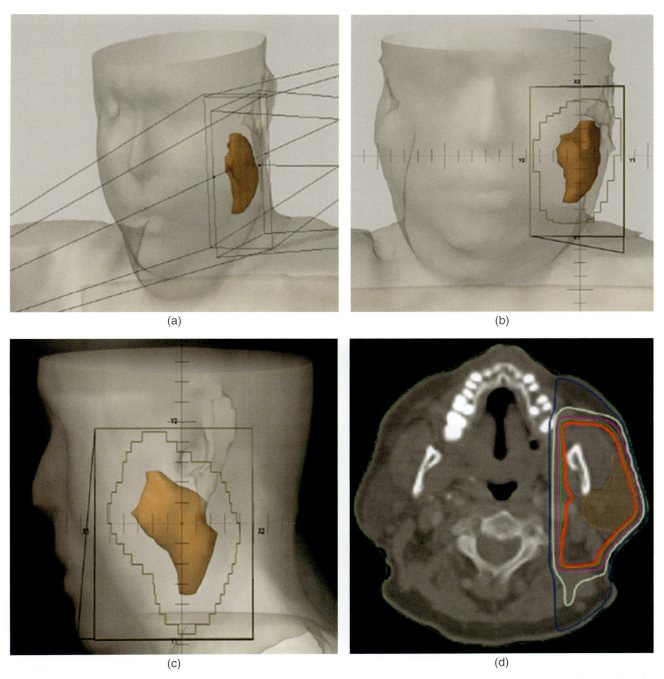

Figure 13.5. A 3D-Conformal radiation treatment plan was generated using three beams of radiation each targeting the left parotid gland from different angles. Radiation blocks are used to protect surrounding normal tissue from radiation damage. The anterior beam is shown in panel A. The posterior beam is shown in panel B. The left lateral beam is shown in panel C. The 3D-Conformal radiation plan provides better coverage of the parotid gland compared to a mixed photon-electron plan as shown in panel D. Here the CTV is shown in orange. The radiation prescription dose is shown in red. The 95% isodose line is shown in dark green. The 90% isodose line is shown in purple. The 75% isodose line is shown in light green. The 50% isodose line is shown in blue.

the current standard of care for radiation of head and neck cancer. IMRT focuses five to nine fixed beams with different intensities of dose on the target while avoiding surrounding normal structures (Figure 13.6). VMAT focuses hundreds of beams of radiation onto the tumor using a computer-generated plan that modulates the dose of energy to provide the maximal coverage of the target while protecting the surrounding normal tissues.

IMRT and VMAT allow high doses of radiation to be delivered to the target tumor while respecting uninvolved normal tissue dose constraints and have shown a clear dose response when treating salivary gland tumors. Researchers at UCSF showed that salivary tumors treated to less than 66Gy showed a local control at 5 and 10 years of 53 and 40% respectively (Chen et al. 2006b). However, if salivary gland tumors were treated to doses above 66Gy, then local control at 5 years was 92% and control at 10 years remained at 81%.

This dose escalation improves tumor control but the chief benefit of IMRT/VMAT is lower rates or radiation-related toxicity. There are three major forms of radiation-related adverse effects that should be considered when planning treatment for salivary gland tumors: xerostomia, osteonecrosis of the bone, and dysphagia.

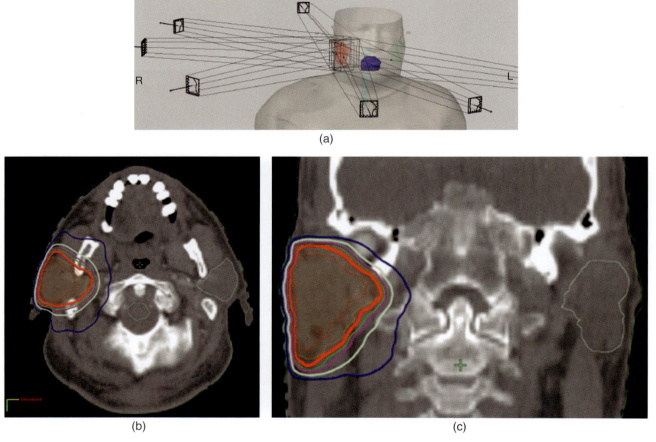

Figure 13.6. Intensity modulated radiation therapy (IMRT) targets the salivary gland tumor from multiple directions. This approach allows radiation to focus on the tumor target while protecting normal tissues in panel A. Here the Clinical Treatment Volume (CTV) is shown in orange. The radiation prescription dose is shown in red. The 95% isodose line is shown in dark green. The 90% isodose line is shown in purple. The 75% isodose line is shown in light green. The 50% isodose line is shown in blue. An axial view of the radiation plan is shown in panel B and a coronal view is shown in panel C. This radiation plan would be a common treatment approach for a patient with moderate-risk salivary gland malignancy.

Complications of Radiation Therapy in Salivary Gland Malignancies

XEROSTOMIA

Salivary glands are exquisitely sensitive to radiation and mild xerostomia begins to develop in patients during the first or second week of radiation therapy. Xerostomia worsens as radiation therapy progresses and can become a severe or even permanent adverse effect to treatment if excessive dose is delivered to the uninvolved salivary glands. Clear dose constraints have been described to prevent injury to uninvolved salivary glands.

The parotid gland is the largest salivary gland and most carefully studied with respect to radiation dose. The parotid gland is composed of serous acinar cells that are extremely sensitive to radiation and mucinous acinar cells that are more resistant to radiation. Parotid tissue treated to more than 26Gy shows rapid and permanent loss of serous function. As a result, modern radiation planning limits the contralateral parotid gland to a mean dose of less than 26Gy (mean < 26Gy). Submandibular glands contain a lower proportion of serous acinar cells and are therefore slightly more resistant to radiation than parotid gland tissue. Sublingual glands contain the highest proportion of mucinous acinar cells and are thus the least sensitive to radiation therapy. In clinical practice, uninvolved submandibular glands are routinely protected to a mean dose of less than 26Gy and sublingual glands rarely need to be considered. A dose volume histogram illustrates how IMRT/VMAT can cover the tumor resection bed and nodes (CTV-60 and CTV-50) while keeping uninvolved salivary glands within dose constraints (Figure 13.7).

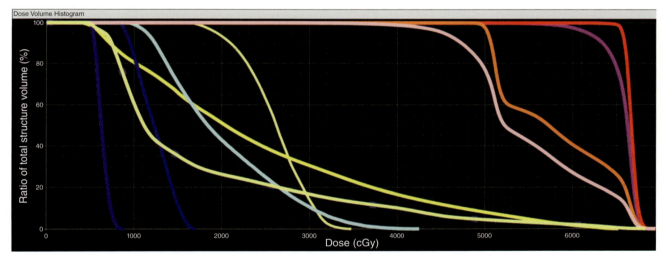

Figure 13.7. Using advanced radiation planning the tumor target can be treated to full dose while protecting the surrounding normal structures. A dose volume histogram plot is shown. The CTV-50Gy and CTV-66Gy are treated to full dose. To prevent xerostomia the contralateral parotid gland and contralateral submandibular gland are protected to a mean dose of less than 26Gy. To decrease the risk of osteonecrosis the mandible and maxilla are kept within normal dose constraints (Mean dose<45Gy, V66Gy<30%). To decrease acute mucositis and late swallow dysfunction, the dose to the superior and middle pharyngeal constrictors is kept within normal dose constraints (Mean dose<50Gy, V50Gy<80%, V60Gy<70%, V65Gy<50%).

Respecting a contralateral parotid mean dose of < 26 Gy, recent studies of IMRT/VMAT for head and neck cancer find that long-term xerostomia is now uncommon. A review from the University of California Los Angeles looked at 158 patients with head and neck cancer treated with IMRT and found long-term xerostomia in only 17% of patients (Duarte et al. 2014).

OSTEORADIONECROSIS

One of the most feared complications of radiation therapy is osteoradionecrosis of the mandible or maxilla. Radiation therapy results in microvascular fibrosis within the treated area of the head and neck. Early radiation techniques did not spare the bone near the CTV and in fact the increased density of bone resulted in "hot spots" of radiation dose in the mandible and maxilla and mastoid adjacent to the target volume. Classically, the vascular damage from radiation develops 12–18 months post-treatment and the resulting hypoxia can lead to osteonecrosis.

IMRT/VMAT now accounts for the increased density of bone and modulate radiation dose to avoid the surrounding normal structures while still covering the tumor target. The dose to bone predicts the risk of radiation-related necrosis and modern planning limits the mandible, maxilla, and mastoid to a maximum point dose less than 70 Gy (V70Gy < 0.02 cc). Typically, the mean dose delivered to the at-risk bone is limited to less than 45 Gy (Mean < 45 Gy). Less than 30% of the mandible, maxilla, or mastoid is treated to a dose of 66 Gy (V66Gy < 30%). Figure 13.7 shows a typical plan covering the at-risk CTV while protecting bone from excessive dose.

In most patients with salivary gland tumors, these bone constraints can be achieved, and the rates of osteonecrosis have declined significantly. A review of patients at UCLA using IMRT limited bone dose to < 70 Gy, and after following 158 patients none developed osteoradionecrosis (Duarte et al. 2014). Another trial of patients treated with IMRT to doses of 65–70 Gy followed patients for 34 months and saw no cases of osteoradionecrosis in 176 treated patients (Ben-David et al. 2007).

DYSPHAGIA

Radiation delivered to the salivary gland tumor resection bed and at-risk nodal regions results in some dose delivery to the lateral mucosa of the oropharynx and oral cavity. This results in mucositis that typically develops during the fifth and sixth week of treatment. Salivary gland tumors pose a risk of nodal spread to the ipsilateral neck only, and as a result, the contralateral neck is not irradiated, and mucositis is generally mild unless treatment is delivered with concurrent chemotherapy. Most patients with salivary gland tumors do not require placement of a feeding tube and mucositis typically resolved one month after completion of radiation. Radiation can result in scarring of the tissue along the lateral oropharynx and treated oral cavity with resulting fibrosis of the swallowing apparatus 12–18 months post-treatment. Studies have found that the superior and middle pharyngeal constrictor muscles must be protected from radiation to minimize acute and late dysphagia from radiation therapy (Christianen et al. 2011; Deantonio et al. 2013; Duprez et al. 2013). A commonly accepted dose constraint for the pharyngeal constrictor muscles keeps the mean dose less than 50 Gy (mean < 50 Gy). The volume of pharyngeal constrictor treated to 50 Gy is limited to less than 80% (V50Gy < 80%). The volume of constrictors treated to 60 Gy is limited to less than 70% (V60Gy < 70%) and the volume of constrictors treated to 65 Gy is limited to less than 50% (V65Gy < 50%). A dose–volume histogram illustrates how IMRT/VMAT can cover the tumor resection bed and nodes (CTV-60 and CTV-50) while keeping pharyngeal constrictor muscles within dose constraints (Figure 13.7).

Salivary gland patients treated with IMRT/VMAT that protects the dose constraints of the superior and middle pharyngeal constrictors have low levels of acute dysphagia or late fibrosis and long-term swallow difficulties. A review of patient reported quality of life metrics after head and neck radiation showed that only 5% of patients reported moderate or greater dysphagia following IMRT/VMAT and the freedom from percutaneous endoscopic gastrostomy tube at two years was 97% (Vainshtein et al. 2015).

Radiation Technique for Low- and Moderate-Risk Salivary Gland Tumors

Low-risk salivary gland tumors such as acinic cell carcinoma or small, low-grade mucoepidermoid carcinomas are often surgically cured when resected with adequate margins. These low-risk patients have only a slight risk of local recurrence and adjuvant radiation is not usually required. However, in the presence of a positive margin or multinodular recurrence, low-grade tumors should be treated with radiation focused on the operative bed. Moderate-risk patients carry a significant risk of local recurrence within the resection bed even after the best surgical management. As a result, adjuvant radiation to the tumor bed improves local control. An IMRT/VMAT plan treating a low- or moderate-risk salivary gland tumor is shown in Figure 13.6 with the surgical bed treated to 60Gy.

Radiation Technique for High-Risk Salivary Gland Tumors

Radiation therapy has an even greater role in high-risk salivary gland patients. After resection, the surgical bed is then defined as a high-risk clinical treatment volume (CTV). The ipsilateral regional lymph nodes are then defined as a low-risk CTV. A typical radiation treatment would deliver 50Gy to the ipsilateral cervical nodes and resection bed. The tumor bed high-risk CTV would then be boosted to a total dose of 60–70Gy. A dose of 60 Gy is administered for a negative margin; 66 Gy is commonly delivered for a close (<5mm) margin; and 70 Gy is administered for a positive margin or gross residual disease. A representative plan of radiation treatment for a patient with a high-risk salivary gland tumor is shown in Figure 13.8.

ADENOID CYSTIC CARCINOMA

Adenoid cystic carcinoma (ACC) is an unusual tumor with a distinct natural history, route of spread, and pattern of local recurrence. As a result, these tumors should be thought of and treated differently from the other histologic tumor types involving the salivary glands. Adenoid cystic carcinomas are common in major salivary glands and often involve the minor

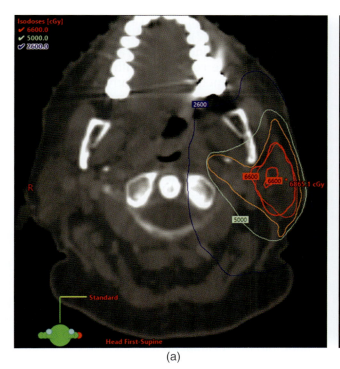 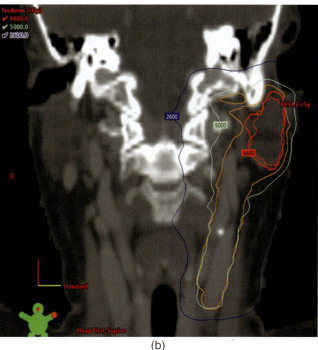

(a)   (b)

Figure 13.8. A representative plan is shown treating a patient with a high-risk salivary gland tumor. The regional nodes are treated at 2Gy per fraction to 50Gy. The tumor bed is then boosted at 2Gy per fraction for an additional 5–10 fractions to a dose of 60–70Gy. 60Gy is delivered for negative margins. 66Gy is delivered for close (<5mm) or positive margins. 70Gy is delivered for gross residual or unresectable disease. An axial view of the treatment plan is shown panel A. A coronal view of the treatment plan is shown in panel B.

salivary glands at the junction of the hard and soft palate but can occur throughout the head and neck. They often present as indolent tumors with a low mitotic rate, making them resistant to treatment. Many adenoid cystic carcinomas demonstrate a slow, relentless pattern of local and distant recurrence decades after initial diagnosis.

Adenoid cystic carcinoma differs from other salivary gland tumors in terms of its treatment. Despite their high risk of local recurrence, these tumors do not carry a high risk of node involvement. Classic texts report nodal involvement by adenoid cystic carcinoma in only 15% of cases in contrast to adenocarcinoma or squamous cell carcinomas that involve the nodes in 40–50% of cases. Given their propensity for recurrence and general poor outcomes, some authors advocate a neck dissection in all adenoid cystic carcinomas. Other groups have shown that a neck dissection is not required. A international review examined 495 patients with adenoid cystic carcinoma treated at nine different centers (Amit et al. 2014). Approximately half of these patients received a neck dissection and 16% were node positive. Patients not treated with neck dissection did not suffer from increased rates of recurrence in the neck and the five-year disease-specific survival for the entire cohort was 80%. Most failures were local or distant not within the regional nodes. Other studies have found the same low rate of nodal recurrence in the absence of neck dissection. Chen et al. (2007) reported on 84 patients with adenoid cystic carcinoma and found no cases of nodal relapse. Pommier et al. (2006) reported on 24 patients with aggressive adenoid cystic carcinoma involving the skull base treated at the Massachusetts General Hospital between 1991 and 2002. None of these patients received a neck dissection, and with a median duration of follow-up of 62 months, none of the patients developed recurrence of disease in the neck.

It appears that T stage may be the most predictive marker for nodal involvement by adenoid cystic carcinoma. The largest study of adenoid cystic carcinoma looked at 2807 patients with clinically node negative disease within the National Cancer Database (Xiao et al. 2019). A subset of these patients was treated with elective node dissection (n = 636, 22.7%) and occult nodal disease was found in 13% of patients. Advanced T stage was correlated with node positivity with 21% of T4 patients harboring an occult node. The site of adenoid cystic carcinoma was also predictive of node involvement. Occult nodes were uncommon in hard/soft palate (9%) or floor of mouth (11%) but increased to 21% in major salivary gland locations with even higher rates of 33% in the oral tongue. Importantly, elective node dissection increased five-year overall survival in patients with T3/T4 disease from 70 to 78%. Elective node dissection with adjuvant radiation gave the best outcomes in patients with locally advanced adenoid cystic carcinoma. An international collaborative study of adenoid cystic patients with clinically node negative necks confirmed the NCD trial results. Occult nodes were found in 17% of patients, with the oral cavity being the most common site for lymph node involvement (Amit et al. 2015).

In a SEER review of 720 patients, age and location of tumor did not correlate with spread to nodes (Megwalu and Sirjani 2017). However, T stage again correlated with outcomes, with T3 patients showing an odds ratio of nodal spread of 4.7 and T4 tumors having an odds ratio of 9.24. A review from South China looked at 228 patients with adenoid cystic carcinoma treated with resection and adjuvant radiation to a mean dose of 59Gy (Ouyang et al. 2017). Overall survival at 5 years was 85% but declined to 71% at 10 years. Again, advanced T stage correlated with poor outcomes. Involvement of nodes significantly decreased disease-specific survival in these studies, suggesting that a neck dissection or elective nodal irradiation is appropriate in patients with locally advanced adenoid cystic carcinoma.

Instead of spreading to regional nodes, adenoid cystic carcinoma grows along nerves. Perineural invasion is pathognomonic for this salivary gland malignancy and these tumors often exhibit perineural spread along named cranial nerves. As a result, radiation therapy should target the tumor bed and follow major cranial nerves from the site of primary tumor up to the neural foramen at the base of skull. This pattern of radiation is opposite to the treatment of other high-risk salivary gland tumors. Most high-grade salivary gland tumors require radiation to track down from the tumor into the regional nodes. Adenoid cystic carcinoma, however, requires adjuvant radiation treatment that tracks up along the nerves (Figure 13.9).

Historically, adenoid cystic carcinoma was difficult to control with radiation therapy and the tumor was thought to be radioresistant. This was a result of inferior radiation techniques and lower

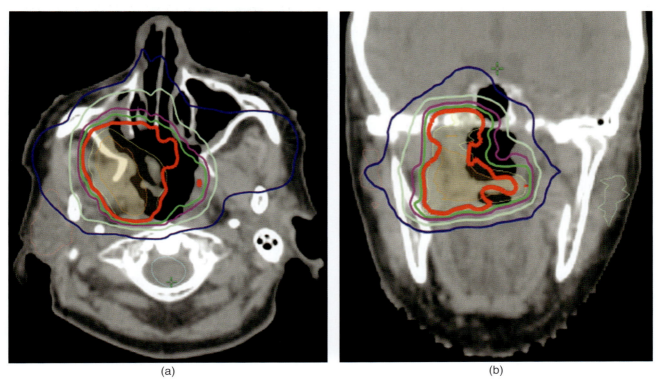

Figure 13.9. An IMRT plan is shown treating a patient with an adenoid cystic carcinoma located at the junction of the soft and hard palate. The tumor was resected with a negative but close margin and contained lymphovascular space invasion. Due to the inherent biology of adenoid cystic carcinoma there is a risk of recurrence within the operative site and along the tract of the V2 cranial nerve. A radiation treatment plan was generated to target the clinical treatment volume (CTV). The patient was treated at 2 Gy per fraction to a dose of 66 Gy. The radiation prescription dose is shown in red. The 95% isodose line is shown in dark green. The 90% isodose line is shown in purple. The 75% isodose line is shown in light green. The 50% isodose line is shown in blue. Panel A shows an axial isodose and Panel B shows a coronal image of the radiation treatment plan.

doses of radiation more than a result of intrinsic resistance on the part of adenoid cystic carcinoma. A large Dutch trial indicated that there is a clear dose-response effect with adenoid cystic carcinoma. When patients received doses of less than 60 Gy, tumor recurrence was common, but at doses greater than 66 Gy, local control of ACC was excellent (Terhaard et al. 2005). Another review of patients treated at the University of Florida with surgery and 66 Gy of adjuvant radiation showed local control at 5 and 10 years as high as 90% (Mendenhall et al. 2005). Overall survival in these patients was low, however, at only 48% at 10 years, with many patients developing distant metastatic disease. A review from the University of Wisconsin followed 70 patients and found local recurrence in only 32% of patients but distant metastatic spread developed in 73% of patients (Jang et al. 2018). This suggests that improvement in systemic therapy will be needed before increases in survival can be shown in adenoid cystic carcinoma. A recent study compared postoperative radiation with postoperative chemoradiation using concurrent cisplatin with adenoid cystic carcinoma. The addition of chemotherapy improved local and regional control at eight years but did not increase distant metastasis-free survival or overall survival (Hsieh et al. 2016). Further clinical studies of systemic therapy are needed.

Advanced Radiation Therapy Techniques

PROTON THERAPY

Just as IMRT/VMAT replaced 3D-conformal radiation and improved outcomes, many groups believe that proton therapy and other heavy particle radiation techniques may further improve outcomes in salivary gland tumors. Protons are positively charged particles that have mass. As a result, when a beam of proton energy strikes a tumor target, it has a characteristic interaction that differs substantially from an X-ray beam (Figure 13.10). The photon of X-ray energy deposits some dose when it initially enters the tissue and then continues to give a low dose of irradiation as it travels through the target. Much of the deposited dose is administered beyond the intended target and is terms "exit dose." A proton beam, however, gives a low amount of deposited dose as it enters the tumor. Then, the proton beam slows down and delivers the vast majority of dose over a short region termed the Bragg peak. Proton beams display a rapid fall off in dose beyond the Bragg peak with no "exit dose" beyond the target. This has an obvious theoretical advantage in focusing the radiation dose on the tumor while further protecting normal tissue beyond the target area.

In the past, proton therapy was limited to only a few centers around the world, but recently there has been a dramatic increase in the availability of proton therapy. There are many examples of theoretical in silico advantages of proton therapy over IMRT/VMAT but, unfortunately, there are only a handful of published reports of actual patient treatment. Pommier et al. (2006) reported on the Massachusetts General Hospital experience with adenoid cystic carcinoma treated with proton therapy in a twice-daily fashion to a median dose of 75.9 Gy equivalents. Despite a very high-risk cohort with positive margins and skull base involvement, they found five-year local control in 93% of patients and eight-year local control in 82%. Disease-free survival was 77 and 59% at five and eight years respectively.

More recently, a retrospective review was published of 41 patients with salivary gland tumors treated between 2001 and 2014 with IMRT or proton therapy (Romesser et al. 2016). Local tumor control and overall survival at one year were identical between groups. This study had some bias in favor of proton therapy with follow-up in the IMRT arm at 16 months with only 8 months of follow-up in proton therapy-treated patients. In addition, 74% of IMRT patients were treated to the tumor bed and ipsilateral neck while only 50% of proton therapy patients received neck irradiation. Furthermore, 30% of IMRT patients received concurrent chemotherapy compared to only 22% in the proton therapy arm. Despite these differences, proton therapy clearly decreased dose to uninvolved normal tissues compared to IMRT. Mean doses to normal structures were: Brainstem 29 Gy with IMRT compared to 0.62 RBE with proton therapy, Spinal Cord 36 Gy with IMRT compared to 1.8 RBE with proton therapy, and mean oral cavity

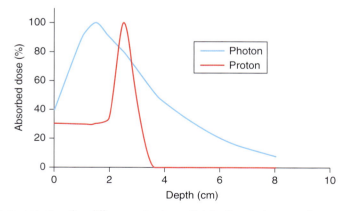

Figure 13.10. The figure demonstrates the difference in dose distribution between a beam of photon energy and a beam of proton energy. The typical behavior of an IMRT photon beam is shown in blue. Note the rapid rise in dose as the beam of energy interacts with the tissue and note the low level of dose that continues through the entire width of tissue. This tail of deposited energy beyond the maximal point is termed "exit dose." In contrast, a proton beam delivers a moderate dose of energy as it enters the tissue and then deposits a large amount of dose at its maximal point. This point of rapid dose delivery is termed the Bragg peak. The sudden fall-off of dose beyond the Bragg peak has an obvious theoretical advantage in limited exit dose to normal tissues that surround the tumor.

dose of 20.6GY with IMRT versus 0.9RBE with proton therapy. This reduction in normal tissue dose led to a decrease in acute grade 2 toxicity in proton therapy-treated patients with a decrease in mucositis from 52.2 to 16.7% and a decline in dysgeusia from 65 to 5.6% likely from the lower mean oral cavity dose. Acute grade 2 nausea was also lower in proton therapy-treated patients at 11% compared to 56% likely due to the lower brainstem dose with less effect on the area post-treatment. Interestingly, proton therapy resulted in an increase in skin toxicity with grade 2 acute dermatitis in 100% of proton therapy-treated patients and only 74% of IMRT patients. This study used a spread-out Bragg peak approach in proton therapy that does not allow skin sparing. More advanced proton delivery using a pencil beam scanning approach or intensity-modulated proton therapy (IMPT) allow skin sparing and should further improve the side effect profile for proton therapy.

NEUTRON THERAPY

Neutron therapy was studied as a means of increasing radiation dose and thus local control for salivary gland tumors. Neutron radiation therapy differs from traditional photon beam radiation. All radiation therapy is thought to function by inducing DNA damage within tumor cells. The neutron particle has mass, and as a result, it interacts with tumor cell DNA differently than a weightless photon of X-rays from IMRT or traditional radiation treatment. The neutron beam causes a higher rate of DNA damage over a short path length compared to photon DNA damage. This is referred to as a high linear energy transfer (LET) and allows a neutron beam to have a much higher biologically effective dose than photon radiation.

It was hoped that the higher biological effect of neutron radiation would improve outcomes in salivary gland tumors. The University of Washington has extensively studied neutron therapy for salivary gland tumors, treating more than 300 consecutive patients with neutron therapy. More than 94% of these patients harbored gross residual disease and 42% of them had T4 lesions. Despite these very high-risk factors, neutron therapy resulted in local control at six years of 59% and a cause-specific survival of 67% (Douglas et al. 2003). Unfortunately, neutron therapy also resulted in higher rates of toxicity with 10% of patients developing late effect grade 3 or grade 4 adverse effects. Four patients developed central nervous system necrosis, three patients developed blindness, and four patients developed osteoradionecrosis.

The neutron treatment experience from the University of Washington was recently updated (Davis et al. 2016). They report a standard treatment of 1.15 neutron Gray (nGy) per day four times per week over four weeks to a dose of 18.4nGy as equivalent to 60–70Gy of photon therapy. Despite a high rate of 63% of patients with a positive margin, they report local control at six years of 72%. Unfortunately, post-treatment trismus was identified in 56% of patients. At 10 years, the local control for treated patients was 79% and the overall survival was 62% (Timoshchuk et al. 2019).

CARBON ION THERAPY

Researchers in Japan and Heidelberg have reported outcomes for salivary gland tumors treated with carbon ion therapy. The heavy mass of a carbon ion results in an even greater biological effect than proton or neutron therapy. Initial reports show good outcomes. In a study of 62 patients with mucoepidermoid carcinoma, dose escalation was achieved from 66Gy with IMRT to 78Gy with carbon ion therapy. Acute toxicity was low with reported grade 3 mucositis of 6%, dermatitis of 3%, and xerostomia in only 3%. Late toxicity was also mild with trismus reported in 3%, hearing loss in 3%, and long-term xerostomia in only 5% of patients. Local control was excellent with local-regional control in 88% of patients at five years (Akbaba et al. 2019).

In a larger study of 289 patients with adenoid cystic carcinoma treated at four Japanese centers, carbon ion therapy was delivered in a hypofractionated approach of 4Gy over 16 fractions to a dose of 64Gy. This resulted in local control at two and five years of 88 and 68% respectively. Overall survival was reported at 94 and 74% at two and five years respectively (Sulaiman et al. 2018).

Summary

- Low-risk salivary gland tumors are most often cured by effective surgical resection with negative surgical margins, and do not frequently require adjuvant therapy.

- Moderate-risk salivary gland tumors have a significant risk of local recurrence even after optimal surgery and benefit from adjuvant radiation therapy to the tumor bed and occasionally to the first echelon of lymph nodes.
- High-risk salivary gland tumors have high rates of local recurrence and suffer from frequent involvement of the regional lymph nodes. These high-risk patients require postoperative radiation to the ipsilateral neck with high doses of radiation to the tumor bed.
- Adenoid cystic carcinoma frequently exhibits perineural spread resulting in a different radiation technique targeting cranial nerves and treating nodes only in locally advanced disease.
- Advances in radiation technique allow for these much better outcomes in salivary gland tumors.
- IMRT and VMAT deliver a higher dose to the tumor, improving local control and avoiding aggressive surgery in many patients.
- More accurate radiation therapy protects critical structures of the head and neck, decreasing adverse effects of treatment.
- Newer and more advanced radiation techniques such as the growing availability of proton therapy hold the promise to further improve the outcome of our patients.
- Clinical trials are ongoing to examine combination chemotherapy and radiation in management of high-risk salivary gland malignancies. It is hoped that better integration of systemic therapy will decrease distant metastatic recurrence and hence improve survival.

References

Akbaba S, Heusel A, Mock A, et al. 2019. The impact of age on the outcome of patients treated with radiotherapy for mucoepidermoid carcinoma (MEC) of the salivary glands in the head and neck: A 15-year single-center experience. *Oral Oncol* 97:115–123.

Ali SA, Kovatch KJ, Yousif ., et al. 2020. Predictors of distant metastasis in acinic cell carcinoma of the parotid gland. *World J Clin Oncol* 11(1):11–19.

Al-Mamgani A, van Rooij P, Verduijn GM, et al. 2012. Long-term outcomes and quality of life of 186 patients with primary parotid carcinoma treated with surgery and radiotherapy at the Daniel den Hoed Cancer Center. *Int J Radiat Oncol Biol Phys* 84:189–195.

Amit M, Binenbaum Y, Sharma K, et al. 2014. Analysis of failure in patients with adenoid cystic carcinoma of the head and neck. An international collaborative study. *Head Neck* 36(7):998–1004.

Amit M, Na'ara S, Sharma K, et al. 2015. Elective neck dissection in patients with head and neck adenoid cystic carcinoma: An international collaborative study. *Ann Surg Oncol* 22(4):1353–1359.

Armstrong JG, Harrison LB, Spiro RH, et al. 1990. Malignant tumors of major salivary gland origin. A matched-pair analysis of the role of combined surgery and postoperative radiotherapy. *Arch Otolaryngol Head Neck Surg* 116(3):290–293.

Armstrong JG, Harrison LB, Thaler HT, et al. 1992. The indications for elective treatment of the neck in cancer of the major salivary glands. *Cancer* 69(3):615–619.

Bakst RL, Su W, Ozbek U, et al. 2017. Adjuvant radiation for salivary gland malignancies is associated with improved survival: A National Cancer Database analysis. *Adv Radiat Oncol* 2(2):159–166.

Ben-David MA, Diamante M, Radawski JD, et al. 2007. Lack of osteoradionecrosis of the mandible after intensity-modulated radiotherapy for head and neck cancer: Likely contributions of both dental care and improved dose distributions. *Int J Radiat Oncol Biol Phys* 68(2):396–402.

Breen JT, Carlson ML, Link MJ, et al. 2012. Skull base involvement by acinic cell carcinoma of the parotid gland. *J Neurol Surg B Skull Base* 73(6):371–378.

Chen AM, Bucci MK, Quivey JM, et al. 2006b. Long-term outcome of patients treated by radiation therapy alone for salivary gland carcinomas. *Int J Radiat Oncol Biol Phys* 66(4):1044–1050.

Chen AM, Garcia J, Bucci MK, et al. 2006a. Recurrent pleomorphic adenoma of the parotid gland: Long-term outcome of patients treated with radiation therapy. *Int J Radiat Oncol Biol Phys* 66(4):1031–1035.

Chen AM, Garcia J, Lee NY, et al. 2007. Patterns of nodal relapse after surgery and postoperative radiation therapy for carcinomas of the major and minor salivary glands: What is the role of elective neck irradiation? *Int J Radiat Oncol Biol Phys* 67(4):988–994.

Chintakuntlawar AV, Shon W, Erickson-Johnson M., et al. 2016. High-grade transformation of acinic cell carcinoma: An inadequately treated entity? *Oral Surg Oral Med Oral Pathol Oral Radiol* 121(5):542–549.e1.

Cho JK, Lim BW, Kim EH, et al. 2016. Low-grade salivary gland cancers: Treatment outcomes, extent of surgery and indications for postoperative adjuvant radiation therapy. *Ann Surg Oncol* 23(13):4368–4375.

Christianen ME, Langendijk JA, Westerlaan HE, et al. 2011. Delineation of organs at risk involved in swallowing for radiotherapy treatment planning. *Radiother Oncol* 101(3):394–402.

Davis C, Sikes J, Namaranian P, et al. 2016. Neutron beam radiation therapy: An overview of treatment and oral complications when treating salivary gland malignancies. *J Oral Maxillofac Surg* 74(4):830–835.

Deantonio L, Masini L, Brambilla M, et al. 2013. Dysphagia after definitive radiotherapy for head and neck cancer. Correlation of dose-volume parameters of the pharyngeal constrictor muscles. *Strahlenther Onkol* 189(3):230–236.

Douglas JG, Koh WJ, Austin-Seymour M, et al. 2003. Treatment of salivary gland neoplasms with fast neutron radiotherapy. *Arch Otolaryngol Head Neck Surg* 129(9):944–948.

Duarte VM, Liy YF, Rafizadeh S, et al. 2014. Comparison of dental health of patients with head and neck cancer receiving IMRT vs conventional radiation. *Otolaryngol Head Neck Surg* 150(1):81–86.

Duprez F, Madani I, De Potter B, et al. 2013. Systematic review of dose – Volume correlates for structures related to late swallowing disturbances after radiotherapy for head and neck cancer. *Dysphagia* 28(3):337–349.

Gomez DR, Katabi N, Zhung J, et al. 2009. Clinical and pathologic prognostic features in acinic cell carcinoma of the parotid gland. *Cancer* 115(10):2128–2137.

Harrison LB, Armstrong JG, Spiro RH, et al. 1990. Postoperative radiation therapy for major salivary gland malignancies. *J Surg Oncol* 45(1):52–55.

Herman MP, Werning JW, Morris CG, et al. 2013. Elective neck management for high-grade salivary gland carcinoma. *Am J Otolaryngol* 34(3):205–208.

Hsieh CE, Lin CW., Lee LY, et al. 2016. Adding concurrent chemotherapy to postoperative radiotherapy improves locoregional control but not overall survival in patients with salivary gland adenoid cystic carcinoma-a propensity score matched study. *Radiat Oncol* 11:47.

Jang JY, Choi N, Ko YH, et al. 2018. Treatment outcomes in metastatic and localized high-grade salivary gland cancer: High chance of cure with surgery and post-operative radiation in T1-2 N0 high-grade salivary gland cancer. *BMC Cancer* 18(1):672.

Johnston ML, Huang SH, Waldron JN, et al. 2016. Salivary duct carcinoma: Treatment, outcomes, and patterns of failure. *Head Neck* 38 Suppl 1:E820–E826.

Lau VH, Aouad R, Farwell DG, et al. 2014. Patterns of nodal involvement for clinically N0 salivary gland carcinoma: Refining the role of elective neck irradiation. *Head Neck* 36(10):1435–1439.

Liu Y, Su M, Yang Y, et al. 2017. Prognostic factors associated with decreased survival in patients with acinic cell carcinoma of the parotid gland. *J Oral Maxillofac Surg* 75(2):416–422.

Lloyd S, Yu JB, Ross DA, et al. 2010. A prognostic index for predicting lymph node metastasis in minor salivary gland cancer. *Int J Radiat Oncol Biol Phys* 76(1):169–175.

Mahmood U, Koshy M, Goloubeva O, et al. 2011. Adjuvant radiation therapy for high-grade and/or locally advanced major salivary gland tumors. *Arch Otolaryngol Head Neck Surg* 137(10):1025–1030.

Megwalu UC and Sirjani D. 2017. Risk of nodal metastasis in major salivary gland adenoid cystic carcinoma. *Otolaryngol Head Neck Surg* 156(4):660–664.

Mendenhall WM, Morris CG, Amdur RJ, et al. 2005. Radiotherapy alone or combined with surgery for salivary gland carcinoma. *Cancer* 103(12):2544–2550.

Mendenhall WM, Mendenhall CM, Werning JW, et al. 2008. Salivary gland pleomorphic adenoma. *Am J Clin Oncol* 31(1):95–99.

Mifsud MJ, Tanvetyanon T, McCaffrey JC, et al. 2016. Adjuvant radiotherapy versus concurrent chemoradiotherapy for the management of high-risk salivary gland carcinomas. *Head Neck* 38(11):1628–1633.

North CA, Lee DJ, Piantadosi S, et al. 1990. Carcinoma of the major salivary glands treated by surgery or surgery plus post-operative radiotherapy. *Int J Radiat Oncol Biol Phys* 18(6):1319–1326.

O'Brien CJ. 2003. Current management of benign parotid tumors – The role of limited superficial parotidectomy. *Head Neck* 25(11):946–952.

Ouyang DQ, Liang LZ, Zheng GS, et al. 2017. Risk factors and prognosis for salivary gland adenoid cystic carcinoma in southern China: A 25-year retrospective study. *Medicine (Baltimore)* 96(5):e5964.

Patel NR, Sanghvi S, Khan MN, et al. 2014. Demographic trends and disease-specific survival in salivary acinic cell carcinoma: An analysis of 1129 cases. *Laryngoscope* 124(1):172–178.

Pohar S, Gay H, Rosenbaum P, et al. 2005. Malignant parotid tumors: Presentation, clinical/pathologic prognostic factors, and treatment outcomes. *Int J Radiat Oncol Biol Phys* 61(1):112–118.

Pommier P, Liebsch NJ, Deschler DG, et al. 2006. Proton beam radiation therapy for skull base adenoid cystic carcinoma. *Arch Otolaryngol Head Neck Surg* 132(11):1242–1249.

Ravasz LA, Terhaard CH, and Hordijk GJ, et al. 1990. Radiotherapy in epithelial tumors of the parotid gland: Case presentation and literature review. *Int J Radiat Oncol Biol Phys* 19(1):55–59.

Regis De Brito Santos I, Kowalski LP, Cavalcante De Araujo V, et al. 2001. Multivariate analysis of risk factors for neck metastases in surgically treated parotid carcinomas. *Arch Otolaryngol Head Neck Surg* 127(1):56–60.

Romesser PB, Cahlon O, Scher E, et al. 2016. Proton beam radiation therapy results in significantly reduced toxicity compared with intensity-modulated radiation therapy for head and neck tumors that require ipsilateral radiation. *Radiother Oncol* 118(2):286–292.

Scherl C, Kato MG, Erkul E, et al. 2018. Outcomes and prognostic factors for parotid acinic cell carcinoma: A National Cancer Database study of 2362 cases. *Oral Oncol* 82:53–60.

Stennert E, Kisner D, Jungehuelsing M, et al. 2003. High incidence of lymph node metastasis in major salivary gland cancer. *Arch Otolaryngol Head Neck Surg* 129(7):720–723.

Sulaiman NS, Demizu Y, Koto M, et al. 2018. Multicenter study of carbon-ion radiation therapy for adenoid cystic carcinoma of the head and neck: Subanalysis of the Japan Carbon-Ion Radiation Oncology Study Group (J-CROS) Study (1402 HN). *Int J Radiat Oncol Biol Phys* 100(3):639–646.

Szewczyk M, Golusinski J, Pazdrowski J, et al. 2018. Patterns of treatment failure in salivary gland cancers. *Rep Pract Oncol Radiother* 23(4):260–265.

Terhaard CH, Lubsen H, Rash CR et al. 2005. The role of radiotherapy in the treatment of malignant salivary gland tumors. *Int J Radiat Oncol Biol Phys* 61(1):103–111.

Timoshchuk MA, Dekker P, Hippe DS, et al. 2019. The efficacy of neutron radiation therapy in treating salivary gland malignancies. *Oral Oncol* 88:51–57.

Vainshtein JM, Moon DH, Feng FY, et al. 2015. Long-term quality of life after swallowing and salivary-sparing chemo-intensity modulated radiation therapy in survivors of human papillomavirus-related oropharyngeal cancer. *Int J Radiat Oncol Biol Phys* 91(5):925–933.

Xiao R, Sethi RKV, Feng AL, et al. 2019. The role of elective neck dissection in patients with adenoid cystic carcinoma of the head and neck. *Laryngoscope* 129(9):2094–2104.

Chapter 14
Systemic Therapy for Salivary Gland Cancer

Janakiraman Subramanian MD, MPH and Lara Kujtan MD, MSc
Department of Medicine, University of Missouri at Kansas City, Kansas City, Missouri

Outline

Introduction
Epidemiology and Risk Factors
Molecular Biology of Salivary Gland Tumors
Clinical Presentation
Treatment
  Adjuvant Treatment
  Treatment of Metastatic Disease
  Targeted Therapy
    Targeting *C-KIT*
    EGFR Inhibition
    Her2 Inhibition
    Multi Kinase Inhibition
    Proteasome Inhibition
    Androgen Receptor Inhibition
    NTRK Inhibition
    Immune Checkpoint Inhibition
Summary
  Case Presentation – *Well, If It Works for Breast Cancer!!*
References

Introduction

Salivary gland tumors are a group of heterogeneous neoplasms that constitute less than 1% of all cancers diagnosed globally (American Cancer Society 2018). The behavior of these tumors varies widely depending on their location, histology, and tumor biology. The tumors can involve both the major salivary glands (parotid, submandibular, and sublingual) and the minor salivary glands (Barnes et al. 2005). The most common location is the parotid gland, which accounts for approximately 80% of all the salivary gland tumors (Guzzo et al. 2010). Tumors involving the minor salivary glands are rare but are also more likely to be malignant. Salivary gland tumors include both benign and malignant neoplasms and they are classified according to the Seethala and Stenman (2017). This chapter will focus on the use of systemic therapy in the treatment of salivary gland cancers.

Epidemiology and Risk Factors

The global annual incidence rates for salivary gland cancers (SGCs) vary between 1.7 and 0.1 per 100,000 (Bray et al. 2017). It has been suggested that radiation exposure, viral infections, diet, and genetic predisposition may play a role in the development of these rare cancers. The association between radiation exposure and SGC was first identified in atomic bomb survivors in Hiroshima (Saku et al. 1997). Subsequently, SGC has been reported in patients receiving radiation to the head and neck region for both cancers and benign conditions (Schneider et al. 1998).

Viral infections have been shown to be associated with the development of SGCs. Lymphoepithelial carcinoma is an SGC that is strongly associated with Epstein-Barr Virus (EBV) infection in areas endemic to the virus (2005). Epidemiologic studies have shown that patients with the human immunodeficiency virus (HIV) are also more likely to develop SGCs (Serraino et al. 2000). The human papillomavirus (HPV) has been identified in some mucoepidermoid carcinomas (Brunner et al. 2012; Isayeva et al. 2013); however, this has not been a

---

Salivary Gland Pathology: Diagnosis and Management, Third Edition. Edited by Eric R. Carlson and Robert A. Ord.
© 2022 John Wiley & Sons, Inc. Published 2022 by John Wiley & Sons, Inc.
Companion website: www.wiley.com/go/carlson/salivary

consistent finding (Jour et al. 2013). Similarly, HPV has been rarely identified in other SGCs (Hafed et al. 2012). It is not currently clear if there is a significant association between HPV and SGCs.

Environmental carcinogens are also associated with SGCs. Tobacco smoke exposure is associated with the development of Warthin tumor (Pinkston and Cole 1996). Exposure to nickel and rubber manufacturing are also risk factors for SGCs (Horn-Ross et al. 1997). In addition, professionals such as hair dressers and beauticians are reported to have higher risk for developing SGCs (Swanson and Burns 1997).

Molecular Biology of Salivary Gland Tumors

SGCs consist of variety of different tumors and there is considerable variation in the type of molecular changes identified in these tumors. These molecular changes include fusion genes, oncogenic mutations, and alterations in gene amplification or expression. Some of these molecular alterations are specific to the tumor type and could help establish the diagnosis in the absence of a histologic diagnosis; others have been identified as potential therapeutic targets.

Fusion genes are relatively rare molecular events in malignant epithelial tumors. The *MYB-NFIB* fusion gene has been identified in adenoid cystic carcinoma (ACC) and appears to be specific to this tumor type (Persson et al. 2009). The *MYB-NFIB* fusion gene activates the transcription of a variety of genes downstream to *MYB*, which includes *BCL2*, *KIT*, *CD34*, *BIRC3*, and *MYC* (Stenman 2013). These genes are important in activation of cell proliferation, differentiation, and apoptosis. The *MYB* gene has been reported to be activated in the most (80%) ACCs either by gene fusion or by other mechanisms. Mucoepidermoid carcinoma (MEC) is characterized by the *CRTC-MAML2* fusion gene and both constituent genes have role in cell cycle (Enlund et al. 2004). The *CRTC1* is a cAMP response element binding protein (CREB) co-activator that regulates genes involved in cell proliferation and differentiation in response to stimulus from growth factors and cytokines (Coxon et al. 2005). The *MAML2* gene is a co-activator for the *NOTCH* gene, which also plays a major role in cell cycle as well as in oncogenesis. The oncoprotein resulting from this gene fusion has transforming activity in both in vitro; and in vivo; experiments. Recently, the *ETV6-NTRK3* gene fusion was identified in mammary analog secretory carcinoma (MASC) and the chimeric tyrosine kinase resulting from this fusion has shown transforming activity as well (Skalova et al. 2010). Targeting the IGF1R pathway has been shown to effectively inhibit the transforming activity of this fusion kinase (Tognon et al. 2011).

Overexpression of the epidermal growth factor receptor (*EGFR*) gene is the most common genomic abnormality reported in SGCs, it is identified in approximately 70% of all SGCs (Locati et al. 2009b). However, activating mutations involving the tyrosine kinase domain of the *EGFR* gene are rare. Other genes that have been reported to be overexpressed or amplified in SGC include *HER2*, *VEGF*, and *C-Kit* (Press et al. 1994; Lim et al. 2003; Skalova et al. 2003; Dagrada et al. 2004; Freier et al. 2005). VEGF expression is an independent prognostic factor and high expression is associated with inferior outcomes. C-Kit expression is found in most high-grade ACCs (90%). Expression of estrogen and progesterone receptors has been reported in some SGCs though this is a rare finding.

Clinical Presentation

The clinical presentation for SGC depends on the site of origin and involvement of adjacent structures. Approximately half of all major SGCs arise in the parotid gland and they usually present as a painless mass arising in the parotid, submandibular, or sublingual gland. Around 90% of all salivary gland tumors arise in the parotid gland and about 25% of them are malignant (2005). In the case of submandibular salivary gland, the proportion of SGCs is about 45%, 70–90% in sublingual gland tumors and 50–75% in minor salivary gland tumors (Guzzo et al. 2010). If the mass is associated with facial nerve palsy, then it is likely to be a malignant SGC. Similarly, the presence of associated lymphadenopathy also indicates malignant SGC.

Tumors arising from minor salivary glands are more likely to be malignant than tumors arising in major salivary glands. More than half of all minor salivary gland tumors arise within the oral cavity. Symptoms for minor SGCs vary according the location, oral tumors may present as a painless submucosal tumor, minor SGCs in the nasopharynx can cause facial pain, nasal obstruction, and bleeding and tumors in the hypopharynx can result in hoarseness of voice and dyspnea. Minor SGCs in the nasopharynx are also more likely to present at an advanced stage with invasion of the skull base, intracranial and cranial nerve involvement (Schramm and Imola 2001). A through initial assessment with history and physical exam could help estimate the extent of the disease and the likelihood of it being a malignant tumor. Tissue diagnosis must be established and this can be achieved in most cases with fine needle aspiration cytology. Imaging scans such as computerized tomography (CT) and/or magnetic resonance imaging (MRI) may be needed to establish the TNM stage of the disease.

Treatment

Treatment of SGCs depends on the location, tumor histology, and the extent of disease involvement. Whenever possible, a complete surgical resection with clear margins is the preferred treatment approach for SGCs. In patients with SGCs that are non-resectable or medically inoperable, definitive radiation remains the treatment of choice. Concurrent chemotherapy with a platinum agent can be considered in patients with good performance status; however, there is insufficient evidence to support this approach over definitive radiation alone.

ADJUVANT TREATMENT

There is no established role for adjuvant chemotherapy alone in patients with resected SGCs though this approach may be considered with concomitant adjuvant radiation. Adjuvant radiotherapy is indicated in patients with high risk features such as high-grade tumors, advanced disease stage, adenoid cystic carcinoma histology, and skin or nerve invasion. In addition, patients with T2 or greater SGCs involving the submandibular, sublingual, and minor salivary glands are potential candidates for adjuvant radiotherapy. The role for concomitant chemotherapy with adjuvant radiation has not been established but has been evaluated by the RTOG 1008 clinical trial (Rodriguez et al. 2008; Caudell et al. 2014). This randomized phase II trial will compare adjuvant radiotherapy with concurrent cisplatin chemotherapy to adjuvant radiotherapy alone in patients with resected SGCs. Retrospective data from the National Cancer Data Base suggest that concurrent chemoradiation does not add survival benefit compared to adjuvant radiation therapy alone in these patients (Amini et al. 2016).

TREATMENT OF METASTATIC DISEASE

Cytotoxic chemotherapy is primarily used in the treatment of advanced stage disease that cannot be treated with definitive surgical resection or radiation. However, the optimal chemotherapy regimen in the treatment of SGCs has not been established. Given the rarity of these tumors, there have been no large randomized trials to establish the survival benefit from cytotoxic chemotherapy treatment. The primary role for chemotherapy treatment is to palliate symptoms in patients with metastatic SGC. Small phase II trials and case series have studied the use of both monotherapy and combination chemotherapy in the treatment of SGCs. In addition, tumor histology in SGCs appears to determine sensitivity to chemotherapy treatment. Treatment with single agent paclitaxel appears to be effective in patients with mucoepidermoid carcinomas and adenocarcinoma but it has not shown activity against ACC (Gilbert et al. 2006; Laurie et al. 2011). Similarly, treatment with cisplatin is associated with increased toxicity but no better efficacy than mitoxantrone, epirubicin, or vinorelbine in patients with ACCs (Table 14.1).

Single agent paclitaxel, cisplatin, doxorubicin, mitoxantrone, vinorelbine, and methotrexate have all shown activity in the treatment of SGCs. The response rate is modest and ranges between 10 and 40% (Schramm et al. 1981; Licitra et al. 1991; Vermorken et al. 1993; Verweij et al. 1996; Airoldi et al. 2001). The choice of agent will depend on the tumor histology and the patient's ability to tolerate the agent. In general, any one of these agents can be considered for the treatment of SGCs except in the case of ACCs where paclitaxel is not particularly effective.

Combination chemotherapy is generally associated with better tumor response rate compared to single agent chemotherapy, but it is also associated with a higher incidence of adverse effects (Table 14.1). Several different combinations of platinum, anthracycline with or without other agents including cyclophosphamide and 5-fluorouracil have been evaluated in the treatment of advanced stage SGCs. The most common regimen being cyclophosphamide, doxorubicin, and cisplatin (CAP) given on day 1 of a 28-day cycle (Dreyfuss et al. 1987; Licitra et al. 1996). The overall response rate ranges between 30 and 40% for all patients with advanced stage SGCs. In addition, the response rates may vary according to the histologic type with some histologic types such as adenocarcinomas showing a better response rate of approximately 60%.

Our approach has generally been to use combination chemotherapy in patients who are symptomatic from the disease and single agent

Table 14.1. Chemotherapy in the treatment of metastatic or recurrent salivary gland cancers.

Agent(s)	ACC		MEC		ADC	
	N	No. of objective responses	N	No. of objective responses	N	No. of objective responses
Cisplatin (Schramm et al. 1981; Suen and Johns 1982; Kaplan et al. 1986; Licitra et al. 1991; de Haan et al. 1992; Jones et al. 1993)	66	28	7	2	8	0
Paclitaxel (Gilbert et al. 2006)	14	0	14	3	17	5
Gemcitabine (van Herpen et al. 2008)	21	0	–	–	–	–
Vinorelbine (Airoldi et al. 2001)	13	2	–	–	5	2
Mitoxantrone (Mattox et al. 1990; Verweij et al. 1996)	50	5	–	–	–	–
Epirubicin (Vermorken et al. 1993)	20	2	–	–	–	–
CAP (Alberts et al. 1981; Kaplan et al. 1986; Dreyfuss et al. 1987; Belani et al. 1988; Creagan et al. 1988; Licitra et al. 1996)	36	9	16	8	29	19
CAP+5FU (Dimery et al. 1990)	7	3	1	1	9	4
Carboplatin/paclitaxel (Ruzich et al. 2002)	10	2	1	0	2	1
Cisplatin/vinorelbine (Airoldi et al. 2001)	9	4	1	0	4	3
Cisplatin/gemcitabine (Laurie et al. 2010)	10	2	4	1	8	3
Cisplatin/5FU (Hill et al. 1997)	11	0	–	–	–	–

ACC = adenoid cystic carcinoma; ADC = adenocarcinoma; MEC = mucoepidermoid carcinoma.

chemotherapy in all other patients. In patients who have an indolent disease that is asymptomatic, close monitoring without any systemic therapy would be appropriate.

TARGETED THERAPY

The field of oncology was revolutionized by the advent of molecularly targeted therapy (Figure 14.1). Some of these agents have been evaluated in patients with SGC. Most of these studies involve agents targeting receptor tyrosine kinases in advanced stage salivary gland cancers. Molecularly targeted treatment approaches are beginning to show significant response and survival benefit in this patient population (Kurzrock et al. 2019; Table 14.2).

Targeting C-KIT

ACCs have been reported to have C-Kit expression and individual case studies have reported response to treatment with imatinib (Mino et al. 2003). Phase II trials evaluating single agent imatinib for the treatment of ACCs did not report any significant treatment response (Pfeffer et al. 2007). The combination of imatinib with cisplatin in a phase II trial was reported to have a partial response in 5 out of 28 evaluable patients with ACC and 19 had stable disease (Ghosal et al. 2011). Overall, prospective studies have not shown any significant treatment benefit with imatinib for patients with ACC.

EGFR Inhibition

Gefitinib is an EGFR tyrosine kinase (TK) inhibitor and has shown activity in patients with lung and pancreatic cancers. EGFR overexpression has been reported in patients with MEC and ACCs. Treatment with gefitinib in a phase II trial did not report any significant objective response in patients with advanced stage SGCs. Stable disease was reported in 10 (34%) patients (Jakob et al. 2015).

EGFR inhibition can also be achieved by cetuximab, which is an anti-EGFR monoclonal antibody. Treatment with cetuximab was not associated with treatment response in a phase II trial with 30 patients with SGCs (Locati et al. 2009a). Disease stabilization was reported in 24 (80%) patients and 15 (50%) patients had disease stabilization for at least six months.

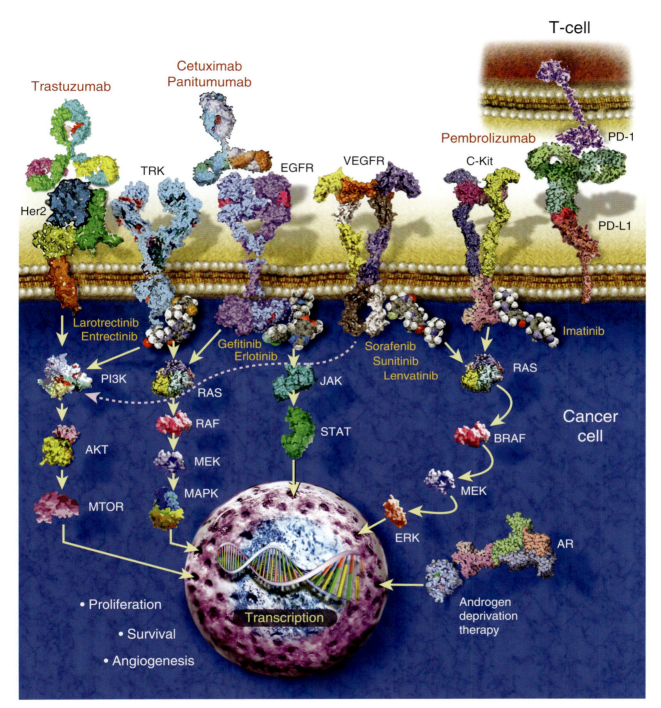

Figure 14.1. Activated signaling pathways and their inhibitory agents in advanced salivary gland cancers. AKT = protein kinase B; AR = androgen receptor; BRAF = B-rapidly accelerated fibrosarcoma protein; C-Kit = receptor tyrosine kinase; EGFR = epidermal growth factor receptor; JAK = Janus tyrosine kinase; MAPK = mitogen-activated protein kinase; MEK = MAPK/ERK (extracellular signal-related kinase) kinase; MTOR = mammalian target of rapamycin; PD-1 = programmed death receptor 1; PD-L1 = programmed death receptor 1 ligand; PI3K = phosphoinositide 3-kinase; RAF = rapidly accelerated fibrosarcoma protein; RAS = rat sarcoma protein; STAT = signal transducer and activator of transcription protein; TRK = tropomyosin receptor kinase; VEGRF = vascular endothelial growth factor receptor.

Table 14.2. Targeted therapy in the treatment of metastatic or recurrent salivary gland cancers.

Agent	Molecular target	N	Tumor type	Response rate	Comment
Imatinib (Pfeffer et al. 2007)	CKIT	26	ACC	–	No significant activity
Gefitinib (Jakob et al. 2014)	EGFR	29	SGC	–	No significant activity
Cetuximab (Locati et al. 2009a)	EGFR	30	SGC	–	No significant activity
Trastuzumab (Haddad et al. 2003)	HER2	15	SGC	–	No significant activity
Lapatinib (Agulnik et al. 2007)	HER2	40	SGC	–	No significant activity
Sorafenib (Thomson et al. 2013)	VEGFR	23	ACC	8.3%	Significant toxicity
Sunitinib (Chau et al. 2012)	VEGFR	14	ACC	–	No significant activity
Bortezomib (Argiris et al. 2011)	Proteasome	25	ACC	–	No significant activity

ACC = adenoid cystic carcinoma; ADC = adenocarcinoma; MEC = mucoepidermoid carcinoma; SGC = salivary gland cancer.
Source: Based on Kurzrock et al. (2019).

Her2 Inhibition

Her2 expression has been reported in MEC and salivary duct cancers (Glisson et al. 2004; Jaehne et al. 2005). A phase II trial was initiated to evaluate trastuzumab, a monoclonal antibody targeting Her2 for patients with Her2 expression positive SGCs (Haddad et al. 2003). The study closed early due to low rates for Her2 expression positive tumors. In one patient with Her2 positive MEC, partial response was reported which lasted for over two years. However, recent studies with trastuzumab in combination with chemotherapy for patients with SGC are encouraging (Limaye et al. 2013). A phase II trial of fifty-seven patients reported an overall response rate of 70.2%, with a median overall survival of 39.7 months when trastuzumab was combined with docetaxel (Takahashi et al. 2018). Her2 testing should be performed in all SGC patients with metastatic disease. Lapatinib is a small molecule dual kinase inhibitor for *Her2* and *EGFR* that was evaluated in a phase II trial for patients with metastatic SGCs (Agulnik et al. 2007). Of the 40 patients enrolled in the multicenter phase II trial, none of them had a treatment response, 15 patients with ACC had stable disease and 8 patients with non-ACC had stable disease. The treatment outcomes did not correlate with either EGFR or Her2 expression in this study.

Multi Kinase Inhibition

Sorafenib, sunitinib, and lenvatinib are multi kinase inhibitors that have been evaluated in patients with advanced stage ACCs. Sorafenib was evaluated in 23 patients with ACC and two patients had partial response with a median progression-free survival of 13 months (Thomson et al. 2015). In another study, 14 patients with ACC were treated with sunitinib and no treatment responses were reported but 5 patients had disease stabilization (Chau et al. 2012). In a phase II trial of lenvatinib in 33 patients with relapsed or metastatic ACC, 5 patients had a partial response and 24 patients had stable disease, with a median progression-free survival of 17.5 months (Tchekmedyian et al. 2019).

All of these treatments were difficult to tolerate; more than half the patients receiving sorafenib developed grade 3 or higher toxicity. The authors did not recommend further evaluation of sorafenib in this patient population. Similarly, sunitinib also had a significant toxicity profile with 3 patients removed from the study due to toxicity and 10 patients required dose reductions. In the lenvatinib study, 23 patients required at least one dose modification, and 56% of patients discontinued lenvatinib due to drug-related issues. Of these three agents, only lenvatinib has a category 2B recommendation for use in patients with metastatic ACC. Sorafenib and sunitinib are not recommended in the treatment of these patients.

Proteasome Inhibition

Bortezomib is a 26S proteasome and *NF-κB* inhibitor that had shown preclinical activity against ACC tumors in combination with doxorubicin. A phase II trial evaluated treatment with both single agent bortezomib and in combination with doxorubicin in the treatment of patients with incurable ACC (Argiris et al. 2011). Of the 24 patients treated with single agent bortezomib, none had an objective response and stable disease was reported in 15 patients. One patient out of 10 receiving the combination therapy had a partial response.

Androgen Receptor Inhibition

Androgen receptor (AR) expression is common in salivary duct carcinomas, ranging anywhere from

71 to 100% of tumors. AR blockade is typically achieved through androgen deprivation therapy (ADT). A retrospective single institution analysis of 58 patients compared first-line ADT with chemotherapy in recurrent or metastatic SGC and reported a median overall survival of 25 months for both arms. The response rate with ADT was 45% compared to 14% for first-line chemotherapy (Viscuse et al. 2019). A single-arm phase II prospective trial showed similar findings with androgen blockade, with a median overall survival of 30.5 months and response rate of 41.7% (Fushimi et al. 2017). ADT is also less toxic than traditional chemotherapy regimens. Testing for androgen receptor expression is now recommended for all metastatic SGC.

NTRK Inhibition

Tropomyosin receptor kinases (TRK) are transmembrane tyrosine kinases encoded by *NTRK* genes. Constitutive activation of these kinases can occur via fusion of the C-terminal kinase domain with a N-terminal partner. Two inhibitors of these fusion products, larotrectinib and entrectinib, have good overall response rates in cancers with NTRK fusions. In a study of 55 adults and children with 12 different tumor types, larotrectinib had a 75% overall response rate (Drilon et al. 2018). A combined analysis of three trials studying entrectinib, with 54 total adult patients across more than 10 tumor types, reported a 57.4% overall response rate, with four complete responses (Demetri et al. 2018). While NTRK fusions are rare (<1%) in most other cancers, it is relatively more common in salivary gland carcinomas, and testing for NTRK is recommended in the metastatic setting.

Immune Checkpoint Inhibition

Immunotherapy, and specifically immune checkpoint inhibition, has transformed the landscape of medical oncology over the past decade. These agents have fewer toxicities and, importantly, provide efficacious treatment for patients. Programmed death receptor ligand (PD-L1) expression is present in 17% of SGC (Vital et al. 2019). Pembrolizumab, a monoclonal antibody directed against PD-1, is approved for all solid tumors with mismatch repair deficiency or high microsatellite instability (Le et al. 2015). In SGC, a phase I trial with pembrolizumab of 26 patients reported an objective response rate of 12% at 20 months, with three partial responses and no complete responses (Cohen et al. 2018).

Summary

- Systemic therapy in the treatment of SGCs is primarily limited to patients with metastatic or recurrent disease.
- The role for chemotherapy in the adjuvant setting is unclear and may be considered in patients with high risk features after tumor resection. However, recent retrospective studies have failed to show benefit for adding concurrent chemotherapy to adjuvant radiation. The RTOG 1008 trial may help shed more light on this issue when results from this study become available.
- In patients with metastatic or recurrent SGCs, the choice of chemotherapy is dependent on several factors including clinical course and histology. Some patients have an indolent course and can be observed without any systemic therapy. In patients with symptomatic and/or progressive disease, both combination and single agent cytotoxic chemotherapy can be considered.
- In patients with ACC, both paclitaxel and gemcitabine have not shown activity and should be avoided.
- The CAP regimen has shown activity against ACC, acinic cell carcinoma, adenocarcinomas, and malignant mixed tumors.
- Agents such as cisplatin, 5-FU, and methotrexate seem to provide better response in patients with MEC and undifferentiated tumors.
- Molecularly targeted therapy holds significant promise in the treatment of SGCs, and several novel agents are now available for use in clinical practice.
- A better understanding of the molecular biology of salivary gland cancers could lead to better treatment options in the future. The rarity and heterogeneity of SGCs pose major challenges to achieving this goal but persistent efforts are needed to achieve better outcomes for the patients.

Case Presentation – *Well, If It Works for Breast Cancer!!*

A 49-year-old man presented in October 2015 with a complaint of left parotid swelling which had increased in size and had become visible two months earlier, but since then had been stable. He had some headaches and earache with a sensation that his left ear was blocked. He also had some restriction in mouth opening. Prior to his appointment, another physician had performed a core needle ultrasound-guided biopsy, which was reported as showing malignant epithelial cells with a differential diagnosis of mucoepidermoid carcinoma, salivary duct adenocarcinoma, squamous cell carcinoma, or adenoid cystic carcinoma. The cells stained positive for CK AE1/2 and were negative for CK5/6 and S-100.

According to the patient, imaging ordered by his primary care physician had apparently shown nodes at levels II and IV. He had multiple pulmonary nodules on chest CT but these had been stable since 2008.

Past Medical History
He had no serious illness and he had never had surgery. He was not taking any medications and had no allergies.

Social History
The patient smoked one pack of cigarettes a day × 20 years.

Examination
On examination, the patient had an obvious left parotid mass, 3.5 × 3 cm that was hard to palpation. The overlying skin did not appear to be involved, but the mass was fixed deeply. He had a slight weakness of the left mandibular branch of the facial nerve. His neck had hard, mobile, palpable nodes at level II, 2 × 1.5 cm; level IV, 1 × 1 cm; and level V, 1 × 1 cm. There were no intraoral findings.

On review of his scans which he had brought with him, his CT showed an extensive mass with invasion of the masseter muscle (Figure 14.2a and b). The mandible was not involved. His MR confirmed multiple enlarged nodes in the neck at levels II, III, and V.

Diagnosis
TIV, N2b, M0 high-grade malignant parotid tumor.

The patient was informed that he would need a total parotidectomy, with the masseter muscle, possible resection of the facial nerve, modified radical neck dissection, and possible soft tissue flap for the resultant hollowing. He was sent for a PET scan to rule out distant metastases, and FNAB of the parotid mass and a cervical node was also ordered.

The patient was reviewed with his PET scans in one week. The PET scan showed a high SUV in the whole parotid region. There were multiple "hot spots" in the neck, but no evidence of distant metastases (Figure 14.2c and d). None of the known pulmonary nodules were FDG avid.

The FNA of the parotid and cervical node was reviewed. Both cytology specimens were positive for high-grade adenocarcinoma (Figure 14.2e). The cells were positive for cytokeratin 7 and negative for p40 and estrogen receptor (ER). Mucicarmine was negative. The profile ruled out SCC and favored a primary adenocarcinoma (the lack of ER staining mitigated against but does not exclude salivary duct carcinoma).

The plan for resection remained the same with the likelihood of sacrifice of the facial nerve being very high given the infiltration of the masseter muscle and deep lobe extension. The reconstruction plan was an anterior lateral thigh flap for replacement of bulk and possible replacement of the overlying skin. The facial nerve would be primarily reconstructed if sacrificed with the femoral motor nerve (from the ALT), or sural nerve or allogenic nerve conduit. A platinum weight was planned for the upper eyelid.

He underwent surgery on November 13, 2015 (Figure 14.2f and g). Histopathology showed a poorly differentiated adenocarcinoma 8.1 × 7.1 × 3.8 cm. There was extensive infiltration into muscle and extensive perineural invasion (the facial nerve was sacrificed) (Figure 14.2h and i). The superior and anterior margins were positive for cancer. One extraparotid node was negative for tumor. Thirty-one of thirty-six lymph nodes were positive for tumor; 1/4 in level I, 5/5 with ENE in level II, 12/12 with ENE in level III, 8/8 with ENE in level IV, and 5/7 in level V (Figure 14.2j and k). There was lympho-vascular invasion. The tumor was positive for HER2/neu overexpression (Figure 14.2l).

In view of his multiple poor prognostic factors including multiple nodes at levels I–V with ENE, positive margins, extensive PNI, he was recommended for chemoradiation by our multidisciplinary tumor board. We also recommend off-label use of Herceptin given the tumors' overexpression of Her2 and some reports of good response in salivary cancers with this profile. He underwent chemoradiation with weekly cis-platinum which was completed on February 11, 2016, followed by one year of monthly Herceptin.

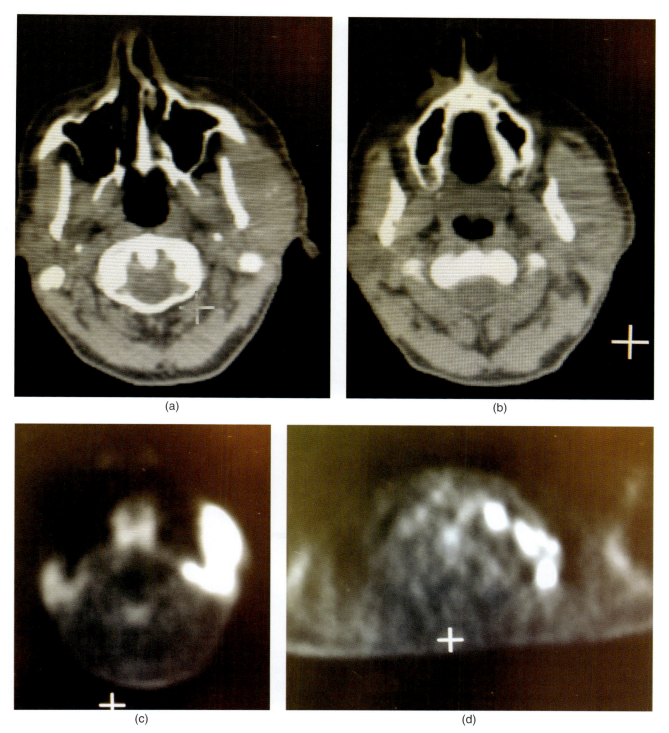

Figure 14.2. (a) Axial CT scan shows a large mass in the left parotid 5.8 × 2.6 cm, confluent with the left masseter muscle. The mass extends beneath the malar arch but the fat plane in the area of the stylomastoid foramen was not involved by tumor. There is a small central area of calcification within the mass. (b) The mass involves both the masseter and the area of the temporalis tendon but the bony mandible is spared. This would account for the patient's history of increased difficulty opening his mouth. Posteriorly, the tumor extends to the sternocleidomastoid muscle. (c) The scan shows intense uptake of the FDG in the entire parotid including the deep lobe extending toward the parapharyngeal area. (d) Axial PET scan of the neck at inferior end level II junction with level III. There are at least five lymph nodes with increased uptake seen on this view.

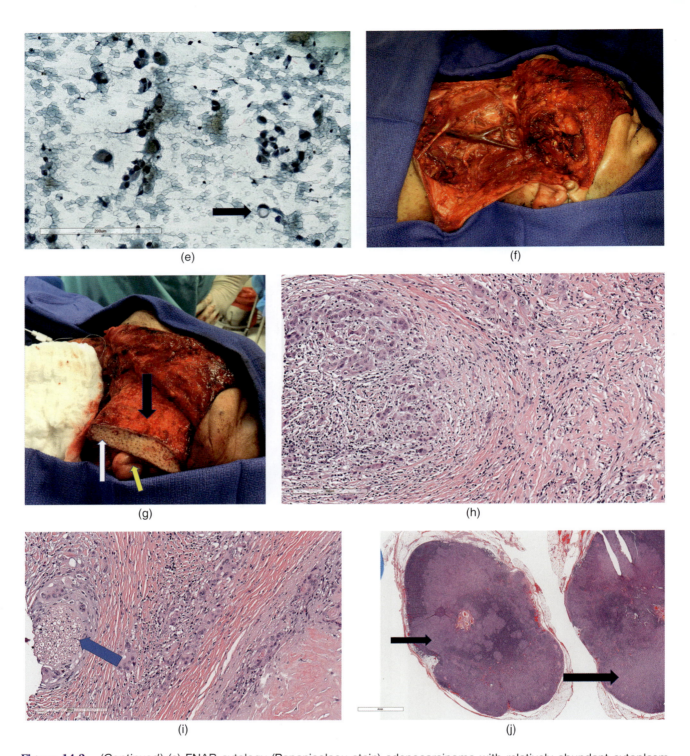

Figure 14.2. (*Continued*) (e) FNAB cytology (Papanicolaou stain) adenocarcinoma with relatively abundant cytoplasm and hyperchromatic nuclei. Occasional signet ring cells are seen (indicated by the blue arrow). Source: By courtesy of Dr. John Papadimitriou, Professor of Pathology, University of Maryland. (f) Post resection intraoperative view. Left modified radical neck dissection with sacrifice of the sternocleidomastoid muscle and accessory nerve, preserving the internal jugular and common facial vein. Left radical parotidectomy with sacrifice of the facial nerve, which was primarily grafted. The left masseter muscle is largely resected. (g) Post resection reconstruction with anterior lateral thigh (ALT) microvascular flap to prevent gross hollowing. The figure shows the insetting of the flap. Yellow arrow shows the left ear lobe. The white arrow points to the thin strip of skin from the thigh that will be sutured preauricularly as a skin monitor for the vascular supply. The black arrow points to the dermis/fascial/fat portion of the de-epithelialized skin paddle used to "bulk out the defect." Source: Reconstruction by Dr. Joshua Lubek, Associate Professor OMFS, University of Maryland. (h) Parotid tumor shows poorly differentiated adenocarcinoma showing cuboidal tumor cells with eosinophilic cytoplasm and vesicular nuclei with prominent nucleoli, arranged in cords or occasionally single cells. Source: By courtesy of Dr. John Papadimitriou, Professor of Pathology, University of Maryland. (i) Shows facial nerve with perineural invasion, completely encapsulated by poorly differentiated adenocarcinoma. Source: By courtesy of Dr. John Papadimitriou, Professor of Pathology, University of Maryland. (j) Bisected cervical lymph node arrows show gross deposits of metastatic adenocarcinoma. Source: By courtesy of Dr. John Papadimitriou, Professor of Pathology, University of Maryland.

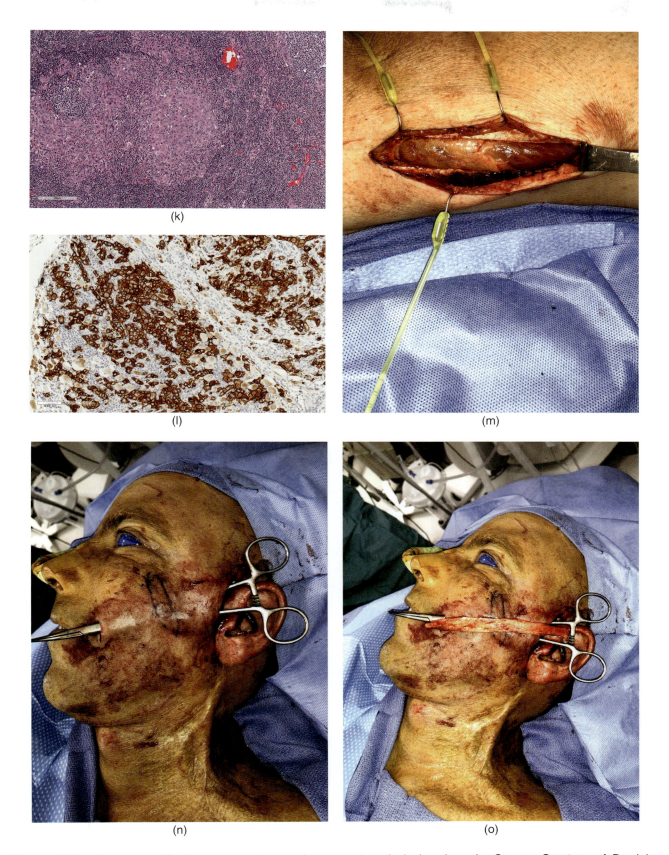

Figure 14.2. (*Continued*) (k) High-power adenocarcinoma metastatic in lymph node. Source: Courtesy of Dr. John Papadimitriou, Professor of Pathology, University of Maryland. (l) Adenocarcinoma HER2/neu immunostain with strong membranous tumor cell staining. Source: By courtesy of Dr. John Papadimitriou, Professor of Pathology, University of Maryland. (m) Harvesting fascia lata strip through lateral thigh incision. Source: Reconstruction by Dr. Joshua Lubek, Associate Professor OMFS, University of Maryland. (n) Subcutaneous tunnel from zygomatic arch/temporalis muscle tendon to commissure of lips. Source: Reconstruction by Dr. Joshua Lubek, Associate Professor OMFS, University of Maryland. (o) Intraoperative view shows how fascia lata strip will be sutured and oriented within the subcutaneous tunnel for a dynamic fascia lata sling. Source: Reconstruction by Dr. Joshua Lubek, Associate Professor OMFS, University of Maryland.

In October 2016, one-year post-surgery, he could achieve lid closure due to his platinum weight but his face still showed total paralysis House Brackmann 6/6 despite his nerve graft. He also had epiphora from a lower lid ectropion and brow sag. The reconstructive plan was for facial reanimation with an endoscopic brow lift and lower lid ectropion repair (oculoplastic surgeon – Dr. Hirschbein), and temporalis adynamic flap and a dynamic fascia lata suspension flap (oral and maxillofacial surgeon – Dr. Lubek). Surgery was performed on October 26, 2016 (Figure 14.2m–o). Four months post-surgery, his speech was good, his epiphora greatly resolved, and he was happy with his facial appearance.

He was last seen on December 4, 2019 four years two months since his original surgery and has had no clinical or imaging sign of cancer.

TAKE-HOME POINTS

1. This case represents an advanced stage IV disease with multiple very poor prognostic features. However, the tumor was positive for Her2 overexpression and the use of off-label Herceptin was attempted. The drug has been successfully used for Her2 overexpression in breast cancer but its use in salivary gland disease is restricted to case reports and small series of high-grade salivary duct adenocarcinoma (some with distant metastasis). Although cis-platinum was used in this case, there is little evidence that it is effective for salivary gland malignancies or in preventing distant metastases. This patient was considered extremely high risk for developing distant disease and had a one-year course of adjuvant Herceptin. Amazingly, he is alive with no evidence of disease four plus years since his original surgery.
2. The other aspect of this case of interest is the facial reanimation surgery that was performed. A platinum eyelid weight and a nerve graft were undertaken primarily in this patient. The nerve graft showed no recovery and secondary reanimation techniques that were used included ectropion repair, endoscopic brow lift, temporalis adynamic flap, and fascia lata facial suspension flap (Figures 16.36–16.38). There are numerous other techniques advocated for dynamic reanimation including the free gracilis transfer, facial nerve to hypoglossal or masseteric nerves, cross facial nerve grafts, and temporalis muscle transfers. In this case, the resection of masseter with its nerve, scarring from the radical radiation, and resection of a large section of the nerve trunk and branches limit choices and add to the complexity.

References

Agulnik M, Cohen EW, Cohen RB et al. 2007. Phase II study of lapatinib in recurrent or metastatic epidermal growth factor receptor and/or erbB2 expressing adenoid cystic carcinoma and non adenoid cystic carcinoma malignant tumors of the salivary glands. *J Clin Oncol* 25:3978–3984.

Airoldi M, Pedani F, Succo G et al. 2001. Phase II randomized trial comparing vinorelbine versus vinorelbine plus cisplatin in patients with recurrent salivary gland malignancies. *Cancer* 91:541–547.

Alberts DS, Manning MR, Coulthard SW, Koopmann CF, Jr, Herman TS. 1981. Adriamycin/cis-platinum/cyclophosphamide combination chemotherapy for advanced carcinoma of the parotid gland. *Cancer* 47:645–648.

American Cancer Society. 2018. *Global Cancer Facts & Figures*, 4th edn. Atlanta, American Cancer Society.

Amini A, Waxweiler TV, Brower JV et al. 2016. Association of adjuvant chemoradiotherapy vs radiotherapy alone with survival in patients with resected major salivary gland carcinoma – Data from the national cancer data base. *JAMA Otolaryngol Head Neck Surg* 142:1100–1110.

Argiris A, Ghebremichael M, Burtness B, Axelrod RS, Deconti RC, Forastiere AA. 2011. A phase 2 trial of bortezomib followed by the addition of doxorubicin at progression in patients with recurrent or metastatic adenoid cystic carcinoma of the head and neck: A trial of the Eastern Cooperative Oncology Group (E1303). *Cancer* 117:3374–3382.

Barnes L, Eveson JW, Reichart P, Sidransky D (eds.). (2005). Tumors of the Salivary Glands. In: *Pathology and Genetics of Head and Neck Tumours*. Lyon, World Health Organization.

Belani CP, Eisenberger MA, Gray WC 1988. Preliminary experience with chemotherapy in advanced salivary gland neoplasms. *Med Pediatr Oncol* 16:197–202.

Bray F, Colombet M, Mery L et al. 2017. *Cancer Incidence in Five Continent*, vol. Xi. Lyon, International Agency for Research on Cancer.

Brunner M, Koperek O, Wrba F et al. 2012. HPV infection and p16 expression in carcinomas of the minor salivary glands. *Eur Arch Otorhinolaryngol* 269:2265–2269.

Caudell JJ, Mifsud M, Rao NG et al. 2014. Postoperative chemoradiation therapy in high-risk salivary gland cancers. *Int J Radiat Oncol* 90:S182–S183.

Chau NG, Hotte SJ, Chen EX et al. 2012. A phase II study of sunitinib in recurrent and/or metastatic adenoid cystic carcinoma (Acc) of the salivary glands: Current progress and challenges in evaluating molecularly targeted agents in Acc. *Ann Oncol* 23:1562–1570.

Cohen RB, Delord J-P, Doi T et al. 2018. Pembrolizumab for the treatment of advanced salivary gland carcinoma. *Am J Clin Oncol* 41:1083–1088.

Coxon A, Rozenblum E, Park YS et al. 2005. Mect1-Maml2 fusion oncogene linked to the aberrant activation of cyclic AMP/CREB regulated genes. *Cancer Res* 65:7137–7144.

Creagan ET, Woods JE, Rubin J, Schaid DJ. 1988. Cisplatin-based chemotherapy for neoplasms arising from salivary glands and contiguous structures in the head and neck. *Cancer* 62:2313–2319.

Dagrada GP, Negri T, Tamborini E, Pierotti MA, Pilotti S. 2004. Expression of HER-2/neu gene and protein in salivary duct carcinomas of parotid gland as revealed by fluorescence in-situ hybridization and immunohistochemistry. *Histopathology* 44:301–302.

De Haan LD, De Mulder PH, Vermorken JB, Schornagel JH, Vermey A, Verweij J. 1992. Cisplatin-based chemotherapy in advanced adenoid cystic carcinoma of the head and neck. *Head Neck* 14:273–277.

Demetri GD, Paz-Ares LG, Farago AF et al. 2018. Efficacy and safety of entrectinib in patients with NTRK fusion-positive (NTRK-fp) tumors: Pooled analysis of STARTRK-2, STARTRK-1 and ALKA-372-001. ESMO Congress 2018.

Dimery IW, Legha SS, Shirinian M, Hong WK. 1990. Fluorouracil, doxorubicin, cyclophosphamide, and cisplatin combination chemotherapy in advanced or recurrent salivary gland carcinoma. *J Clin Oncol* 8:1056–1062.

Dreyfuss AI, Clark JR, Fallon BG, Posner MR, Norris CM, Jr., Miller D. 1987. Cyclophosphamide, doxorubicin, and cisplatin combination chemotherapy for advanced carcinomas of salivary gland origin. *Cancer* 60:2869–2872.

Drilon A, Laetsch TW, Kummar S et al. 2018. Efficacy of larotrectinib in TRK fusion-positive cancers in adults and children. *NEJM* 378:731–739.

Enlund F, Behboudi A, Andren Y et al. 2004. Altered Notch signaling resulting from expression of a Wamtp1-Maml2 gene fusion in mucoepidermoid carcinomas and benign Warthin's tumors. *Exp Cell Res* 292:21–28.

Freier K, Flechtenmacher C, Walch A et al. 2005. Differential Kit expression in histological subtypes of adenoid cystic carcinoma (Acc) of the salivary gland. *Oral Oncol* 41:934–939.

Fushimi C, Tada Y, Takahashi H et al. 2017. A prospective phase Ii study of combined androgen blockade in patients with androgen receptor-positive metastatic or locally advanced unresectable salivary gland carcinoma. *Ann Oncol* 29:979–984.

Ghosal N, Mais K, Shenjere P et al. 2011. Phase II study of cisplatin and imatinib in advanced salivary adenoid cystic carcinoma. *Br J Oral Maxillofac Surg* 49:510–515.

Gilbert J, Li Y, Pinto HA et al. 2006. Phase Ii trial of taxol in salivary gland malignancies (E1394): A trial of the Eastern Cooperative Oncology Group. *Head Neck* 28:197–204.

Glisson B, Colevas AD, Haddad R et al. 2004. Her2 expression in salivary gland carcinomas: Dependence on histological subtype. *Clin Cancer Res* 10:944–946.

Guzzo M, Locati LD, Prott FJ, Gatta G, Mcgurk M, Licitra L. 2010. Major and minor salivary gland tumors. *Crit Rev Oncol Hematol* 74:134–148.

Haddad R, Colevas AD, Krane JF et al. 2003. Herceptin in patients with advanced or metastatic salivary gland carcinomas. A phase Ii study. *Oral Oncol* 39:724–727.

Hafed L, Farag H, Shaker O, El-Rouby D. 2012. Is human papilloma virus associated with salivary gland neoplasms? An in situ-hybridization study. *Arch Oral Biol* 57:1194–1199.

Hill ME, Constenla DO, A'hern RP et al. 1997. Cisplatin and 5-fluorouracil for symptom control in advanced salivary adenoid cystic carcinoma. *Oral Oncol* 33:275–278.

Horn-Ross PL, Ljung BM, Morrow M 1997. Environmental factors and the risk of salivary gland cancer. *Epidemiology* 8:414–419.

Isayeva T, Said-Al-Naief N, Ren Z, Li R, Gnepp D, Brandwein-Gensler M. 2013. Salivary mucoepidermoid carcinoma: Demonstration of transcriptionally active human papillomavirus 16/18. *Head Neck Pathol* 7:135–148.

Jaehne M, Roeser K, Jaekel T, Schepers JD, Albert N, Loning T. 2005. Clinical and immunohistologic typing of salivary duct carcinoma: A report of 50 cases. *Cancer* 103:2526–2533.

Jakob JA, Kies MS, Glisson BS et al. 2015. A phase Ii study of gefitinib in patients with advanced salivary gland cancers. *Head Neck* 37:644–649.

Jones AS, Phillips DE, Cook JA, Helliwell TR. 1993. A randomised phase II trial of epirubicin and 5-fluorouracil versus cisplatinum in the palliation of advanced and recurrent malignant tumour of the salivary glands. *Br J Cancer* 67:112–114.

Jour G, West K, Ghali V, Shank D, Ephrem G, Wenig BM. 2013. Differential expression of p16(INK4A) and cyclin D1 in benign and malignant salivary gland tumors: A study of 44 Cases. *Head Neck Pathol* 7:224–231.

Kaplan MJ, Johns ME, Cantrell RW. 1986. Chemotherapy for salivary gland cancer. *Otolaryngol Head Neck Surg* 95:165–170.

Kurzrock R, Bowles DW, Kang H et al. 2019. Targeted therapy for advanced salivary gland carcinoma based on molecular profiling: Results from MyPathway, a phase IIa multiple basket study. *Ann Oncol* 31:412–421.

Laurie SA, Siu LL, Winquist E et al. 2010. A phase 2 study of platinum and gemcitabine in patients with advanced salivary gland cancer: A trial of the NCIC Clinical Trials Group. *Cancer* 116:362–368.

Laurie SA, Ho AL, Fury MG, Sherman E, Pfister DG. 2011. Systemic therapy in the management of metastatic or locally recurrent adenoid cystic carcinoma of the salivary glands: A systematic review. *Lancet Oncol* 12:815–824.

Le DT, Uram JN, Wang H et al. 2015. PD-1 blockade in tumors with mismatch-repair deficiency. *N Engl J Med* 372:2509–2520.

Licitra L, Marchini S, Spinazze S et al. 1991. Cisplatin in advanced salivary gland carcinoma. A phase II study of 25 patients. *Cancer* 68:1874–1877.

Licitra L, Cavina R, Grandi C et al. 1996. Cisplatin, doxorubicin and cyclophosphamide in advanced salivary gland carcinoma. A phase II trial of 22 patients. *Ann Oncol* 7:640–642.

Lim JJ, Kang S, Lee MR et al. 2003. Expression of vascular endothelial growth factor in salivary gland carcinomas and its relation to p53, Ki-67 and prognosis. *J Oral Pathol Med* 32:552–561.

Limaye SA, Posner MR, Krane JF et al. 2013. Trastuzumab for the treatment of salivary duct carcinoma. *Oncologist* 18:294–300.

Locati LD, Bossi P, Perrone F et al. 2009a. Cetuximab in recurrent and/or metastatic salivary gland carcinomas: A phase II study. *Oral Oncol* 45:574–578.

Locati LD, Perrone F, Losa M et al. 2009b. Treatment relevant target immunophenotyping of 139 salivary gland carcinomas (SGCs). *Oral Oncol* 45:986–990.

Mattox DE, Von Hoff DD, Balcerzak SP. 1990. Southwest Oncology Group study of mitoxantrone for treatment of patients with advanced adenoid cystic carcinoma of the head and neck. *Invest New Drugs* 8:105–107.

Mino M, Pilch BZ, Faquin WC. 2003. Expression of KIT (Cd117) in neoplasms of the head and neck: An ancillary marker for adenoid cystic carcinoma. *Mod Pathol* 16:1224–1231.

Persson M, Andren Y, Mark J, Horlings HM, Persson F, Stenman G. 2009. Recurrent fusion of Myb and Nfib transcription factor genes in carcinomas of the breast and head and neck. *Proc Natl Acad Sci U S A* 106:18740–18744.

Pfeffer MR, Talmi Y, Catane R, Symon Z, Yosepovitch A, Levitt M. 2007. A phase II study of Imatinib for advanced adenoid cystic carcinoma of head and neck salivary glands. *Oral Oncol* 43:33–36.

Pinkston JA, Cole P. 1996. Cigarette smoking and Warthin's tumor. *Am J Epidemiol* 144:183–187.

Press MF, Pike MC, Hung G et al. 1994. Amplification and overexpression of HER-2/neu in carcinomas of the salivary gland: Correlation with poor prognosis. *Cancer Res* 54:5675–5682.

Rodriguez C, El-Naggar A, Adelstein DJ et al. 2008. Radiation therapy oncology group RTOG 1008 a randomized Phase II study of adjuvant concurrent radiation and chemotherapy versus radiation alone in resected high-risk malignant salivary gland tumors. Update. RTOG 1008.

Ruzich JC, Ciesla MC, Clark JI. 2002. Response to paclitaxel and carboplatin in metastatic salivary gland cancer: A case report. *Head Neck* 24:406–410.

Saku T, Hayashi Y, Takahara O et al. 1997. Salivary gland tumors among atomic bomb survivors, 1950-1987. *Cancer* 79:1465–1475.

Schneider AB, Lubin J, Ron E et al. 1998. Salivary gland tumors after childhood radiation treatment for benign conditions of the head and neck: Dose-response relationships. *Radiat Res* 149:625–630.

Schramm VL, Jr., Imola MJ 2001. Management of nasopharyngeal salivary gland malignancy. *Laryngoscope* 111:1533–1544.

Schramm VL, Jr., Srodes C, Myers EN 1981. Cisplatin therapy for adenoid cystic carcinoma. *Arch Otolaryngol* 107:739–741.

Serraino D, Boschini A, Carrieri P et al. 2000. Cancer risk among men with, or at risk of, HIV infection in southern Europe, *AIDS* 14:553–559.

Seethala RR, Stenman G. 2017. Update from the 4th edition of the World Health Organization classification of head and neck tumours: tumors of the salivary gland. *Head and Neck Pathol* 11:55–67.

Skalova A, Starek I, Vanecek T et al. 2003. Expression of HER-2/neu gene and protein in salivary duct carcinomas of parotid gland as revealed by fluorescence in-situ hybridization and immunohistochemistry. *Histopathology* 42:348–356.

Skalova A, Vanecek T, Sima R et al. 2010. Mammary analogue secretory carcinoma of salivary glands, containing the ETV6-NTRK3 fusion gene: A hitherto undescribed salivary gland tumor entity. *Am J Surg Pathol* 34:599–608.

Stenman GR. 2013. Fusion oncogenes in salivary gland tumors: Molecular and clinical consequences. *Head Neck Pathol* 7:12–19.

Suen JY, Johns ME. 1982. Chemotherapy for salivary gland cancer. *Laryngoscope* 92:235–239.

Swanson GM, Burns PB. 1997. Cancers of the salivary gland: Workplace risks among women and men. *Ann Epidemiol* 7:369–374.

Takahashi H, Tada Y, Saotome T et al. 2018. Patients with human epidermal growth factor receptor 2-positive salivary duct carcinoma. *J Clin Oncol* 37:125–134.

Tchekmedyian V, Sherman EJ, Dunn L, et al. 2019. Phase II study of lenvatinib in patients with progressive, recurrent or metastatic adenoid cystic carcinoma. *J Clin Oncol* 37:1529–1537.

Thomson DJ, Silva P, Denton K et al. 2015. Phase Ii trial of sorafenib in advanced salivary adenoid cystic carcinoma of the head and neck. *Head Neck* 37:182–187.

Tognon CE, Somasiri AM, Evdokimova VE et al. 2011. ETV6-NTRK3-mediated breast epithelial cell transformation is blocked by targeting the IGF1R signaling pathway. *Cancer Res* 71:1060–1070.

Van Herpen CM, Locati LD, Buter J et al. 2008. Phase II study on gemcitabine in recurrent and/or metastatic adenoid cystic carcinoma of the head and neck (EORTC 24982). *Eur J Cancer* 44:2542–2545.

Vermorken JB, Verweij J, De Mulder PH et al. 1993. Epirubicin in patients with advanced or recurrent adenoid cystic carcinoma of the head and neck: A phase II study of the EORTC Head and Neck Cancer Cooperative Group. *Ann Oncol* 4:785–788.

Verweij J, De Mulder PH, De Graeff A et al. 1996. Phase II study on mitoxantrone in adenoid cystic carcinomas of the head and neck. EORTC Head and Neck Cancer Cooperative Group. *Ann Oncol* 7:867–869.

Viscuse PV, Price KA, Garcia JJ, Schembri-Wismayer DJ, Chintakuntlawar AV 2019. First line androgen deprivation therapy vs. chemotherapy for patients with androgen receptor positive recurrent or metastatic salivary gland carcinoma – A retrospective study. *Front Oncol* 9:701.

Vital D, Ikenberg K, Moch H, Rössle M, Huber GF. 2019. The expression of PD-L1 in salivary gland carcinomas. *Sci Rep* 9:12724.

Chapter 15
Non-salivary Tumors of the Salivary Glands

Outline

Introduction
Mesenchymal Tumors
  Benign Mesenchymal Tumors
    Hemangiomas
    Lymphangiomas
    Neural Tumors
    Lipomas
  Malignant Mesenchymal Tumors
    Sarcomas
Epithelial Non-salivary Tumors
  Direct Involvement by Skin Cancers
Tumors of Salivary Gland Lymph Nodes
  Primary Lymph Node Tumors
    Lymphomas
  Secondary Lymph Node Tumors
    Mucosal Primary Cancer of the Head and Neck Metastasizing to Salivary Glands
    Cutaneous Cancer Metastasizing to Parotid Nodes
    Distant Metastases to Salivary Glands
Miscellaneous
Summary
Case Presentation – *From One Salivary Gland to Another*
References

Introduction

This chapter discusses the non-salivary tumors that occur in the major salivary glands. Epithelial salivary gland tumors have been discussed in Chapters 10–12. This chapter will be divided into primary benign and malignant mesenchymal tumors and metastatic lesions mostly epithelial in the lymph nodes or substance of the major glands. As the epidemiology and etiology of these tumors are very variable it will be discussed in relation to individual tumors and groups of tumors. Wherever possible, recent references will encompass prospective trials, systematic reviews, meta-analysis, and large series based on population databases, e.g., SEER, NCDB to improve the scientific evidence base for the recommendations given.

Mesenchymal Tumors

BENIGN MESENCHYMAL TUMORS

Hemangiomas

Hemangiomas and hemangioendotheliomas are most commonly seen in the parotid gland and in children where they account for up to 35% of salivary tumors. (Ord 2004) These tumors are most commonly seen under the age of one year and may be present at birth where they may exhibit aggressive growth. Hemangioendotheliomas are more aggressive and rapidly growing and occur in the <6-month infant, while the older children tend to present with the slower growing cavernous lesions (Figure 15.1). The diagnosis can usually be made reliably on clinical examination. Ultrasound can give a firm diagnosis of a vascular lesion with pulsatile fast-flow seen on Doppler. If the diagnosis is not certain or there is doubt regarding the extent of the lesion then MR will show hyperintense T2-weighted images, isointense T1, with intense enhancement post-contrast (Weber et al. 2017). In the past, surgical removal was advocated but as most tumors involute over time and because of the morbidity of surgery in infants this has largely been abandoned in favor of medical therapy. Older papers indicated that vascular malformations of the parotid respond poorly to medical therapy, and

---

Salivary Gland Pathology: Diagnosis and Management, Third Edition. Edited by Eric R. Carlson and Robert A. Ord.
© 2022 John Wiley & Sons, Inc. Published 2022 by John Wiley & Sons, Inc.
Companion website: www.wiley.com/go/carlson/salivary

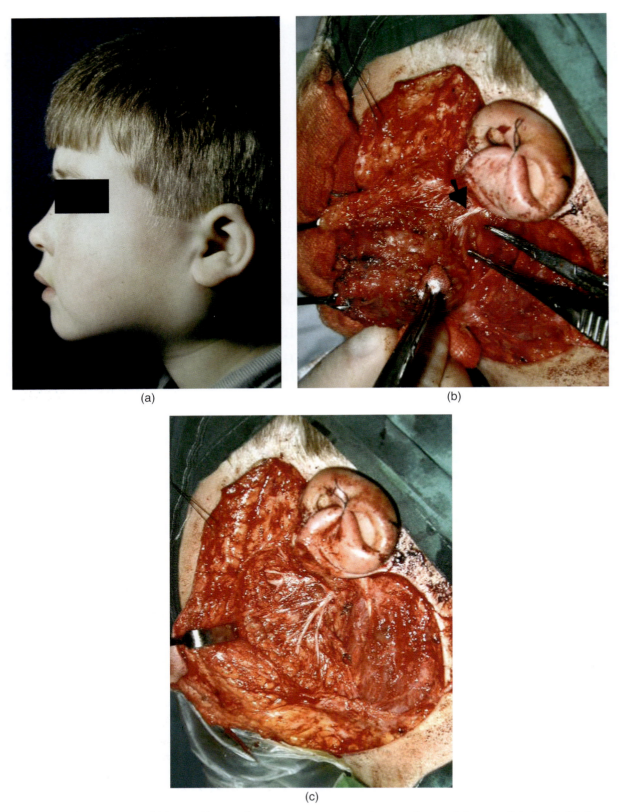

Figure 15.1. (a) three-year-old boy with prominent cavernous vascular neoplasm of the parotid gland. (b) Operative sequence shows the neoplasm is mobilized forward after tying off feeding vessels and is being peeled of the trunk of the facial nerve (arrow). (c) The vascular neoplasm is removed in total with the superficial lobe of the parotid gland after complete facial nerve dissection.

however, this was disproved in the paper by Greene et al. (2004). These authors reviewed 100 consecutive children with a 4.5:1 female-to-male ratio with 59% ulcerating during the proliferating phase and 89% involved nearby structures. Seventy of the patients were treated medically 67 primarily with corticosteroids and 3 with interferon. Initially, 56/67 of the patients treated with steroids showed regression or stabilization but 18 required further treatment with interferon. The overall response to steroids/alfa-2a or -2b interferon was 98% and the authors conclude that parotid gland vascular tumors respond in the same way as hemangiomas elsewhere. Interestingly, 66% of the children required some form of reconstructive surgery during the involuted phase.

In the last 10 years, there has been increased interest in the use of oral Propranolol for head and neck hemangiomas in children. In one study of 39 children (all head/neck sites), including parotid, propranolol therapy resulted in lightening and reduction of hemangioma in 37 of 39. There were no complications but in five patients acebutolol was substituted due to sleep disturbance with propranolol (Fuchsmann et al. 2011). In a retrospective review of 56 patients treated for parotid hemangiomas, 22 patients had steroid therapy and initially responded but 68% rebounded after steroid cessation. Overall, 16 patients had good results with surgery. Ten patients had oral propranolol and 8 of 10 had significant shrinkage within the first month with no side effects. The authors conclude that propranolol seemed a promising new modality for managing parotid hemangiomas (Weiss et al. 2011). Mantadakis et al. (2012) reviewed the current literature and concluded that oral propranolol at therapeutic doses of 2–3 mg/kg per day in divided doses was safe for the management of children with symptomatic hemangiomas and felt it should be considered as the first-line agent in all infants with symptomatic hemangiomas who do not have a pulmonary or cardiovascular contraindication to it. In a follow-up of 15 cases female: male 4:1 with an average age of 8.75 months, 14 were treated with propranolol. 66.&% had complete response and 20% partial response. The average duration of treatment was 9.9 ± 8.45 months. After treatment was completed, two patients relapsed two to three months later and were restarted on therapy (Harris and Phillips 2019). In a large prospective study of 87 patients treated with propranolol, response overall was excellent in 28 (32%), good in 53 (61%), stable in 4 (6%), and poor in 2 (2.3%). Regrowth was seen in

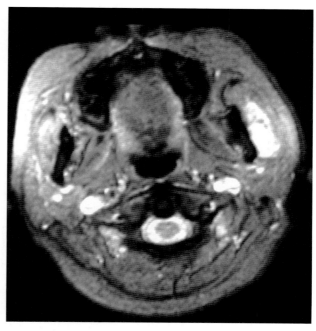

Figure 15.2. MR shows vascular malformation is located intramuscularly in the masseter muscle deep to the parotid.

12.6%. Ten patients had pretreatment Doppler which measured depths, vessel densities, and resistance indices, and these were altered following treatment. The authors concluded that hemodynamic changes might play an important role in propranolol treatment (Chang et al. 2016).

In adults, vascular lesions of the parotid are less common but intramuscular hemangiomas of the masseter muscle can be a diagnostic challenge (Figure 15.2). High-resolution ultrasound and MRI have been suggested for accurate diagnosis of vascular lesions of the parotid in adults (Wong et al. 2004). Vascular lesions of the submandibular gland are seen rarely and like vascular lesions elsewhere will be treated depending on their flow characteristics and the vessel(s) affected (Figure 15.3).

Lymphangiomas

Lymphangiomas may be capillary or cavernous (and associated with vascular malformations) or be cystic in nature. They are common in the neck and seen more in the submandibular (37%) than parotid glands (31%) (Orvidas and Kasperbauer 2000). They may be prominent at birth as cystic hygromas and may pose a threat to the airway (Figure 15.4). In children, they can increase considerably in size during upper respiratory tract infections. Some authors have documented the posterior triangle to be a more common site in the neck than the submandibular space

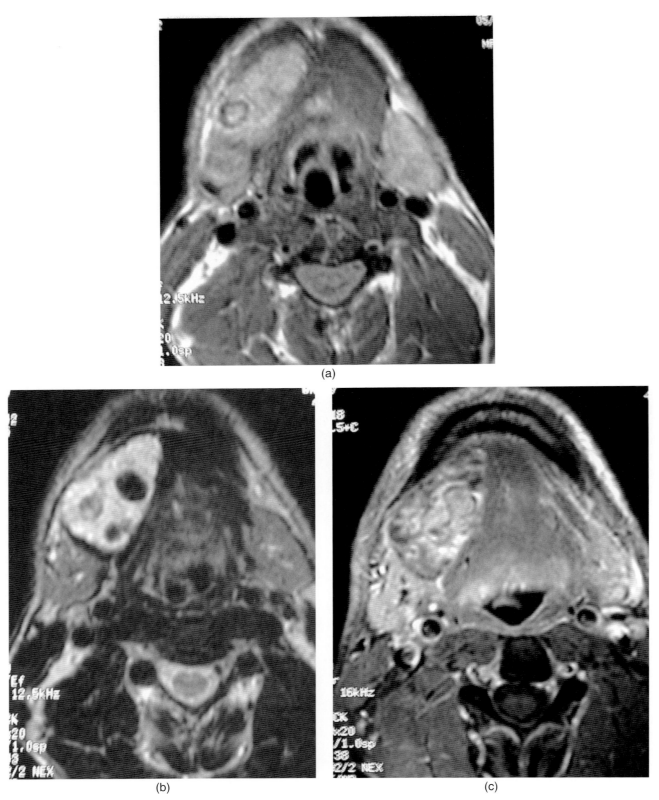

Figure 15.3. (a–c) Vascular malformation in the submandibular region. At the time of surgery, this was found to be cavernous and primarily venous.

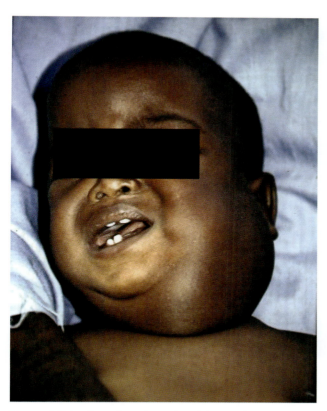

Figure 15.4. Lymphangioma involving both parotid and submandibular glad in an eight-month-old infant.

54% versus 17%, respectively (Fageeh et al. 1997). In 25 cases of cystic hygroma reported in 2012, 12 (48%) were in the posterior triangle, 7 (28%) submandibular, and 3 (12%) in the parotid (Zainine et al. 2012). In a series of 324 pediatric patients with salivary gland masses, 89 (27.5%) were lymphangiomas compared to 192 (59.2%) of hemangiomas (Bentz et al. 2000). Many of these lesions are treated surgically but persistence and recurrence are problematic (Orvidas and Kasperbauer 2000). Especially in the infiltrating lesions, complete excision may be impossible and debulking is performed. Surgery can be combined with sclerosing injections or these can be used as a single modality. Sclerosants are most effective in macro-cystic lymphangiomas, and in 54 of these cases, 49% had excellent results, 35% good, and 16% poor using sclerosant injection (Emran et al. 2006).

A systematic review on the use of doxycycline sclerotherapy in children with head and neck lymphangiomas found five studies all of which were retrospective with a high risk of bias. In this study, 32/38 of children (84.2%) were successfully treated, with 23 (60.5%) of cases having only one treatment. The type of lymphangioma was not related to success (Cheng 2015). Another retrospective study of 38 children with head and neck lymphangiomas treated with doxycycline and sodium tetradecyl sulfate sclerotherapy also found it to be safe and effective. Site of involvement was the face 61.3%, posterior neck 48.4%, submental area 45.2%, and anterior neck 35.5%. Twenty-nine subjects had good follow-up data with 51.7% showing complete resolution, 27.6% moderate improvement, and 20.7% no response. Macrocystic lesions had a significantly higher resolution rate (95.2%) than micro-cystic or mixed lesions (Farnoosh et al. 2015).

A systematic review on treatment of lymphatic malformations with the mTOR inhibitor Sirolimus reviewed 20 studies with 71 patients. Forty-five patients had lymphatic malformations and the rest mixed lymphatic-vascular malformations. Partial remission was seen in 60 cases (84.5%) (Wiegand et al. 2018).

Neural Tumors

In Siefert and Oehne's (1986) review of 150 benign mesenchymal tumors of the salivary glands, 16% were neurogenic in origin distributed over the fourth to seventh decade. These were divided into neurilemmomas (neurinomas) 12 of 27 cases, neurofibromas 12 of 27 cases, and neurofibromatosis 3 of 27 cases. There was a predominance of males 75% for neurofibromas and for females 65% for neurilemmomas. Four out of five salivary neurofibromas in one small series arose in a background of neurofibromatosis type 1 (Guraya and Prayson 2016). Both MR and CT scan may be useful in imaging. In the parotid gland, extension of the tumor in the gland and in the petrous bone is well defined by MR imaging, while CT scan shows bone erosion and relationship to the inner ear. A combination of CT and MR is recommended when surgical resection is planned (Martin et al. 1992).

Complete removal of these lesions especially the plexiform neurofibroma can be extremely difficult due to their infiltrating nature and often increased vascularity (Figure 15.5).

Although approximately one third of neurilemmomas occur in the head and neck (Almeyda et al. 2004), they are comparatively rare in the salivary glands usually published as isolated case reports. However, as they may be mistaken for a malignant parotid tumor due to facial nerve dysfunction, e.g., progressive weakness, sudden facial

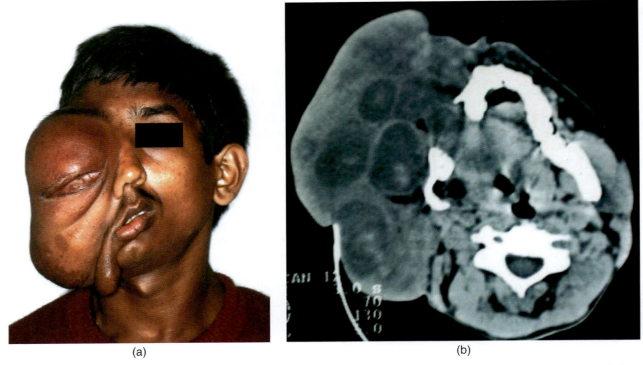

Figure 15.5. (a) Massive plexiform neurofibroma involving the parotid and orbit. (b) CT scan shows extensive soft tissue involvement.

paralysis, hemifacial spasm, and pain (Balle and Greisen 1984), it is important to make the diagnosis to avoid inappropriate radical surgery. Forty-two intra-parotid facial nerve neurilemmomas were found in a series of 5977 parotid tumor cases (0.7%). The authors concluded that tumors involving the main trunk of the facial nerve lead to unsatisfactory nerve outcomes. They recommended that facial nerve preservation was essential and that stripping surgery or intracapsular enucleation could be the preferred method of surgery (Li et al. 2019).

Regarding intraparotid neurofibromas, a "conservative course of treatment with limited tumor excision and emphasis on retaining facial nerve function" is advocated (McGuirt et al. 2003). Indeed, once the histologic diagnosis is made because of the slow growth of the tumor and the unlikelihood of malignant change conservative treatment of leaving the tumor in situ to preserve the nerve has been recommended (Fierke et al. 2006).

Lipomas

Approximately 15–20% of lipomas occur in the head and neck region (Weiss and Goldblum 2001), and in reviewing 125 lipomas in the oral and maxillofacial region, 30 (24%) were parotid and 17 (13.6%) were submandibular (Furlong et al. 2004). In this series, there was a 3:1 male to female gender ratio and a mean age of 51.9 years. Histologically, almost half 62/125 were classic lipomas, while 59 were spindle cell/pleomorphic, 2 were fibrolipomas, and 2 chondroid lipomas. Spindle cell lipomas comprised most of parotid lipomas. In a review of 167 mesenchymal salivary gland tumors, Seifert and Oehne (1986) found lipomas comprised 22.5% of 150 benign tumors and 95% were in the parotid. Again 85% occurred in males. A more recent report of 660 parotid neoplasms found only 8 patients had lipomatous tumors (1.3%), 5 with focal lipoma and 3 with diffuse lipomatosis (Ethunandan et al. 2006). Only one tumor of eight was in the deep lobe but small series of parotid lipomas in the deep lobe are reported (Gooskens and Mann 2006). The largest series of 70 lipomas of the parotid showed 70% male, with 63.2% intra-parotid and 36.8% peri-parotid (Starkman et al. 2013).

Lipomas are comparatively rare in the oral cavity, but in one paper with 46 cases, two patients were classified as having minor salivary gland lipomas (Fregnani et al. 2003). Salivary lipomas usually present as slow growing painless masses and their appearance on CT or MR is diagnostic (Figure 15.6).

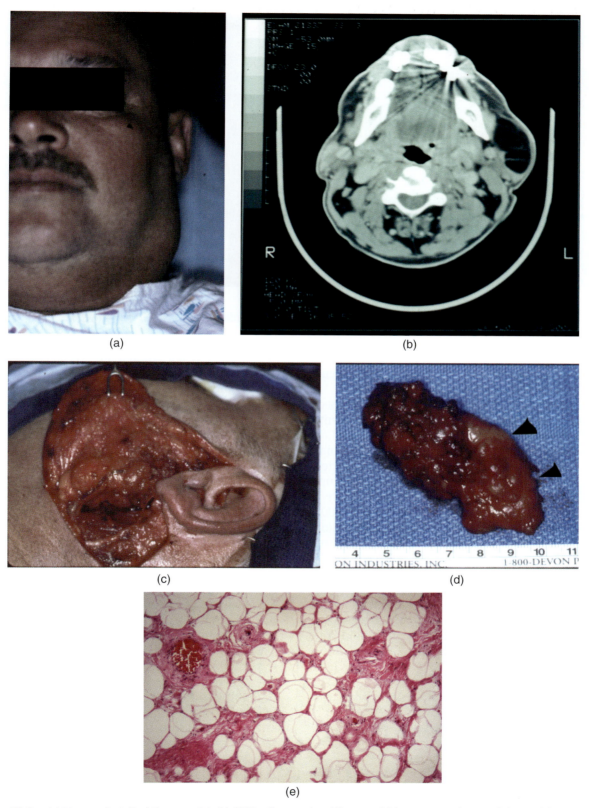

Figure 15.6. (a) Lipoma in tail of the parotid. (b) CT is diagnostic of lipoma. (c) Intra-operative partial parotidectomy with parotid tail lipoma. (d) Specimen with arrows to lipoma. (e) Specimen confirms the lipoma.

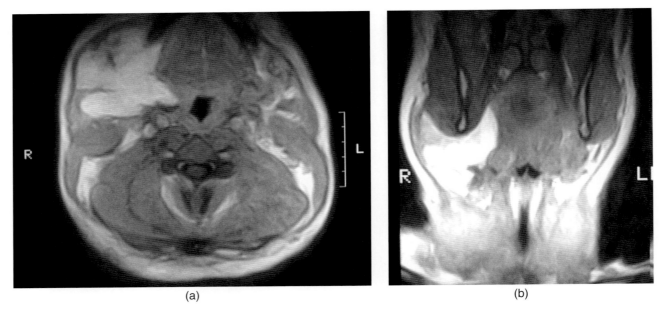

Figure 15.7. (a) and (b) MR images of infiltrating lipoma of submandibular region.

Surgical excision is the treatment of choice, and although easy in classic lipoma, it can be challenging in the infiltrating variety (Figure 15.7).

Recently, a designation of sialolipoma has been proposed for lipomas containing glandular elements, e.g., ductal or acinar tissue (Nagao et al. 2001). In their series of 2051 salivary tumors, 7 sialolipomas, 5 in the parotid, and 2 palatal tumors were reported. Excision of sialolipoma as for classic lipoma is curative. Since the initial report, other cases both in major and minor glands are published Lin et al. 2004; Michaelidis et al. 2006). In a case report of a sialolipoma of the submandibular gland, the literature review found 27 total cases. The parotid was the commonest location 17/27 (60.7%) followed by the palate 4/27 (14.2%) (Jang et al. 2009). A 2013 review of 31 lipomatous lesions of the parotid/submandibular gland found 20 ordinary lipomas, 6 oncocytic lipomas, 4 non-oncocytic sialolipoma, and one microcystic lipoadenoma (Agaimy et al. 2013). Congenital sialolipoma of the parotid have been rarely reported in infants (Mazlumoglu et al. 2015b).

MALIGNANT MESENCHYMAL TUMORS

Sarcomas

Sarcomas of the salivary glands are very rare and case reports of virtually all histologic types have been reported. In Siefert and Oehne's 1986 review of 167 mesenchymal tumors of the salivary glands, only 17 were sarcomas (10%). In this series, 5 cases were malignant fibrous histiocytomas, 5 cases malignant schwannomas, 4 cases embryonal rhabdomyosarcoma, and single cases of myxoid liposarcoma, leiomyosarcoma, and malignant hemangioendothelioma. An 18-year retrospective study from the MD Anderson found only 17 cases, primarily in the parotid. All cases were treated surgically and 76% had adjuvant therapy, 41% of cases recurred and 5-year and 10-year survival was 42% and 20%, respectively. The authors reviewed the literature and found 187 cases of salivary gland sarcoma reported. The commonest sarcomas identified were rhabdomyosarcoma 12.8%, hemangiopericytoma 8.5%, angiosarcoma 7.5%, liposarcoma 7.5%, malignant fibrous histiocytoma 7.5%, and Synovial sarcoma 5.3% (Cockerill et al. 2013). In a study of 184 secondary non-lymphomatous malignancies of the salivary glands, only 4 were sarcomas (2.2%) (Wang et al. 2017).

In reviewing salivary masses in children, rhabdomyosarcomas were the most common malignant mesenchymal tumor 7% (Bentz et al. 2000), and in 137 children with rhabdomyosarcomas of the head and neck, the parotid was the site for 6% of these tumors (Hicks and Flaitz 2002). In a recent report of 140 children with non-parameningeal, rhabdomyosarcomas of the head and neck, 14% were in the salivary glands.

Radiation therapy as first-line treatment was independently prognostic for event-free survival for the entire cohort (Orbach et al. 2017). Obviously, treatment plans will be dictated by the individual sarcoma type with initial chemotherapy for rhabdomyosarcoma in children followed by radiation therapy or surgery for residual disease. Rhabdomyosarcoma of the salivary glands appears locally aggressive with a poor prognosis (BenJelloun et al. 2005).

In malignant fibrous histiocytoma, clear surgical margins appear to be the most important prognostic factor (Sachse et al. 2006). Angiosarcoma may affect the parotid as a primary or metastatic tumor, and in a series of 29 angiosarcomas of the oral and salivary gland region, there were 4 primary parotid and 3 primary submandibular gland angiosarcomas with a further 3 metastatic to the parotid (Fanburg-Smith et al. 2003). All patients with metastatic disease died but patients with primary salivary gland angiosarcoma appear to have a better prognosis than cutaneous or deep tissue angiosarcomas. Malignant neural sarcomas are treated with wide excision and facial nerve grafting or reanimation (McGuirt et al. 2003). Other sarcomas of the salivary glands are rare, e.g., Chadan et al. (2004) found only 11 reported cases of salivary gland liposarcoma in the literature.

Salivary gland swelling is not infrequent in HIV positive and AIDS patients (see Chapter 4). Although rare, Kaposi's sarcoma can be the underlying cause. One series of six cases found four in the submandibular gland and two in the parotid (Castle and Thompson 2000).

The adamantinoma-like Ewing sarcoma (ALES) of the salivary glands has been recognized as a distinct entity. This is an important diagnosis as ALES mimics other small blue round cell tumors especially basaloid salivary carcinomas. It shows the classic EWSR-FLI1 translocation of Ewing's despite expressing epithelial markers such as cytokeratins and p40. In a recent review of 10 cases, (8 parotid, 2 submandibular), nine were initially misdiagnosed. The authors concluded that monotonous cytology despite a highly infiltrative growth pattern when combined with positive p40 and synaptophysin can alert the pathologist to the true diagnosis. ALES can be confirmed by the EWSR translocation (Rooper et al. 2019). Other papers have advocated using CD99 in round cell malignancy, as a screen, even when the tumor shows strong expression of cytokeratins. If CD99 is strongly positive, then testing for the EWSR1 gene rearrangement is indicated (Bishop et al. 2015). Sarcomas can involve any of the major salivary glands although the parotid gland is most common and due to their rarity, treatment is usually on an individual and empiric basis (Figure 15.8).

Epithelial Non-salivary Tumors

DIRECT INVOLVEMENT BY SKIN CANCERS

The major salivary glands may be infiltrated by squamous cell carcinoma from the overlying skin or be primarily involved by melanoma. Surgical resection with a margin of normal tissue preserving the facial nerve and utilizing neck dissection and adjuvant radiotherapy as indicated by the tumor stage is the appropriate treatment (Figure 15.9). Depending on stage and molecular biomarkers immunotherapy with check point inhibitors may be indicated for melanomas.

Tumors of Salivary Gland Lymph Nodes

PRIMARY LYMPH NODE TUMORS

Lymphomas

Since the last edition of this book, there has been a significant revision of the World Health Organization Classification of Head and Neck Hematolymphoid Tumors. In addition to the inclusion of CD30-Positive T-cell lymphoproliferative disorders which typically affect the oral cavity and other mucosal surfaces, there has been updating of the increased understanding in the molecular biology for many of the lymphomas. Space does not allow an in-depth review of all these changes. Those readers who are interested in reviewing the new classification can read the comprehensive article by Brown and Elenitoba-Johnson (2017).

Primary lymphoma of the salivary glands is rare and comprises primarily non-Hodgkin Lymphoma (NHL), only 3.5% of parotid lymphoma is due to Hodgkin lymphoma (HL) (Feinstein et al. 2013). Interestingly, when found in the parotid gland HL is mostly intra-nodal, (Agaimy et al. 2015), whereas NHL tends to be extra-nodal

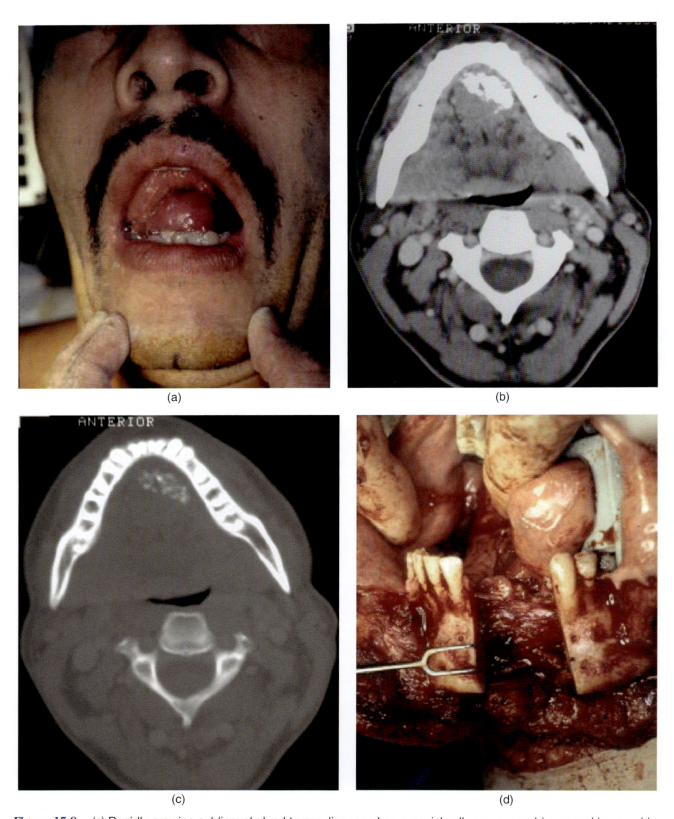

Figure 15.8. (a) Rapidly growing sublingual gland tumor diagnosed as synovial cell sarcoma on biopsy and immunohistochemistry. (b) and (c) CT images reveal calcification in the mass leading to an initial clinic diagnosis of a high-grade malignant carcinoma ex-pleomorphic adenoma. (d) Access via a lip split and mandibulotomy. (e) Bilateral selective neck dissections in continuity with resection of the floor of mouth and partial glossectomy. (f) Surgical specimen. (g) Post-resection the reconstruction will be a microvascular forearm flap. (h) Four weeks post-surgery. (i) intraoral view showing the forearm flap reconstruction of the floor of mouth.

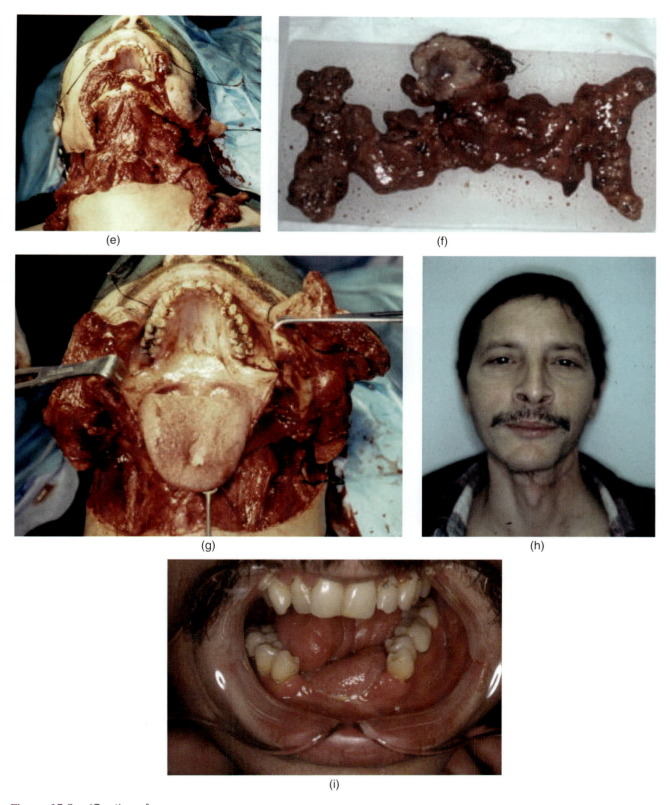

Figure 15.8. (Continued).

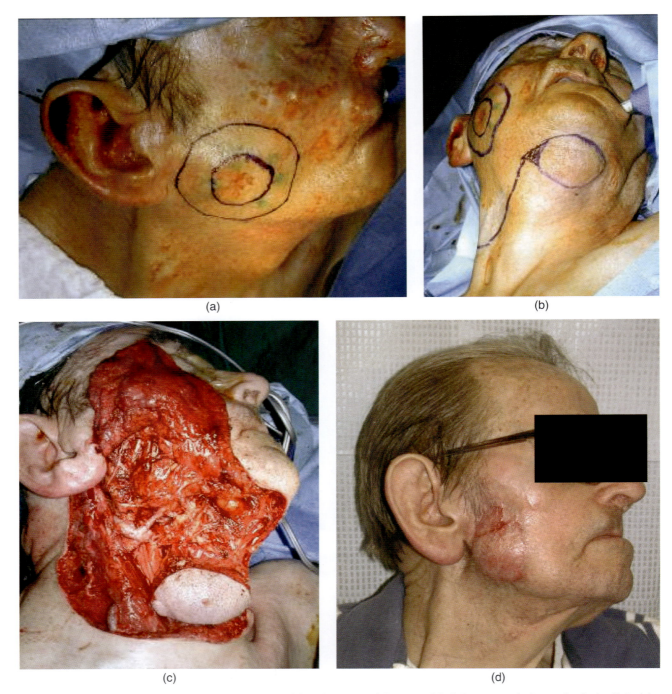

Figure 15.9. (a) Elderly man with primary desmoid melanoma of the parotid. A 2 cm margin is marked, the light blue staining of the skin around the lesion is from dye injection for sentinel node biopsy (patient has had lymphoscintigraphy immediately preoperative). (b) Markings for the proposed surgery which is a total parotidectomy with left supraomohyoid neck dissection (unless sentinel nodes are found at Levels IV or V). Reconstruction with a submental flap based on the submental vessels. (c) The neck dissection and parotidectomy with preservation of the facial nerve is complete, the submental flap is pedicled on its vascular supply prior to be rotated into the defect. (d) Three months postoperative.

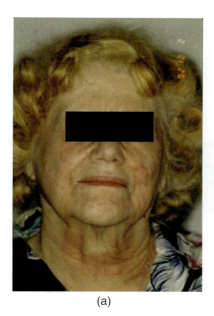
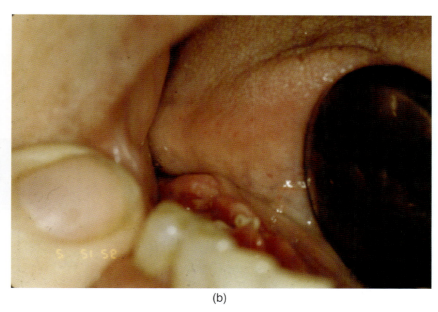

Figure 15.10. (a) Elderly lady with itchy facial and neck rash who complains of an intraoral swelling. (b) The patient's finger is retracting the commissure and the mouth mirror the tongue and a red fleshy swelling of the sublingual gland can just be appreciated. Biopsy showed a non-Hodgkin lymphoma of the sublingual gland.

in the gland parenchymal lymphoid tissue. In a series of 580 cases of extranodal lymphomas, 190 (33%) were present in the head and neck. The most common site was tonsil 34% followed by salivary glands (16%) (Hart et al. 2004).

Primary lymphoma of the salivary glands is found 80% of the time in the parotid gland and 20% in the submandibular gland with only case reports of sublingual and minor gland involvement (Eraso et al. 2005) (Figure 15.10). The authors in 1013 cases of salivary gland tumors have only diagnosed 3 sublingual gland lymphomas. All three were non-Hodgkin lymphoma, one was a marginal zone B-cell lymphoma, one a large B-cell lymphoma, and the other non-specified non-Hodgkin lymphoma. The largest series of sublingual gland lymphomas appears to be four reported in the Chinese literature (Li et al. 2009). Other authors have found a higher incidence of submandibular involvement (39%) (Dunn et al. 2004). In 121 parotid tumors, 8.3% were lymphomas (Shine et al. 2006), and in 51 submandibular tumors, 14% were lymphomas (Preuss et al. 2007). Patients with Sjögren syndrome, AIDS, and hepatitis C have an increased risk of developing salivary lymphomas. In a review of 463 cases of Sjögren's syndrome (SS), 27 patients had a diagnosis of lymphoma (5.8%) (Tonami et al. 2003). In this series, 26 of the 27 patients had non-Hodgkin lymphoma (including 6 mucosa-associated lymphoid tissue MALT lymphomas) and only 1 patient had Hodgkin lymphoma. At the initial presentation, 14 (52%) of patients had extra-nodal disease, with 9 of 27 (33%) in the salivary glands. However, 21 patients (78%) had nodal involvement mostly in the cervical nodes. Masaki and Sugai (2004) also give a figure of 5% of Stage III Sjogren patients developing lymphomas which are thought to arise from lymphoepithelial lesions. The B cells in these lesions become activated by interactions between CD40L and CD40 with progression from polyclonal lymphoproliferation to monoclonal lymphoproliferation to MALT lymphoma and finally to high grade lymphoma as a multistep process. Other authors have highlighted the difficulty diagnosing true lymphoma from the other lymphoproliferative disorders occurring in Sjögren's syndrome although there is a 40-fold increased risk in developing B-cell lymphomas (Prochorec-Sobieszek and Wagner 2005). In a Swedish population study, 105 patients with SS and lymphoma were identified 32% had diffuse large B-cell lymphoma (DLBCL) and 31% marginal zone lymphoma including MALT lymphoma. The proportion of DLBCL was equivalent to the general non-SS population, in contrast marginal zone lymphoma was significantly increased (general population 5%). Men accounted for 15% of the SS lymphomas twice the proportion in the general SS population. Men had shorter time from SS diagnosis to developing lymphoma (one vs eight years $p = 0.0003$) and were more likely to have their lymphomas in the salivary glands (56 vs 29% $p = 0.04$) (Vasaitis et al. 2020).

Clinical features associated with lymphoma include persistent major salivary enlargement (>2 months), persistent lymphadenopathy or splenomegaly, monoclonal gammopathy, and type II mixed cryoglobulinemia. In a systematic review of studies exploring biomarkers attempting to predict development, course and effect of treatment for lymphomas developing in Sjögren syndrome 58 studies were eligible for inclusion. Parotid enlargement, mixed monoclonal cryoglobulins, and low C4 levels were the strongest predictor of lymphoma development. The role of histological biomarkers and specifically germinal centers remains controversial (Delli et al. 2019). Recently, there is evidence that shear wave elastography combined with gray-scale ultrasound may be useful to identify parotid lymphoma in Sjögren syndrome (SS). In this study of 35 patients with SS, 8 were found to have MALT lymphomas. When shear wave elastography findings of high stiffness were added to ultrasound findings of hyperechoic bands in more than half the parenchyma, large hyperechoic area > 20 mm and traced gland area > 5 cm², the sensitivity was 92.3%, specificity was 100%, PPV 100% and NPV 98.3% for the diagnosis of non-Hodgkin lymphoma. The authors conclude that the higher stiffness of parotid NHL can be used for early diagnosis, biopsy guidance, and possible treatment monitoring (Bădărinză et al. 2020).

Hepatitis C is also associated with MALT lymphomas of the salivary glands. In a series of 33 cases of primary salivary, MALT lymphomas 15 patients had a history of Sjögren's syndrome (42%), 2(6%) other autoimmune disease, and 7(21%) hepatitis C infection (Ambrossetti et al. 2004). There is an increase in lymphoma in AIDS; however, although 51% of patients in a study of 100 patients who died with AIDS with no salivary gland symptoms showed histologic signs of parotid disease, only one case of lymphoma was found (Vargas et al. 2003) (Figure 15.11).

Not all primary salivary lymphomas fall into the MALT group and Follicular lymphomas

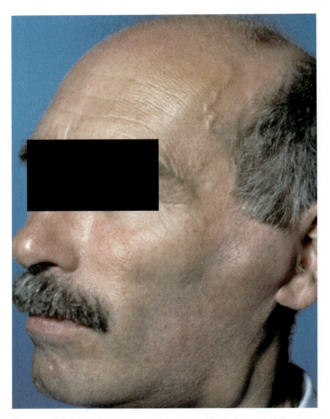

Figure 15.11. 52-year-old man with left parotid mass and firm Level II node who has a salivary lymphoma as a presenting sign of previously undiagnosed AIDS.

comprise 30 and 22% of two published series (Kojima et al. 2001; Nakamura et al. 2006). (Figure 15.12) These lymphomas have a younger age of onset than MALT lymphomas, do not occur in patients with autoimmune disease, and appear relatively more common in the submandibular gland.

Most salivary lymphomas present as unilateral, painless masses, usually with a history of <4 months and although CT scans show poorly defined indistinct margins there is no pathognomonic sign for salivary lymphoma (Shine et al. 2006; Shum et al. 2014). The lesions may be multiple in the ipsilateral gland and lymphadenopathy can be associated. The use of FNAB in diagnosing salivary lymphoma is questioned as inaccurate with high rates of false-negative results. Zurrida et al. (1993) were only able to identify 2 of 7 lymphomas (28.6%), and Hughes et al. (2005) found a 57% false-negative rate in salivary lymphomas in reviewing the data from the College of American Pathologists Interlaboratory Comparison

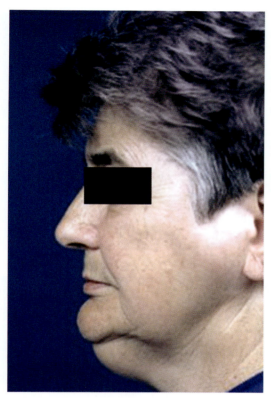

Figure 15.12. Non-Hodgkin lymphoma of the left parotid and submental node.

Program in Non-gynecologic cytology. In a review of FNAB versus core needle biopsy (CNB) of the cervical nodes and salivary glands, the FNAB gave false negatives for all cases of lymphoma (Park et al. 2018). In a study of 237 lymphoma patients who had CNB, the CNB was 97% fully diagnostic 230/237 (Skelton et al. 2015). However, a systematic review of the effectiveness of fine-needle aspiration biopsy and/or core needle biopsy for subclassifying lymphoma looked at 42 studies which showed the median sub-type specific diagnosis of lymphoma was 74%. They concluded that 25–35% of fine needle or core aspirates had to be followed by an excisional node biopsy (Frederiksen et al. 2015).

In the absence of Sjögren syndrome or clinical suspicion of lymphoma, these lesions are frequently diagnosed following surgical removal.

Treatment of salivary lymphoma is by chemotherapy, medical therapy, and radiation therapy depending on the histologic diagnosis and the clinical staging. MALT lymphomas of salivary gland appear to have a low-grade indolent course with 5-year overall survival, cause-specific survival, and progression-free survival of 85% (±8%), 94% (±6%) and 65% (±10%), respectively (Ambrossetti et al. 2004). These results were despite 42% of their patients being stage IV, and local therapy was often adequate (Figure 15.13). In their series of 23 primary salivary lymphomas, 19 MALT, 3 diffuse large cell and 1 follicular, Dunn et al. (2004) found overall 5-year survival of 94.7% and relapse-free survival of 51.4%. Only two patients died, one patient with MALT lymphoma transformed into diffuse large cell lymphoma and died. In a series of 63 patients with MALT lymphoma involving the salivary glands, 41 received multimodal therapy (37 with surgery as a treatment and 9 by surgery alone. Five-year disease-free survival was 54.4%, disease-specific survival 93.2%, and overall survival 81.7%. Factors significant for disease-free survival were the use of RT, stage, and residual tumor. Factors significant in disease-specific survival were stage, recurrence, and residual tumor. The authors concluded that recurrence can occur in up to 35% at 5 years although survival is not affected and that radiotherapy is the only modality that improves disease specific survival (Anacak et al. 2012).

A large study of extra-nodal marginal zone MALT lymphoma of the salivary glands using the SEER database with 577 cases available for frequency/incidence analysis and 712 for relative survival. The parotid gland was the site of 80.9% of cases and 73% of patients were female. Fifteen-year relative survival was 78.4% worse in blacks and advanced stage disease. There was no survival difference between cases treated with surgery, RT, or both. The study concludes that early-stage disease could be treated by unimodality therapy and that even advanced stage disease has a relatively high survival (Vazquez et al. 2015). An updated SEER review of 2140 cases of parotid lymphoma found that 72% had some type of surgery. Survival decreased with age > 50 years, advanced stage, male gender, non-Hodgkin-lymphoma and unmarried status (Feinstein et al. 2013).

A study of MALT lymphoma (isolated extra-nodal mantle cell lymphoma) showed 17.13% of 127 patients to have tumors located in the oral cavity or salivary glands. These MALT MCL patients showed better PFS and OS than classical nodal mantle cell lymphomas and had a more indolent course (Morello et al. 2019). In 105 patients with MALT lymphoma in the oro-maxillofacial region, 81% involved the major salivary glands and 52% of patients had long-term

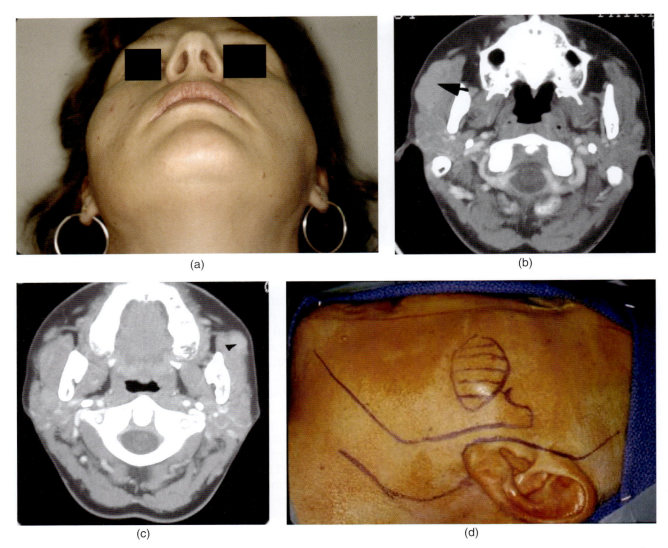

Figure 15.13. (a) 35-year-old lady with MALT lymphoma of Waldeyer's ring controlled by chem.otherapy. Now has bilateral parotid involvement which is not responding to medical therapy and she is concerned regarding her appearance. (b) and (c) CT scans show bilateral parotid involvement which has slowly increased in size over a 3-year period. (d) Proposed parotidectomy and excision of MALT lymphoma.

xerostomia, autoimmune disease, or chronic parotitis. The study suggested a satisfactory outcome after initial treatment and that MALT lymphoma progresses slowly (Zhang et al. 2020.)

Kojima et al. (2001) noted that follicular lymphomas arising from salivary glands appeared to share some of the characteristics of MALT lymphoma with an indolent prognosis. A meta-analysis of treatment of non-Hodgkin lymphoma of the parotid found radiation therapy was a valid treatment for early-stage NHL, and surgery (parotidectomy), had a similar outcome for early-stage MALT lymphoma. In diffuse large B-cell lymphoma combination treatment afforded a better survival outcome than single modality (Jamal 2017).

SECONDARY LYMPH NODE TUMORS

Mucosal Primary Cancer of the Head and Neck Metastasizing to Salivary Glands

The lymph nodes associated with the major salivary glands may be involved by regional metastases from mucosal primary SCC in the head and neck. The risk of oral cavity and oropharyngeal primary SCC metastasizing to lymph nodes, in or related to, the major salivary glands will be reviewed in this section. Embryologically, the parotid gland develops earlier than the submandibular and sublingual glands. However, between the 18th and 25th week in utero when the glands become encapsulated the parotid gland is encapsulated last. This is important because the lymphatic system develops within the mesenchyme after the submandibular and sublingual glands have developed their capsules. This means that the submandibular and sublingual glands do not normally have intraglandular nodes, whereas the lymphatic system develops prior to the encapsulation of the parotid (Goldenberg et al. 2000). It is the parotid that has the potential for metastases to intraglandular nodes whereas the nodes associated with the other major glands are outside the capsule. Most of the parotid nodes are inferior in the parotid tail region. The parotid tail has always been a recognized part of the radical neck dissection.

The submandibular gland has traditionally been taken in neck dissections that encompass level I. Given that the associated lymph nodes are separate from the gland itself, there has been much discussion on whether it can be preserved in early oral cancer (Cakir Cretin et al. 2018). In one paper, the literature review showed metastasis to the submandibular gland was rare and found in only 2/2074 cases (0.096%) (Panda et al. 2015).

Selective neck dissections have become increasingly more common for early-stage OSCC with a N0 neck, so that the neck dissection is usually performed separately from the primary, not as a composite in-continuity resection. This means that the sublingual gland and its associated nodes are not routinely removed for tongue and floor of mouth primary OSCC. If these nodes were the sentinel node in some oral cancers, it would explain why recurrence sometimes occurs "locally," despite excellent margins (see discussion below).

Parotid node metastasis from primary oral squamous cell carcinoma OSCC is unusual, mostly documented in short series and case reports. In a review of 1358 OSCC cases, only 10 patients with parotid metastases were identified (0.74%). All parotid metastases were poorly differentiated with T3/4 primaries. These metastases were frequently following neck dissection and radiation therapy. Five-year survival was 38.9% (Zhang et al. 2019a, b). A series of 253 cases who had undergone 289 neck dissections in which the tail of the parotid had been resected, is reported. From 183 of the neck dissections, 539 parotid nodes (222 extraglandular and 317 intraglandular) were collected. Ten patients of the 253 cases had positive parotid nodes (4%), and the rate in OSCC was 2.5% (Harada and Omura 2009). Another small series identified 12 cases of parotid metastases from the oral cavity and the oropharynx. Nine of these arose from oropharyngeal primary sites and three from the oral cavity. Again, in this series all tumors were grade 3 or 4 (Olsen et al. 2011). Metastases to the parotid from the oral cavity are more common if the usual lymphatic drainage pattern has been disrupted by previous neck dissection or radiation therapy (Ord et al. 1989). It is also possible for oral mucosal melanoma to metastasize to the parotid region (see Figure 15.18). Although the parotid tail is the most common site, there are nodes in the superficial and deep parotid lobes which have the potential to be involved in metastatic disease (Garatea-Creglo et al. 1993).

It is very rare indeed for non-squamous cell carcinoma of the oral cavity to metastasize to the parotid lymph nodes (see case presentation).

There are fewer reports of the submandibular gland being directly involved by lymph node metastases despite its routine removal during neck dissection. A few cases of secondary involvement of the gland due to extra nodal extension of overlying nodes have been published, but more commonly involvement is due to direct invasion from large T4 floor of mouth OSCC (Cetin et al. 2018). As previously stated, lymph nodes are not usually found within the submandibular gland's capsule, however, Preuss et al. (2007) found that in 24 malignant submandibular gland tumors, 33% were metastatic, 3 from the oropharynx, 2 from the nasopharynx, and 2 with unknown primaries.

Metastatic spread from tongue cancer to sublingual nodes is not common and was first reported in three cases in 1985 (Ozeki et al. 1985). In one study of 253 patients with 326 neck dissections, 5 cases of lingual lymph node metastases were found, and in all these cases, additional bilateral cervical nodes were found (Woolgar 1999). In a multi-center study between the University of Maryland and Peking Union Medical College, we were only able to identify two cases (Zhang et al. 2011). Whether these may explain some cases of "local" recurrence with previous negative margins is unclear. Certainly, these lingual nodes would be removed in composite or "commando" resections where the tongue primary is removed in continuity with the neck dissection, but they may be left in cases where the primary is resected from an intraoral approach and the neck dissection is done separately. One study reports a five-year actuarial survival of 80% for patients treated with in-continuity neck dissection compared to 63% for those with discontinuity dissection (Leemans et al. 1991). However, these findings were contradicted in a later study which retrospectively studied 193 patients grouped into three cohorts of in-continuity, discontinuous resection, and delayed discontinuous neck dissection. There was no difference in disease-free survival, cancer-specific survival, or between early-stage and late-stage disease in the three cohorts (Tesseroli et al. 2006).

Another mucosal primary site with a propensity to metastasize to the parotid lymph nodes is the nasopharynx (NPC). This cancer is more common in Chinese populations, related to EBV infection, and most large series are reported from the Far East. An MRI study of 2221 patients with untreated non-metastatic NPC, who were treated with intensity-modulated radiation therapy (IMRT), found 64 patients developed parotid metastases (2.9%). Interestingly, 34 had parotid sparing IMRT and 30 had parotid-radical IMRT. Parotid nodes were associated with retropharyngeal nodes, level II nodes with ENE, N3 nodes, and parapharyngeal extension. Parotid sparing IMRT was not an independent prognostic factor. OS at five years was 70.4%, and most deaths were associated with distant metastases (Xu et al. 2016). In the largest study from a single center of 10 126 patients with nasopharyngeal cancers (2009–2016), only 43 (0.4%) were identified as having parotid node metastases. 38/43 (88.4%) also had cervical nodes at level II and 15/43 (34.9%) nodes at level Ib. The three-year DFS was 70%, and distant metastasis-free survival was 74.8% which was equivalent to patients with N3 disease (Zhang et al. 2019c).

Cutaneous Cancer Metastasizing to Parotid Nodes

Skin cancers particularly squamous cell carcinoma (SCC) and malignant melanoma (MM) of the scalp, forehead, temple, upper lip, cheek, and ear are most common although Merkel cell tumors, malignant syringomas, and other more unusual skin cancers may metastasize to parotid nodes (Figure 15.14). The largest experience with these tumors is in Australia where squamous cell carcinoma and melanoma of the facial skin are epidemic and

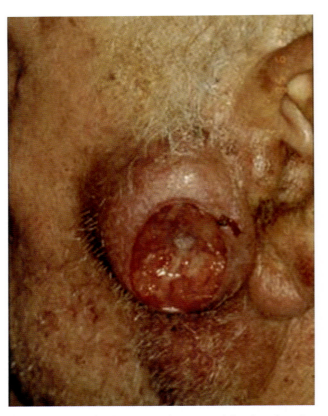

Figure 15.14. Malignant syringoma of forehead metastatic to left parotid and fungating through preauricular skin.

metastatic cutaneous cancer is the commonest parotid malignancy (O'Brien et al. 2002).

Although fewer than 5% of patients with cutaneous, SCC do metastasize to lymph nodes certain features may make these tumors at increased risk of metastasizing. In a review of 266 patients, 61% having parotid lymph node involvement ± cervical involvement; tumor thickness > 4–5 mm., and proximity to the parotid (temple/forehead, cheek, or ear) were high risks, and increasing tumor size and recurrence contribute to an increased risk (Vaness et al. 2006). In 2002, O'Brien et al. suggested that the TNM system of designating all nodal metastases from cutaneous cancer N1 was limited and did not accurately delineate the extent of disease. They suggested separating disease in the parotid P1 < 3 cm, P2 > 3 cm. and < 6 cm. P3 > 6 cm. from neck disease: N0 no nodal disease, N1 a single node < 3 cm, N2 multiple nodes or any node > 3 cm. for staging. In a multivariate analysis of 87 patients, they found that increasing P Stage, positive margins, and lack of adjuvant RT independently predicted for decreased local control in the parotid. Clinical and pathologic N stage both significantly impacted survival. They concluded that patients with positive nodes in both parotid and neck had the worst prognosis and that prognosis was worse for nodal disease > N1 (Figure 15.15). A much smaller study

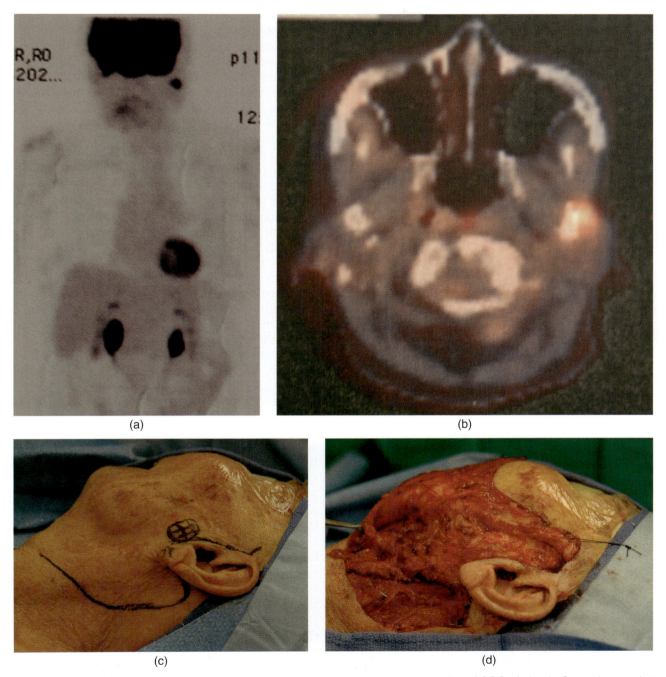

Figure 15.15. (a) PET scan of elderly lady with left preauricular mass post-resection of SCC of cheek. Scan shows a hot spot SUV 6.7. (b) Fused PET/CT confirms positive node in the parotid. (c) Proposed surgery of superficial parotidectomy with extended Blair incision to allow for supraomohyoid neck dissection. (d) Incision allows wide access down to level III. (e) Postoperative patient has no nerve weakness.

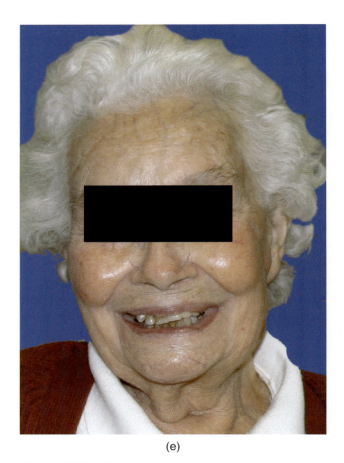

(e)

Figure 15.15. (*Continued*).

from Israel showed a 0% overall survival for patients with both parotid and cervical nodes positive for metastatic cutaneous SCC (Barzilai et al. 2005). Using the separate staging system for parotid disease (P) and neck disease (N) proposed by O'Brien et al. (2002), two further studies have been published. One series of 67 patients from New Zealand found again that the extent of parotid disease was an independent prognostic factor and that patients with both parotid and neck disease did worst although interestingly adjuvant RT did not influence survival in their data (Ch'ng et al. 2006). The second paper was a retrospective multi-center trial from 3 Australian and 3 US centers with 322 patients with metastatic cutaneous SCC to the parotid and/or neck. Results from this study show a significantly worse five-year survival for patients with advanced P stage 69% vs 82% for early P stage; and 61% with parotid + neck disease vs 79% for parotid alone. This study supported the adoption of the new staging system separating parotid and neck disease (Andruchow et al. 2006).

In terms of treatment of metastatic cancer to the parotid, Bron et al. (2003) reviewed 232 cases of which 54 were primary parotid cancers, 101 were metastatic cutaneous SCC, 69 MM and 8 with other metastatic cancers. Patients were treated with primary surgery sparing the facial nerve where indicated, with 54 therapeutic and 110 elective neck dissections and 78% of the patients had adjuvant RT. Five-year survival rates were 77% for primary cancers, 65% for metastatic SCC, 46% for MM, and 56% for other metastatic cancers. As expected, local failure was highest in metastatic SCC and distant failure in MM.

In treating patients with nodal involvement of the parotid, superficial parotidectomy with wide excision to obtain negative margins is indicated with facial nerve sacrifice if it is infiltrated. When the neck is also involved level II is the commonest site and, in these cases, a comprehensive neck dissection recommended. If the neck is clinically uninvolved (N0), and the primary cancer anterolateral to the parotid then a supraomohyoid neck dissection including the external jugular nodes is indicated, (Figure 15.15), with positive cervical nodes a modified radical or radical neck dissection is indicated, (Figure 15.16) and with a posterior primary, level V should be dissected as well (Figure 15.17) (Vauterin et al. 2006). Adjuvant RT is given in node-positive necks for close margins or perineural invasion. In the case of MM where sentinel lymph nodes are identified in the parotid by scintigraphy, intraparotid sentinel lymph node biopsy is a reliable, accurate, and safe procedure (Loree et al. 2006) (see Figure 15.9). SPECT/CT has been used to evaluate sentinel nodes in the parotid and external jugular chain with a specificity of 88.9%, sensitivity of 69.2%, and PPV of 85.7% (Sethi et al. 2018). In two recent comprehensive reviews of the management of regional nodes from squamous cell carcinoma and malignant melanoma of the skin, the authors examined the role of surgery in the neck and parotid gland. In malignant melanoma for P0/N0, the authors do not recommend elective neck dissection but sentinel node biopsy. Even in positive sentinel node biopsy, the authors provide evidence that a completion neck dissection does not confer a five-year survival benefit over a watch and wait policy. In P + N0 therapeutic parotidectomy and neck dissection levels, I-V is recommended, and in P0 N+ if

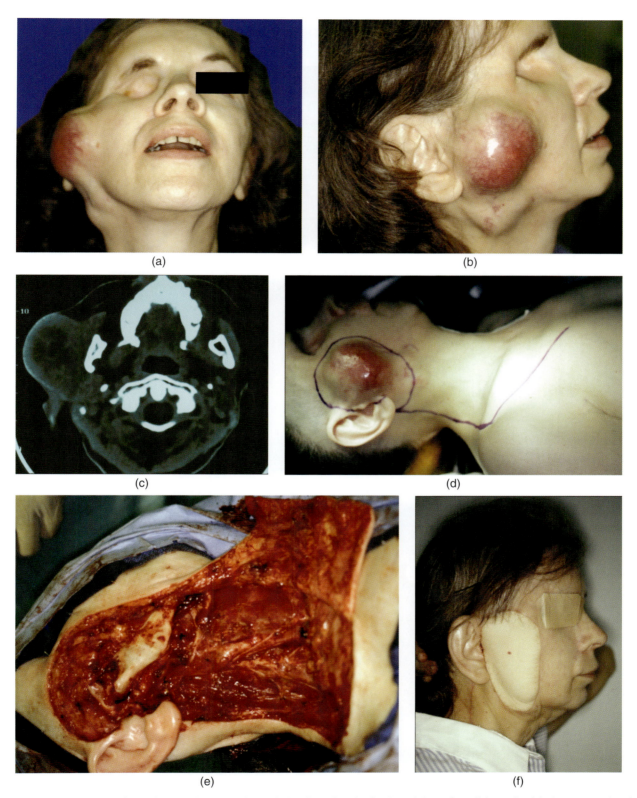

Figure 15.16. (a and b) Full face and lateral view of elderly lady who had excision of eyelids and orbital exenteration for advanced squamous cell carcinoma of the lids. She was lost to follow up and now presents with massive disease in the parotid nodes (P3) and Level II neck nodes (N2). (c) CT scan shows huge parotid mass. (d) Proposed surgery with radical parotidectomy and radical neck dissection. (e) Post-resection the masseter muscle is sacrificed along with the facial nerve and a total parotidectomy. The mandible was uninvolved by tumor and was preserved. (f) Reconstruction is with a latissimus dorsi flap. Patient developed chest metastases 18 months post-surgery.

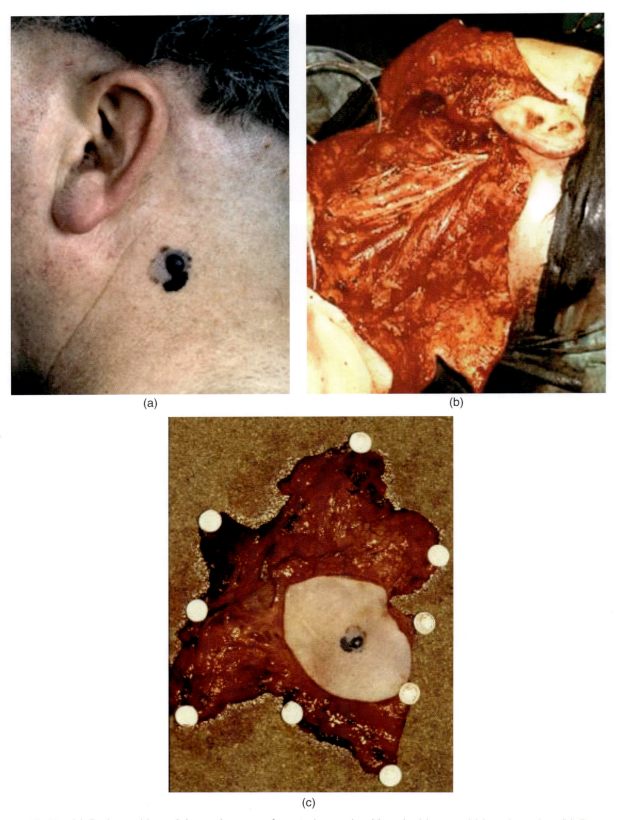

Figure 15.17. (a) Patient with nodular melanoma of posterior neck with palpable parotid lymph nodes. (b) Post-total parotidectomy and radical neck dissection (c) Surgical specimen with 5 cm skin margin. Patient developed lung metastases within six months and died of disease.

the cutaneous primary is likely to have drained through the parotid, then superficial parotidectomy should be done with a I-V neck dissection. Similarly, for cutaneous squamous cell carcinoma, the authors recommend no role for elective neck dissection in P0 N0 disease. Whether sentinel node biopsy is useful for high-risk cutaneous SCC is currently under investigation. In P+/N0 disease, parotidectomy and a selective regional approach to the elective neck is recommended (Gurney and Newlands 2014; Newlands and Gurney 2014). In a study of 276 P+ MM patients, identified from two prospective databases, all underwent neck dissection and histologic outcomes were analyzed, 185 necks were cN0 and 82 CN+, 36/185 elective neck dissections were positive for occult nodes (19.5%). Occult nodes were located in level I (16.7%), II (58.3%), III (36.1%), IV (13.9%), and V (30.6%). In addition, 32 patients with cN0 had regional recurrence. The authors concluded that elective comprehensive neck dissection reduced regional failure rates and provided accurate staging and prognostic information. Based on their analysis of levels involved by occult disease, they propose that it is probably safe to omit levels I and IV from the neck dissection (Den Hondt et al. 2019). There is much less evidence for the management of the neck for mucosal melanoma (Figure 15.18). This is generally thought to have a poor prognosis with five-year survival of 20%. Despite its different biology, it is treated in the same way as cutaneous melanoma (Ascierto et al. 2017). The effect of immunotherapies such as anti-CTLA-4 and anti-PD-1/PDL1 antibodies has not yet been clearly defined in mucosal melanoma due to its rarity.

Different recommendations in the elective management of cervical and parotid lymph nodes in N0 cutaneous SCC were given following a decision analysis approach. In this study, the authors concluded using a decision tree and probabilities of recurrence and salvage from the literature, that a wait and see approach is justified when the probability of occult metastasis is <19%. When the probability of metastasis exceeds 25%, elective neck dissection has a higher utility than observation (Wong and Morton 2013).

Distant Metastases to Salivary Glands

The major salivary glands can also be a site for distant metastatic disease especially the parotid gland although these cases are rare. In a literature review of over 800 patients with metastatic disease in the parotid, 80% were from cutaneous SCC or melanoma (as described above) while 66 were non-cutaneous head and neck tumors and 87 from a distant primary site (Pisani et al. 1993). In their personal series of 38 patients, 10 had non-cutaneous head and neck cancers while 4 were from distant sites (2 renal and 2 lung). In a review of 10 944 cases from the Salivary Gland Register (1965–1985), there were 21 cases from distant site primaries (0.19%). There were 7 cases from lung, 6 renal, 6 breast, and 1 case from colon and uterus (Seifert et al. 1986). Nuyens et al. (2006) found 34 of 520 parotid tumors to be metastatic 31 from cutaneous primaries 2 from ductal breast cancer and 1 from a limb rhabdomyosarcoma. In a review of 184 metastatic tumors to the salivary glands, (171 parotid and 13 submandibular), 16 cases were from distant metastatic sites. These sites included breast, lung, kidney, thyroid, pancreaticobiliary, prostate, and bladder (Wang et al. 2017). Although rare these distant metastases can provide a diagnostic challenge as the commonest primary sites appear to be breast, lung, and kidney. Small cell lung cancer is very difficult to differentiate from primary small cell carcinoma of the salivary gland so CT scan of the lungs is an essential part of the work-up (Figure 15.19). In one review of the literature, a total of seven cases metastatic to the parotid from primary small cell lung cancer were found (Yu et al. 2019).

Primary small cell neuroendocrine carcinomas of the salivary glands are rare comprising 1,85–2.8% of salivary gland tumors (Gnepp and Wick 1990; Baca et al. 2011). In a small series of five cases of neuroendocrine and small cell carcinomas of the parotid, one of the authors (RAO) found only one primary parotid cancer. Salivary glands are the second commonest head and neck site for primary small cell carcinomas (Figure 15.20), with larynx being the most common, and they are aggressive tumors with an overall poor prognosis (Renner 2007). They are divided into neuroendocrine and ductal types, and according to cytokeratin, 20 immunoreactivity the ductal sites can be subdivided into pulmonary and Merkel types (Nagao et al. 2004). This study indicated that negative immune-stain for cytokeratin 20 could be a marker for poor prognosis and that salivary gland small cell carcinoma may have a better prognosis than extra-salivary sites. A later study has shown absence of Merkel cell polyoma virus in these

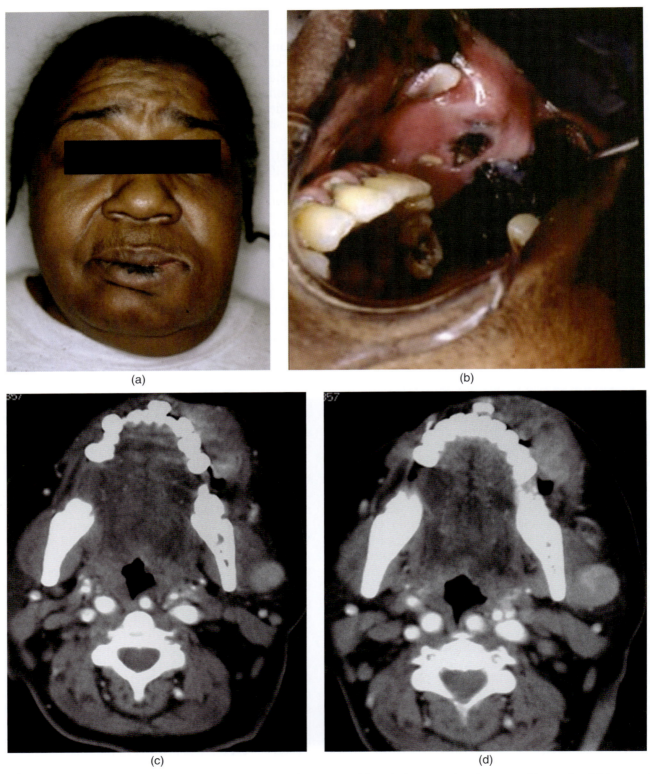

Figure 15.18. (a) Patient with large lymph node swelling at level I and pigmented melanoma of lower lip. (b) Intraoral examination shows deeply pigmented melanoma involving the buccal mucosa and extending to the retromolar region. (c) and (d) CT scans show primary melanoma as thickening of the left cheek and lip with nodal involvement of the parotid. (e) CT scan at a more cephalad level now shows multiple positive nodes in the parotid gland. (f) and (g) Hematoxylin and eosin stain of the tumor(f) and HMB-45 stain (g) confirming the diagnosis of mucosal melanoma.

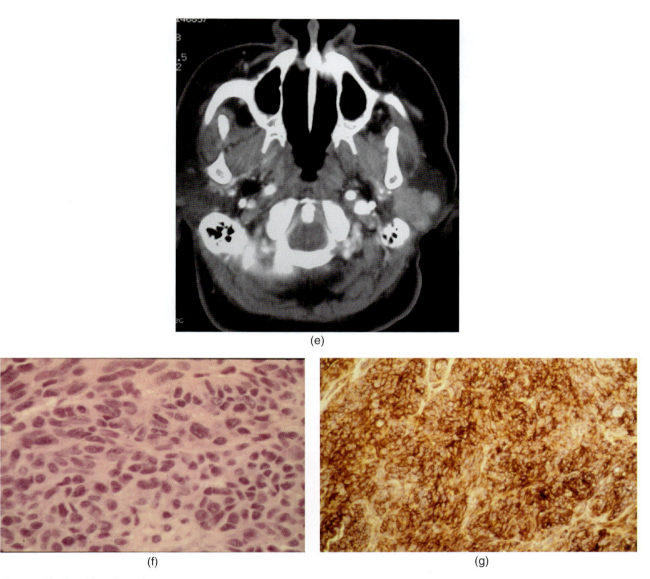

Figure 15.18. (Continued).

parotid tumors irrespective of the cytokeratin 20 status (Chernock et al. 2011).

In a single case report, immunohistochemical study of estrogen receptors was used to identify a parotid tumor as a breast metastasis (Perez-Fidalgo et al. 2007). Regarding distant metastases from renal cell cancer, the same problem is found. Most of these will be from clear cell renal carcinoma and mimic the salivary clear cell adenocarcinoma or clear cell variant of MECA which are both primary salivary gland cancers. The recognition of EWSR1-AFT translocations allows recognition of the more recently described hyalinizing clear cell carcinoma of salivary glands found in soft tissue (Hsieh et al. 2017). An identical gene re-arrangement is seen in clear cell odontogenic carcinoma, which is found in bone. In a case report and review of the literature, Park and Hlivko (2002) found 25 cases of metastatic renal cell carcinoma to the parotid gland. In 14 of these cases (56%), the metastasis was the initial presenting sign of a previously undiagnosed renal carcinoma. None of the cases presented with facial paralysis and the authors could make the diagnosis in 3 of 6 cases with FNAB. In a

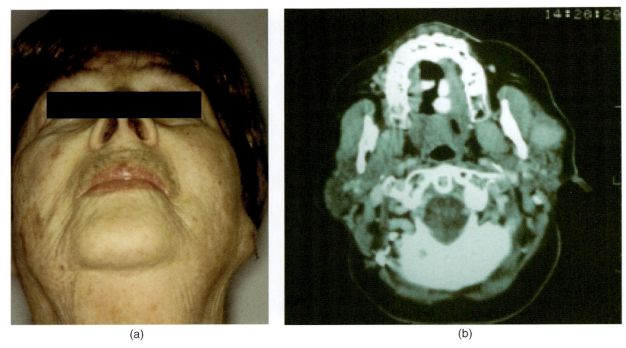

Figure 15.19. (a) An 80-year-old woman with known small cell carcinoma of the lung presenting with metastatic mass in the left parotid gland. (b) CT scan of the patient showing parotid mass.

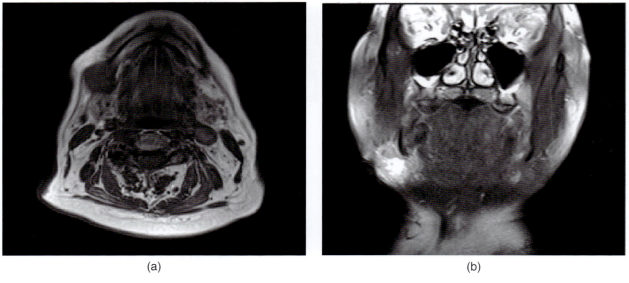

Figure 15.20. (a) and (b) MR of submandibular gland mass fixed to the lower border of the mandible. FNAB small blue round cell tumor. Following neck dissection and marginal resection of the mandible with the mass histopathology shows a primary small cell neuroendocrine tumor of the submandibular gland. Postoperative radiation therapy was given. (c) Cytology from FNAB reported as small blue round tumor with neuroendocrine features. (d) H+E stain shows SCC with neuroendocrine features. (e) Synaptophysin stain and (f) 14.20f DD56 immunohistochemical stain shows positivity and confirms the neuroendocrine nature of this tumor. Source: Dr. John C. Papadimitriou Professor of Pathology University of Maryland reproduced with permission Dr. Papadimitriou.

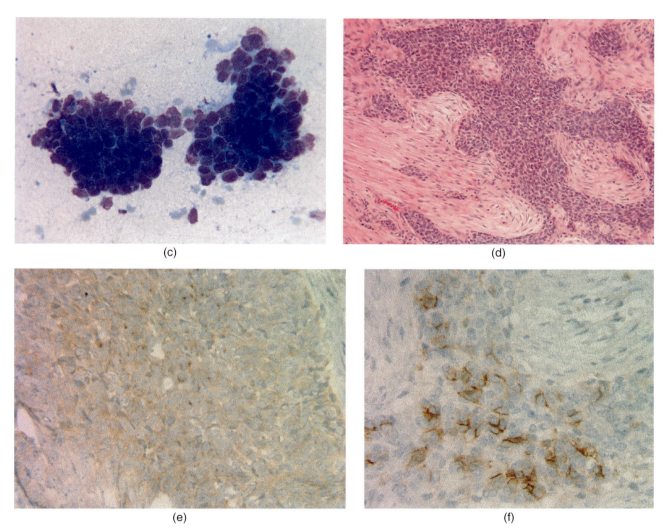

Figure 15.20. (Continued).

small series of our own patients, we could differentiate renal cell carcinoma from monomorphic clear cell salivary adenocarcinoma by immunohistochemistry and electron microscopic ultrastructural differences (Rezende et al. 1997).

Distant metastasis to salivary glands other than the parotid appears to be extremely unusual, although a unique case of bilateral submandibular gland metastases from breast carcinoma was published in 2001, (Cain et al. 2001).

Miscellaneous

It is difficult to include every disease process that can present rarely in the parotid gland. A case of unicentric Castleman's disease in the parotid gland that we surgically resected has been published (Reece et al. 2012). It appears that the unicentric type is benign in nature and can be cured by simple excision or parotidectomy. An analysis of 10 cases of Castleman's disease in the parotid and neck also concluded that surgical resection is the choice of treatment with excellent results (Zhong et al. 2009).

Summary

- The commonest parotid tumors in children are hemangiomas and hemagioendotheliomas.
- In vascular parotid lesions in children medical therapy with steroids, alpha/beta interferon or oral propranolol is preferred.

- In salivary lymphangiomas, a combination of debulking and sclerosing injections to macrocystic areas is used for management.
- Parotid lymphomas are usually associated with Sjögren syndrome, hepatitis C, or AIDS.
- Most salivary lymphomas are MALT lymphomas which follow an indolent course.
- The parotid lymph node bed may be the first echelon nodes for cutaneous cancers of the cheek, ear, scalp, forehead, and temple.
- Metastatic parotid nodes (P) and neck nodes (N) should be staged separately when involved by primary cutaneous cancers.
- Patients with both neck nodes and parotid nodes have the worst prognosis.
- Radiation therapy is given for close margins, perineural spread, and more than one positive node.
- In small cell carcinomas of the salivary gland, a full work-up must be done to determine whether the tumor is a salivary primary or metastatic from a distant site.

Case Presentation – *From One Salivary Gland to Another*

A 41-year-old Caucasian lady presented in July 2002 with a 1–1.5 cm raised submucosal swelling of the left palate, which had been present for two years. It was intermittently painful. Biopsy by an OMFS showed adenocarcinoma NOS.

PAST MEDICAL HISTORY
Meningitis in 1983.
   Heart murmur on ECHO
   She had knee replacement surgery × 6, and bunionectomy.
   She was taking Phentermine, Vioxx for arthritis, Valtrex for recurrent herpes, and she disclosed no known drug allergies.

SOCIAL HISTORY
She was a nonsmoker.

EXAMINATION
Clinical examination showed no palpable cervical nodes. Intraoral examination revealed a firm nontender mass in the left palate which was smooth and non-ulcerated (Figure 15.21). The lesion was located at the junction of the hard and soft palate near the greater palatine foramen. There was a slight bluish discoloration.

The provisional clinical diagnosis was a minor salivary gland tumor, and because of the cystic appearance, a low-grade mucoepidermoid carcinoma was the favored diagnosis. Other possibilities in the differential diagnosis at that time were a cystic pleomorphic adenoma or adenoid cystic carcinoma. She was recommended for biopsy and imaging.

Biopsy revealed a low-grade adenocarcinoma.
Her imaging shows no enlarged lymph nodes and no bone involvement.

She underwent a wide local excision with 1 cm margins of the palatal mucosa and removal of the tumor. The periosteum was uninvolved, and the underlying bony hard palate was preserved.

Postoperatively the patient did well without any complications. Histopathology showed a moderately differentiated ductal type adenocarcinoma. The deep margin was close < 1 mm. The MD H + N Tumor Board recommended close follow-up

The patient was followed regularly until November 2004, (two years and five months), when she was noted to have a bluish discoloration at the junction of the hard/soft palate, which had been a little sore. MRI was reported as normal in February 2005, but on reviewing the films, I felt that she had a mass extending into the floor of the nose. Clinically, the blue area was still present. Biopsy at that time showed an adenocarcinoma. CT confirmed destruction of the bone of the posterior palate with involvement of the inferior turbinate and nasal septum (Figure 15.21b and c).

In March, the patient underwent a partial maxillectomy with again 1 cm. margins around the lesion encompassing bone of the palate, maxilla, and lateral nasal wall. Her postoperative final pathology showed a 2-mm deep margin and 3 mm anterior margin. The multidisciplinary tumor board recommended re-resection or radiation. The patient elected for re-excision of the anterior margin area, which was carried out in May 2005. Histology was negative for tumor.

Again, the patient was followed regularly and she did well for three years and eight months, but in January 2009, she was found to have a granular area in the maxillectomy cavity and swollen nasal

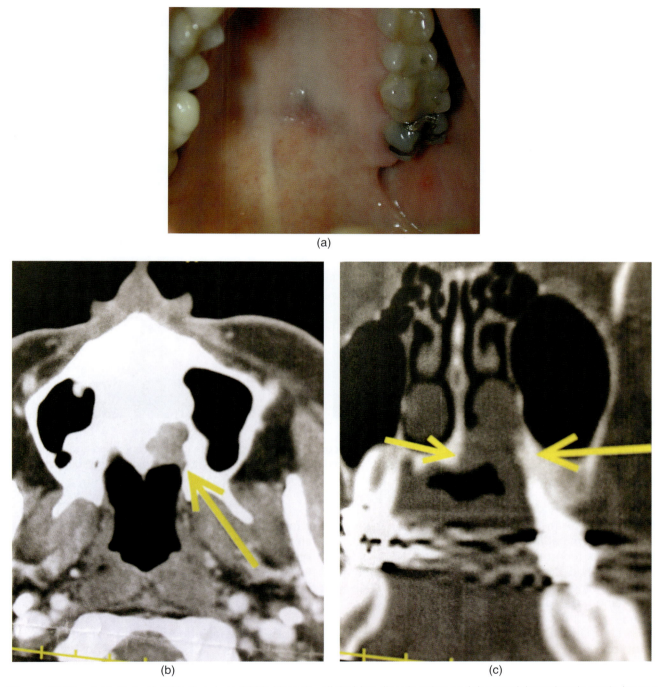

Figure 15.21. (a) Initial palatal lesion June 2002. Note the slight blue discoloration and the overlying telangiectasia (tumor vessels) of the palatal mucosa. (b) Axial CT Scan 2005 shows destruction of posterior palatal bone. (c) Coronal CT scan 2005 shows invasion of the floor of the left nose with involvement of the inferior turbinate.

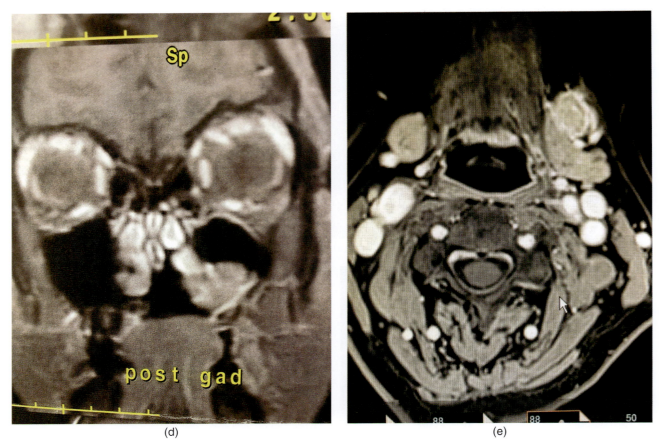

Figure 15.21. *(Continued)* (d) Coronal MR 2009 shows recurrent tumor involves inferior maxillary sinus and left inferior nasal wall. (e) Axial MR 2019 shows enhancing 2 cm. lymph node superficial to the anterior portion of the submandibular gland.

tissues. MRI scan showed recurrent tumor in the left inferior maxilla into the nose (Figure 15.21d). Biopsy was reported as adenocarcinoma NOS.

She had a further salvage maxillectomy. Histopathology showed an intermediate-grade adenocarcinoma. Again, margins were clear but close laterally, <1 mm.

The patient was followed with no problems until June 2016 (seven-years and four months since her last surgery) and then was lost to follow-up. She returned to our clinic in December 2019, (9 years 10 months since her last surgery) with some swelling of the left retromolar area and tenderness when wearing her obturator. She was also noted to have a firm palpable 2 cm lymph node in the left submandibular triangle. Her mouth opening was somewhat restricted to about two finger breadths maximum. There was a 1–2 cm area of granulation tissue on the inside of the remaining lateral wall of the left sinus. The tissues of her retromolar fossa on the left side were full to inspection. On lingual palpation of this area, it felt firm in the area of the lateral pterygoid muscle.

A biopsy of the granulation tissue was performed, and the patient was sent for an MRI with contrast of the facial bones and neck.

The biopsy was reported as positive for an intermediate grade adenocarcinoma.

The MRI showed an enlarged enhancing lymph node in the left submandibular region (Figure 15.21e) and a 1 cm nodule in the left parotid (Figure 15.21f). In addition, three seemingly separate areas of contrast enhancing lesions suspicious for tumor recurrence were seen in the left maxillary area. One was located in the left pterygoid muscle, one in the maxillary sinus where the

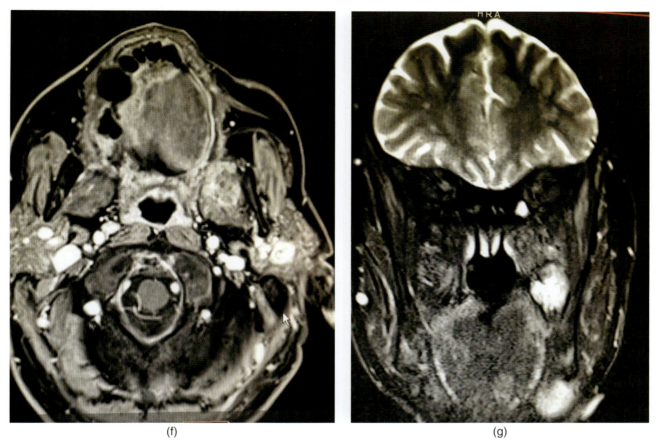

Figure 15.21. (*Continued*) (f) Axial MR shows enhancing ovoid mass in the left parotid gland. (g) Coronal CT shows enhancing mass 2.5 cm within the substance of the medial pterygoid muscle. The enhancing Level I node is also well visualized.

biopsy was taken and one lateral to the sinus deep to the malar arch in the inferior part of the infratemporal fossa (Figures 15.21g and h).

An ultrasound guided fine-needle aspiration biopsy of the parotid mass confirmed salivary adenocarcinoma.

DIAGNOSIS

Recurrent intermediate adenocarcinoma T1 (× 3), N2 M0, Stage Iva.

The surgical plan due to her poor mouth opening and scarring from her three previous surgeries was an in-continuity parotidectomy and neck dissection levels I–IV, with a lip split and mandibulotomy and malar osteotomy/ostectomy for access to the primary tumor. Reconstruction was planned with a fibular flap (Figures 15.21i–k). The expectation was that adjuvant radiation therapy would be required.

Surgery was technically difficult due to scar tissue. The final pathology showed a 6.3 cm polymorphous adenocarcinoma, intermediate grade (Figure 15.21l and m) and confirmed a positive node in the parotid (Figures 15.21n and o) and at level I (total 2/23). No other lymph nodes were positive. Margins were close (< 1 mm) in the muscle. The pathologists felt that the three "separate" foci of tumor were microscopically connected to each other.

Postoperatively the patient had some facial nerve weakness, but otherwise made a good recovery (Figure 15.21p and q). The multidisciplinary tumor board recommended adjuvant radiation therapy.

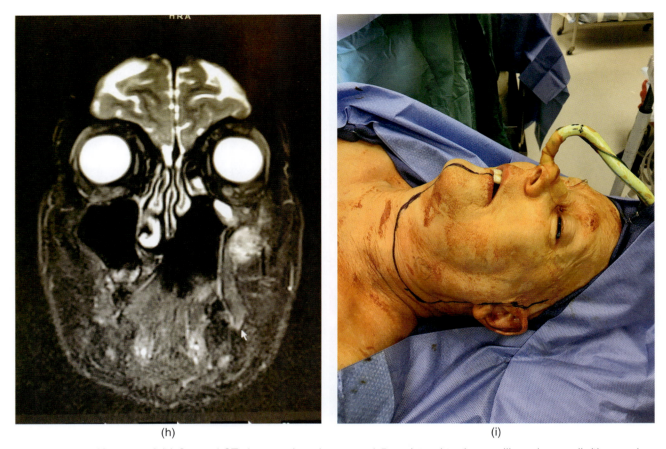

Figure 15.21. (*Continued*) (h) Coronal CT shows enhancing mass 1.5 cm lateral to the maxillary sinus wall, (the previous maxillectomy with resection of the inferior turbinate is appreciated). This mass lies deep to the anterior malar arch. (i) Intraoperative view of extended lip split incision marked on skin. The cervical incision extends inferiorly to just above the clavicle to allow access to level IV and V. The preauricular extension is for the parotidectomy.

TAKE HOME POINTS

1. This case firstly emphasizes that many salivary gland pathologies need to be followed for a long period of time to observe their real behavior and evolution. Tumors such as adenoid cystic carcinoma, and mucoepidermoid carcinoma can take many years before they are clinically seen to have recurred or metastasized. Even pleomorphic adenomas may have a considerable period of time prior to local recurrence. In this case, it took 17 years and 6 months from initial presentation for the tumor to reveal its true potential.

2. The final diagnosis was polymorphous adenocarcinoma, (formerly polymorphous low-grade adenocarcinoma PLGA). As the name implies this tumor can present with many histological forms, often within the same tumor. Because of this, the tumor can be easily misdiagnosed most commonly as adenoid cystic carcinoma or pleomorphic adenoma. If the diagnosis had been made initially in 2002, it would still have been regarded as low-grade and treatment would have been the same. At that time, the papillary variant was regarded as having higher potential for aggressive behavior and metastasis. Effective with the World Health Organization 4th edition of head and neck

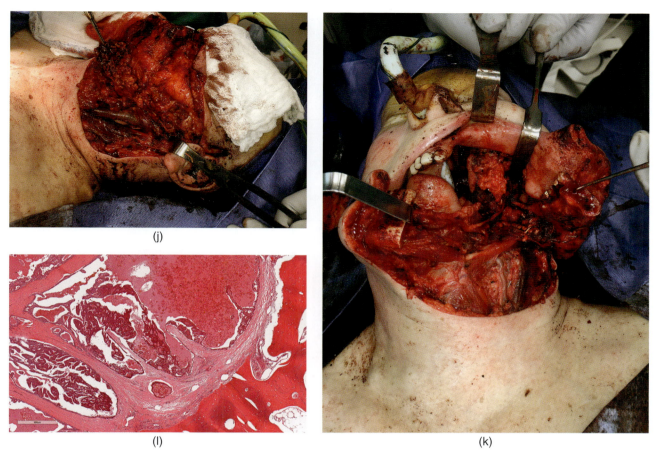

Figure 15.21. (*Continued*) (j) The parotidectomy in-continuity with the neck dissection has been mobilized anteriorly with an Allis clamp. The facial nerve is preserved. (k) The lip split mandibulotomy allows good access for the en-bloc excision of the maxilla pterygoid muscles and part of the malar arch. (l) Polymorphous adenocarcinoma of the maxilla, papillary/cystic and cribriform patterns maxillary bone invasion is seen at the right inferior portion of the figure.

tumors, the cribriform adenocarcinoma of minor salivary glands (CAMSG) is also recognized as behaving more aggressively. This type may be classified as a distinct entity from the polymorphous adenocarcinoma in the next WHO revision and update. The polymorphous adenocarcinoma in this case shows both papillary and cribriform histologic variants. Polymorphous adenocarcinoma does show a propensity for perineural invasion and looking at the initial location of the tumor, over the greater palatine foramen it is a possibility that one of the reasons for the initial recurrence was perineural spread.

3. The most interesting perhaps unique facet of this case is the regional metastasis to the parotid. It is well known that a primary carcinoma of the parotid can metastasize to intraparotid nodes and cervical nodes. As documented in Chapter 15, metastasis from skin cancers and from mucosal SCC in the Head and Neck can occur. Very rarely metastasis from distant cancers can also be seen. However, metastasis to the parotid from another salivary gland site, in this case a minor salivary gland tumor of the oral cavity, is a singular event.

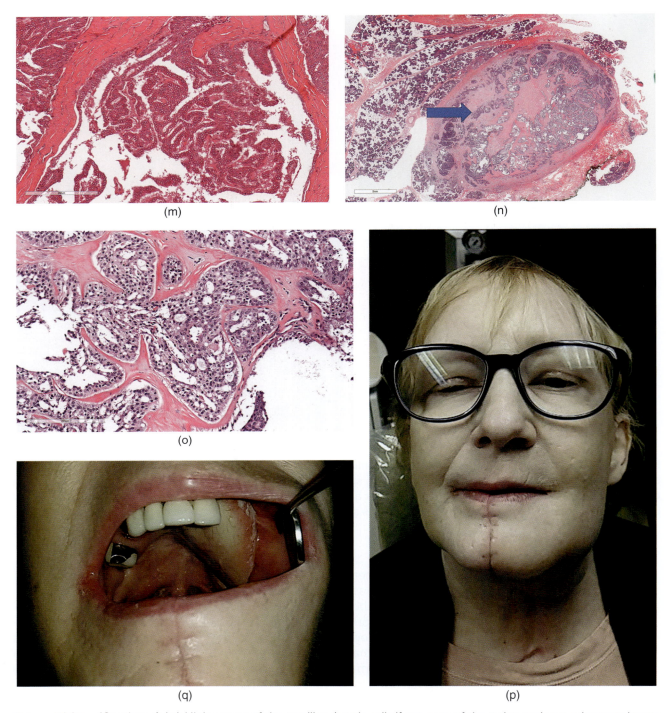

Figure 15.21. (*Continued*) (m) High power of the papillary/cystic cribriform area of the polymorphous adenocarcinoma shows pale, optically clear/vesicular nuclei reminiscent of papillary thyroid carcinoma. (n) Polymorphous adenocarcinoma metastatic to a parotid node indicated by blue arrow. (o) High power of parotid metastasis mostly cribriform pattern. Source: Courtesy of Dr. John Papadimitriou Professor of Pathology University of Maryland. (p) Three weeks postoperative. The patient has some facial nerve weakness. (q) Intraoral view of fibular flap reconstruction of the maxilla. Source: Reconstruction undertaken by Dr. Joshua Lubek.

References

Agaimy A, Ihrier S, Märki B, et al. 2013. Lipomatous salivary gland tumors; a series of 31 cases spanning their morphologic spectrum with emphasis on sialolipoma and oncocytic lipoadenoma. *Am J Surg Pathol* 37(1);128–137

Agaimy A, Wild V, Märkl B, et al. 2015 Intraparotid classical and nodular lymphocyte-predominant Hodgkin lymphoma: Pattern analysis with emphasis on associated lymphadenoma-like proliferations. *Am J Surg Pathol* 39(9):1206–1212.

Almeyda R, Kothari P, Chau H, Cumberworth V. 2004 Submandibular neurilemmoma; a diagnostic dilemma. *J Laryngol Otol* 118(2):156–158

Ambrossetti A, Zanotti R, Passaro C, et al. 2004 Most cases of primary salivary mucosa-associated lymphoid tissue lymphoma are associated either with Sjögren syndrome or hepatitis C virus infection. *Br J Haematol* 126(1):43–49

Anacak Y, Miller RC, Constantinou N, et al. 2012. Primary mucosa-associated lymphoid tissue lymphoma of the salivary glands: A multicenter rare cancer network study. *Int J Radiat Oncol Biol Phys* 82(1):315–320

Andruchow JL, Veness MJ, Morgan GJ, et al. 2006 Implications for clinical staging of metastatic cutaneous carcinoma of the head and neck based on a multicenter study of treatment outcomes. *Cancer* 106(5):1078–1083

Ascierto PA, Accorona R, Botti G, et al. 2017. Mucosal melanoma of the head and neck. *Crit Rev Oncol Hematol* 112:136–152.

Baca JM, Chiara JA, Strenge KS, et al. 2011. Small cell carcinoma of the parotid gland. *J Clin Oncol* 29(2):e34–e36

Bădărinză M, Serban O, Maghear L, et al. 2020. Shear wave elastography as a new method to identify parotid lymphoma in primary Sjögren's syndrome. *Rheumatology Int* 40(8):1275–1281. doi:10.1007/s00296-020-04548-x (Epub ahead of print).

Balle VH, Greisen O. 1984. Neurilemmomas of the facial nerve presenting as parotid tumors. *Ann Otol Rhinol Laryngol* 93:70–72

Barzilai G, Greenberg E, Cohen-Kermen R, Doweck I. 2005. Pattern of regional metastases from cutaneous squamous cell carcinoma of the head and neck. *Otolaryngol Head Neck Surg* 132(6):852–856

BenJelloun H, Jouhadi H, Maazouzi A, et al. 2005 Rhabdomyosarcoma of the salivary glands. Report of 3 cases. (article in French) *Cancer Radiother* 9(5):316–321

Bentz BG, Hughes CA, Ludemann JP, Maddalozzo J. 2000. Masses of the salivary gland region in children. *Arch Otolaryngol Head Neck Surg* 126(12):1435–1439.

Bishop JA, Alaggio R, Zhang L, et al. 2015.Adamantinoma-like Ewing family tumors of the head and neck: A pitfall in the differential diagnosis of basaloid and myoepithelial carcinomas. *Am J Surg Pathol* 39(9):1267–1274.

Bron LP, Traynor SJ, McNeil EB, O'Brien CJ. 2003. Primary and metastatic cancer of the parotid; comparison of clinical behavior in 232 cases. *Laryngoscope* 113(6):1070–1075

Brown NE, Elenitoba-Johnson KSJ, 2017. Update from the 4th edition of the World Health Organization classification of head and neck tumors: Hematolymphoid tumors. *Head Neck Pathol* 11(1):68–77.

Cain AJ, Goodland J, Denholm SW. 2001 Metachronous bilateral submandibular gland metastases from carcinoma of the breast. *J Laryngol Otol* 115(8):683–684

Cakir Cretin A, Dogan E, Ozay H, et al. 2018. Submandibular gland invasion and feasibility of gland-sparing neck dissection in oral cavity carcinoma. *J Laryngol Otol* 132950;446–451

Castle JT, Thompson LD. 2000. Kaposi's sarcoma of major salivary gland origin: A clinicopathologic series of six cases. *Cancer* 88(1):15–23.

Cetin AC, Dogan E, Ozay H, et al. 2018. Submandibular gland invasion and feasibility of gland-sparing neck dissection in oral cavity carcinoma. *J Laryngol Otol* 132(5):446–451.

Chadan VS, Fung EK, Woods CI, et al. 2004. Primary pleomorphic liposarcoma of the parotid gland: a case report and review of the literature. *Am J Otolaryngol* 25(6):432–437.s

Chang L, Jin Y, Lv D, et al. 2016. Use of propranolol for parotid hemangioma. *Head Neck* 38(Suppl 1):E1730–E1376.

Cheng C. 2015. Doxycycline sclerotherapy in children with head and neck lymphatic malformations. *J Pediatr Surg* 50(12):2143–2146.

Chernock RD, Duncavage EJ, Gnepp DR, et al. 2011. Absence of Merkle cell polyoma virus in primary parotid high grade neuroendocrine carcinomas regardless of cytokeratin 20 immunophenotype. *Am J Surg Pathol* 35(12):1806–1811.

Ch'ng S, Maitra A Lea R, et al 2006 Parotid metastasis-an independent prognostic factor for head and neck cutaneous squamous cell carcinoma. *J Plast Reconstr Aesthet Surg* 59(12):1288–1293

Cockerill CC, Daram S, El-Naggar AK, et al. 2013. Primary sarcomas of the salivary glands; case series and literature review. *Head Neck* 35(11):1551–1557

Delli K, Villa A, Farah CS, et al. 2019. World workshop on oral medicine VII: Biomarkers predicting lymphoma in the salivary glands of patients with Sjögren's syndrome-a systematic review. *Oral Dis* 25 (Suppl 1):49–63.

Den Hondt M, Starr MW, Millet M, et al. 2019. Surgical management of the neck in patients with metastatic melanoma in parotid lymph nodes. *J Surg Oncol* 120(8):1462–1469.

Dunn P, Kuo TT, Shih LY, et al. 2004. Primary salivary gland lymphoma: A clinicopathologic study of 23 cases in Taiwan. *Acta Hematol* 112(4):203–208

Emran MA, Dubois J, Laberge L, et al. 2006 Alcoholic solution of zein (Ethibloc) sclerotherapy for treatment of lymphangiomas in children. *J Pediatr Surg* 41(5):975–979

Eraso A, Lorusso G, Palacios E. 2005 Primary lymphoma of the parotid gland. *ENT-Ear Nose Throat J* 84(4)198–199

Ethunandan M, Vura G, Umar T, et al. 2006 Lipomatous lesions of the parotid gland *J Oral Maxillofac Surg* 64(11):1583–6

Fageeh N, Manoukian J, Tewfik T, et al. 1997 Management of head and neck lymphatic malformations in children *J Otolaryngol* 26(4):253–258

Fanburg-Smith JC, Furlong JC, Childers EL. 2003. Oral and salivary gland angiosarcoma: A clinicopathologic study of 29 cases. *Mod Pathol* 16(3):263–271

Farnoosh S, Don D, Koempel J, et al. 2015.Efficacy of doxycycline and sodium tetradecyl sulfate sclerotherapy in pediatric head and neck lymphatic malformations. *Int J Pediatr Otolaryngol* 79(6):883–887.

Feinstein AJ, Ciarleglio MM, Cong X, et al. 2013.Parotid lymphoma: Prognostic analysis of 2140 patients. *Laryngoscope* 123(5):1199–1203.

Fierke O, Laskawi R, Kunze E. 2006 Solitary intraparotid neurofibroma of the facial nerve. Symptomatology, bioplogy and management. (in German) *HNO* 54(10):772–777

Frederiksen JK, Sharma M, Casulo C Burack WR. 2015. Systematic review of the effectiveness of fine-needle aspiration biopsy for subclassifying lymphoma. *Arch Pathol Lab Med* 139(2):245–251.

Fregnani ER Pires FR, Falzoni R, et al. 2003 Lipomas of the oral cavity: Clinical findings, histological classification and proliferative activity of 46 cases. *Int J Oral Maxillofac Surg* 32(1):49–53

Fuchsmann C, Quintal MC, Giguere C,et al. 2011. Propranolol as a first-line treatment of head and neck hemangiomas. *Arch Otolaryngol Head Neck Surg* 137(5):471–478.

Furlong MA, Fanburg-Smith JC, Cnilders EL. 2004 Lipomas of the oral and maxillofacial region: Site and subclassification of 125 cases. *Oral Surg Oral Med Oral Pathol Oral Radiol Endod* 98(4):441–450

Garatea-Creglo J, Gay-Escoda C, Bermejo B, Buenechea-Imaz R. 1993. Morphological study of the parotid lymph nodes *J Craniomaxillofac Surg* 21(5):207–209.

Gnepp DR, Wick MR 1990. Small cell carcinoma of the major salivary glands. An immunohistochemical study. *Cancer* 66(1):185–192

Goldenberg D, Flax-Goldenberg R, Joachims HZ, Peled N. 2000. Misplaced parotid glands: Bilateral agenesis of parotid glands associated with bilateral accessory parotid tissue. *J Laryngol Otol* 114:883–885.

Gooskens I, Mann JJ, 2006 Lipoma of the deep lobe of the parotid gland: Report of 3 cases. *ORL J Otorhinolaryngol Relat Spec* 68(5):290–295.

Greene AK, Rogers GF, Mulliken JB. 2004 Management of parotid hemangiomas in 100 children. *Plast Reconstr Surg.* 113(1):53–60

Guraya S, Prayson RA. 2016. Peripheral nerve sheath tumors arising in salivary glands: A clinicopathologic study. *Ann Diag Pathol* 23:38–42.

Gurney B, Newlands C. 2014 Management of regional metastatic disease in head and neck cutaneous malignancy 1 cutaneous squamous cell carcinoma. *Br J Oral and Maxillofac Surg* 52(4):294–300

Harada H, Omura K. 2009.Metastasis of oral cancer to the parotid node. *Eur J Surg Oncol* 35(8):890–894.

Harris J, Phillips DP. 2019. Evaluating the clinical outcomes of parotid hemangiomas in the pediatric population. *Ear Nose Throat J* 145561319877760. doi:101177/0145561319877760 (Online ahead of print).

Hart S, Horsman JM, Radstone CR, et al. 2004.Localised extra nodal lymphoma of the head and neck: The Sheffield lymphoma group experience (1971–2000). *Clin Oncol (R Coll Radiol)* 16(3):186–192.

Hicks J, Flaitz C. 2002 Rhabdomyosarcoma of the head and neck in children. *Oral Oncol* 38(5):450–459

Hsieh M-S, Wang H, Lee Y-H, et al 2017. Reevaluation of MAML2 fusion -negative mucoepidermoid carcinoma: A subgroup being actually hyalizing clear cell carcinoma of the salivary gland with EWSR1 translocation. *Hum Pathol* 61:9–18.

Hughes JH, Volk EE Wilbur DC. 2005.Pitfalls in salivary gland fine-needle aspiration cytology: Lessons from the College of American Pathologists Interlaboratory Comparison Program in nongynecologic cytology. *Arch Pathol Lab Med* 129(1):26–31

Jamal. 2017. Treatment of parotid non-Hodgkin lymphoma: A meta-analysis. *J Glob Oncol* 4:1–6.

Jang Y-W, Kim S-G, Pai H, et al 2009. Sialolipoma: Case report and review of 27 cases. *Oral Maxillofac Surg* 13(2):109–113.

Kojima M, Nakamura S, Ichimura K, et al. 2001, Follicular lymphoma of the salivary gland: A clinicopathologic and molecular study of six cases. *Int J Surg Pathol* 94(4):287–293

Leemans CR, Tiwari R, Nauta JJ, Snow GB. 1991 Discontinuous vs in-continuity neck dissection in carcinoma of the oral cavity. *Arch Otolaryngol Head Neck Surg* 117(9):1003–1006.

Li B-Z, Yu C-J, Xu J-J, et al. 2009. Clinicopathologic characteristics and chromosomal abnormalities in salivary mucosa associated lymphoid tissue lymphomas. *Zhonghua Er Bi Yan Hou Tou jing Wai Ke Za Zhi* 44(8):651–656.

Li S, Lu X, Xie S, et al. 2019. Intra-parotid facial nerve schwannoma: A 17-year, single-institution experience of diagnosis and management. *Acta Otolaryngol* 139(5):444–450

Lin YJ, Lin LM, Chen YK, et al. 2004 Sialolipoma of the floor of the mouth: A case report. *Kaohsiung J Med Sci* 20(8):410–414.

Loree TR, Tomljanovich PI, Cheney RT, et al. 2006 Intraparotid sentinel lymph node biopsy for head and neck melanoma. *Laryngoscope* 116(8):1461–1464

Mantadakis E, Tsouvala E, Deftereos S, et al. 2012. Involution of a large parotid hemangioma with oral propranolol: An illustrative report and review of the literature. *Case Reports in Pediatrics* 2012:353812

Martin N, Sterkers O, Mompoint D, Nahum H. 1992 Facial nerve neuromas: MR imaging. Report of four cases. *Neuroradiology* 34(1):62–67

Masaki Y, Sugai S. (2004). Lymphoproliferative disorders in Sjögren's syndrome. *Autoimmun Rev* 3(3):175–182

Mazlumoglu, AE, Atlas E, Oner F, et al. 2015a.FNA biopsy of secondary nonlymphomatous malignancies in salivary glands: A multi-institutional study of 184 cases. *Cancer Cytopathol* 125(2):91–103.

Mazlumoglu, AE, Atlas E, Oner F, et al. 2015b. Congenital sialolipoma in an infant. *J Craniofac Surg* 26(8):e696–e697.

McGuirt WF Sr, Johnson PE, McGuirt WT. 2003 Intraparotid facial nerve neurofibromas. *Laryngoscope* 113(10:82–84

Michaelidis IG, Stefanopoulos PK, Sambaziotis D, et al. 2006 Sialolipoma of the parotid gland. *J Craniomaxillofac Surg* 34(1):43–46.

Morello L, Rattotti S, Giodarno L, et al. 2019. Mantle cell lymphoma of mucosa-associated lymphoid tissue: A European mantle cell lymphoma network study. *Hemasphere* 4(1):e302.

Nagao T, Sugano I, Ishida Y, et al 2001. Sialolipoma: a report of seven cases of a new variant of salivary gland lipoma. *Histopathology* 38: 30–36.

Nagao T, Gaffey TA, Olsen KD, et al. 2004 Small cell carcinomas of the major salivary glands: Clinicopathologic study with emphasis on cytokeratin 20 immunoreactivity and clinical outcomes. *Am J Surg Pathol* 28(6):762–770

Nakamura S, Ichimura K, Sato Y, et al. 2006 Follicular lymphoma frequently originates in the salivary gland *Pathol Int* 56(10):576–583.

Newlands C, Gurney B. 2014 Management of regional metastatic disease in head and neck cutaneous malignancy 2 cutaneous malignant melanoma. *Br J Oral and Maxillofac Surg* 52(4):301–307

Nuyens M, Schupbach J, Stauffer E, Zbaren P. 2006 Metastatic disease to the parotid gland. *Otolaryngol Head Neck Surg* 135(6):844–848

O'Brien CJ, McNeil EB, McMahon JD, et al. 2002. Significance of clinical stage, extent of surgery, and pathologic findings in metastatic cutaneous squamous cell carcinoma of the parotid gland. *Head Neck* 24(5):417–422

Olsen SM, Moore EJ, Koch CA, et al. 2011. Oral cavity and oropharynx squamous cell carcinoma with metastasis to the parotid lymph nodes. *Oral Oncol* 47(2):142–144.

Orbach D, Mosseri V,Gallego S, et al. 2017. Nonparamenigeal head and neck rhabdomyosarcoma in children and adolescents: Lessons from the consecutive international society of pediatric oncology malignant mesenchymal tumor studies. *Head Neck* 39(1):24–31.

Ord RA. 2004. Salivary gland tumors in children. In: Kaban, LA, Roulis, MJ (eds), *Pediatric Oral and Maxillofacial Surgery*. Philadelphia, Saunders, pp. 202.

Ord RA, Ward-Booth RP, Avery BS. 1989. Parotid lymph node metastases from primary intraoral carcinomas. *Int J Oral Maxillofac Surg* 18:104–106

Orvidas LJ, Kasperbauer JL. 2000. Pediatric lymphangiomas of the head and neck. *Ann Otol Rhinol Laryngol* 109(4):411–421.

Ozeki S, Tashiro H, Okamoto M, Matsushima T. 1985 Metastasis to the lingual lymph nodes in carcinoma of the tongue. *J Maxillofac Surg* 13(6):277–281.

Panda NK, Patro SK, Bashi J, et al. 2015.Metastasis to submandibular glands in oral cavity cancers: Can we preserve the gland safely? *Auris Nasus Larynx* 42(4):322–325.

Park YW, Hlivko TJ, 2002 Parotid gland metastasis from renal cell carcinoma. *Laryngoscope* 112(3):453–456.

Park YM, Oh KH, Cho JG, et al. 2018. Analysis of efficacy and safety of core-needle biopsy versus fine-needle aspiration cytology in patients with cervical lymphadenopathy and salivary gland tumor. *Int J Oral Maxillofac Surg* 47(10):1229–1235.

Perez-Fidalgo JA, Chirivella I, Laforga J, et al. 2007 Parotid gland metastasis of a breast cancer. *Clin Transl Oncol* 9(4):264–265

Pisani P, Krengeli M, Ramponi A, Pia F. 1993 Parotid metastases: A review of the literature and case reports. *Acta Otorhinolaryngol Ital* 12(Suppl 37):1–28.

Preuss SF, Klussman JP, Wittekindt C, et al, 2007 Submandibular gland excision: 15 years of experience. *J Oral Maxillofac Surg* 65(5):953–957

Prochorec-Sobieszek M, Wagner T. 2005 Lymphoproliferative disorders in Sjögren's syndrome (article in polish) *Otolaryngol Pol* 59(4):559–564

Reece B, Ord R, Papadimitrou J. 2012. Rare presentation of unicentric Castleman's disease in the parotid gland. *J Oral Maxillofac Surg* 70(9):2114–2117

Renner G. 2007 Small cell carcinomas of the head and neck: A review. *Semin Oncol* 34(1):3–14

Rezende RB, Drachenberg CB, Kumar D, et al, 1997 Differential diagnosis between monomorphic adenocarcinoma of the salivary glands and renal (clear) cell carcinoma. *AM J Surg Path* 23:1532–1538

Rooper LM, Jo VY, Antonescu CR, et al. 2019.Adamantinoma-like Ewing sarcoma of the salivary glands: A newly recognized mimicker of basaloid salivary carcinomas. *Am Jn Surg Pathol* 43(2):187–194.

Sachse F, August C, Alberty J. 2006 Malignant fibrous histiocytoma in the parotid gland. Case series and literature review. (article in German) *HNO* 54(2):116–120

Seifert G, Oehne H. 1986. Mesenchymal (non-epithelial) salivary gland tumors. Analysis of 167 tumor cases of the salivary gland register. *Laryngol Rhinol Otol (Stuttg)* 65(9):485–491

Seifert G, Hennings J, Caselitz J. 1986. Metastatic tumors to the parotid and submandibular glands – Analysis and differential diagnosis of 108 cases. *Pathol Res Pract* 181(6):684–692.

Sethi RK, Abt NB, Remenschneider A, et al.2018.Value of SPECT/CT for sentinel lymph node localization in the parotid and external jugular chain. *Otolaryngol Head Neck Surg* 159(5):866–870.

Shine NP, O'Leary G, Blake SP. 2006 Parotid lymphomas-clinical and computed tomographic features *S Afr J Surg* 44(2):60,62–64

Shum JW, Emmerling M, Lubek JE, Ord RA. 2014. Parotid lymphoma: A review of clinical presentation and management. *Oral Surg Oral Med Oral Pathol Oral Radiol* 118991)e1–e5

Skelton E, Jewison A, Okpalupa C, et al. 2015. Image-guided core needle biopsy in the diagnosis of malignant lymphoma. *Eur J Surg Oncol* 41(7):852–858.

Starkman SJ, Olsen SM, Lewis JE, et al. 2013.Lipomatous lesions of the parotid gland; analysis of 70 cases. *Laryngoscope* 123(3):651–656

Tesseroli MA, Calabrese L, Carvalho AL, et al. 2006. Discontinuous vs in-continuity dissection in carcinoma of the oral cavity. Experience of two oncologic chospitals. *Acta Otolaryngol Ital* 26(6):350–355

Tonami H, Matoba M, Kuginuki Y, et al. 2003. Clinical and imaging findings of lymphoma in patients with Sjögren syndrome. *J Comput Assist Tomogr* 27(4):517–524.

Vaness MJ, Palme CE, Morgan GJ. 2006 High-risk cutaneous squamous cell ca4rcinoma of the head and neck: Results from 266 treated patients with metastatic lymph node disease. *Cancer* 106(11):2389–2396.

Vargas PA, Mauad T, Bohm GM, et al. 2003 Parotid gland involvement in advanced AIDS *Oral Dis* 9(2):55–61

Vasaitis L, Nordmark G, Theander E, et al. 2020. Population-based study of patients with primary Sjögren's syndrome and lymphoma: lymphoma subtypes: Clinical characteristics and gender differences. *Scand J Rheumatol.* 2020:1–8.

Vauterin TJ, Veness MJ, Morgan GJ, et al. 2006. Patterns of lymph node spread of cutaneous squamous cell carcinoma of the head and neck *Head Neck* 28:785–791.

Vazquez A, Khan MA, Sanghvi S, et al. 2015. Extranodal marginal zone lymphoma of mucosa-associated lymphoid tissue of the salivary glands: a population-based study from 1994 to 2009. *Head Neck* 37(1):18–22.

Wang H, Hoda RS, Faquin W. 2017. FNA biopsy of secondary non-lymphomatous malignancies in salivary glands: A multi-institutional study of 184 cases. *Cancer Cytopathol* 125(2):91–103.

Weber FC, Greene AK, Adams DM, et al. 2017. Role of imaging in the diagnosis of parotid infantile hemangiomas. *Int J Pediatr Otolaryngol* 102:61–66.

Weiss SW, Goldblum JR. 2001. In: Enzinger, FM, Weiss, SW (eds), Neural tumors *Soft Tissue Tumors*, 4th edn. St Louis, Mosby, pp. 571.

Weiss I, O TM, Lipari BA, et al. 2011. Current management of parotid hemangiomas. *Laryngoscope* 121(80; 1642–1650

Wiegand S, Wichmann G, Dietz A, 2018. Treatment of lymphatic malformations with the mTOR inhibitor Sirolimus: A systematic review. *Lymphat Res Biol* 16(4):330–339.

Wong WK, Morton RP. 2013. Elective management of cervical and parotid lymph nodes in stage N0 cutaneous squamous cell carcinoma of the head and neck: a decision analysis. *Eur Arch Otorhinolaryngol* 271(11):3011–3019.

Wong KT, Ahula AT, King AD, et al. 2004. Vascular lesions of parotid gland in adult patients: Diagnosis with high-resolution ultrasound and MRI. *Br J Radiol* 77(919):600–606

Woolgar JA. 1999. Histological distribution of cervical lymph node metastases from intraoral/oropharyngeal squamous cell carcinomas. *Br J Oral Maxillofac Surg* 37(3):175–180

Xu Y, Zhang M, Xiao Y, et al. 2016. Parotid area lymph node metastases from preliminarily diagnosed patients with nasopharyngeal carcinoma: Report on tumor characteristics and oncologic outcomes. *Oncotarget* 7(15):19654–19565.

Yu C, Cui X-Y, Wu Y, et al. 2019. A case of metastasis of small cell lung cancer to the parotid gland. *J Int Med Res* 47(11):5824–5830.

Zainine R, El Aoud C, Sellami M, et al. 2012. Cystic hygroma: report of 25 cases. *Tunis Med* 90(1):19–24

Zhang T, Ord RA, Wei WI, Zhao J. 2011. Sublingual lymph node metastasis of early tongue cancer: Report of two cases and review of the literature. *Int J Oral Maxillofac Surg* 40(6):597–600.

Zhang WB, Wang Y, Mao C, et al. 2019a. Oral cavity and oropharynx squamous cell carcinoma with metastasis to the parotid lymph nodes. *Oral Oncol* 47(2):142–144

Zhang WB, Wang Y, Mao C, et al. 2019b. Oral squamous cell carcinoma with metastasis to the parotid lymph node. *Chin J Dent Res* 22(3):175–179.

Zhang Y, Zhang Z-C, Li W-F, et al 2019c. Prognosis and staging of parotid lymph node metastasis in nasopharyngeal carcinoma: An analysis in 10,126 patients. *Oral Oncol* 95:150–156.

Zhang T, Wu Y, Ju H, et al. 2020. Extranodal marginal zone B-cell lymphoma of the mucosa-associated lymphoid tissue in the oromaxillofacial region: A retrospective analysis of 105 patients. *Cancer Med* 2020(1):194–203.

Zhong LP, Wang LZ, Ji T, et al. 2009. Clinical analysis of Castleman's disease (hyaline vascular Type0 in parotid and neck region). *Oral Surg Oral Med Oral Pathol Pral Radiol Endo* 109(3):432–440

Zurrida S, Alasio L, Tradati N, et al. 1993. Fine needle aspiration of parotid masses *Cancer* 72(8):2306–2311.

Chapter 16
Trauma and Injuries to the Salivary Glands

Outline

Introduction
Penetrating Injuries
  Trauma to the Gland
    Salivary Fistula
    Sialocele
    Facial Nerve Injuries
      Facial nerve injuries in primary trauma
      Facial nerve injuries in elective surgery
    Frey Syndrome
    Hollowing
  Trauma to Salivary Gland Ducts
    Transection of the Salivary Duct
    Stricture of the Salivary Duct
Radiation Injury
  External Beam
  Radioactive Iodine
  PSMA Radioligand Therapy
Barotrauma
Summary
References

Introduction

The salivary glands may be subjected to numerous injuries and insults. Trauma to the parotid is relatively rare, 0.21% of patients in a trauma unit (Lewis and Knottenbelt 1991). Penetrating trauma may be truly uncontrolled or accidental in nature; however, identical complications and injuries are seen after the intentionally controlled trauma of surgery. This chapter will therefore deal with the complications of both salivary gland surgery and true traumatic injury. The injurious effects of radiation and barotraumas will be reviewed.

Penetrating Injuries

TRAUMA TO THE GLAND

Salivary Fistula

Penetrating injury to the substance of a major gland e.g. the parotid or submandibular gland will cause direct damage to the gland and possible related structures and may lead to the formation of an external salivary fistula to the skin (Figure 16.1). When the substance of the gland is injured suture of the parenchyma is recommended (Lewkowicz et al. 2002). In addition to direct closure of the parotid capsule, a pressure dressing for 48 hours is applied to reduce the chances of sialocele formation. In 51 cases of parotid complications following trauma, 15 (30%) developed parotid fistula, treated by intravenous fluids and nil by mouth, with faster healing of parenchymal injuries alone than when the ductal system was involved (Parkeh et al. 1989). Similarly, Ananthakrishnan and Parkash (1982), reported that their three cases of fistula from the parotid gland parenchyma resolved without treatment unlike the 14 fistulae related to the parotid ductal injury. In a study of 13 patients with traumatic parotid fistulae, 54% resolved with conservative management within three weeks and the remaining patients were cured by internal drainage with a catheter (Cant and Campbell 1991). Landau and Stewart (1985) advocated conservative management of post-traumatic parotid fistulae and sialoceles found that parenchymal injuries alone resolved in five days whereas ductal injuries took 14 days. While Morestin (1917), in a series of 62 war injuries with parotid fistula, 30 glandular and 32 ductal, reported good success with the creation of an intraoral fistula. In a literature review,

---

Salivary Gland Pathology: Diagnosis and Management, Third Edition. Edited by Eric R. Carlson and Robert A. Ord.
© 2022 John Wiley & Sons, Inc. Published 2022 by John Wiley & Sons, Inc.
Companion website: www.wiley.com/go/carlson/salivary

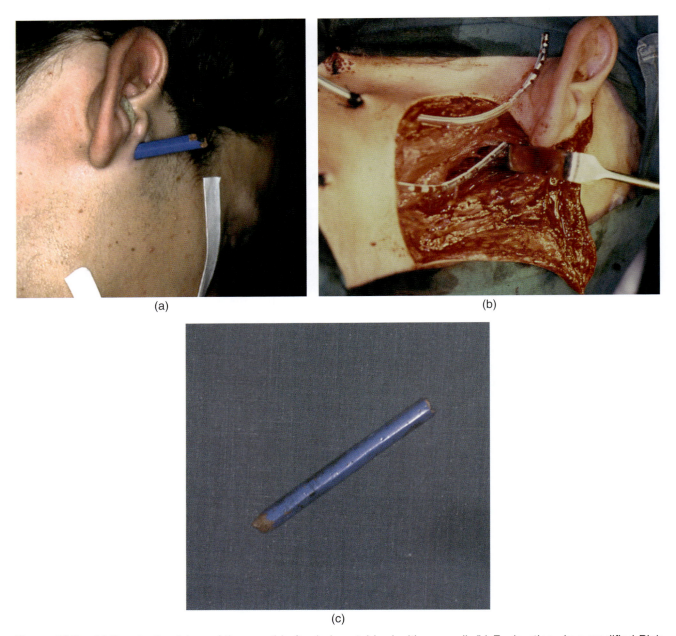

Figure 16.1. (a) Penetrating injury of the parotid after being stabbed with a pencil. (b) Exploration via a modified Blair incision to check for damage to the external carotid artery, facial nerve and suture the capsule. (c) The length of the recovered pencil illustrates the depth of the wound.

70 cases of parotid trauma were identified. Assault was responsible for 90% of cases and sialoceles and fistulae were the main sequelae. In all 54% were managed conservatively (Akinbami 2009).

In more extensive avulsive injuries with gross scarring conservative treatment may be less successful (Figure 16.2) and established epithelialized fistulae may require excision with the repair of the parotid capsule and closure.

The submandibular gland is less liable to be involved in the development of traumatic fistulae perhaps because it is protected by the mandible and its smaller size. Few cases are reported; and in 1995, a published case report of a submandibular

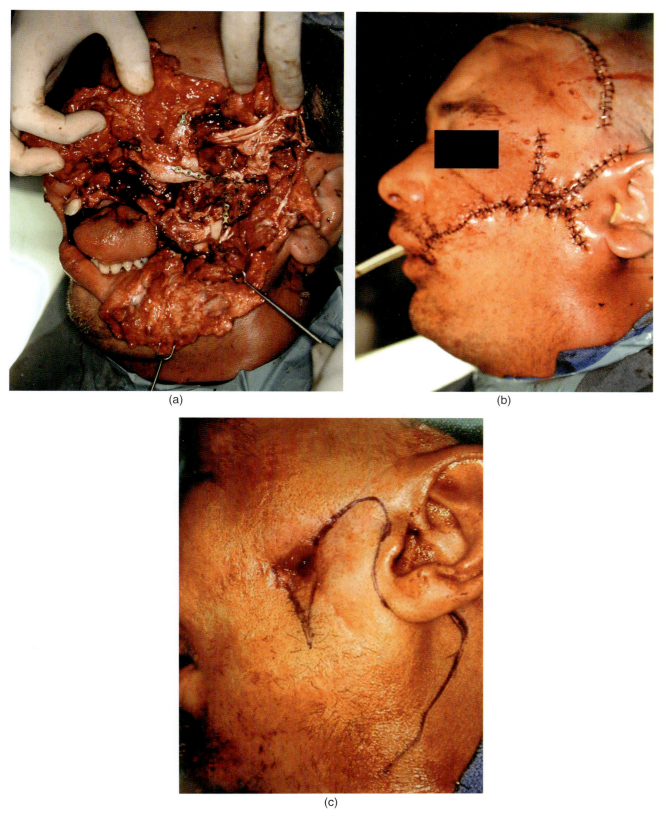

Figure 16.2. (a) Extensive avulsive injury from self-inflicted shotgun wound. (b) Post-surgical reduction of facial fractures and wound closure. (c) The patient developed a salivary fistula which was treated by excision resuturing and a rotation flap as outlined.

gland fistula secondary to a gunshot wound, which reviewed the literature found only one other case from 1976 (Singh and Shaha 1995). In their 1995 case, the fistula resolved without active treatment in 10 days.

Rarely internal parotid fistulae can occur presenting as rhinorrhea or rhinorrhea related to food usually resulting from maxillary fracture with parotid fistula into the maxillary antrum (Scher and Poe 1988; Faussat et al. 1993). In a recent report of parotid fistula into the maxillary antrum (and a very rare case of a sublingual gland fistula to the skin), excellent results were achieved with Botulinum toxin injection (Breuer et al. 2006). Although the authors state that primary surgical repair should be carefully considered they found the injection of Botulinum toxin to be effective, shorten fistula closure time, and be minimally invasive.

The current management of fistulae from the parotid gland parenchyma is therefore conservative as cases not involving the duct will resolve. In recalcitrant cases, Botulinum toxin appears a good option. True fistulas post-surgery e.g. superficial parotidectomy, are not common but may occur through the surgical skin incision. Usually, management with antisialogogues, nil by mouth, or Botulinum toxin will lead to resolution. In a report of three cases post-parotidectomy treated with an injection of botulinum toxin under electromyographic control, all resolved with no recurrence 14–21 months after therapy (Marchese-Ragona et al. 2006). In a small series of six post-traumatic parotid fistulas treated by Abobotulinum toxin, all fistulas closed after one injection session without the need for other conservative treatment (Costan et al. 2019).

In reviewing the literature for iatrogenic parotid fistulae and sialoceles as a postoperative complication of parotid surgery a rate of 1.7% of the salivary fistula was identified for superficial parotidectomy and 0–11% for total parotidectomy (Nahlieli 2017).

Sialocele

A sialocele is formed by the extravasation of saliva into glandular or periglandular tissues due to disruption of the parenchymal or ductal structures of the saliva gland. This is most commonly seen following trauma and the usual sites are the sublingual gland (ranula) or minor salivary glands (mucocele). Ranulae and mucoceles have been

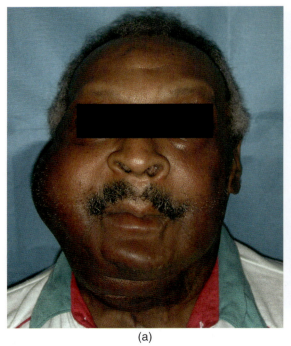
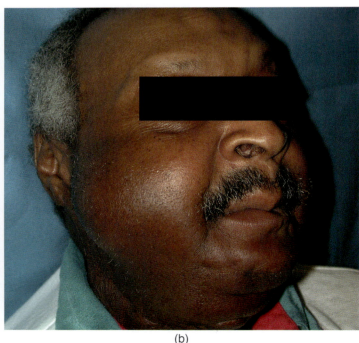

(a)   (b)

Figure 16.3. (a and b) Frontal and three-quarter views of patient with right parotid sialocele post-surgery. (c) MR views of sialocele with enhancing capsule.

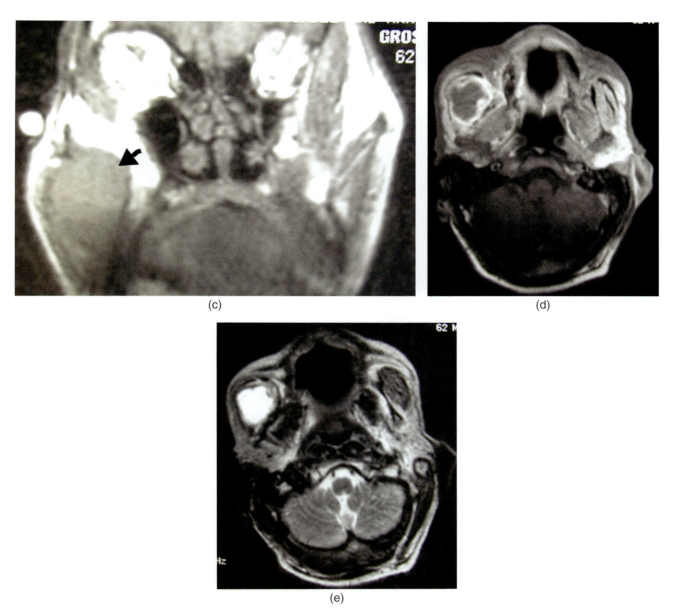

Figure 16.3. *(Continued)*.

discussed in Chapter 4 and this section will concentrate largely on parotid sialoceles. Parotid sialocoeles are usually seen after penetrating trauma to the parotid region and will present as painless, cystic swellings that are gradually increasing in size. They may reach giant size (Júnior et al. 2012). Aspiration of the sialocele with fluid positive for amylase > 10,000 units/l will confirm the diagnosis. CT scan will show a cystic mass with smooth margins and a density lower than the surrounding tissues. After two weeks, CT scans will show enhancing borders due to the development of a capsule (Cholankeril and Scioscia 1993) (Figure 16.3).

Traditional management has been conservative the same as for parotid parenchymal fistulae (Landau and Stewart 1985; Parkeh et al. 1989; Cant and Campbell 1991) with resolution reported in approximately the same time period as for fistulae. Most sialoceles develop 8–14 days post-injury and the development of a late capsulated sialocele is more difficult to treat. Literature reviews show that treatments proposed include multiple aspirations, pressure dressings, secondary duct repair if duct injury is the etiology, creation of an intraoral fistula, sectioning the auriculotemporal nerve, the use of antisialogogues (atropine, probanthine, glycopyrrolate), duct ligation, and even radiation or parotidectomy (Canosa and Cohen 1999; Lewkowicz et al. 2002) (Figures 16.4 and 16.5).

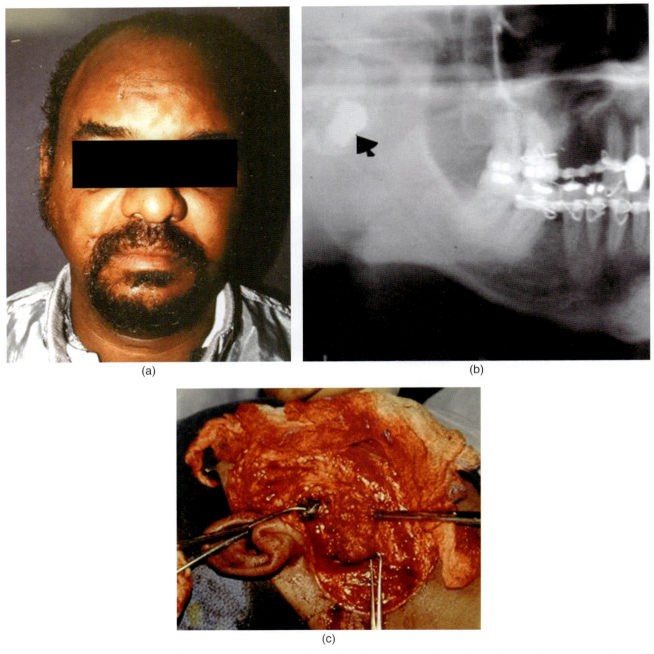

Figure 16.4. (a) 41-year-old male post a gunshot wound which entered in the left parotid region and traversed to the right parotid region with fracture of both left and right condyles developed an increasing sialocele in the right parotid gland. (b) Panoramic film shows the retained bullet in the right parotid gland (arrow). (c) Modified Blair incision and partial parotidectomy, with mosquito forceps indicating the bullet. The bullet was located between the superior and inferior branches of the facial nerve which was intact with no weakness. The capsule of the parotid was repaired and the sialocele resolved.

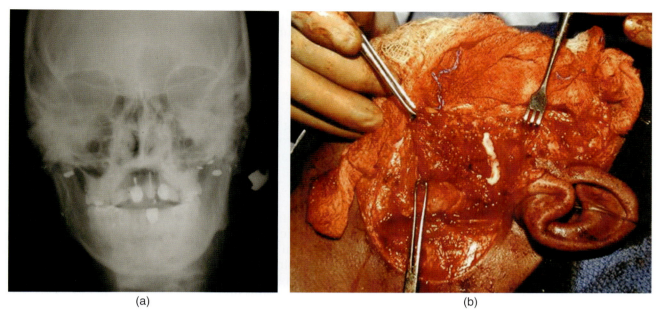

Figure 16.5. (a) Plain film of 20-year old boy following a gunshot wound shows bullet "floating" in parotid. sialocele. (b) Surgical exploration to remove the bullet revealed an abscess cavity where the bullet had lodged. Note pus draining.

In recent years, the use of botulinum toxin has caused a paradigm shift in the way these injuries can be managed. In 1999, Ragona et al. reported a case of post-traumatic parotid sialocele resistant to conservative therapy that was successfully cured using botulinum injection. These authors used botulinum F due to its earlier and shorter efficacy compared to botulinum A and injected the gland with electromyographic control. Botulinum toxin works by causing chemical denervation of the gland by blocking the cholinergic neurotransmitter. Following this paper, a report of four cases of recurrent post-parotidectomy sialoceles treated with botulinum A toxin injected subcutaneously with 100% success was published (Vargas et al. 2000) as well as other case reports (Chow and Kwok 2003). There is a single case of a submandibular sialocele treated with resolution using botulinum toxin A (Capaccio et al. 2006).

Another novel approach to these injuries has been the use of sialo-endoscopy. In a review of salivary trauma related to facial rejuvenation procedures, Nahlieli et al. (2008a) classified the injuries into four types; compression of the ducts by temporary swelling, laceration of the gland capsule, stretching and compression of the duct with penetration of the duct capsule leading to sialocele/long term swelling (a combination of the first two) and a complete cut or penetration of the main duct/or main branch resulting in sialocele. In 14 cases of these injuries, endoscopic treatment was 100% successful (Nahlieli et al. 2008a). Bilateral parotid duct obstruction has been reported following "facelift" surgery (Mandel and Silver 2012).

The data for sialoceles following parotidectomy surgery are 0–26% for superficial parotidectomy, 0–1% for deep lobe excision only, and 0–16% for total parotidectomy (Nahlieli 2017).

Facial Nerve Injuries
Facial nerve injury in primary trauma
The facial nerve is at risk from penetrating injury to the facial region both in the parotid and in the distribution of its peripheral branches to the facial musculature. It is stated that damage to branches distal to a line drawn from the lateral canthus to the commissure does not require repair and may be managed expectantly. All patients with facial wounds should have a careful clinical examination of the facial nerve function. Where this is not possible e.g. in the unconscious patient or the uncooperative infant (Figure 16.6), the wound should be carefully explored at the time of surgery to exclude transaction of the branches of the facial nerve. Primary repair soon after the injury with end to end anastomosis is the ideal scenario, as paralysis

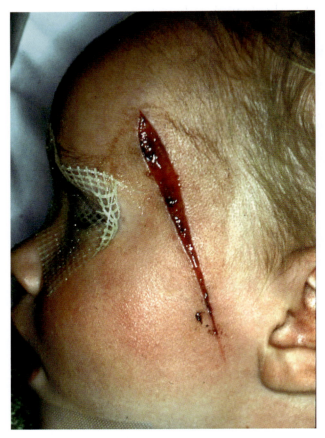

Figure 16.6. Infant with laceration from broken glass. No facial nerve damage.

of the facial nerve is a devastating injury for the patient, and even when "successful" nerve repair has been carried out with satisfying results (based on House-Brackmann, Stennert, and May grading) patients experienced a reduced quality of life (Guntinas-Lichius et al. 2007) (Figures 16.7 and 16.8). Early repair is emphasized as early repairs have better outcomes, but function will continue to evolve following repair for a year or longer (Condie and Tolkachjov 2019). This section will discuss the management of the primary nerve injury and will not discuss the techniques for facial reanimation or static slings which are beyond the scope of this text. The interested reader will find many recent review articles addressing these topics (Malik et al. 2005; Guntinas-Lichius et al. 2006). The management of a patient with established facial nerve paralysis will be discussed in the case presented at the end of Chapter 14.

Classically, the nerve is sutured under the microscope using 9-0 or 10-0 nylon sutures attempting to coapt the nerve ends without tension (Figure 16.9). The suturing can be epineural or fascicular. In epineural suturing, less damage is caused to the neural bundles with less foreign body reaction in the fascicles due to the suture materials; however, fascicular suturing should allow better adaptation of the fascicles and trimming back the epineurium to prevent fibrous tissue in-growth. However, anatomic studies have shown the fascicular and connective tissue anatomy of the facial nerve to be complex with the number of fascicles increasing in a proximo-distal way from the geniculate ganglion with diminishing diameter (Figure 16.10). This variability in the number of fascicles and structure along the extratemporal facial nerve constitutes a difficulty in facial nerve repair (Captier et al. 2005). The use of tubes e.g. collagen, to support the anastomosis and prevent connective tissue ingrowth and tissue glues e.g. fibrin, to replace sutures and their foreign body reactions have been advocated. However, the tubes can themselves cause foreign body reactions and possible compression. Regarding the tissue glues, animal experiments appear to show sutures to be superior. In the rabbit model, axonal growth was faster and greater with epineural suture than fibrin adhesive (Junior et al. 2004). Although the rate and amount of reduction in conduction velocity was equivalent between the two methods the authors concluded that epineural suture appears the method of choice. In another study in the rat model looking at suture and the effects of platelet-rich plasma (PRP) and fibrin sealant, the best return of function for the facial nerve was again with suture (Farrag et al. 2007). The authors did note a favorable neurotropic effect for the PRP but no benefit for the fibrin sealant.

As it is vital that the anastomosis be tension-free, the difficulty is encountered when a gap between the nerve ends exists. In a cadaver study, Gardetto et al. (2002) showed that removal of the superficial part of the parotid gland could allow an overlap of the cut branches of the facial nerve. They found it possible to bridge gaps of 15 mm in the temporo-zygomatic branches, 23 mm in the buccal-mandibular branches, and 17 mm in the nerve trunk. Following this experimental work, the authors reported successful clinical results on three patients recommending the technique for gaps up to 15 mm but cautioning against its use in the presence of infection or nerve defects (Piza-Katzer et al. 2004). In another approach, the use of a rapid

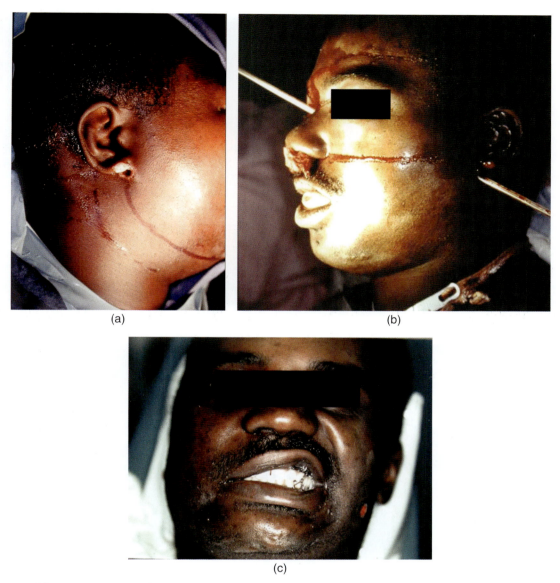

Figure 16.7. (a) Entrance wound for bullet below ear lobe. (b) Bougie placed through track of bullet to demonstrate entrance and exit. (c) Frontal, and buccal facial nerve paralysis.

nerve expander (2 cm/30 minutes) was used to bridge gaps up to 3 cm (Ya et al. 2007). In nine patients, five achieved good results with EMG peak value of mimetic muscles 82–95% of the normal side, three cases were fair EMG 60–90%, and one case poor EMG 55%. Other surgical options in this situation are the use of a tube as a conduit and grafting. In seven patients with post-traumatic defects up to 3 cm, the use of a bioabsorbable polyglycolic acid tube was reported as giving very good results in one case, good in four and fair in two (Navissano et al. 2005). The two commonest sites for donor's nerves for the facial nerve are the greater auricular which is adjacent to the surgical field and the sural nerve (Figure 16.11). The greater auricular nerve may already be exposed by the existing traumatic injuries. If not, it is easily located as it crosses the sternocleidomastoid muscle. Its surface markings are located by bisecting a line drawn between the tip of the mastoid and the angle of the mandible. The sural nerve is identified just posterior to the lateral malleolus. The use of a specially designed instrument allows tunneling/ dissection and cutting of a 25 cm. graft through a

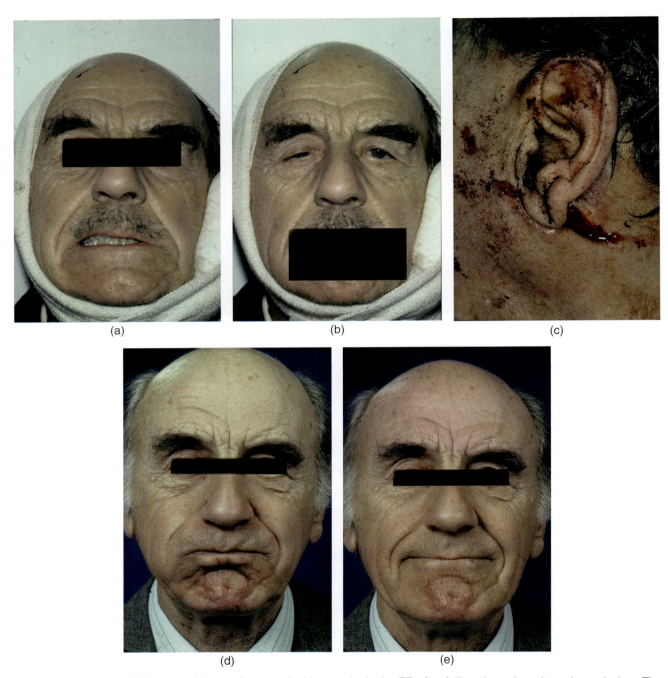

Figure 16.8. (a and b) 72-year-old man diagnosed with a stroke in the ER after falling through a plate glass window. The diagnosis was made due to the dense facial nerve palsy. (c) After removing the dressings, the deep penetrating wound in the region of the facial nerve trunk is appreciated. (d and e) One-year post repair of nerve trunk and microneural suture the patient still has some weakness of the upper lid and cannot "blow out" his cheek on the left side, but has good facial symmetry and function.

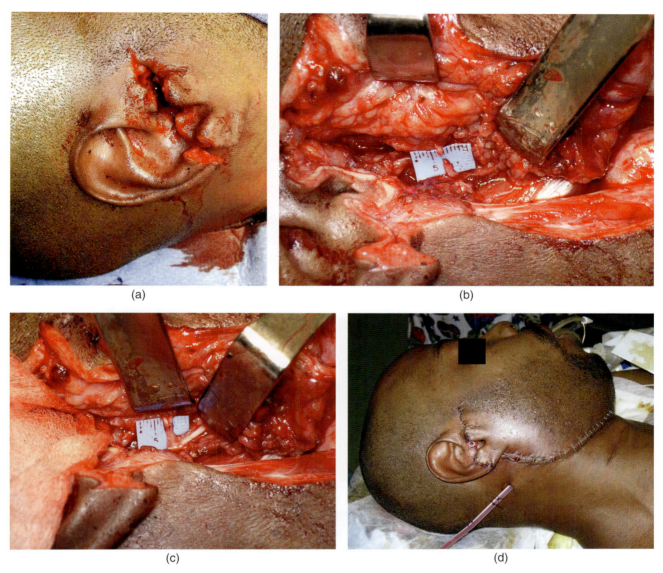

Figure 16.9. (a) Penetrating wound through ear and parotid. (b) Exploration of wound reveals transaction of the superior branch of the facial nerve. (Ruler from surgical margin makes a good background for microsuture if custom microsurgical background material is unavailable). (c) Post-microsurgical repair. (d) Post-suturing of wounds. Source: This case was treated by Dr. J. Caccamese, Department of OMS University of Maryland.

single incision at the lateral malleolus. The patient will be left with anesthesia on a small area of the lateral foot and ankle.

Surgical principles for repair follow those for direct anastomosis. As expected, facial nerve function from cable nerve graft interposition is not as favorable as an end-to-end anastomosis (Malik et al. 2005). If there is widespread destruction of multiple branches from an injury such as a gunshot the entire superficial cervical plexus can be used to supply multiple grafts. In the animal model, a peptide amphiphile nanofiber nerve graft has been shown to be equivalent to an autogenous nerve graft (Greene et al. 2018). We have used acellular nerve allografts for repair, mostly for the inferior alveolar nerve (Figure 16.12).

It should be remembered that the facial nerve lies superficial to the external carotid artery, which may be damaged in penetrating Zone III neck injuries. A report of emergency parotidectomy due to massive bleeding from such an injury, necessitated subsequent facial nerve repair (Morris et al. 2007).

Facial nerve injury in elective surgery

In elective surgery, the facial nerve may be damaged accidentally (iatrogenic trauma) or there may be a preplanned need to resect a portion of the nerve usually due to tumor involvement by cancer or for surgical access. In most of these cases, a decision on whether to perform a repair, an early reanimation procedure or to elect for no primary treatment of the nerve and consider delayed reanimation will have been discussed with the patient preoperatively.

In 285 cases of total parotidectomy with facial nerve sacrifice 89 patients, 31.2% underwent a concurrent intraoperative reanimation procedure. In 41 cases, the nerve was repaired, in 31 a sling procedure was performed and in 17 cases a combination of the two procedures was undertaken. Patients having nerve repair were significantly younger 57.6 vs. 72.1 years. In addition, 49 patients had microvascular free tissue and 49% had facial reanimation procedures whereas only 28% of those who did not have soft tissue reconstruction had reanimation procedures ($p = 0.003$) (Lu et al. 2019). In another study of 17 patients with radical parotidectomy, the reconstruction

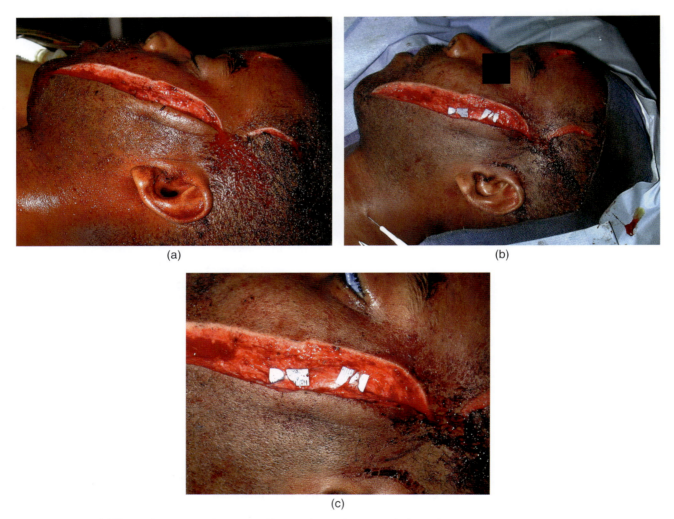

Figure 16.10. (a) Extensive penetrating wound is anterior to the parotid gland that involves the peripheral branches of the nerve. (b) Nerve branches identified for microneural repair. (c) High power view of the completed repair. (d, e, f, and g) Post repair note upper branch weakness persists. Source: This case was treated by Dr. J Caccamese, Department OMS University of Maryland.

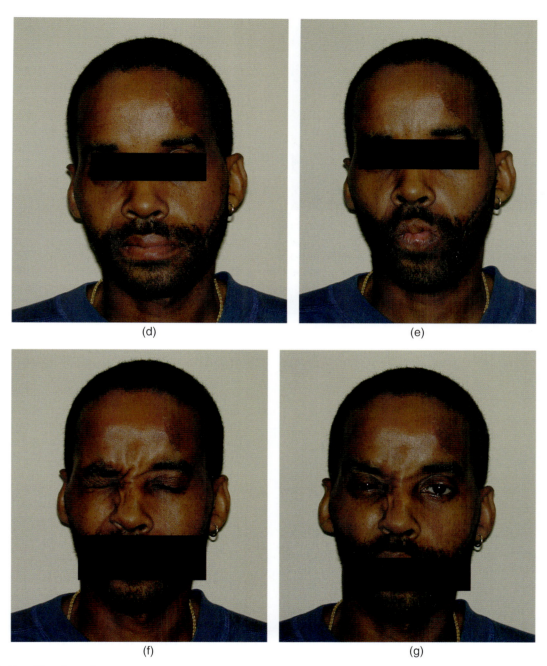

Figure 16.10. *(Continued).*

included antero-lateral thigh flap with the nerve to the vastus lateralis and a fascia lata sling from the lower lip to the temporalis tendon. All patients achieved oral competence and a dynamic smile with activation of the tendon sling. Facial nerve recovery was only seen in eight patients (47%) and five reached a House Brackman score of 3 (Ciolek et al. 2018). A study of primary nerve grafting in total parotidectomy with either sural nerve in 12 patients or greater auricular nerve in 10 patients showed House Brackman grade V (four cases), grade IV (seven cases), grade III (eight cases), and grade II (three cases) (Rashid et al. 2019).

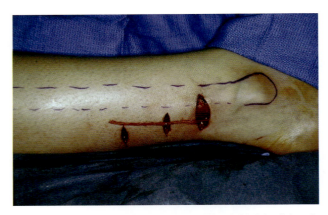

Figure 16.11. Sural nerve graft. The initial incision is made close to the lateral malleolus to locate the sural nerve. The nerve can be dissected free superiorly up to 25 cm in length. In this case, small step-ladder incisions were made to aid access.

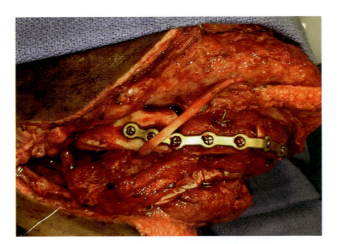

Figure 16.12. Avance nerve graft used to reconstruct resected inferior alveolar nerve following segmental mandibular resection for ameloblastoma. Source: Case of Dr. Donita Dyalram, with permission from Dr. Dyalram.

In oncologic parotid surgery with facial nerve sacrifice surgery will usually be followed by postoperative radiation therapy (PORT). In a study of 39 patients who underwent primary facial nerve repair, there was a trend towards better function in patients who did not receive radiation but this was not significant. The authors concluded that PORT appeared not to prevent achieving good facial nerve function after primary repair of the facial nerve (Gidley et al. 2010). In 53 patients with PORT given by external beam and brachytherapy, the functional outcomes of immediate facial nerve repair with grafts were not affected (Hontanilla et al. 2014).

During lateral skull base surgery, the facial nerve may be sacrificed both for access or tumor involvement. In a study of 213 patients with cable graft repair of the facial nerve in lateral skull-base surgeries, 108 (50.7%) had recovered to a House-Brackman (HB) grade III nerve function. Preoperative HB status had a significant effect on the outcome. The authors found that the stitch-less fibrin glue-aided coaptation gave the best results (Prasad et al. 2018).

In facial transplantation surgery, problems with managing salivary glands have emerged as a postoperative challenge according to a review of the 35 cases worldwide published in 2015. The authors reviewed 25/35 cases finding 48% had undesirable salivary problems 42% parotid, 25% parotid and submandibular glands, and 33% minor salivary glands. Sialoceles were treated successfully with botulinum. The facial nerve was managed by repair at the level of the trunk/primary divisions in 66% of patients or the terminal branches in 34%. When the parotid gland was included in the transplant the facial nerve was anastomosed at the trunk, and when the gland was excluded the terminal branches were repaired. The authors felt that exclusion of the gland was the preferable method (Frautschi et al. 2015).

Finally, as discussed earlier in this chapter (see penetrating injuries) the parotid gland and facial nerve may be damaged during esthetic facial surgery. In these cases, there is of course a higher risk of medico-legal consequences.

Frey Syndrome

Although Frey syndrome is now most commonly seen in relation to parotid surgery, it was originally described after a shotgun injury to the parotid gland (Frey 1923), however, despite Frey's landmark paper, gustatory sweating was probably first described by Baillarger in 1853 (Dulguerov et al. 1999). In the trauma arena, the obvious problem is management and treatment of the condition post-surgery, whereas in post-parotidectomy cases much work has been done on prevention. Frey syndrome is also a recognized entity in children. A multicenter study in France identified 48 cases of which 35 were unilateral and 13 bilateral. Although these children exhibited gustatory flushing, which defined the Frey syndrome diagnosis, only 10%

had associated sweating. The diagnosis was only made in 20% of children at the first consultation, it was often mistaken for food allergies. The unilateral form was significantly associated with "instrumented vaginal delivery," presumably blunt trauma to the parotid region during forceps delivery. The condition had a favorable course in the pediatric population with 57% regression, 20% recovery, and only 23% persistence. Regression was seen in 69% of unilateral cases at a median age of 27 months, and recovery in 58% of bilateral forms at the median age of eight months (Blanc et al. 2016).

Previously reported treatments of Frey syndrome have included topical and systemic anticholinergics, tympanic neurectomy, sectioning of the auriculotemporal or glossopharyngeal nerves, or interposition of a layer between the parotid gland and the skin, e.g. fascia lata, temporalis fascia, or dermal allografts (see Chapter 18). Currently, the use of botulinum toxin is the most frequently reported therapeutic modality for Frey syndrome. A report of 33 patients with Frey syndrome treated by intracutaneous injection of 16–80 IU of botulinum toxin A showed all symptoms to resolve within a week (Eckardt and Kuettner 2003). In a prospective non-randomized, non-blinded study of 11 patients treated with botulinum toxin A with follow-up 6–23 months, only one patient recurred and was successfully retreated (Kyrmizakis et al. 2004). A prospective randomized trial to establish the ideal dosage and length of effect of botulinum toxin A was carried out on 20 patients divided into two groups receiving either 2 or 3 MU/cm. In the 3 MU/cm group, a single injection resulted in a nearly complete absence of gustatory sweating during the 12-month follow-up period. In the 2 MU/cm group, 44% of the total skin areas were still sweating and required a second injection, and the authors concluded that 3 MU/cm^2 is the recommended dose (Nolte et al. 2004). Some authors have cautioned that the effect of botulinum in Frey syndrome is often temporary and further injections may be necessary depending upon the initial dose and the length of time followed (Ferraro et al. 2005). However, when considering the evidence base for treatment of Frey syndrome a Cochrane database systematic review found only eight possible studies for inclusion. All studies had to be excluded due to lack of randomization or other major flaws. The authors concluded that they were unable to establish the efficacy and safety of the different methods used for the treatment of Frey syndromes such as topical application of anticholinergics, antiperspirants, and botulinum toxin (Li et al. 2015).

In regards to parotidectomy patients, probably 100% of patients will have gustatory sweating if tested with starch and iodine (Laage-Hellman 1957) (Figure 16.13). However, few patients clinically notice this problem and most do not wish for treatment so that this condition will be underestimated in clinical reports. Although the gustatory sweating usually occurs directly over the parotidectomy site, it may occur beyond the parotid bed distal to the gland. In a report of seven cases, the authors postulate the mechanism is either regeneration of severed postganglionic fibers into sympathetic targets along the course of the auriculotemporal nerve or by regeneration into fibers of the sympathetic plexus along the superficial temporal artery (Wood and Netterville 2019).

Frey syndrome is rarely reported after submandibular gland removal. Berini-Aytes and Gay-Escoda (1992) reviewed 206 submandibular gland excisions and found only one case of Frey syndrome. While Teague et al. (1998) reviewed the literature and could find seven reported cases since 1934. Only occasional case reports are seen (Lee and Yoon 2010; Hong and Hong 2020). Frey syndrome in the submandibular region has also been reported after neck dissection (Yoshimura et al. 2012). A case of bilateral gustatory sweating following bilateral neck dissection which was successfully treated with Botulinum toxin is also described (Philouze et al. 2014).

The techniques described for the prevention of Frey syndrome depend upon placing a barrier between the parotid bed and skin to prevent the growth of the secretory parasympathetic nerves from the parotid into the sweat glands causing a paradoxical innervation. The acellular dermis has been used with success but a higher complication rate (Govindaraj et al. 2001). Temporoparietal flaps and the superficial musculoaponeurotic system (SMAS) have been used with good outcomes in 146 parotidectomy patients (Cesteleyn et al. 2002). No cases of Frey syndrome were encountered in reviewing 160 patients followed from 5 to 22 years treated with an interpositional SMAS layer at the time of parotidectomy and tested with starch/iodine during follow-up (Bonanno et al. 2000). Other reported barriers have been the use of parotid gland fascia (Zumeng et al. 2006), and

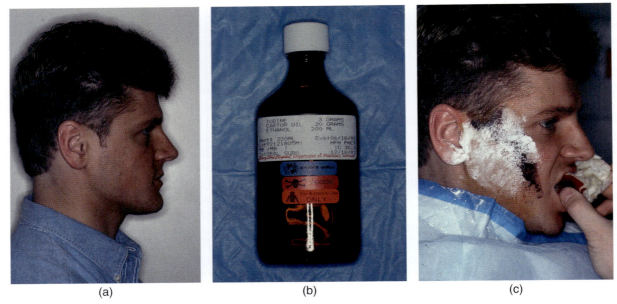

Figure 16.13. (a) Lateral view of face of patient complaining of gustatory sweating (Frey syndrome). (b) Bottle of iodine solution that is painted on the face and then covered with corn starch. (c) While the patient ate an apple the corn starch is colored blue-black, indicative of gustatory sweating.

sternocleidomastoid flaps with mixed results (Kerawala et al. 2002; Filho et al. 2004). Fascia lata, free fat, polyglycolic felt, or acellular dermis have all been inserted between the parotid bed and overlying skin (Aizawa et al. 2018; Hojjat et al. 2018). It would appear that Frey syndrome is preventable in most cases and perhaps the use of the SMAS layer is the most convenient for the surgeon intraoperatively.

Hollowing

Hollowing is a complication seen in patients following parotidectomy rather than trauma and can be managed in a variety of ways. Reconstruction at the time of surgery to prevent the defect from occurring is preferable to secondary reconstruction when scarring and the superficial position of the facial nerve post-parotidectomy increase the risk of nerve damage. Various techniques have been used some of which have been discussed in this chapter in relation to Frey syndrome and Chapter 10. Techniques include the use of layered acellular dermis, free fat grafts (see Figure 10.4), use of the SMAS layer, temporalis and sternocleidomastoid flaps as well as microvascular free flaps including fascial forearm flaps and anterior lateral thigh flaps for larger defects (See case presentation at the end of the chapter). Choice of technique will depend on the size of the defect, the surgeon's own experience, and the wishes of the patient.

TRAUMA TO SALIVARY GLAND DUCTS

Transection of the Salivary Duct

As has already been discussed above in the sections on fistulae and sialoceles related to parenchymal trauma, conservative management is usually satisfactory except in those cases where the injury involves the partial or complete transaction of the duct. Under these circumstances, most papers have indicated that resolution is less certain and takes longer with active management frequently required. There are studies that support conservative measures in duct injuries and one report, 19 patients with duct injury confirmed by methylene blue dye injection in a retrograde fashion through Stensen duct who were treated non-operatively, 9 (47%) healed without complications. Although seven patients (36.8%) developed salivary fistulas and 4 (21.4%) developed sialoceles, these were described as short term and resolved without the need for surgery (Lewis and Knottenbelt 1991). Van Sickels (1981), divided the parotid duct anatomically into three sites of injury, based on implications for treatment. Site A is the intra-glandular portion of the duct and ductal injuries in this location are treated as described above for parenchymal trauma. Site B represents the duct as it overlies the masseter muscle and site C the duct's course anterior to the masseter muscle through the deep tissues of the cheek into the mouth. Injuries at both these sites require exploration and direct repair of the duct if possible. If repair is impossible, creating a direct fistula into the mouth is the treatment of choice for site C injuries (Lazaridou et al. 2012). However, in most cases, current management is directed toward primary repair and the clinician must therefore have a high level of suspicion for injuries involving the region of the parotid duct. There may be accompanying damage to the buccal branch of the facial nerve, but the absence of saliva on "milking" the gland does not confirm injury neither does saliva at the papilla rule it out (Lazaridou et al. 2012). The classic anatomic surface markings of the duct are illustrated in Figure 16.14. However, an ultrasound study has shown that 92% of ducts were below the classic anatomic surface markings, although 93% of the ducts were within 1.5 cm of the middle half of a line between the tragus and the cheilion (Stringer et al. 2012). In this study, the mean internal caliber of the duct was 0.6 ± 0.2 mm. Toure et al. (2015) point out that in their anatomic study that the duct follows a curved trajectory before it penetrates the buccinator muscle. A rare anatomic variation of a duplication of the duct has been described. In one study of 35 hemifacial cadaver dissections, the authors found three cases of duplication of the duct (Tsai et al. 2019).

Confirmatory evidence for the transaction is obtained by cannulating the distal portion of the duct through Stensen papilla and observing the catheter in the wound (Figure 16.15) or by injecting saline or a small (1 cc) amount of methylene blue through Stensen papilla. Van Sickels (2009) cautions against injecting too much dye which can stain the tissues and increase the difficulty of the dissection. A technique using fluorescein to identify duct injuries is also described (Montag et al. 2016). Identification of the proximal end may be technically difficult as it can retract into the gland substance. Milking the gland to obtain salivary flow is helpful in these circumstances and the anesthesiologist must be cautioned preoperatively against the use of anti-parasympathetic agents. If the proximal and distal ends of the duct are

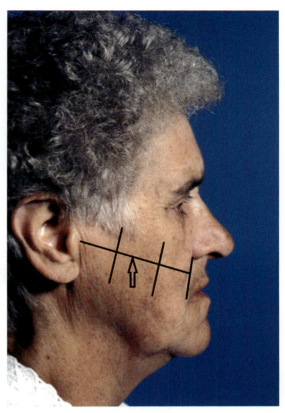

Figure 16.14. Surface markings of the parotid duct are shown by a line drawn from the tragus of the ear to bisect a line drawn from the alar base to the commissure. The middle third of this line (arrow) is surface marking of the parotid duct.

identified and can be coapted then the microsurgical repair can be carried out (Hallock 1992) (Figure 16.16).

The use of stents (usually indwelling catheters) for 10–14 days to prevent stenosis is advocated by some and appears a reasonable hypothesis although no long-term studies of these injuries with and without stenting have been published. A technique of using a 4F Foley embolectomy catheter for identification of the transaction and then left in place as a stent is described (Etoz et al. 2006). When the proximal and distal ends of the duct cannot be coapted due to tissue loss, repair using a vein graft has been reported (Heymans et al. 1999). Steinberg and Herréra (2005) recommended the use of sialography postoperatively to assess the result of duct repair, stating this technique may not always be practical or possible in the acute setting. However, we have used sialography

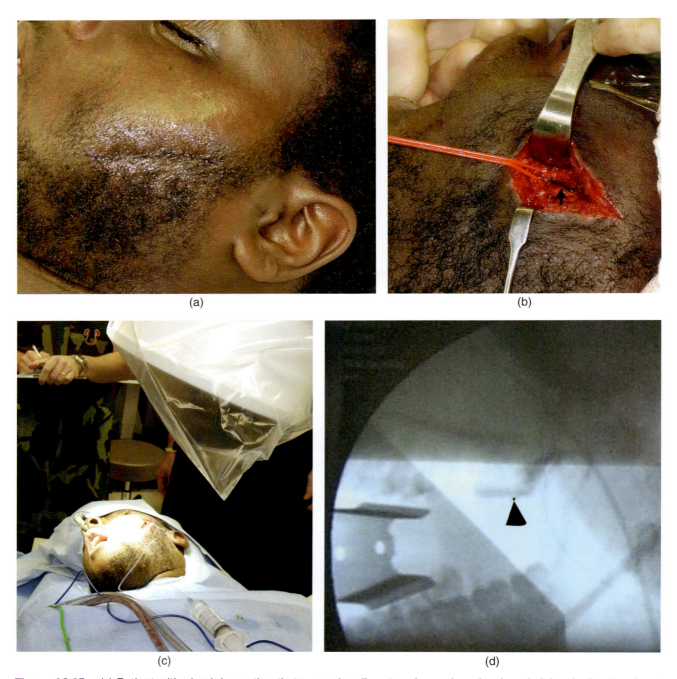

Figure 16.15. (a) Patient with cheek laceration that was primarily sutured, now has developed sialocele due to missed duct injury. (b) Wound reopened for re-exploration at which point the duct was noted to be transected. Vessel loop around distal end of duct. Lacrimal probe passed from intra-oral through Stensen's duct into the wound (short arrow). (c) The duct is approximated after locating the proximal end of the duct by milking the gland. The duct is cannulated and contrast dye injected for intra-operative sialogram. (d) Fluoroscopic image of intra-operative sialogram with repaired duct (arrow).

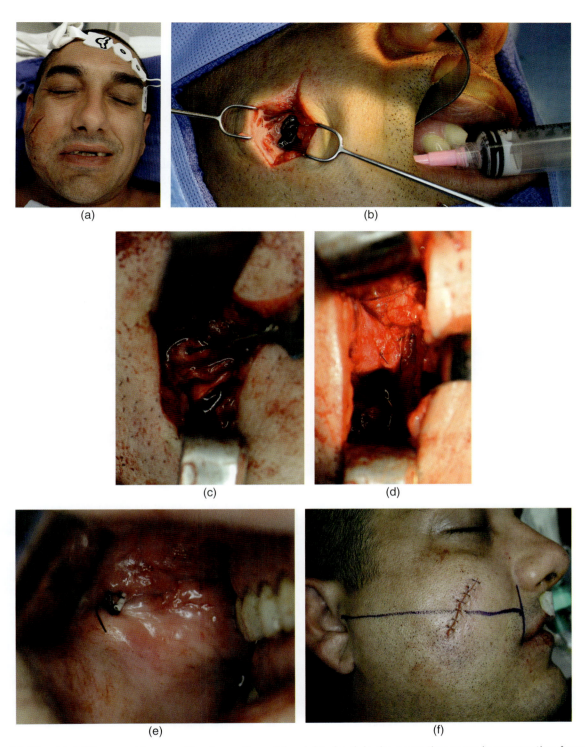

Figure 16.16. (a) A 38-year-old man with a laceration of the right cheek in the operating room in preparation for primary closure and exploration of Stensen duct due to the depth and anatomic location of the laceration. (b) Sterile milk was injected in the distal aspect of Stensen duct that permitted the identification of its laceration. (c) The proximal end of the lacerated Stensen duct is cannulated with a lacrimal probe. (d) The proximal and distal ends of the Stensen duct are primarily closed with 6-0 Prolene sutures with an indwelling catheter in place. (e) The catheter is sutured to the oral mucosa and maintained in place for two weeks. (f) The cheek wound is primarily closed in anatomic layers. The location of the laceration is appreciated to exist along with the middle third of the line denoting the surface marking of the Stensen duct. Source: Courtesy of Dr. J. Greg Anderson and Dr. Michael Foster, University of Tennessee Medical Center Department of Oral and Maxillofacial Surgery.

intraoperatively (Figure 16.15). Further development in the repair of ductal injuries has been the utilization of the sialendoscope in some centers, for both repair and follow-up assessment (Kopeć et al. 2013; Koch et al. 2013).

When the injury is too proximal, the wound is avulsive or the duct cannot be identified, the clinician can either create an intraoral fistula or ligate the proximal duct. A controlled fistula can be created by suturing the proximal duct through the buccinator into the oral cavity if enough length is present or by placing a catheter or drain from the area of the wound into the mouth and leaving it to fistulize (Figure 16.17). Although ligating the proximal duct to cause eventual atrophy has been proposed (Van Sickels 1981), in the author's experience this is unpredictable, and even with the use of pressure and antisialogogues, these patients can have considerable swelling and pain. Chemical denervation using Botulinum toxin A may be used to achieve a good outcome in these circumstances (Arnaud et al. 2006).

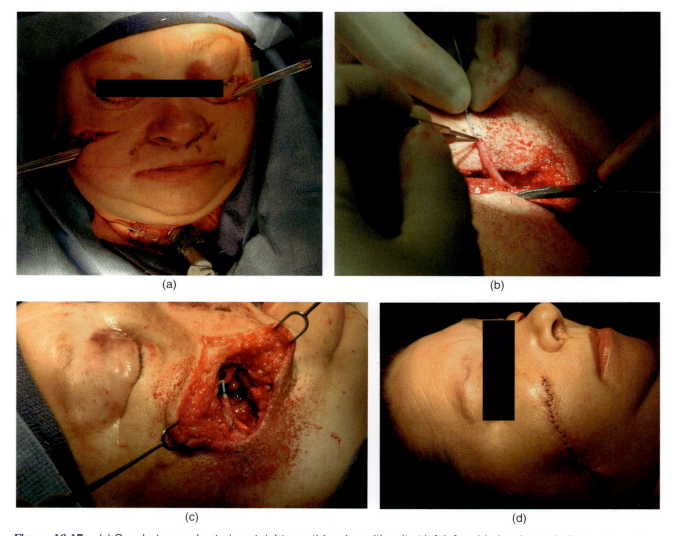

Figure 16.17. (a) Gunshot wound entering at right parotid region with exit at left infraorbital region as indicated by suction tubing. (b) The parotid duct is identified and dissected from the wound to be cannulated as shown. (c) The duct is diverted intraorally via the cannula. Note powder burn at entrance wound. (d) Final repair. Source: This case was treated by Dr. J. Caccamese, Department of Oral and Maxillofacial Surgery, University of Maryland.

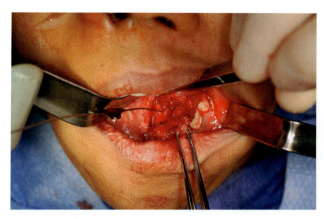

Figure 16.18. Degloving injury of the floor of mouth with a torn left Wharton duct. The duct lumen has been identified and cannulated with a lacrimal probe prior to repositioning and sialodochoplasty.

In the case of the submandibular duct, transection is usually iatrogenic resulting from surgery on the sublingual gland, sialolithotomy from the Wharton duct, or resection of floor of mouth cancer. Injury and obstruction have been reported following dental implant placement (Nahlieli et al. 2008b). It can occur in trauma usually associated with mandibular fracture and degloving injuries of the lingual mucosa. In this case, sialodochoplasty with repositioning of the duct posteriorly is all that is required (Figure 16.18). A catheter has been used as a stent (Ord and Lee 1996), following reposition of Wharton duct in the floor of mouth cancer, however, our current practice is to identify the duct lumen and insert one blade of sharp iris scissors and cut vertically through one wall of the duct. The duct is now "fish-tailed" and sutured to a newly created hole in the oral mucosa with 6-0 nylon sutures. Stenosis and stricture have not been a problem with this technique.

An alternative technique for ductal injuries is the use of sialendoscopy as referenced in the section of this chapter on sialocele, (above) (Nahlieli et al. 2008a; Koch et al. 2013; Man et al. 2017).

Stricture of the Salivary Duct

When ductal injuries are not surgically repaired immediately, complications such as fistulae and sialoceles may arise and their management has been discussed. If the duct has not been surgically repaired by 72 hours, conservative or medical therapy is recommended (Arnaud et al. 2006). In the long-term stricture of the duct may occur, although most strictures are secondary to inflammatory or infective conditions. In cases of intraductal salivary gland obstruction, 22.6% of 642 cases were due to strictures which were more common in females (Ngu et al. 2007) (Figure 16.19). When this occurs at the distal end of the Stensen duct, excision and diversion of the duct into the oral cavity may be feasible. When the main duct is involved with strictures sialoendoscopy may be useful to dilate the strictures using saline pressure, balloon dilatation, or the mini forceps grasper, and even the insertion of a stent to the duct lumen (Nahlieli et al. 2004). Simple balloon angioplasty was successful in seven/nine patients and five of these patients remained asymptomatic on follow-up (Salerno et al. 2007). If this is unsuccessful and the patient continues to have recurrent swelling and sialadenitis denervation with botulinum toxin or even parotidectomy may be required.

In the submandibular gland, the stricture can be excised and sialodochoplasty performed as described above. The most recent approaches to the problem of submandibular duct stenosis have been with the use of sialendoscopy. In a study of 47 patients with salivary stenosis pre-endoscopic, work-up included subjective symptoms, salivary flow rate, scintigraphy, and MR-sialography. Sialendoscopic grading of stenosis severity was grade I in 17 cases, grade II in 18, and grade III in 12. Outcomes at three months post-sialendoscopy were that symptoms completely resolved 44.7%, partially improved 40.4 and 14.9% (seven cases) showed no improvement or were worse. In multivariate analysis, T_{min} (time from stimulation to minimal count on scintigraphy), stenosis type on MR-sialography, and sialendoscopic grade were significantly associated with outcomes (Choi et al. 2018).

With the increased use of sialendoscopy for elective salivary gland surgery there may be an increase in iatrogenic duct injuries associated with the use of the endoscope. In Nahlieli's review of the literature, he found an incidence of stricture 2–4% in the parotid and 1–2% in the submandibular gland post-sialendoscopy (Nahlieli 2017).

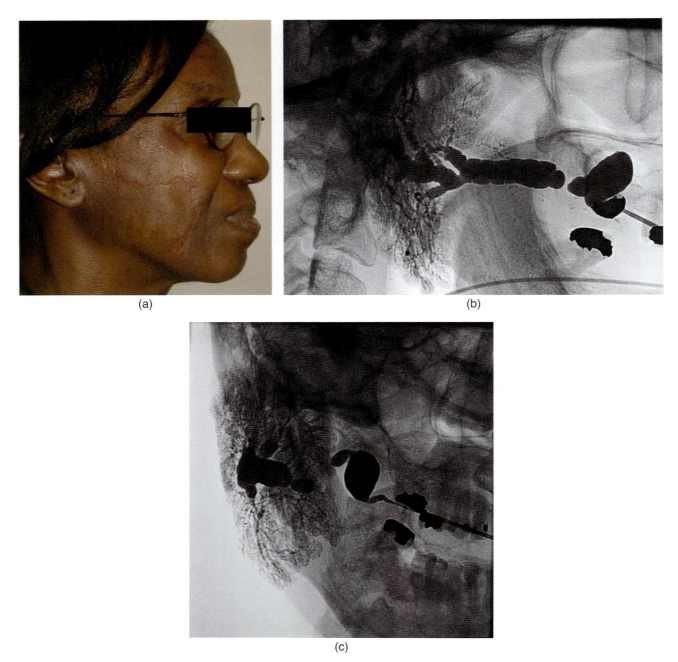

Figure 16.19. (a) Patient with soft-tissue scarring from penetrating wounds caused by a road traffic accident 10 years previously. She now has a seven-year history of parotid and cheek swelling. (b and c) Sialogram shows stricture of duct with proximal dilatation of Stensen duct and secondary ducts and a large cystic swelling distal to the structure.

Radiation Injury

EXTERNAL BEAM

Radiotherapy is commonly administered to patients with head and neck cancer, however, the injurious effect that this treatment modality has on the salivary glands leading to profound xerostomia, which may be permanent, is well-known. The serous cells found in the parotid gland are extremely sensitive to apoptotic death following even moderate doses of radiation. Indeed, permanent loss of salivary function is seen after doses approximately larger than 3500 cGy with little in the way of

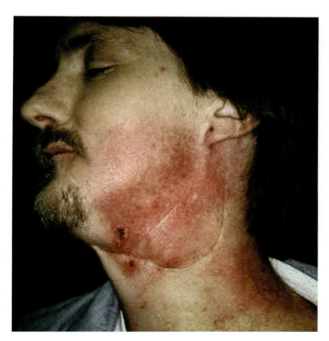

Figure 16.20. Marked skin reaction over parotid and submandibular region following 65 Gy external beam radiation given postoperatively.

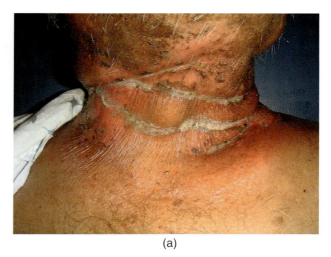

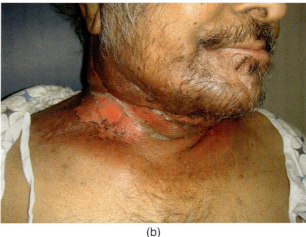

Figure 16.21. (a) Bilateral acute reaction with redness and exudation involving both submandibular regions. (b) Close-up view of the right neck shows skin sloughing and peeling.

measurable parotid saliva, and 5% of patients will demonstrate a sialadenitis with gland swelling and raised amylase within 12 hours of their first treatment (Parsons 1994). However, although it is known that damage to the salivary glands will increase with radiation dose and volume of gland irradiated there is no universal agreement over the dose required to produce xerostomia. Someya et al. (2003) found the gradual recovery of function over time with doses of less than 5000 cGy, while no significant recovery was seen in patients who received greater than 5800 cGy (Figure 16.20). The minor salivary/sublingual glands do not seem to play much of a role in the development of xerostomia which seems to depend mainly on the mean dose to both the parotid and submandibular glands (Jellema et al. 2005) (Figure 16.21). These authors also found that the stickiness of saliva post-radiation depended mainly on the mean dose to the submandibular glands.

The exact pathogenesis and mechanism of injury to the saliva glands resulting from radiation therapy is also controversial with no universal agreement as to cause. Based on animal studies on the rat model a mechanism of delayed serious cell death due to sublethal DNA damage, which results in death during a reproductive phase due to highly redox-reactive metal ions, e.g. iron, copper associated with secretion granules has been proposed (Nagler 2002, 2003). Another study showed a significant increase in cytotoxic T cells in irradiated submandibular glands suggesting cell-mediated mechanisms may be responsible for the sialadenitis with subsequent acinar cell destruction/atrophy (Teymoortash et al. 2005). The use of FDG-PET-CT to measure the fractional loss of parotid FDG uptake has been proposed to predict post-radiation therapy parotid toxicity (Cannon et al. 2012).

The ductal cells are thought to be more resistant to radiation damage and to maintain the gland architecture and potential for regeneration (May et al. 2018). There is also a great deal of animal work and interest in stem cells and gene transfer therapy in treating salivary glands damaged by PORT (Vissink et al. 2015; Pringle et al. 2016).

Obviously, once established, the effects of radiation damage are difficult to treat or reverse, so that much effort has been aimed at prevention. Important advances in the delivery of radiation therapy using 3-D conformal planning and intensity-modulated radiation therapy (IMRT), combined with drugs such as growth factors, cholinergic agonists and cytoprotective agents (Amifostine) are currently the preferred modalities of prevention (Garden et al. 2006).

It has been shown with conventional radiation therapy that the ability to spare the contralateral major salivary glands or to spare the parotid by the positioning of the portals can significantly increase salivary flow and reduce xerostomia (Beer et al. 2002; Malouf et al. 2003). The sophistication of 3-D conformal planning and IMRT allows the radiotherapist to give more radiation to the tumor target with increased sparing of normal tissue. In one study, only 12% of patients developed xerostomia following IMRT for head and neck cancer, and there were no locoregional recurrences with a median follow up of 24 months (Saarilahti et al. 2005). Jen et al. (2005) compared 108 patients treated with conventional RT to 72 treated with 3-D conformal radiation therapy finding 3-D conformal radiation therapy delivered a higher dose to the tumor with better local control in T4 patients and improved survival with significantly better parotid function. IMRT has also been used to spare the submandibular glands to prevent radiation-induced xerostomia (Saarilahti et al. 2006). The ability to use 3-D conformal RT and IMRT to spare the opposite parotid by excluding the contralateral level II nodes from the field was not shown to be associated with any loco-regional recurrence and no recurrence occurred in the spared area (Bussels et al. 2004).

Several studies have shown that IMRT is superior to 3-D conformal radiotherapy in regards to late toxicity from xerostomia (Kouloulias et al. 2013; Lambrecht et al. 2013). In a study on 159 patients with oropharyngeal cancer 3D-CRT vs IMRT, the IMRT cohort had significant improvement in PEG tube and toxicity-related outcomes (Lohia et al. 2014). In all of these studies, there was no difference in tumor control. Further trials to include sparing both parotid and submandibular glands with IMRT have shown both better patient-reported outcomes (Hawkins et al. 2018) and patient + observer reported outcomes (Little et al. 2012).

A Meta-analysis of seven RTCs with 1155 patients of IMRT vs conventional ± 3D RT found consistent moderately-quality evidence that IMRT reduced the risk of moderate -severe acute and late xerostomia (Gupta et al. 2018). A similar systematic review and meta-analysis of 5 RCTs with 871 patients confirmed a reduced incidence of grade 2–4 xerostomia without compromise in locoregional control or OS (Marta et al. 2014).

Numerous drugs have been investigated for preventing radiation damage. A phase III prospective randomized trial of Amifostine (Ethyol) with 315 patients showed a significant reduction in grade 2 or greater xerostomia and chronic xerostomia with no effect on locoregional control, disease-free survival, or overall survival. In this study, however, 53% of patients experienced nausea and/or vomiting (Brizel et al. 2000). A follow-up study to review results of this study after two years, found a significant decrease in grade 2 or > xerostomia had been maintained as well as an increase in the proportion of patients with meaningful unstimulated saliva and reduced mouth dryness. There was no compromise of locoregional control, progression-free, or disease-free survival (Wasseman et al. 2005). In this study, the Amifostine was given intravenously, and a recent phase II study has shown a similar radioprotective benefit for Amifostine given subcutaneously as a simpler alternative (Anne et al. 2007). Another approach has been to use pilocarpine which has been used to treat xerostomia during radiotherapy as a chemopreventive agent. A randomized, double-blind, placebo-controlled trial of pilocarpine on 60 patients only 39 of whom were evaluable indicated that pilocarpine used with radiotherapy could lead to a significant diminishment in subsequent xerostomia (Haddad and Karimi 2002). Another randomized trial with 66 patients also concluded that patients with stimulated glands from pilocarpine during radiation had less decrease in the salivary flow which reduced radiation side-effects (Nyarady et al. 2006). However, the RTOG study 97–09 which was a phase III trial with 245 patients showed that although there was a significantly increased unstimulated salivary flow in the pilocarpine group, there was no difference in parotid stimulated salivary flow, in the amelioration of mucositis or quality of life between the two groups (Scarantino et al. 2006).

In a systematic review and meta-analysis of 1732 patients from 20 studies treatment interventions studied included pilocarpine, cevimeline, saliva substitutes/mouth care systems, hypothermic humidification, acupuncture, transcutaneous electrical nerve stimulation, low-level laser therapy, and herbal medications. The metanalysis of six studies suggests pilocarpine and cevimeline reduce xerostomia symptoms and increase salivary flow vs. placebo and should represent the first line of therapy in radiation-induced xerostomia (Mercadante et al. 2017). Another, systematic review of pilocarpine with 6 PRCTs concluded that pilocarpine increased unstimulated salivary flow and reduced clinician-rated xerostomia. But they found no effect on stimulated salivary flow (Yang et al. 2016).

Other novel approaches to the problem have been the use of gene therapy which has yielded promising results in animal models (Thula et al. 2005; Cotrim et al. 2006). Future directions may lie in the use of stem cells to regenerate damaged salivary glands (Stiubea-Cohen et al. 2013). A translational approach to radiation-induced xerostomia of the submandibular glands post-cancer radiation therapy is the transplantation of adipose tissue-derived stem cells. There was a 33% increase in salivary flow at one month post the stem cells rising to 50% by four months (Grönhöj et al. 2018).

Finally, a surgical approach to the prevention of xerostomia has been the transfer of the submandibular glands into the submental triangle out of the radiation field prior to the commencement of radiation therapy. In a phase II trial of patients who had primary surgery for oropharyngeal cancer followed by adjuvant RT, with or without submandibular gland transfer 24 of 51 patients were evaluated for swallowing. The cohort with preservation of one gland (13 patients) had significantly increased saliva and swallowing function (Rieger et al. 2005). Similar results are reported in a small series of patients undergoing chemoradiation (Al-Qahtani et al. 2006). Regarding long-term results in 26 patients followed for two years, normal amounts of saliva were reported in 83% (Seikaly et al. 2004). A further study by the same group showed this surgical technique of submandibular gland transfer to be reproducible in a multicenter setting with 74% of patients prevented from XRT-induced acute xerostomia (Jha et al. 2012). In a Chinese study of 38 patients, 92.3% of patients had no or minimal xerostomia two years following radiation therapy (Zhang et al. 2012). A combination of submandibular gland transfer and IMRT in 40 patients having 60 Gy postoperative radiation therapy showed 0-mild xerostomia at one year in 89% of patients. Salivary flow rates were 75% of pre-radiation levels at one year (Scrimger et al. 2018).

RADIOACTIVE IODINE

Radioactive iodine is used in the treatment of thyroid cancer but is also concentrated in the salivary glands particularly the parotid and may cause sialadenitis which is immediate or begins a few months after treatment (Mandel and Mandel 2003). In a prospective study of 76 patients receiving radioactive iodine, 20 patients (26%) developed salivary gland toxicity, 11 patients developed toxicity within 48 hours, and nine patients not until three months post-therapy. A total of 16 patients had chronic toxicity typically xerostomia at 12 months (Hyer et al. 2007). In seeking to quantitate salivary gland dysfunction using scintigraphy in 50 patients, 46% and 42% were found to have decreased maximum secretion and uptake ratio, respectively (Raza et al. 2006). The damage was seen more in the parotid and was dependant on the radioiodine dose. The damage and symptoms may be permanent (Mandel and Mandel 1999). The damage is most likely related to an oxidation injury indicated by an increase in prostaglandin levels (Wolfram et al. 2004). Salivary gland dysfunction is present in as many as two-thirds of patients treated with radioiodine ablation.

A randomized placebo-controlled study using vitamin E found a significant protective effect against radiation-induced dysfunction in salivary glands. In this trial, the salivary function was assessed using salivary gland scintigraphy, and although the control group had significantly reduced salivary secretion following the radioactive iodine, the group receiving Vitamin E had no reduced function (Fallahi et al. 2013).

Current management is symptomatic as for sialadenitis and xerostomia from other causes. Animal studies using the rabbit model indicate that Amifostine can significantly reduce radioiodine-induced parenchymal damage (Kutta et al. 2005).

The use of sialendoscopy in this condition for patients with partial duct stenosis has also been reported (Kim et al. 2007). In one series of sialendoscopy with dilation and irrigation, 54% of patients reported complete resolution of symptoms, 36% partial improvement and 10% no improvement at a mean follow-up of 18 months (Prendes et al. 2012). Sialendoscopy improved 89% of patients partially or completely following radioiodine induced sialadenitis. In 86% of cases, there were mucous plugs or ductal stenosis (Canzi et al. 2017). Sialendoscopy was also found to be more cost-effective than diagnostic ultrasound and medical management, which was, in turn, more cost-effective than medical management with diagnostic CT and MR sialography (Kowalczyk et al. 2018). A systematic review of eight studies, 122 patients, showed most centers only employed sialendoscopy after the failure of conservative measures but that sialendoscopy gave a clinical improvement of 75–100% (Cung et al. 2017).

PSMA Radioligand Therapy

The use of labeled prostate-specific membrane antigen (PSMA) for the treatment of metastatic castration-resistant prostate disease has had an impressive effect on the disease (Langbein et al. 2018). However, xerostomia has been a significant side effect with all these new agents ^{131}I-labeled PMSA, ^{177}Lu-labeled compounds, and ^{225}Ac-PSMA radioligand therapy. The salivary toxicity may limit the usefulness of these compounds. In one series of 40 patients, 4(10%) patients had to discontinue therapy due to xerostomia (Kratochwil et al. 2018). In Langbein et al.'s paper (2018), he reviews the ways to reduce or deal with this toxicity. Amongst these were reducing radionuclide uptake, labeling PSMA-targeting antibodies, sialendoscopy (as discussed for radioiodine induced sialadenitis above), and stem cell therapy to regenerate salivary glands.

Barotrauma

Air can be forced in a retrograde fashion into the parotid duct by a rise in intraoral pressure and cause parotid emphysema or pneumoparotid. This condition may occur in glassblowers and

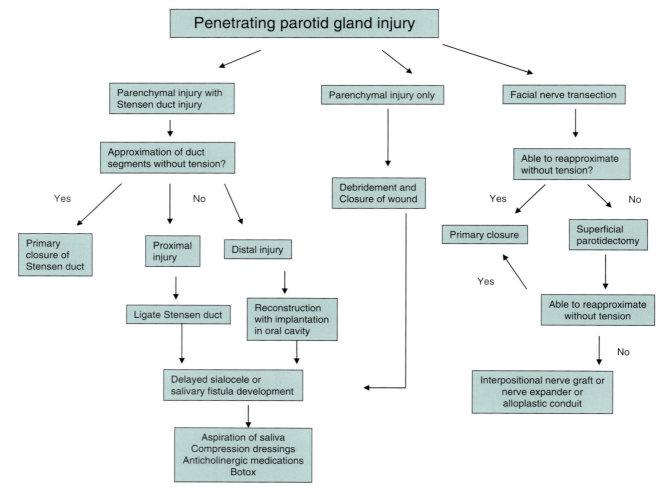

Figure 16.22. Algorithm for management of penetrating trauma to the parotid gland.

musicians who play woodwind or brass instruments (Mukundan Jenkins 2009). It is usually a benign condition but can cause recurrent sialadenitis or even progress to subcutaneous emphysema. The condition has also been reported in conjunction with the use of an air syringe during routine dentistry (Takenoshite et al. 1991), secondary to coughing with chronic obstructive airways disease (Cook and Layton 1993), and self-induced in children and adults (Goguen et al. 1995; Gudlaugsson et al. 1998; Yamazaki et al. 2018). The condition can be diagnosed by palpation of emphysema in the parotid and the escape of frothy saliva from the duct. Sialography, and CT scans have been used for diagnosis (Gudlaugsson et al. 1998; Maehara et al. 2005). In one case with subcutaneous emphysema extending to the mediastinum, parotid duct ligation was used for the cure (Han and Isaacson 2004).

Summary (Figures 16.22 and 16.23)

- Most parenchymal penetrating injuries of the parotid gland will resolve with conservative treatment.
- Parotid fistulas and sialocele due to parenchymal injury will also resolve with conservative therapy.
- Chemical denervation of the gland with botulinum A toxin injected subcutaneously appears a safe way of treating fistulae and sialoceles.
- It is important to recognize the possibility of duct injury early as the immediate repair is indicated.
- Microneural repair of facial nerve injuries primarily without tension is the ideal management for a transected facial nerve or its branches.
- At present, the use of tissue glues for nerve repair does not appear to improve results.

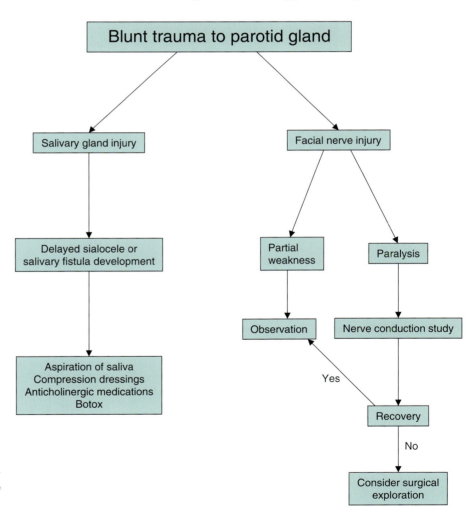

Figure 16.23. Algorithm for management of blunt trauma to the parotid gland.

- Most cases of Frey syndrome following parotidectomy are subclinical.
- Botulinum toxin is useful in the treatment of Frey syndrome.
- A variety of barrier techniques to prevent Frey syndrome have been described with the use of the SAMAS layer appearing to give good results.
- IMRT and 3-D conformal planning show great promise in preventing radiation damage to the salivary glands.
- Amifostine and pilocarpine used during radiation may act as radioprotectants.
- Sialendoscopy appears to be the best approach to radioiodine induced sialadenitis.

References

Aizawa T, Kuwabara M, Kubo S et al. 2018. Polyglycolic acid felt for prevention of Frey syndrome after parotidectomy. *Ann Plast Surg* 81(4):438–440.

Akinbami BO. 2009. Traumatic diseases of the parotid gland and sequelae. Review of the literature and case reports. *Niger J Clin Pract* 12(2):212–215.

Al-Qahtani K, Hier MP, Sultanum K, Black MJ. 2006. The role of submandibular salivary gland transfer in preventing xerostomia in the chemoradiotherapy patient. *Oral Surg Oral Med Oral Pathol Oral Radiol Endod* 101(6):753–756.

Ananthakrishnan N, Parkash S. 1982. Parotid fistuas: A review. *Br J Surg* 69:641–644.

Anne PR, Machtay M, Rosenthal DI et al. 2007. A phase II trial of subcutaneous amifostine and radiation therapy in patients with head and neck cancer. *Int J Radiat Oncol Biol Phys* 67(2):445–452.

Arnaud S, Batifol D, Goudot P, Yachouh J 2006. Nonsurgical management of traumatic injuries of the parotid gland using type a botulinum toxin. *Plast Reconstr Surg* 117(7):2426–2430.

Beer KT, Zehnder D, Lussi A, Greiner RH. 2002. Sparing of contralateral major salivary glands has a significant effect on oral health in patients treated with radical radiotherapy of head and neck tumors. *Strahlenther Onkol* 178(12):722–726.

Berini-Aytes L, Gay-Escoda C. 1992. Morbidity associated with removal of the submandibular gland. *J Craniomaxillofac Surg* 20(5):216–219.

Blanc S, Bourrier T, Borralevi F et al. 2016. Frey syndrome. *J Pediatr* 174:211–217.e2.

Bonanno PC, Palaia D, Rosenberg M, Casson P. 2000. Prophylaxis against Frey's syndrome in parotid surgery. *Ann Plast Surg* 44(5):498–501.

Breuer T, Ferrazzini A, Grossenberger R. 2006. Botulinum toxin A as a treatment of traumatic salivary gland fistulas. (In German) *HNO* 54(4):385–390.

Brizel DM, Wasserman TH, Henke M et al. 2000. Phase III randomized trial of Amifostine as a radioprotector in head and neck cancer. *J Clin Oncol* 18(19):3339–3345.

Bussels B, Maes A, Hermans R et al. 2004. Recurrences after conformal parotid sparing radiotherapy for head and neck cancer. *Radiother Oncol* 72(2):119–127.

Cannon B, Schwartz DL, Dong L. 2012. Metabolic imaging of postradiotherapy xerostomia. *Int J Radiol Oncol Biol Phys* 83(5):1609–1616.

Canosa A, Cohen MA. 1999. Post-traumatic parotid sialocele: Report of two cases. *J Oral Maxillofac Surg* 57(6):742–745.

Cant PJ, Campbell JA. 1991. Management of traumatic parotid sialoceleles and fistulae: A prospective study. *Aust N Z J Surg* 61(10):742–743.

Canzi P, Cacciola S, Capaccio P et al. 2017. Interventional sialendoscopy for radioiodine-induced sialadenitis: Quo vadis? *Acta Otorhinolaryngol Ital* 37:155–159.

Capaccio P, Cuccarini V, Benicchio V et al. 2006. Treatment of iatrogenic submandibular sialocele with botulinum toxin. Case report. *Br J Oral Maxillofac Surg* 45(5):415–417.

Captier G, Canovas F, Bonnel F, et al. 2005. Organization and microscopic anatomy of the adult human facial nerve: anatomical and histologic basis for surgery. *Plast Reconstr Surg* 115(6):1457–1465.

Cesteleyn L, Helman J, King S, Van de Vyvere G. 2002. Temporoparietal fascia flaps and superficial musculoaponeurotic system placation in parotid surgery reduces Frey's syndrome. *J Oral Maxillofac Surg* 60(11):1284–1297.

Choi J-S, Choi Y-G, Kim Y-M, Lim J-Y. 2018. Clinical outcomes and prognostic factors of sialendoscopy in salivary duct stenosis. *Laryngoscope* 128(4):878–884.

Cholankeril JV, Scioscia PA. 1993. Post-traumatic sialoceles and mucoceles of the salivary glands *Clin Imaging* 17(1):41–45.

Chow TL, Kwok SP. 2003. Use of botulinum type A in a case of persistent parotid sialocele. *Hong Kong Med J* 9(4):293–294.

Ciolek PJ, Prendes BL, Fritz MA. 2018. Comprehensive approach to reestablishing form and function after radical parotidectomy. *Am J Otolaryngol* 39(5):542–547.

Condie D, Tolkachjov SN. 2019. Facial nerve injury and repair: A practical review for cutaneous surgery. *Dermatol Surg* 45(3):340–357.

Cook JN, Layton SA. 1993. Bilateral parotid swelling associated with chronic obstructive pulmonary disease. A case of pneumoparotid. *Oral Surg Oral Med Oral Pathol* 76(2):157–158.

Costan V-V, Dabija MG, Ciofu ML et al. 2019. A functional approach to post-traumatic salivary fistula treatment: The use of botulinum toxin. *J Craniofac Surg* 30(3):871–875.

Cotrim AP, Mineshiba F, Sugito T et al. 2006. Salivary gland gene therapy 2006. *Dent Clin North Am* 50(2): 157–173.

Cung T-D, Lai L, Svider PF et al. 2017. Sialendoscopy in the management of radioiodine induced sialadenitis. A systematic review. *Am J Otol Laryngol,* 126(11):768–773.

Dulguerov P, Marchal F, Gusin C. 1999. Frey syndrome before Frey: The correct history. *Laryngoscope* 109(9):1471–1473.

Eckardt A, Kuettner C. 2003. Treatment of gustatory sweating (Frey's syndrome) with botulinum toxin A. *Head Neck* 25(8):624–628.

Etoz A, Tuncel U, Ozcan M. 2006. Parotid duct repair by use of an embolectomy catheter with a microvascular clamp. *Plast Reconstr Surg* 117(10):330–331.

Fallahi B, Beiki D, Abedi SM et al. 2013. Does vitamin E protect salivary glands from I-131 radiation damage in patients with thyroid cancer? *Nucl Med Commun* 34(8):777–786.

Farrag TY, Lehar M, Verhaegen P et al. 2007. Effect of platelet rich plasma and fibrin sealant on facial nerve regeneration in a rat model. *Laryngoscope* 117(1):157–165.

Faussat JM, Ghiassi B, Princ G. 1993. Rhinorrhea of parotid origin. Apropos of a case. *Rev Stomatol Chir Maxillofac* 94(6):363–365.

Ferraro G, Altieri A, Grella E, D'Andrea F. 2005. Botulinum toxin: 28 patients affected by Frey's syndrome treated with intradermal injections. *Plast Reconstr Surg* 115(1):344–345.

Filho WQ, Dedivitis RA, Rapoport A, Guimaraes AV. 2004. Sternocleidomastoid muscle flap in preventing Frey's syndrome following parotidectomy. *World J Surg* 28(4):361–364.

Frautschi R, Rampazzo A, Bernard S et al. 2015. Management of the salivary glands and facial nerve in face transplantation. *Plast Reconstr Surg* 137(6):1887–1889.

Frey L. 1923. Le Syndrome du nerf auriculo-temporal. *Rev Neurol* 2:97.

Garden AS, Lewin JS, Chambers MS. 2006. How to reduce radiation-related toxicity in patients with cancer of the head and neck. *Curr Oncol Rep* 8(2):140–145.

Gardetto A, Kovacs P, Piegger J et al. 2002. Direct coaptation of extensive facial nerve defects after removal of the superficial part of the parotid gland: An anatomic study. *Head Neck* 24(12):1047–1053.

Gidley PW, Herrera SJ, Hanasono MM et al. 2010. The impact of radiation therapy on facial nerve repair. *Laryngoscope* 120(10):1985–1989.

Goguen LA, April MM, Karmody CS, Carter BL. 1995. Self-induced pneumoparotitis. *Arch Otolaryngol Head Neck Surg* 121(12):1426–1429.

Govindaraj S, Cohen M, Genden EM et al. 2001. The use of acellular dermis in the prevention of Frey's syndrome. *Laryngoscope* 111(11 Pt 1):1993–1998.

Greene JJ, McClendon MT, Stephanopoulos N et al. 2018. Electrophysiological assessment of a peptide amphiphile nanofiber nerve graft for facial nerve repair. *J Tissue Eng Regen Med* 12(6):1389–1401.

Grönhöj C, Jensen DH, Vester-Glowinski P et al. 2018. Safety and efficacy of mesenchymal stem cells for radiation-induced xerostomia: A randomised, placebo-controlled phase ½ trial (MESRIX). *Int J Radiol Oncol Biol Phys* 101:581–592.

Gudlaugsson O, Geirsson AJ, Benediktsdottir K. 1998. Pneumoparotitis: A new diagnostic technique and a case report. *Ann Otol Rhinol Laryngol* 107(4):356–358.

Guntinas-Lichius O, Streppel M, Stennert E. 2006. Postoperative functional evaluation of different reanimation techniques for facial nerve repair. *Am J Surg* 191(1):61–67.

Guntinas-Lichius O, Straesser A, Streppel M. 2007. Quality of life after facial nerve repair. *Laryngoscope* 117(3):421–426.

Gupta T, Kannan S, Ghosh-Laskar S, Agarwal JP. 2018. Systematic review and meta-analysis of intensity modulated radiation therapy versus conventional two-dimensional and/or three-dimensional radiotherapy in curative-intent management of head and neck squamous carcinomas. *PLoS One*, 13(7), e0200137.

Haddad P, Karimi M. 2002. A randomized, double-blind, placebo-controlled trial of concomitant pilocarpine with head and neck irradiation for prevention of radiation-induced xerostomia. *Radiother Oncol* 64(1):29–32.

Hallock GG. 1992. Microsurgical repair of the parotid duct. *Microsurgery* 13(5):243–246.

Han S, Isaacson G. 2004. Recurrent pneumparotid: Cause and treatment. *Otolaryngol Head Neck Surg* 131(5):758–761.

Hawkins PG, Lee JY, Mao Y et al. 2018. Sparing all salivary glands with IMRT for head and neck cancer: Longitudinal study of patient-reported xerostomia and head and neck quality of life. *Radiother Oncol* 126(1):68–74.

Heymans O, Nelissen X, Medot M, Fissette J. 1999. Microsurgical repair of Stensen's duct using an interposition vein graft. *J Reconstr Microsurg* 15(2):105–107.

Hojjat H, Svider PE, Raza SN et al. 2018. Economic analysis of using free fat graft or acellular dermis to prevent post-parotidectomy Frey syndrome. *Facial Plast Surg* 34(4):423–428.

Hong YT, Hong KH. 2020. Submandibular Frey syndrome following submandibular gland excision. *Ear Nose Throat J* 99(3):185–186.

Hontanilla B, Qui S-S, Marré D. 2014. Effect of postoperative brachytherapy and external beam radiotherapy on functional outcomes of immediate facial nerve repair after radical parotidectomy. *Head Neck* 36(1):113–119.

Hyer S, Kong A, Pratt B, Harmer C. 2007. Salivary gland toxicity after radioiodine therapy for thyroid cancer. *Clin Oncol (R Coll Radiol)* 19(1):83–86.

Jellema AP, Doornaert P, Slotman BJ et al. 2005. Does radiation dose to the salivary glands and oral cavity predict patient-rated xerostomia and sticky saliva in head and neck cancer patients treated with curative radiotherapy? *Radiother Oncol* 77(2):164–171.

Jen YM, Shih R, Lin YS et al. 2005. Parotid gland-sparing 3-dimmensional conformal radiotherapy results in less severe dry mouth in nasopharyngeal cancer patients: A dosimetric and clinical comparison with conventional radiotherapy. *Radiother Oncol* 75(2):204–209.

Jha N, Harris J, Seikaly H et al. 2012. A phase II study of submandibular gland transfer prior to radiation for prevention of radiation-induced xerostomia in head and neck cancer (RTOG 0244) *Int J Radiol Oncol Biol Phys* 84(2):437–442.

Junior EDP, Valmaseda-Castellon E, Gay-Escoda C. 2004. Facial nerve repair with epineural suture and anastomosis using fibrin adhesive: An experimental study in the rabbit. *J Oral Maxillofac Surg* 62(12):1524–1529.

Júnior RM, da Rocha Neto AM, Queiroz IV et al. 2012. Giant sialocele following facial trauma. *Braz Dent J* 23(1):82–86.

Kerawala CJ, McAloney N, Stassen LF. 2002. Prospective randomized trial of the benefits of a sternocleidomastoid flap after superficial parotidectomy. *Br J Oral Maxillofac Surg* 40(6):468–472.

Kim JW, Han GS, Lee SH et al. 2007. Sialoendoscopic treatment for radioiodine induced sialadenitis. *Laryngoscope* 117(1):133–136.

Koch M, Bozzato IH, Zenk J. 2013. Sialendoscopy-assisted microsurgical repair of traumatic transection of Stensen's duct. *Laryngoscope* 123(12):3074–3077.

Kopeć T, Wierzbicka M, Szyfter W. 2013. Stensen's duct injuries: The role of sialoendoscopy and adjuvant botulinum toxin injection. *Wideochir Inne Tech Malo Inwazyine* 8:112–116.

Kouloulias V, Thalassinou S, Platoni K et al. 2013. The treatment outcome and radiation-induced toxicity for patients with head and neck carcinoma in the IMRT era: A systematic review with dosimetric and clinical parameters. *Biomed Res Int* 2013:401261.

Kowalczyk DM, Jordan JR, Stringer SP. 2018. Cost-effectiveness of sialendoscopy versus medical management for radioiodine-induced sialadenitis. *Laryngoscope* 128(8):1822–1828.

Kratochwil C, Bruchertseifer F, Rathka H et al. 2018. Targeted α-therapy of metastatic castration resistant prostate cancer with ^{225}Ac-PSMA-617: Swimmer plot analysis suggests efficacy regarding duration of tumor control. *J Nucl Med* 59:795–802.

Kutta H, Kampen U, Sagowski C et al. 2005. Amifostine is a potent radioprotector of salivary glands in radioiodine therapy. Structural and ultrastructural findings. *Strahlenther Onkol* 181(4):237–245.

Kyrmizakis DE, Pangalos A, Papadakis CE et al. 2004. The use of botulinum toxin type A in the treatment of Frey and crocodile tears syndromes. *J Oral Maxillofac Surg* 62(7):840–844.

Laage-Hellman J-E. 1957. Gustatory sweating and flushing after conservative parotidectomy. *Acta Otolaryngol (Stokh)* 48:234.

Lambrecht M, Nevens D, Nuyts S. 2013. Intensity-modulated radiotherapy vs parotid-sparing 3D conformal radiotherapy. Effect on outcome and toxicity in locally advanced head and neck cancer. *Strahlenther Onkol* 189(3):223–229.

Landau R, Stewart M. 1985. Conservative management of post-traumatic parotid fistulae and sialoceles: A prospective study. *Br J Surg* 72:42.

Langbein T, Chausse G, Baum RP. 2018. Salivary gland toxicity of PSMA radioligand therapy: Relevance and preventative strategies. *J Nucl Med* 59(8):1172–1173.

Lazaridou M, Liopoulos C, Antoniades K et al. 2012. Salivary gland trauma: A review of diagnosis and treatment. *Craniomaxillofac Trauma Reconstr* 5(4):189–196.

Lee JW, Yoon YH. 2010. Gustatory sweating after submandibular gland excision. *Otolaryngol Head Neck Surg* 143(6):845–846.

Lewis G, Knottenbelt JD. 1991. Parotid duct injury: Is immediate surgical repair necessary? *Injury* 22:407.

Lewkowicz AA, Hasson O, Nablieli O. 2002. Traumatic injuries to the parotid gland and duct. *J Oral Maxillofac Surg* 60(6):676–680.

Li C, Wu F, Zhang Q, et al. 2015. Interventions for the treatment of Frey's syndrome. *Cochrane Database Syst Rev* (3):CD009959. doi:10.1002/14651858. PMID: 25781421.

Little M, Schipper M, Feng FY et al. 2012. Reducing xerostomia after chemo-IMRT for head and neck cancer: Beyond sparing the parotid glands. *Int J Radiat Oncol Biol Phys* 83(3):1007–1014.

Lohia S, Rajapurkar M, Nguyen S et al. 2014. A comparison of outcomes using intensity-modulated radiation therapy and 3-dimensional conformal radiation therapy in treatment of oropharyngeal cancer. *JAMA Otolaryngol Head Neck Surg* 140(4):331–337.

Lu GN, Villwock MR, Humphrey CD et al. 2019. Analysis of facial reanimation procedures performed concurrently with total parotidectomy and facial nerve sacrifice. *JAMA Facial Plast Surg* 21(1):50–55.

Maehara M, Ikeda K, Ohmura N et al. 2005. Multislice computed tomography of pneumoparotid: A case report. *Radiat Med* 23(2):147–150.

Malik TH, Kelly G, Ahmed A et al. 2005. A comparison of surgical techniques used in dynamic reanimation of the paralyzed face. *Otol Neurotol* 26(2):284–291.

Malouf JG, Aragon C, Henson BS et al. 2003. Influence of parotid-sparing radiotherapy on xerostomia in head and neck cancer patients. *Cancer Detect Prev* 27(4): 305–310.

Man C-B, Patel R, Karavidas K. 2017. Intraoperative sialendoscopy to assist with and confirm repair of Stensen's duct. *Br J Oral Maxillofac Surg* 55(7):e45–e46.

Mandel SJ, Mandel L. 1999. Persistent sialadenitis after radioactive iodine therapy: Report of two cases. *J Oral Maxillofac Surg* 57(6):738–741.

Mandel SJ, Mandel L. 2003. Radioactive iodine and the salivary glands. *Thyroid* 13(3):266–271.

Mandel L, Silver A. 2012. Bilateral parotid duct obstruction after rhytidectomies: A case report. *J Oral Maxillofac Surg* 70(2):449–452.

Marchese-Ragona R, Marioni G, Restivo DA, Staffieri A. 2006. The role of botulinum toxin in post-parotidectomy fistula. A technical note. *Am J Otolaryngol* 27(3):221–224.

Marta NM, Silva V, Carvallo HAD et al. 2014. Intensity-modulated radiation therapy for head and neck cancer: A systematic review and meta-analysis. *Radiother Oncol* 110(1):9–15.

May AJ, Cruz-Pacheo N, Emmerson E et al. 2018. Diverse progenitor cells preserve salivary gland ductal architecture after radiation-induced damage. *Development* 145(21: dev166363.doi.

Mercadante V, Hamad AA, Lodi G, et al. 2017. Interventions for the management of radiotherapy induced xerostomia and hyposalivation: A systematic review and meta-analysis. *Oral Oncol* 66:64–74

Montag DT, Jethwa AR, Oland RM. 2016. Novel technique to diagnose parotid duct injuries at the bed side using fluorescein. *Am J Emerg Med* 34(2):308–309

Morestin M. 1917. Contribution a l'etude du traitement des fistules salivaires consecutives aux blessures de guerre. *Bull Mém Soc Chir Paris* 43:845.

Morris LG, Miglietta MA, Sikora AG et al. 2007. Emergency parotidectomy for penetrating Zone III neck trauma. *Arch Surg* 142(12):1206–1208.

Mukundan D, Jenkins O. 2009. Images in clinical medicine. A tuba player with air in the parotid gland. *N Engl J Med* 360(7):710.

Nagler RM. 2002. The enigmatic mechanism of irradiation induced damage to the major salivary glands. *Oral Dis* 8(3):141–146.

Nagler RM. 2003. Effects of head and neck radiotherapy on major salivary glands-animal studies and human implications. *In vivo* 17(4):369–375.

Nahlieli O. 2017. Complications of traditional and modern therapeutic salivary approaches. *Acta Otorhinolaryngol Ital* 37(2):142–147

Nahlieli O, Bar T, Shacham R et al. 2004. Management of chronic recurrent parotitis: Current therapy. *J Oral Maxillofac Surg* 62(9):1150–1155.

Nahlieli O, Abramson A, Shachman R et al. 2008a. Endoscopic treatment of salivary gland injuries due to facial rejuvenation procedures. *Laryngoscope* 118(5): 763–767.

Nahlieli O, Droma EB, Eliav E et al. 2008b. Salivary gland injury subsequent to implant surgery. *Int J Oral Maxillofac Implants* 23(3):556–560.

Navissano M, Malan F, Carnino R, Battiston B. 2005. Neurotube for facial nerve repair. *Micron* 25(4):268–271.

Ngu RK, Brown JE, Whaites EJ et al. 2007. Salivary duct strictures: Nature and incidence in benign salivary obstruction. *Dentomaxillofac Radiol* 36(2):63–67.

Nolte D, Gollmitzer I, Loeffelbein DJ et al. 2004. Botulinum toxin for treatment of gustatory sweating. A prospective randomized study. (In German). *Mund Kiefer Gesichtschir* 8(6):369–375.

Nyarady Z, Nemeth A, Ban A et al. 2006. A randomized study to assess the effectiveness of orally administered pilocarpine during and after radiotherapy of head and neck cancer. *Anticancer Res* 26(2B):1557–1562.

Ord RA, Lee VA. 1996. Submandibular duct repositioning after excision of mouth cancer. *J Oral Maxillofac Surg* 54:1075–1078.

Parkeh D, Glezerson G, Stewart M et al. 1989. Post-traumatic parotid fistulae and sialoceles. A prospective study of conservative management in 51 cases. *Ann Surg* 209(1):105–111.

Parsons JT. 1994. The Effect of Radiation on Normal Tissues of the Head and Neck. In: Million RR, Cassisi NJ (eds.) *Management of Head and Neck Cancer: A Multidisciplinary Approach*. Philadelphia, JB Lippincott Co., pp. 247–250.

Philouze P, Vertu D, Ceruse P. 2014. Bilateral gustatory sweating in the submandibular region after bilateral neck dissection successfully treated with botulinum toxin. *Br J Oral Maxillofac Surg* 52(8):761–763.

Piza-Katzer H, Balough B, Muzika-Herczeg E, Gardetto A. 2004. Secondary end to end repair of extensive facial nerve defects: Surgical technique and postoperative functional results. *Head Neck* 26(9):770–777.

Prasad SC, Balasubramanian K, Piccirillo E et al. 2018. Surgical technique and results of cable graft interpositioning of the facial nerve in lateral skull base surgeries; Experience with 213 consecutive cases. *J Neurosurg* 128(2):631–638.

Prendes BL, Orloff LA, Eisele DW. 2012. Therapeutic sialendoscopy for the management of radioiodine sialadenitis. *Laryngoscope* 138(1):15–19.

Pringle S, Maimets M, van der Zwaag M et al. 2016.Human salivary stem cells functionally restore radiation damaged salivary glands *Stem Cells* 34(3):640–652.

Ragona RM, Blotta P, Pastore A et al. 1999. Management of parotid sialocele with botulinum toxin. *Laryngoscope* 109(8):1344–1346.

Rashid HU, Rehman IU, Rashid M et al, 2019. Results of immediate facial nerve reconstruction in patients undergoing parotid tumor resection. *J Ayub Med Coll Abbottabad* 31(3):340–345.

Raza H, Khan AU, Hameed A, Khan A. 2006. Quantitative evaluation of salivary gland dysfunction after radioiodine therapy using salivary gland scintigraphy. *Nucl Med Commun* 27(6):495–499.

Rieger J, Seikaly H, Jha N et al. 2005. Submandibular gland transfer for prevention of xerostomia after radiation therapy: Swallowing outcomes. *Arch Otolaryngol Head Neck Surg* 131(2):140–145.

Saarilahti K, Kouri M, Collan J et al. 2005. Intensity modulated radiotherapy for head and neck cancer: Evidence for preserved salivary gland function. *Radiother Oncol* 74(3):251–258.

Saarilahti K, Kouri M, Collan et al. 2006. Sparing of the submandibular glands by intensity modulated radiotherapy in the treatment of head and neck cancer. *Radiother Oncol* 78(3):270–275.

Salerno S, Lo Casto A, Comparetto A et al. 2007. Sialodochoplasty in the treatment of salivary duct stricture in chronic sialadenitis: Technique and results. *Radiol Med (Torino)* 112(1):138–144.

Scarantino C, LeVeque F, Swann RS et al. 2006. Effect of pilocarpine during radiation therapy: Results of RTOG 97-09, a phase III randomized study in head and neck cancer patients. *J Support Oncol* 4(5):252–258.

Scher N, Poe DS. 1988. Post-traumatic prandial rhinorrhea. *J Oral Maxillofac Surg* 46(1):63–64.

Scrimger RA, Seikaly H, Vos LJ et al. 2018. Combination of submandibular salivary gland transfer and intensity-modulated radiotherapy to reduce dryness of mouth (xerostomia) in patients with head and neck cancer. *Head Neck* 40(11):2353–2361.

Seikaly H, Jha N, Harris JR et al. 2004. Long term outcomes of submandibular gland transfer for prevention of post radiation xerostomia. *Arch Otolaryngol Head Neck Surg* 130(8):956–961.

Singh B, Shaha A. 1995. Traumatic submandibular salivary gland fistula. *J Oral Maxillofac Surg* 53(3):338–339.

Someya M, Sakata, Nagakura H et al. 2003. The changes in irradiated salivary gland function of patients with head and neck tumors treated with radiotherapy. *Jpn J Clin Oncol* 33(7):336–340.

Steinberg JM, Herréra AF. 2005. Management of parotid duct injuries. *Oral Surg Oral Med Oral Pathol Oral Radiol Endod* 99(2):136–141.

Stiubea-Cohen R, David R, Neumann Y, Palmon A, Aframian D. 2013. Toward salivary gland stem cell regeneration. *Compend Contin Educ Dent* 34 Spec No:14-7; quiz 18.

Stringer MD, Miralili SA, Meredith SJ, Muirhead JC. 2012. Redefining the surface anatomy of the parotid duct: An in vivo ultrasound study. *Plast Reconstr Surg* 130(5):1032–1037.

Takenoshite Y, Kawano Y, Oka M. 1991. Pneumoparotis an unusual occurrence of parotid gland swelling during dental treatment. Report of a case with a review of the literature. *J Craniomaxillofca Surg* 19(8):362–365.

Teague A, Akhtar S, Phillips J. 1998. Frey's syndrome following submandibular gland excision: An unusual post operative complication. *ORL J Otorhinolaryngol Relat Spec* 60(6):346–348.

Teymoortash A, Simolka N, Schrader C et al. 2005. Lymphocyte subsets in irradiation-induced sialadenitis of the submandibular gland. *Histopathology* 47(5):493–500.

Thula TT, Schultz G, Tran-Soy-Tay R, Batich C. 2005. Effects of EGF and bFGF on irradiated parotid glands. *Ann Biomed Eng* 33(5):685–695.

Toure G, Foy J-P, Vacher C. 2015. Surface anatomy of the parotid duct and its clinical relevance. *Clin Anat* 28(4):455–449.

Tsai CH, Ting CC, Wu SY et al. 2019. Clinical significance of buccal branches of the facial nerve and their relationship with the emergence of Stensen's duct. An anatomical study on adult Taiwanese cadavers. *J Craniomaxfac Surg* 47(11):1809–1818.

Van Sickels JE. 1981. Parotid duct injuries. *Oral Surg Oral Med Oral Pathol Oral Radiol Endod* 52(4):364–367.

Van Sickels JE. 2009. Management of parotid gland and duct injuries. *Oral and Maxillofac Clin North Am* 21(2):243–246.

Vargas H, Galati LT, Parnes SM. 2000. A pilot study evaluating the treatment of post parotidectomy sialoceles with botulinum toxin type A. *Arch Otolaryngol Head Neck Surg* 126(3):421–424.

Vissink A, van Luijk P, Langendijk JA, Coppes RP. 2015. Cuttrent ideas to reduce or salvage radiation damage to salivary glands. *Oral Dis* 21(1):e1–1Q.

Wasseman TH, Brizel DM, Henke M et al. 2005. Influence of intravenous amifostine on xerostomia, tumor control, and survival after radiotherapy for head-and –neck cancer: A 2-year follow up of a prospective, randomized phase III trial. *Int J Radiat Oncol Biol Phys* 15(4):985–990.

Wolfram RM, Palumbo B, Chehne F et al. 2004. (iso) Prostaglandins in saliva indicate oxidation injury after radioiodine therapy. *Rev Esp Med Nucl* 23(30):183–188.

Wood CB, Netterville JL. 2019. Temporoparietal Frey syndrome: An uncommon variant of a common syndrome. *Laryngoscope* 129(9):2071–2075.

Ya Z, Gao Z, Wang J. 2007. Primary clinical study on using end to end neurorrhaphy following rapid nerve expansion to repair facial nerve defect. (In Chinese) *Zhongguo Xiu Fu Chong Jian Wai Ke Za Zhi* 21(1):23–25.

Yamazaki H, Kojima R, Nakanishi Y, Kaneko A. 2018. A case of early pneumoparotid presenting with oral noises. *J Oral Maxillofac Surg* 76(1):67–69.

Yang W-F, Liao G-G, Hakim SG et al. 2016. Is pilocarpine effective in preventing radiation-induced xerostomia: A systematic review and meta-analysis. *Int J Radiat Oncol Biol Phys* 94(3):503–511.

Yoshimura H, Tobita T, Kumakiri M et al. 2012. Gustatory sweating in the submandibular region following neck dissection. *J Oral Maxillofac Surg* 70(11):e667–e673.

Zumeng Y, Zhi G, Gang Z, et al. 2006. Modified superficial parotidectomy: preserving both the greater auricular nerve and the parotid gland fascia. *Otolaryngol Head Neck Surg* 135(3):458–462.

Zhang Y, Guo CB, Zhang L et al. 2012. Prevention of radiation-induced xerostomia by submandibular gland transfer. *Head Neck* 34(7):937–942.

Chapter 17
Miscellaneous Pathologic Processes of the Salivary Glands

Outline

Introduction
Hereditary and Congenital Conditions
    Aplasia
    Duct Atresia
    Aberrant Glands
    Polycystic Disease of the Salivary Glands
    First Branchial Cleft Cysts, Fistulae, and Sinuses
    Cystic Fibrosis
Saliva
    Saliva as a Diagnostic Fluid
    Drooling
    Saliva in the Management of Xerophthalmia
Ischemic/Degenerative Changes
    Necrotizing Sialometaplasia
    Age Changes in Salivary Glands
Küttner Tumor
Salivary Gland Biopsy for Systemic Disease
    Amyloid and the Salivary Glands
        Hereditary Amyloidosis
        AL Amyloidosis (Primary Amyloidosis)
        AA Amyloidosis (Secondary Amyloidosis)
    Parkinson Disease
Summary
Case Presentation – *The Great Pretender*
References

Introduction

This chapter reviews a heterogenous group of salivary diseases that are not covered in other chapters of this book. Hereditary and developmental conditions of the glands are rare. The most common conditions are first arch branchial arch anomalies and their clinical management will be emphasized. Under the heading of saliva, the various pathways, (non-medical, medical, and surgical) for treating drooling will be explored. Recent developments in the use of saliva as a diagnostic tool and in the understanding of the mechanisms of IgG4-related disease will be discussed. Wherever possible, recent references will encompass prospective trials, systematic reviews, meta-analyses, and large series based on population databases, e.g. Surveillance, Epidemiology, and End Results (SEER), and the National Cancer Data Base (NCDB), to improve the scientific evidence base for the recommendations given.

Hereditary and Congenital Conditions

APLASIA

Aplasia of one or all of the major salivary glands is a rare condition which may present with severe xerostomia, rampant caries, candidiasis, pharyngitis, and laryngitis. In addition, "dental chipping" (Mandel 2006) and recurrent herpes labialis (Heath et al. 2006) have been described as presenting signs of salivary gland aplasia. The condition is said to be more common in males, (Frydrych and Koong 2014). It is seen mostly in the parotid gland and this may be related to this gland's earlier embryonic development (Goldenberg et al. 2000). There is an estimated incidence of parotid gland aplasia of 1:5000 live births (Togni et al. 2019).

Clinical examination will show the usual signs of severe xerostomia with absence of Stensen

---

Salivary Gland Pathology: Diagnosis and Management, Third Edition. Edited by Eric R. Carlson and Robert A. Ord.
© 2022 John Wiley & Sons, Inc. Published 2022 by John Wiley & Sons, Inc.
Companion website: www.wiley.com/go/carlson/salivary

and/or the Wharton duct. MR imaging may be used to confirm the clinical diagnosis of salivary gland aplasia (Mohan et al. 2013). Ultrasound is an inexpensive modality and gives good visualization of the parotid gland. CT scans should not be used electively in infants and children for "non-essential" head and neck scanning due to a small elevated risk for brain tumor development (Chen et al. 2014; Sheppard et al. 2018).

Salivary gland aplasia may occur as part of a recognized syndrome including Down syndrome (Odeh et al. 2013), associated with other congenital anomalies, or as an isolated phenomenon. In one series of 21 Treacher Collins patients, 19% had aplasia and 29% had dysplasia diagnosed on ultrasound and salivary gland function tests (Østerhus et al. 2012). Aplasia of the lacrimal and salivary glands (ALSG) presenting with irritable eyes and xerostomia is an autosomal dominant condition which appears to be related to mutations in FGF10 (Entesarium et al. 2007). In lacrimo-auriculo-dento-digital syndrome (LADD) agenesis of salivary glands as well as lacrimal glands can be seen and is an autosomal dominant condition with variable expressivity (Inan et al. 2006). Major salivary gland dysplasia has also been associated with Klinfelter syndrome (Togni et al. 2019).

A case of submandibular agenesis with parotid gland hypoplasia in association with ectodermal dysplasia is reported (Singh and Warnakulasuriya 2004). In addition, aplasia in association with hypoplasia of the thyroid (D'Ascanio et al. 2006), accessory parotid tissue (Antoniades et al. 2006), facial cleft (Sun et al. 2013), and cleft lip and palate (Reija et al. 2013) is described.

In a comprehensive review of the literature in 2010 by Pham Dang et al, 35 cases of bilateral major gland aplasia were identified. These authors also documented 10 cases of unilateral submandibular agenesis, 10 cases of aplasia of the salivary glands with absent lacrimal puncta with no family history, and two familial forms of this condition, which have also been studied.

Management of salivary gland aplasia is symptomatic and directed towards treating the xerostomia and other oral health care issues. A regime like that used for radiation-induced xerostomia with regular dental check-ups, low glucose diet, fluoride trays, and artificial saliva substitutes is recommended. Future approaches may be with novel tissue engineering techniques using transplanted salivary gland stem/progenitor cells, non-epithelial cells/bioactive lysates to trigger residual cells, or generate new salivary tissues or biomaterials loaded with glandular cells/bioactive lysates to function as an artificial saliva gland (Lombaert et al. 2017).

DUCT ATRESIA

Duct atresia is rare and in a 2001 review (Hoffrichter et al. 2001) only eight previous case of submandibular duct atresia were found with six unilateral and two bilateral. The condition usually presents in babies or infants as a "ranula" (Aronovitch and Edwards 2014) and is thought to be due to failure of the duct to penetrate the oral mucosa during development. These authors indicated that the penetration of the duct through the floor of mouth mucosa is one of the final stages in the embryonic development of the submandibular gland. The diagnosis can be made by the presence of dilated Wharton duct(s) on CT scans. Management is by sialodochoplasty to create a new duct orifice (Figure 17.1).

ABERRANT GLANDS

Accessory glands are ectopic in position but possess a duct that usually opens into another main duct e.g. the accessory parotid gland whereas aberrant glands have no duct system. Some of these aberrant glands can form fistulae and secrete while the patient is eating others do not secrete but form choristomas. A recent study of children with ectopic accessory parotid gland system (EAPS) fistula postulates that this is a rare syndrome related to the oculo-auriculo-vertebral spectrum (OAVS). In the author's review, 16 patients had been reported in the literature with an average age of 8.3 years, with 44% below the age of five-years. The accessory parotid fistula was always unilateral, 13/16 children had preauricular appendages (microtia) and 25% mandibular hypoplasia. Complete removal of the EAPS intraorally or transposing the fistula into the mouth was the usual management. The author speculates that the condition is due to dysmorphogenesis of the first two pharyngeal arches and relates it to OAVS embryologically and clinically (Dutta 2017). The commonest sites for these aberrant glands are the lateral neck, pharynx, and middle ear (Enoz and Suoglu 2006) presumably from their proximity to the first two branchial arches during development. When fistulas form into the external auditory meatus the diagnosis may be made by testing the fluid for amylase. These

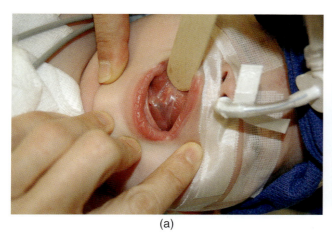
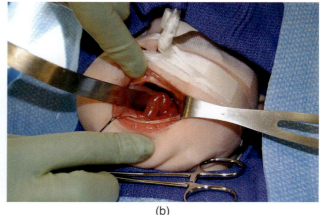

Figure 17.1. (a) Three-month-old baby with a swelling of the left floor of mouth. Pre-operative diagnosis was congenital ranula. (b) Intra-operative exploration revealed a significantly dilated Wharton duct with no evidence of a papilla to the oral mucosa. An imperforate duct was diagnosed and surgical management was by sialodochoplasty. Source: Dr. John Caccamese. Reproduced with permission from Dr. Caccamese.

"choristomas" of the middle ear may be accompanied by other facial anomalies of the facial nerve and ossicles (Chen and Li 2015), and sinus inversus totalis (Toros et al. 2010). These aberrant glands may be involved in neoplastic change and may account for the central salivary tumors of the jaws (usually mucoepidermoid carcinoma of the mandible).

A case of ectopic parotid in conjunction with CHARGE syndrome is reported (Ormitti et al. 2013). Space does not allow for description of all reported developmental abnormalities of the salivary glands and for the interested reader the review and classification by Togni et al. (2019), gives an excellent overview.

POLYCYSTIC DISEASE OF THE SALIVARY GLANDS

This is a rare disease which may be a hereditary condition as familial cases have been reported (Smyth et al. 1993). It is thought to be due to a developmental abnormality of the intercalated duct system. Seifert et al. (1981) reviewed 5739 cases of salivary gland disease and found 360 cases of cystic disease of which two patients were classified with dysgenetic polycystic parotid disease. Although it is usually bilateral, unilateral cases have been described (Seifert et al. 1981) (Figure 17.2). It is said to be always seen in females, however, a case of the condition in the submandibular glands in a male patient is reported (Garcia et al. 1998). Histologically the gland is replaced with multiple cysts which may contain spheroliths or microliths. There is a marked absence of inflammatory change. Parotidectomy may be carried out for esthetic reasons.

Recently two cases involving the minor salivary glands have been reported. In one case the dysgenetic polycystic disease involved a 21-year-old male and involved solely the lower lip (Srikant et al. 2017). The second patient had involvement of both submandibular glands as well as the minor salivary glands (Koudounarakis et al. 2016).

FIRST BRANCHIAL CLEFT CYSTS, FISTULAE, AND SINUSES

Anomalies of the first brachial arch are intimately associated with the parotid gland and the periauricular structures. They are less common than second branchial arch anomalies. In a survey of 183 patients with branchial cleft cysts and fistulae, 148 patients (80.8%) had branchial cysts of which 35 (23.6%) arose from the first arch and 35 (23.6%) had fistulae of which 11 (31.4%) arose from the first arch (Agaton-Bonilla and Gay-Escoda 1996). The usual figure for the incidence of first branchial arch anomalies is 10% (Olsen et al. 1980). There may be a geographical difference in incidence of first arch anomalies as only 12.4% of 105 cases of brachial anomalies were related to the second branchial arch in one Chinese series. There were

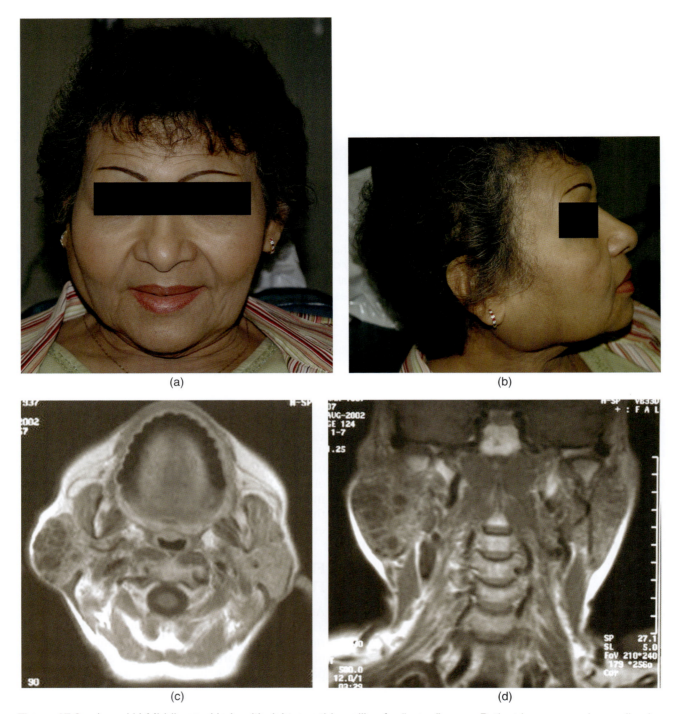

Figure 17.2. (a and b) Middle aged lady with right parotid swelling for "many" years. Patient is concerned regarding her appearance as she has no symptoms. (c, d, e, and f) MRI films show multiple cysts within the gland. At the time of surgery multiple microliths were seen.

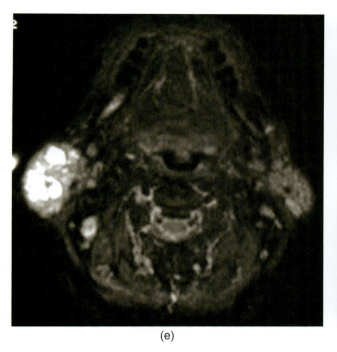
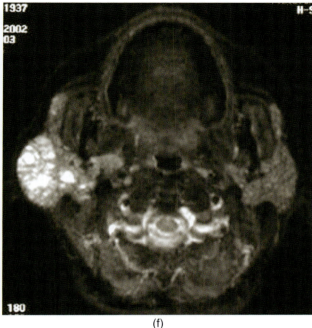

(e)   (f)

Figure 17.2. *(Continued).*

31.4% first arch anomalies and the rest (56.2%) were third and fourth branchial arch anomalies. (Li et al. 2018) Another paper from Singapore showed 23% first arch and only 13.3% of second arch cases (Teo et al. 2015).

Although Work (1972) classified type I cystic lesions as containing only squamous epithelium and type II lesions as containing squamous epithelium with adnexal skin structures plus cartilage, the presence of infection may make it impossible to classify these lesions using these criteria. Olsen et al. (1980) simplified this classification dividing the type II anomaly into cysts, fistulae, and sinuses. Cysts are tracts with no opening, sinuses are a tract with a single opening usually from the external auditory canal and fistulae are tracts with two openings usually from the external auditory meatus to the anterior neck above the hyoid bone. In their series of 39 cases, Triglia et al. (1998), found 20 (51%) sinuses, 11 (28%) fistulas, and 8 (21%) cysts. Similarly, in the series of 10 patients by Solares et al. (2003), 5 (50%) were sinuses, 3 (30%) fistulae, and 2 (20%) cysts.

Presentation is usually with recurrent infection, with discharge of pus or abscess in the anterior neck, a chronic purulent discharge from the ear, or an infected swelling of the parotid region (Figure 17.3). The usual age of presentation is

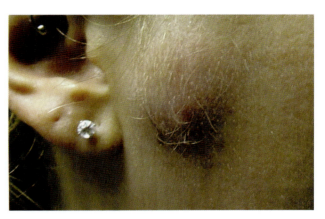

Figure 17.3. Twenty-year-old girl with recurrent localized infection of the parotid and a periparotid sinus.

between birth and twenty years with most cases diagnosed at age two and a half years.

Unfortunately, the infection is often not recognized as a manifestation of a first branchial arch abnormality and is treated with drainage or inadequate limited exploration which will complicate subsequent surgery. In the series of Triglia et al. (1998), 44% of patients had undergone prior surgery. In another paper, 65% of patients had incomplete surgery before referral (Martinez et al. 2007). According to Maddy and Ashram (2013), 50% of their patients had prior abscess drainage and 2 of 18 cases unsuccessful previous excisions. Liu et al. (2017) found that 76.2% of their patients had incision and drainage histories and 16.2% had one or more surgeries at other hospitals.

As the fistulae and sinuses communicate with the external auditory canal and their relationship to the facial nerve is variable a wide parotidectomy exposure with dissection of the nerve is essential for complete removal. In fistulae to the auditory meatus removal of the cartilage surrounding the fistulous tract is recommended (Figure 17.4). Rarely defects of the tympanic membrane in association with first branchial arch fistulae are reported (Pradhu and Ingrams 2011). If the fistula or sinus tract is not completely removed the lesion will recur and although the recurrence rate is small, 3–5% (Stulner et al. 2001) this may increase in patients with previous infection or inadequate surgery. Computed tomography fistulography is best to demonstrate the complete course of the tract if there is a cutaneous opening (Goff et al. 2012).

Branchial cysts will usually appear as parotid masses and are usually clinically diagnosed as cystic parotid tumors. (Figure 17.5). The first branchial lesions are usually superficial to the nerve and Triglia et al. (1998) reviewed 73 cases including their 39 and found that 63% were superficial, 29% deep, and 8% between the nerve (Figure 17.6). In the Solares et al. (2003) small series, however, 7 of 10 lesions were deep to the nerve, and one lay between the branches. A recent review found 72% of cases superficial to the nerve but sometimes adherent, deep to the nerve in 17% and between the nerve branches in 11% (Maddy and Ashram 2013). In a series of 43 cases, patients two years or younger were more likely to have first branchial cleft anomalies deep to the nerve, 33 vs 9.7%. All children with anomalies deep to the nerve had a greater risk of nerve weakness postoperatively (relative risk 7.2). (Brown et al. 2019) Larger cysts deep to the nerve may be difficult to remove as the nerve may be adherent to them and dissection can be slow and tedious (Figure 17.7).

It is very important to recognize the first arch abnormality as its complexity and anatomical variety necessitates wide exposure through a parotidectomy incision and dissection of the facial nerve to minimize the chances of subsequent facial nerve damage. Rarely facial nerve anomalies may occur with first arch anomalies (Hinson et al. 2014).

CYSTIC FIBROSIS

The composition of saliva is changed in cystic fibrosis and the formation of viscous mucus may lead to cystic dilations of the ducts and acini especially in the sublingual gland. The calcium concentration in saliva is also raised and microliths of calcium complexes with the viscous mucous can be seen. There is a positive correlation between raised values of sweat sodium and chloride with raised values in saliva. Saliva can be used for a screening diagnostic tool where sweat cannot be obtained or CFTR mutation screening is difficult (Gonçalves et al. 2019).

Saliva

SALIVA AS A DIAGNOSTIC FLUID

In many ways, saliva represents an ideal fluid for diagnostic analysis being readily available and not requiring invasive techniques. Currently, there is much interest in developing technologies to use saliva to diagnose, monitor progress, and assess treatment and recurrence of oral cancer. However, its mucus nature has made it difficult to analyze. In addition, there is evidence to suggest that the methods of processing saliva prior to analysis may have a significant effect on the results obtained for proteins in proteome analysis (Oshiro et al. 2007). In seeking to analyze the proteome of saliva researchers are hoping to find specific diagnostic biomarkers and develop techniques to discriminate between these biomarkers using proteomic and genomic technologies (Wong 2006). Several different research groups have examined varying aspects of salivary composition and have demonstrated significant differences between saliva in healthy subjects and those with oral cancer. Studies have examined biochemical and immunological parameters (Shpitzer et al. 2007), salivary endothelin levels (Pickering et al. 2007), and reactive nitrogen species and antioxidant profile (Bahar et al. 2007). Using genomic analysis four mRNAs (OAZ, SAT, IL8, IL1b) were identified that collectively had a discriminatory power of 91% sensitivity and specificity for detecting oral cancer (Zimmerman et al. 2007). Nonetheless, despite these promising initial results this technique currently remains a research tool. A review on salivary markers for interested readers is provided by Yakob et al. (2014). A recent review on "salivaomics"

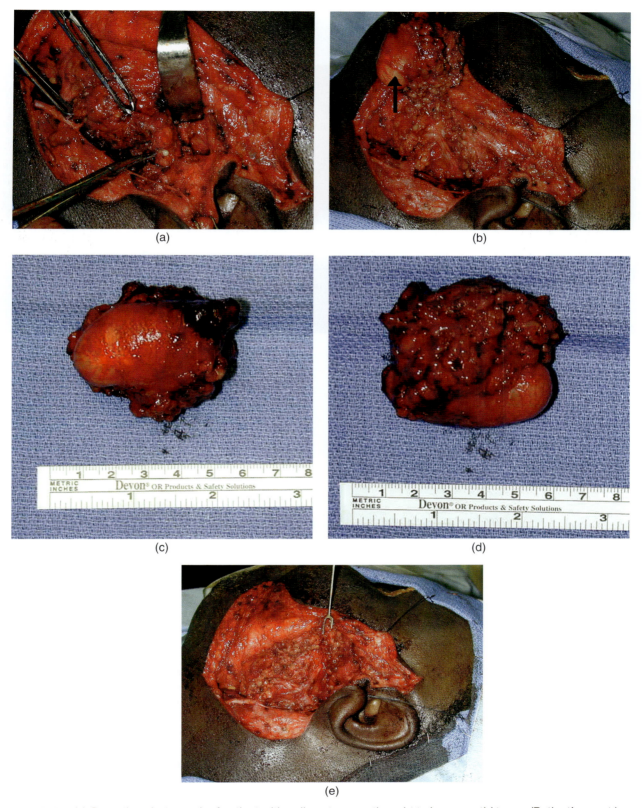

Figure 17.4. (a) Operative photograph of patient with a discrete mass thought to be a parotid tumor (Patient's ear at lower right of image). While dissecting down the external auditory meatus a fistulous tract to the cartilage was identified and the clamp points to a bead of pus from the fistulous tract. (b) The fistula was removed with a rim of the cartilage from the ear canal and a superficial parotidectomy carried out to remove the branchial cyst (arrow). (c and d) The parotidectomy specimen shows the cyst deep in the parotid but it was lying superficial to the facial nerve. (e) Following superficial parotidectomy (the ear lobe is sutured up for surgical retraction).

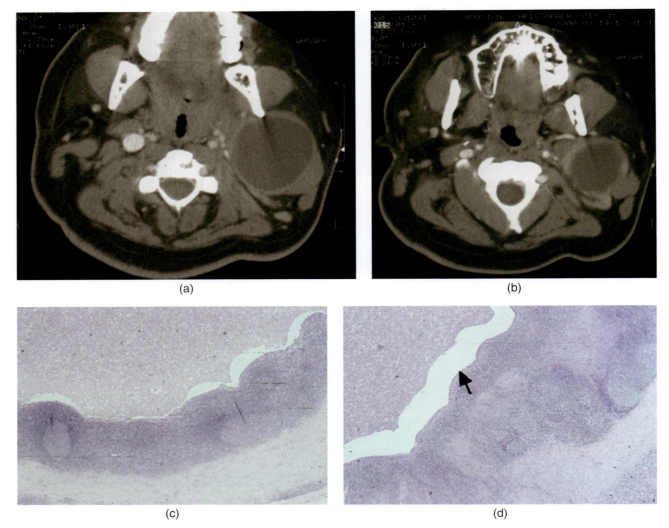

Figure 17.5. (a and b) CT scans of large branchial cyst in the parotid gland. (c and d) Histology of the branchial (lymphoepithelial cyst). The proteinaceous cyst contents are superior and the arrows point to the squamous epithelial lining and its associated lymphoid follicles.

states that many protein and mRNA salivary biomarkers have been identified that can detect oral squamous cell carcinoma, but none so far have been validated for clinical use. They found the most reliable results are gathered with the use of multiple biomarker candidates to improve accuracy (Aro et al. 2019). A further systematic review and meta-analysis conclude that saliva can be used as a diagnostic tool for oral squamous cell carcinoma using two highly sensitive specific markers MMP-9 and Chemerin. (Shree et al. 2019). An earlier systematic review, however, concluded that there was "no sufficient scientific evidence to support the capacity of the identified salivary biomarkers for the early diagnosis of oral cancer (sub-clinical stages of the pathogenic period before cancer phenotypes are manifested)." The authors did conclude that salivary biomarkers could be used to discriminate between patients with clinical oral cancer and healthy individuals (Gualtero and Castillo 2016).

Finally, saliva has been suggested as a means to monitor patients' post-treatment to detect recurrence early. The problem with this approach is that many patients will have xerostomia due to radiation therapy. It is therefore not clear whether the constituents in the residual saliva will have been altered by the treatment itself. There is, however,

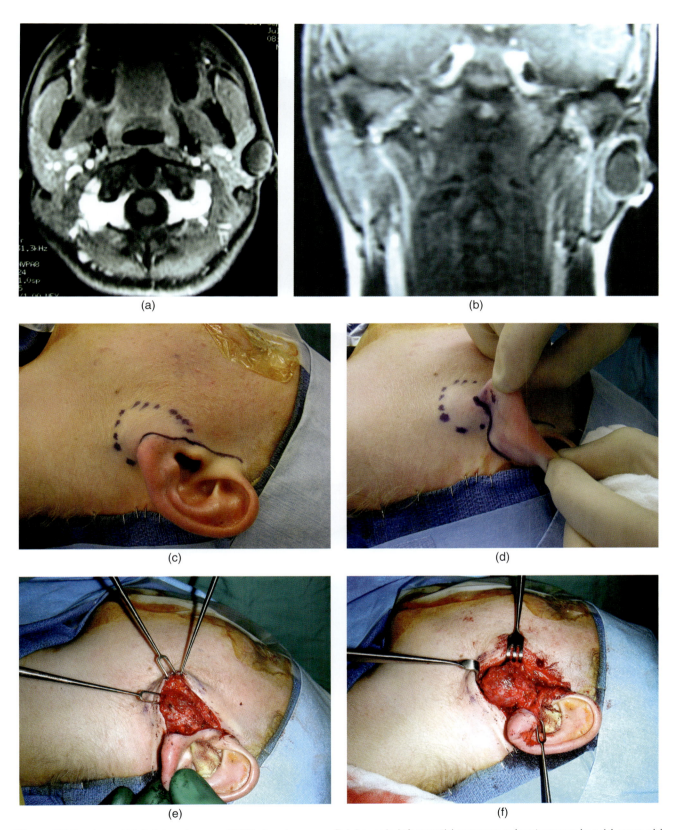

Figure 17.6. (a and b) Axial and coronal MRI showing superficial cyst in left parotid appears subcutaneous in a 14-year-old girl. (c and d) Cyst outlined by dotted line an omega incision will be used. Pre-auricular limb seen in c and retro-auricular portion in figure (d). (e) Cyst lies superficial to the parotid gland. (f) After further dissection, the fistulous attachment of the cyst to the cartilaginous external auditory meatus is revealed. (g) 3 cm cyst removed intact with a portion of the cartilaginous meatus to prevent recurrence. (h) The instrument points to the area where cartilage was removed from the external auditory meatus with the fistula. (i) Closure with subcuticular sutures.

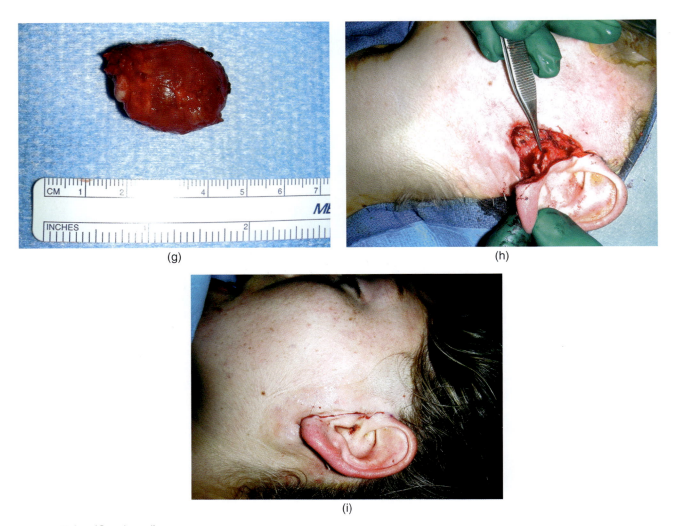

Figure 17.6. (*Continued*).

at least one study that showed a difference in salivary cytokines before and after oral cancer treatment. The authors comment that with the ability to spare salivary glands using intensity-modulated radiation therapy (IMRT) it is possible to collect post-treatment saliva as a monitor (Russo et al. 2016).

Another area of current interest in diagnosis utilizing saliva is the detection of HPV given its now proven status as a causative etiology in oropharyngeal cancer (OPC). In a cohort of patients with oropharyngeal cancer, a research study compared testing for HPV in saliva with PCR, to p16IHC and HPV DNA in situ hybridization (ISH) on surgical biopsies. The sensitivity and sensitivity for saliva were 72.25 and 90% with PPV and NPV of 96.3 and 47.4%. The authors concluded that a positive test could avoid the need for biopsy leading to faster treatment, lower morbidity, and less cost (Qureishi et al. 2018). Similarly, saliva testing with PCR for high-risk HPV in 62 patients showed that patients with high-risk HPV were more likely to have an oropharyngeal primary 76 vs 24%. A positive assay was 100% specific with a PPV of 100% for a p16 positive tumor located in the oropharynx. Again, the authors recommended this test when biopsy is not readily available (Wasserman et al. 2017).

It does not seem that HPV associated with oral cancer has a major etiological role as has been proven for oropharyngeal cancer, and virtually all oral cancers are readily biopsied. It is therefore difficult to see a role for salivary testing for HPV in oral cancer. In a study of 142 consecutive oral SCC

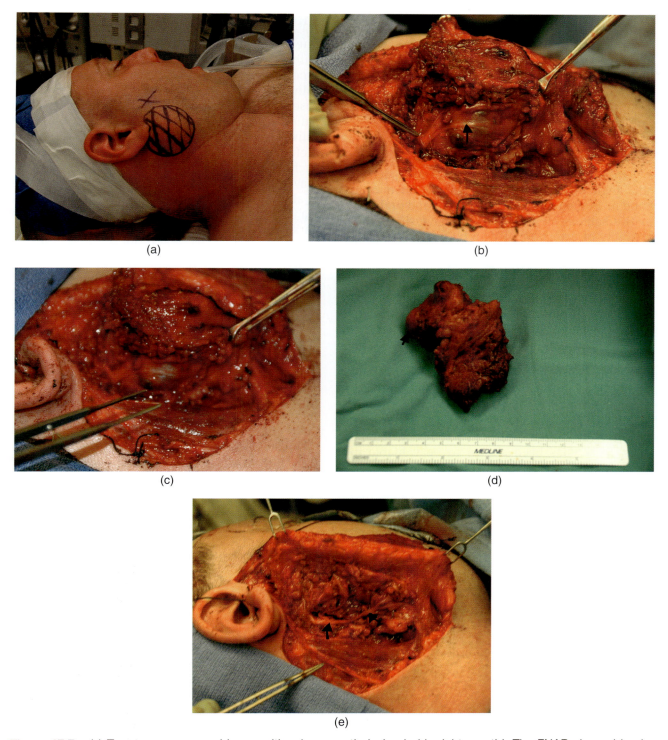

Figure 17.7. (a) Twenty-seven-year-old man with a large cystic lesion in his right parotid. The FNAB showed benign disease. (b) Initial superficial parotidectomy (superficial lobe retracted by an Allis clamp) reveals the cyst lying deep to the cervico-mandibular branch of the facial nerve (arrow). (c) The cervico-mandibular branch is carefully dissected off the cyst capsule and retracted towards the ear. (d) Parotidectomy specimen with deep lobe branchial cyst. (e) The cervico-mandibular trunk (arrow) is stretched over the defect that the deep lobe brachial cyst occupied.

using PCR and Q-PCR on the tumor tissue the HPV sequences were found in only five cases, (2 HPV16 and 2HPV 18 one mixed). The authors concluded that oncogenic HPV is uncommon in oral SCC and routine testing of HPV cannot be advocated (Lopes et al. 2011). Dang and Feng (2016) found a 9% incidence of p16 oral SCC compared to 79% for oropharyngeal SCC. There does not currently appear to be any utility in saliva testing for HPV in oral cancer.

In areas of high rates of oral cancer such as India high levels of HPV 16 and 18 have been found in women with cervical cancer and oral cancer (Kulkarni et al. 2011). Studies have shown the feasibility of detecting HPV 16 by saliva screening in healthy patients (Turner et al. 2011), and those with genital HPV (Peixoto et al. 2011). It is hard at present to see what a positive HPV saliva test means and what diagnostic or therapeutic implications it may have for the patient, unless oropharyngeal cancer is suspected. In view of the higher risk for asymptomatic oral infection in women with genital HPV infection, some authors have postulated that prophylactic HPV vaccination may reduce the burden of HPV-related diseases, (Adamopoulou et al. 2013). Vaccination against high-risk HPV is offered to girls in the USA to prevent cervical cancer, and boys to prevent genital warts. Saliva has been shown to be valuable in testing for HPV antibodies after vaccination (Parker et al. 2018).

Recent publications have suggested that saliva can be used to assess biomarkers inpatients with medication-related osteo necrosis of the jaws. These bone deterioration biomarkers NTX and B-AP were suggested as useful in diagnosis and perhaps to monitor patients (Kolokythas et al. 2015).

HIV is a systemic disease that can be diagnosed by a "spit" test, using a rapid and semi-quantitative lateral flow assay format, saliva and serum samples for HIV anti IgG/secretory IgA correlate. This can allow rapid non-invasive means of diagnosis. (Corsjens et al. 2000) Saliva allows effective HIV population testing as it is non-infectious and as it is noninvasive, it is easier to collect. Recent developments using agglutination-PCR (ADAP) technology have improved sensitivity and enable earlier diagnosis and treatment (Tsai et al. 2018). The oral fluid (saliva) test has also been shown to increase self-testing frequency in persons at high-risk of HIV infection. (Katz et al. 2018).

DROOLING

The term drooling is often used synomonously with sialorrhea, however, virtually all patients who drool do not have an increase in the amount of saliva they produce. Patients with Parkinson's disease with a reduced saliva production can often suffer from drooling as well as silent aspiration of saliva. Although Parkinson's disease results in inefficient oropharyngeal swallowing other factors such as multitasking and distracted attention may play a role in drooling in this disease (Reynolds et al. 2018). Another study confirmed that dysphagia is only weakly associated with drooling in Parkinson's and that it is the voluntary oral phase that is the key. The oral phase is negatively impacted by cognitive defects (Nienstedt et al. 2018). Drooling is the result of a lack of coordinated swallowing with pooling of saliva in the anterior floor of mouth with subsequent drooling as exemplified in conditions such as cerebral palsy and amyotrophic lateral sclerosis. This condition can have a severe impact on the patient's quality of life. In patients with cerebral palsy (CP) a review of 385 children showed a 40% prevalence of drooling, severe in 15%. Poor gross motor function with poor head control, difficulty eating, and lip incompetence were significant factors. Also, in this cohort intellectual disability and epilepsy were significantly associated with drooling (Reid et al. 2012). Many different methods of managing this condition have been proposed and are summarized in an excellent review by Meningaud et al. (2006). These patients benefit from a multidisciplinary team approach and both medical and surgical treatments are used in their management. Medical therapy includes oral motor therapy, orofacial regulation therapy, and behavioral modification via biofeedback. In an analysis of studies from 1970 to 2005 of behavioral treatments of drooling only 17 articles with 57 patients met the inclusion criteria. The evidence base found 15 studies that used a single participant design and two that used an experimental comparison group design. Some studies were poorly designed and methodological flaws identified. Conclusions were that it was not possible to assess the efficacy of behavioral therapy and that further research is needed (Van der Burg et al. 2007). A later systematic review also found only low-level evidence to support the use of behavioral interventions. They also suggest the need for further well-designed studies (McInerney et al. 2019). Anticholinergic drug therapy may be given orally or by botulinum toxin injections. Certain conditions such as glaucoma preclude the use of these oral drugs and side effects are not uncommon. In a systematic review of the literature, only seven papers were found to meet the inclusion criteria and the authors concluded that there was some evidence benztropine, glycopyrrolate and bezhexol hydrochloride were effective in children with drooling (Jongerius et al. 2003). Botulinum toxin A has been injected into the parotid glands solely or with the submandibular glands with good results. However, the effect is only temporary. In a double-blind placebo-controlled study on 20 patients with Parkinsonism, botulinum toxin A injection into the parotid and submandibular glands was found to be an effective and safe treatment for drooling (Mancini et al. 2003). In another prospective, double-blind, placebo-controlled trial of different doses of botulinum toxin A (18.75, 37.5, and 75MU per parotid) the primary end-point was achieved with the highest dose of 75MU without side effects (Lipp et al. 2003). Similarly, in a controlled trial of botulinum against scopolamine in children with cerebral palsy and drooling Botulinum toxin was found to have a significant effect (Jongerius et al. 2004). Although botulinum showed fewer and less severe side effects than transdermal scopolamine general anesthesia was required for the injections. Despite the fact that treatment by botulinum toxin A can improve drooling for up to six months there is currently no data in the literature for optimum or maximum dosage, frequency of injections, and duration of action (Lal and Hotaling 2006). In some syndromes (CHARGE syndrome), excess salivation may be associated with aspiration and intermittent and prospective botulinum injections have proven helpful in managing aspiration (Blake et al. 2012).

Radiation therapy has been used to reduce saliva production but is obviously contraindicated in children due to its effects on growth and the possibility of radiation-induced sarcoma. Even in adults, its long-term side effects may preclude its use. An exception may be in patients such as those with poor life expectancy, including those with as amyotrophic lateral sclerosis (ALS), where radiation may be of benefit in reducing salivary production. In a systematic review of patients with either Parkinson's disease or ALS treated by external beam radiotherapy, 10 studies (four prospective) with 216 patients were reviewed. Overall 81% of patients benefitted with symptomatic improvement. The commonest target was bilateral submandibular glands and tail of the parotid. However, 40% of patients had acute toxicity and 12% experienced long-term toxicity (Hawkey et al. 2016).

Surgery encompasses both sectioning of secretory nerves as well as operations on the glands and ducts. Sectioning of Jacobson's nerve in the middle ear has fallen out of favor and sectioning of the chorda tympani will cause loss of taste. Many different surgical techniques have been described since Wilkie's classic paper advocating excision of the submandibular glands combined with posterior positioning of the parotid ducts (Wilkie 1967). These methods have included duct ligation, duct repositioning, and gland excision of one or more of the major glands. Currently, excellent permanent results have been reported with submandibular duct repositioning and sublingual gland excision. Although submandibular gland excision with parotid duct ligation has also been reported as 87% successful (Manrique et al. 2007), it does give rise to temporary parotid edema which can be significant. Greensmith et al. (2005) reported that bilateral submandibular duct repositioning with sublingual gland excision was superior to this technique. However, some authors have questioned the need for excision of the sublingual glands. In a study to assess submandibular duct reposition alone against duct reposition and sublingual gland removal, a 3% postoperative hemorrhage and 12% of parents expressing concerns of pain was found for the duct reposition only procedure, while 13.7% hemorrhage and 36% concern over postoperative pain was found in the group with sublingual gland excision (Glynn and O'Dwyer 2007). As both procedures were equally effective in controlling drooling, the authors state that they no longer carry out sublingual gland excision. There are few studies that have examined the long-term outcome of surgery for drooling. A study of 62 patients who had bilateral submandibular duct translocation and bilateral excision of the sublingual glands (between 1994 and 2014), were contacted via a questionnaire. The families indicated outcomes as very good with no drooling issues in 21 and 48% had only mild to moderate drooling. However, 9/62 families 14.5% said they would not have surgery again due to the difficult recovery, lack of effectiveness, and subsequent problems with coughing, gagging, and dental decay (Reid et al. 2019) Another study examined 43 children who had bilateral submandibular duct relocation between 2003 and 2017. In this study, 53% of caregivers were very satisfied and 30% satisfied with the results (Sousa et al. 2018).

Due to the number of different causes of drooling and the multiple treatment choices available these patients are best assessed by a multidisciplinary team. As in many other aspects of pediatrics and medicine, simple noninvasive methods of management are attempted first before suggesting surgical management.

SALIVA IN THE MANAGEMENT OF XEROPHTHALMIA

Although dry eyes may occur in relation to dry mouth in conditions such as Sjögren syndrome, keratoconjunctivitis sicca can occur in isolation. Isolated keratoconjunctivitis sicca is not an uncommon condition and currently there is no satisfactory treatment. Transfer of the submandibular gland duct into the lacrimal basin was first undertaken in 1986 (Murube-Del-Castillo 1986). A series of 38 cases with micro-anastomosis of the submandibular gland vessels to the temporal vessels in the temporal fossa and insertion of the Wharton duct into the upper eyelid was reported in 2004 (Yu et al. 2004). In this series, only five cases failed, eight cases had epiphora which required reduction of the size of the submandibular gland and two cases had ductal reconstruction secondary to blockage. The authors stress the use of scintigraphy preoperatively to assess the salivary glands function and rule out Sjogren disease, and also postoperatively to assess revascularization and function. Paniello (2007) reported success in six of seven transfers (86%). Four of five patients had keratoconjunctivitis sicca secondary to Stevens-Johnson syndrome. A larger series with long-term follow-up has been reported recently. In a series of 185 patients (two hundred eyes,) operated between 1999 and 2015 successful transplantation was reported in 90%. In the 20 failures, 15/20 were due to venous thrombosis and 5/20 obstruction of the duct. Follow-up data for 163 eyes showed epiphora in 60.1% which was treated by surgical reduction of the submandibular gland, topical atropine gel, and botulinum injection. Further duct obstruction occurred in 10.6% and was treated with duct reconstruction. Patient satisfaction was 87.7% with improved visual acuity in 56.3% and objective improvement in reduction of corneal staining (Zhang et al. 2019). In dealing with some of the long-term complications of this procedure one study found that 25-U of botulinum toxin A was a suitable dose to treat epiphora from the transplanted submandibular gland (Shan et al. 2019). Another study proved the feasibility of sialography to diagnose obstructive sialadenitis in the transplanted sub mandibular gland (Su et al. 2014).

Note that it will be important in the future to test these patients for IgG4-related disease (see later section) as steroid therapy may be indicated rather than surgery in some of these cases. Novel approaches to the problem of xerostomia and keratoconjunctivitis sicca include the use of stem cells. Promising research is being done in animal models (Abughanam et al. 2019).

Ischemic/Degenerative Changes

NECROTIZING SIALOMETAPLASIA

Necrotizing sialometaplasia can be seen in any of the salivary glands but is most commonly diagnosed in the minor salivary glands of the palate (Figure 17.8). Very rarely it may be bilateral (Kandula et al. 2016). It occurs in major glands in about 10% of cases (Kaplan et al. 2012).

It is thought to be secondary to local ischemia with secondary necrosis of the gland and may be secondary to trauma or surgery, but is usually spontaneous. It is more frequent in smokers but can also be associated with cocaine use and bulimia. Initially, there is swelling quickly followed by ulceration which may be deep down to the bone. Healing may take 2–3 months. Biopsy may be necessary to distinguish this lesion from a malignancy and the histology may be misinterpreted. Both clinical and histopathologic appearance can mimic malignancy. In one case reported in the parotid, facial nerve palsy was seen (Haen et al. 2017). There is lobular necrosis of the salivary gland with squamous metaplasia of the ducts and this can be misdiagnosed as mucoepidermoid carcinoma or squamous cell carcinoma. In addition, the epithelium adjacent to the ulcer can display pseudo-epitheliomatous hyperplasia which can also be mistaken for squamous cell carcinoma. If the patient keeps the lesion clean with mouthwashes healing will occur and recurrence is not

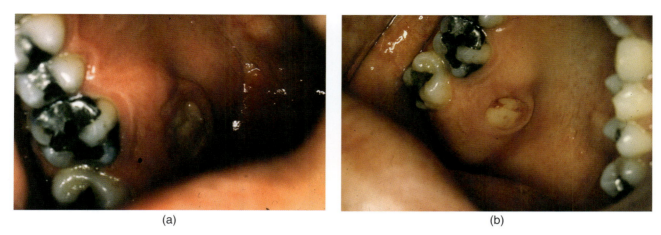

Figure 17.8. (a) Necrotizing sialometaplasia of palate with rolled edge and granular base clinically resembling squamous cell carcinoma. (b) Necrotizing sialometaplasia at a later stage with exposed palatal bone.

seen. Biopsy will often be required to rule out malignancy and histologic interpretation by an experienced pathologist is essential.

AGE CHANGES IN SALIVARY GLANDS

Generalized acinar atrophy can occur in the major salivary glands with age. Frequently the glandular tissue is replaced with fat. In addition, oncocytic metaplasia increases in older patients. Oncocytes are large granular eosinophilic cells. Their granular cytoplasm appears to be secondary to numerous mitochondria. A diffuse oncocytosis of the salivary glands can occur. These changes are not clinically relevant although oncocytes can give rise to an oncocytoma which is usually benign but may occasionally be a malignant type. Oncocytomas are of interest as they are similar to Warthin tumors in appearing as "hot" spots on technetium scans.

Focal lymphocytic infiltration occurs in minor salivary glands in the palate in older patients and is significantly less seen in labial salivary glands (Vered et al. 2001). Decreases in the volume of saliva and change in constituents have been reported in the elderly. It is difficult to interpret some of the literature, as many elderly patients are taking medication which can cause xerostomia.

Küttner Tumor

In the 1992 WHO classification, Küttner tumor (chronic sclerosing sialadenitis of the submandibular gland) was included in the new designation of tumor-like lesions to be distinguished from true tumors (Seifert 1992). Clinically the "tumor" described by Küttner in 1896 cannot be distinguished from a true neoplasm (Williams et al. 2000) (see case presentation). A sclerosing variant of mucoepidermoid carcinoma can make the diagnosis even more difficult. This variant is rarely reported and of the 31 cases in the literature only 6 have occurred in the submandibular gland (Heptinstall et al. 2017). Early work by Seifert and Donath (1977) reviewing 349 cases of chronic sialadenitis had caused them to postulate that two factors were important in the etiology of Küttner Tumor. There was an initial disturbance of secretion with an obstructive electrolyte sialadenitis and an immune reaction of the salivary duct system with the final phase of an obstructive progressive immune-sialadenitis. By 2003 numerous studies emphasized that this was an under-recognized entity and was a specific entity with a possible immunologic background (Blanco et al. 2003). In 2008 Machado de Sousa et al. (2008) using immunohistochemical markers concluded that Küttner tumor was more in keeping with an inflammatory induced degenerative disease. However, by 2010 after the recognition of Mikulicz disease as being an IgG4- related disease, comparison to Küttner tumor also revealed serologic and histopathologic findings implicating Küttner tumor as an immunoglobulin G4 disease (Takano et al. 2010). These findings have been validated and the high expression of IgG4 confirms that it belongs in the spectrum of immunoglobulin G4 diseases and differentiates Küttner tumor from Sjögren syndrome, lymphoepithelial sialadenitis, and non-specified chronic sialadenitis (Gever et al. 2010). This has led to the realization that Küttner tumor is not just a solitary tumor of the submandibular gland seen in the fifth to seventh decade of life but represents a more systemic disease. This disease has now been reported in children and the importance of recognition is because it may be treated by steroids to prevent other IgG4 complications (Melo et al. 2012.) Not surprisingly reports of Küttner tumor with involvement of lacrimal glands are now increasingly reported (Shin et al. 2012).

Currently, the spectrum of IgG4-related diseases in the head and neck is thought to include idiopathic orbital inflammatory syndrome (inflammatory pseudotumor), orbital lymphoid hyperplasia, Mikulicz disease, Küttner tumor, Hashimoto's thyroiditis, Reidel thyroiditis, and pituitary hypophysitis. The disease not only affects the submandibular and lacrimal gland, but the parotid and minor salivary glands (Godbehere et al. 2019). IgG4-related disease isolated to the head and neck alone may be more common in Asians and women. (Wallace et al. 2019).

Because multiple site involvement is common in IgG4-related disease, the pancreas, bile ducts, gallbladder, kidneys, retroperitoneum, mesentery, lungs, GI tract and blood vessels all may show manifestations. Diagnosis is important as IgG4) disease may show a dramatic response to corticosteroid therapy, and radiologic diagnosis may be possible (Fujita et al. 2012). Salivary gland enlargement, with marked enhancement and restricted diffusion has been suggested as MR features favoring this diagnosis (de Cocker et al. 2014) Ultrasound has also be found by numerous authors to be a useful imaging for diagnosis of IgG4 related-disease (Shimizu et al. 2015). As the disease often affects multiple organ systems PET scanning is useful to look for systematic disease at other sites (Maehara et al. 2020). Biopsy is essential for diagnosis to show the sclerosing sialadenitis, lymphocytic infiltration, fibrosis, phlebitis, and the infiltration by IgG4-plasma cells. The serum IgG4 is usually raised but does not always correlate with what is seen histologically. FNAB does not seem to be as useful as a diagnostic tool in this condition (Leon et al. 2016).

It does not appear that IgG4 has a central role in the disease manifestations which seem to be related to an antigen-antibody immune response mechanism. B cells are important in this antigen response, and T cells particularly CD4 + T cells play an important role. There is also evidence that follicular helper T cells are involved in the pathogenesis (Maehara et al. 2020).

Steroids remain the primary initial therapy (Kamisawa et al. 2009; Masaki et al. 2017) Response is usually rapid with maintenance steroid therapy to prevent recurrence. In patients who fail to respond to steroid therapy, rituximab has been used. This appears to have its effect by depleting B cells.

Salivary Gland Biopsy for Systemic Disease

Just as saliva has been used as a diagnostic test for systemic disease such as HIV, salivary gland biopsy can also be used for this purpose. The use of labial gland biopsy for diagnosing diseases that primarily affect the salivary glands, such as Sjögren syndrome, is well described and discussed in chapter 6. There are numerous other systemic conditions that effect the salivary gland secondarily, however, that can also be diagnosed from salivary biopsy, specifically the various manifestations of amyloid disease and Parkinson's disease.

AMYLOID AND THE SALIVARY GLANDS

Amyloid is an abnormal protein which can be laid down in many different body tissues and this may be a result of an AL amyloidosis (primary amyloidosis), an AA amyloidosis (secondary amyloidosis), or a rare hereditary syndrome with amyloidosis. The salivary glands may play a role in the diagnosis in all scenarios. Labial minor salivary gland biopsy will often be essential for diagnosis, and signs of salivary disease may be a part of the clinical picture (Figure 17.9).

Hereditary Amyloidosis

The hereditary forms of amyloidosis are rare. Familial amyloid polyneuropathy (FAP)has an autosomal transmission. It is caused by a mutation of the transthyretin gene (TTR). It is fatal if not treated but is often diagnosed late due to a slow diverse onset and lack of a family history in half of late-onset cases. The most sensitive biopsies for diagnosis are labial salivary gland or skin biopsy (Adams et al. 2016). In one series of

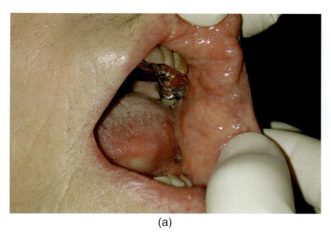 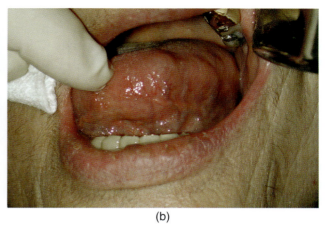

Figure 17.9. (a) Seventy-year-old lady with "lumps" in her mouth. Clinical photograph shows firm to hard submucosal mass inside the lower lip at the commissure. Biopsy showed amyloid. (b) Left lateral tongue also shows numerous raised submucosal nodules, which are positive for amyloid.

seventeen patients with FAP, none of whom had symptoms of xerostomia, minor salivary biopsy was undertaken. Nine of twelve patients with neurologic symptoms were positive for amyloid on salivary biopsy (75%). The test was significantly more accurate in patients with neurologic dysfunction (de Paula Eduardo et al. 2017). It has also been shown that labial gland biopsy can not only confirm a diagnosis of amyloidosis but that the histologic pattern of distribution combined with its semi-quantification using Congo-red fluorescence can accurately distinguish the subtypes of the amyloid deposit. In a retrospective study of 92 cases the type of amyloidosis was AL in 51 cases, non-V30M mutant ATTR in 10 cases, V30M mutant ATTR in 8, serum amyloid A-derived amyloidosis (AA) in 6, wild -type ATTR in 4, gelsolin in 3 and unclassified in 10 patients (Jamet et al. 2015).

Lysozyme amyloidosis (ALys) is an autosomal dominant (p.Trp82Arg variant) amyloidosis that may present as Sicca syndrome due to deposition of amyloid in the major salivary glands (Benyamine et al. 2017). There are about fifty cases reported, and Sicca syndrome may precede the actual diagnosis by many years. The disease is progressive and renal and liver transplant may be required (Scafi et al. 2019).

AL Amyloidosis (Primary Amyloidosis)

Primary amyloidosis is the commonest type of amyloidosis and clinical presentation is very diverse as any organ except the brain can be involved by the monoclonal immunoglobulin light chain. Early diagnosis is necessary to prevent amyloid cardiomyopathy and either biopsy by abdominal fat aspiration or minor salivary gland lip biopsy is recommended to make the diagnosis (Jaccard et al. 2015). Gertz (2018) stated that invasive organ biopsy is not required for the diagnosis for immunoglobulin light chain amyloidosis as amyloid deposits are found in 85% of bone marrow aspirate, salivary gland biopsy, or subcutaneous fat aspirates. Furthermore, salivary gland lip biopsy is a more effective technique for the diagnosis of systemic amyloid than biopsy of clinically normal skin (Lecadet et al. 2018). A series of 34 patients with suspected amyloidosis was submitted to labial salivary gland, bone marrow, and skin biopsies. Eighteen patients were positive with labial gland being the most sensitive (89%) compared to 77% for bone marrow and 72% for skin (Suzuki et al. 2016). In a major gland like the submandibular gland FNAB has also been successful in diagnosing systemic amyloidosis (Giorgadze et al. 2004). ^{11}C-PiB PET scanning can accurately demonstrate both submandibular and sublingual gland involvement in systemic amyloidosis (Ezawa et al. 2018).

AA Amyloidosis (Secondary Amyloidosis)

Amyloid can be related to many other primary diseases including multiple myeloma, renal disease, and pulmonary disease. In myeloma, the classic head and neck presentation is macroglossia but salivary gland involvement can also be seen (Mateo

Arias et al. 2003). Amyloid can also be seen in relation to MALT lymphoma related to the salivary glands particularly the minor salivary glands (Odell et al. 1998; Kojima et al. 2006; Flaig and Ihrier 2009). This phenomenon has been reported in the lip of an 11-year old boy, where initial biopsy was felt to be amyloidosis. Eventually, the diagnosis of low-grade B-cell lymphoma surrounded by AL $_k$-type amyloid was established (Gabali et al. 2013). The submandibular gland may also present with amyloidosis in relation to low-grade marginal zone B-cell lymphoma (Perera et al. 2010). The clinician should suspect an underlying lymphoma in cases of unexplained amyloid deposition in relation to salivary glands.

In 2001 a case of primary Sjögren syndrome was found to have amyloid deposits on her lip biopsy of minor salivary glands. Further investigation showed primary systemic amyloidosis. A recent paper reviewed patients with amyloidosis and primary Sjögren syndrome. Most cases were localized AL amyloidosis most frequently found in skin and lung. Salivary glands were involved and seven cases had an associated lymphoma (Hernandez-Molina et al. 2018). Sicca syndrome with alopecia and nail changes in conjunction with AL amyloidosis is also reported (Renker et al. 2014). The ultrasound appearance of Sjögren syndrome cannot reliably be distinguished from AL amyloid or sarcoidosis, but their common features do distinguish these patients from patients without systemic rheumatologic disease (Law et al. 2019).

The parotid gland and other major salivary gland can be involved with local amyloid deposits without any sign of systemic disease (Nandapalan et al. 1998; Gareb et al. 2018). A rare case of amyloid deposits in the sublingual glands causing sleep apnea is reported from China (Hu et al. 2013).

PARKINSON DISEASE

The early diagnosis of Parkinson disease can be made by detecting the presence of Lewy type α-synucleinopathy (LTS) on biopsied tissue. A small study of 15 patients underwent biopsy of minor salivary glands of the lower lip and core needle biopsy (CNB) of the submandibular gland. Only 1/15 of the labial biopsies were positive for LTS (6.75%). Twelve of fifteen of the CNB had salivary tissue in the specimen and of these 9/12 (75%) were positive for LTS. Overall, including specimens without suitable tissue, 9/15 of the submandibular CNB were diagnostic for LTS (60%) (Adler et al. 2014). In another study of 25 patients, submandibular needle biopsy was diagnostic for LTS in 74% of cases. The authors felt that false positives may be true false positives or represent prodromal disease. Again six of the 25 patients had inadequate specimens (Adler et al. 2016). The most compelling evidence for the use of submandibular gland CNB comes from a 2014 systematic review which looked at 49 studies of the use of peripheral tissues and body fluids as biomarkers for Parkinson disease. The study showed that of the three peripheral tissues that have been biopsied most commonly, colonic mucosa had a sensitivity of 42-90% and a specificity of 100%, skin biopsy sensitivity 19% and specificity of 80%, and submandibular gland had sensitivity and specificity of 100%. Neither plasma nor CSF alpha-synuclein was a reliable marker (Malek et al. 2014).

Summary

- Fistulae and sinuses above the hyoid bone in the periparotid region should be suspected of being first arch anomalies.
- In managing first branchial arch anomalies wide exposure with complete dissection of the facial nerve is mandatory because of the complex and unpredictable relationship of the sinuses, fistulae, and cysts to the nerve.
- In managing drooling, a multidisciplinary team is optimum.
- Surgery for drooling is used when other less invasive therapies have been tried and failed. Posterior repositioning of the submandibular ducts with or without sublingual gland excision appears to give good results.
- Saliva can be used to diagnose/confirm the presence of oropharyngeal SCC and is useful in HIV screening. Its role in diagnosing oral SCC is not yet defined.
- Necrotizing sialometaplasia should be considered in the diagnosis of ulcerative palatal lesions and may be mistaken clinically and histologically for a malignancy
- IgG4 disease of the head and neck is important to recognize as it may be a manifestation of systemic disease and requires medical therapy.

Case Presentation – *The Great Pretender*

A 59-year old woman was evaluated in September 2017 complaining of a mass in the neck. She had woken one morning three months ago and felt a lump under her right jaw. She had some pain which radiated to her ear but this was not severe. She saw her primary care physician who referred her to an otolaryngologist who ordered an ultrasound guided FNAB and an MRI. Her FNAB showed benign salivary tissue with a focal zone of acinar dropout and stromal fibrosis with chronic inflammation. There was no atypical acinar or ductal proliferation.

Her MRI revealed a 16 × 15 mm. enhancing mass in the lower aspect of the right submandibular gland (Figure 17.10a–c).

Past Medical History
Bilateral narrow-angle glaucoma- treated by Iridotomy
History of idiopathic thrombocytopenic purpura
Lyme disease
CIS of the skin of her arm-treated by excision.
She had a caesarian section.
She takes Flonase and MCG/ACT nasal spray and Estrace vaginal cream

Social History
Quit smoking 38 years ago
Drinks 4.2 oz. of alcohol a week

Examination
There were no palpable cervical nodes. In the right submandibular triangle, there was a hard, discrete, mass which felt like the submandibular gland. It was discrete and mobile. Intraoral exam was normal.

In view of the three-month history, with no decrease in size, and the findings of the MRI we recommended a repeat of the US-guided FNAB to attempt to get a tissue diagnosis. This was performed on October 9, 2017. The ultrasound showed a peripheral sharply marginated area of decreased echogenicity at the inferior aspect of the right submandibular gland. There was preservation of the color flow and ductal branching. The lesion was very tender and firm on aspiration. The appearance of the ultrasound was felt to favor inflammation rather than a mass (Figure 17.10d and e).

The FNAB showed a basaloid cell salivary neoplasm, adenoid cystic carcinoma vs pleomorphic adenoma.

Diagnosis
Given the MRI report and the FNAB findings, the provisional diagnosis was submandibular gland tumor rule out adenoid cystic carcinoma.

The patient was recommended for an en-bloc excision combined with an elective supraomohyoid neck dissection. She underwent surgery in October and final pathology showed no neoplasm but focal chronic fibrosing sialadenitis (Figure 17.10f and g). The final diagnosis was Küttner tumor. Serum IgG4 was not raised and staining for IgG4 on the specimen was negative (Figure 17.10h). Surprisingly there was no evidence to support that the disease was caused by IgG4 in this case.

Post-operatively the patient had slight weakness of the marginal mandibular branch of the facial nerve. This began to improve within four weeks. At her 1-year follow-up, her scar had healed well and her facial nerve function was normal.

TAKE-HOME POINTS
This case illustrates why Küttner tumor is called a tumor. It is extremely difficult to distinguish this inflammatory/immune condition from a true neoplasm. There was very little indication of an inflammatory condition from the history. The mass did not increase or decrease with eating. Although there was some pain radiating to the ear the patient had similar symptoms on the contralateral side. Both the MRI and the false-positive FNAB pointed in the direction of a submandibular tumor most likely an adenoid cystic carcinoma. The final diagnosis was histologically a benign inflammatory condition. All testing for IgG4 was negative in this patient. Although the patient had an elective neck dissection there is very little extra morbidity from this procedure in the absence of any permanent nerve injury. The cervical scar for neck dissection is obviously larger than for a submandibular gland removal. The Küttner tumor remains the great pretender and a diagnostic challenge.

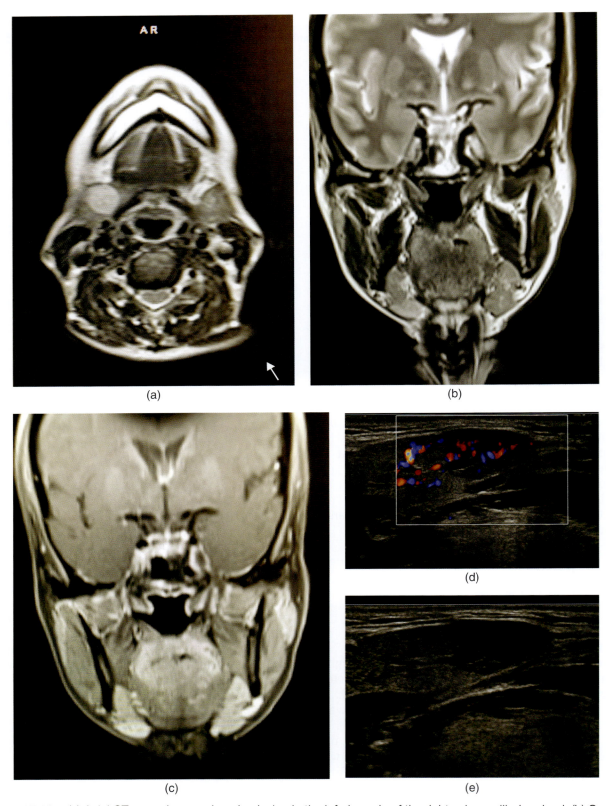

Figure 17.10. (a) Axial CT scan shows enhancing lesion in the inferior pole of the right submandibular gland. (b) Coronal scan shows well-defined mass at the inferior of the submandibular gland. (c) The mass shows enhancement on T2 image. (d) Color Doppler Ultrasound shows well-defined area of decreased echogenicity. (e) Ultrasound shows sharply marginated lesion. Source: Courtesy of Dr. J. Wong, Professor of Radiology, University of Maryland. (f) Low power hematoxylin and eosin-stained submandibular gland shows prominent fibrous bands with chronic inflammation, breakdown, and absence of acinar tissue compatible with fibrosing sialadenitis. (g) Higher power view shows prominent chronic inflammatory infiltration with lymphocytes, fibrosis with isolated islands of glandular tissue. (h) IgG4 immuno-stain shows only very rare IgG4 staining plasma cells (blue arrow points to two positive cells). There is very little staining and no evidence of IgG4 disease.

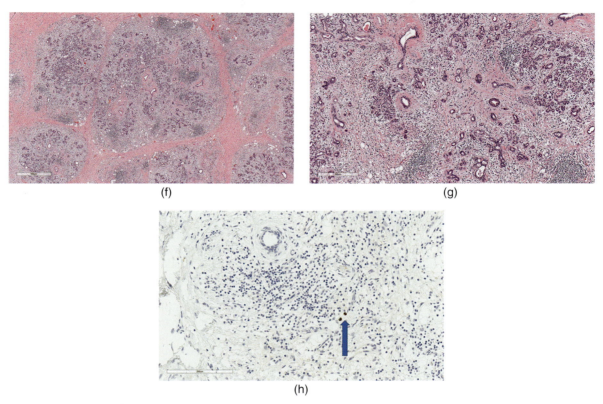

Figure 17.10. (Continued).

References

Abughanam G, Elkashty OA, Liu Y et al. 2019. Mesenchymal stem cells extract (MSCsE)-based therapy alleviates xerostomia and keratoconjunctivitis sicca in Sjogren's syndrome-like disease. *Int J Mol Sci* 20(19):4750.

Adamopoulou M, Vairaktaris E, Nkenke E et al. 2013.Prevelance of human papilloma virus in saliva and cervix of sexually active women. *Gynecol Oncol* 129(2):395-400.

Adams D, Beaudonnet G, Adsam C et al. 2016. Familial amyloid polyneuropathy: When does it stop to be asymptomatic and need a treatment. *Rev Neurol (Paris)* 172(10):642-652.

Adler CH, Dugger BN, Hinni ML et al. 2014. Submandibular gland needle biopsy for the diagnosis of Parkinson's disease. *Neurology* 82(10):858-864.

Adler CH, Dugger BN, Hentz JG et al. 2016. Peripheral synucleinopathy in early Parknson's disease: Submandibular gland needle biopsy *Mov Disord* 31(2):250-256.

Agaton-Bonilla FC, Gay-Escoda C. 1996. Diagnosis and treatment of branchial cleft cysts and fistulae. A retrospective study of 183 patients. *Int J Oral Maxillofac Surg* 25:449-452.

Antoniades DZ, Markopoulos AK, Deligianni E, Andreadis D. 2006. Bilateral aplasia of the parotid glands correlated with accessory parotid tissue. *J Laryngol Otol* 120(4):327-329.

Aro K, Kaczor-Urbanowicz K, Carreras-Presas CM. 2019. Salivaomics in oral cancer. *Curr Opin Otolaryngol Head Neck Surg* 27(2):91-97.

Aronovitch S, Edwards SP. 2014. A case of imperforate Wharton duct. *J Oral Maxillofac Surg* 72(4):744-747

Bahar G, Feimesser R, Shpitzer T et al. 2007. Salivary analysis in oral cancer patients: DNA and protein oxidation, reactive nitrogen species and anti oxidant profile. *Cancer* 109(1):54-59.

Benyamine A, Bernard-Guervilly F, Tummino C, et al. 2017. Hereditary lysozyme amyloidosis with Sicca syndrome, digestive, arterial and tracheobronchial involvement: a case-based review. *Clin Rheumatol* 36(11):2623–2628.

Blake KD, MacCuspie J, Corsten G. 2012. Botulinum toxin injections into salivary glands to decrease oral secretions in CHARGE syndrome: Prospective case study. *Am J Med Genet* 158(4):828-831

Blanco M, Mesko T, Cura M, Cabello-Inchausti B. 2003. Chronic sclerosing sialadenitis (Küttner's tumor): Unusual presentation with bilateral involvement of major and minor salivary glands. *Ann Diagn Pathol* 7(1):25-30

Brown LA, Johnston DR, Rastatter J et al. 2019. Differences in management outcome for first branchial cleft anomalies: A comparison of infants and toddlers to older children. *Int J Pediatr Otorhinolaryngol* 122:161-164.

Chen S, Li Y. 2015. Salivary gland choristoma of the middle ear. *Ear Nose Throat J* 94(2):E9-E12.

Chen JX, Kachniarz B, Gilani S, Shin JJ. 2014. Risk of malignancy associated with head and neck CT in children: A systematic review. *Otolaryngol Head Neck Surg* 151(14):554-566.

de Cocker LJ, D'Arco F, De Beule T, Tousseyn T, Blockmans D, Hermans R. 2014. IgG(4)-related systemic features affecting the parotid and submandibular glands: Magnetic resonance imaging features of IgG(4)-related chronic sclerosing sialadenitis. *Clin Imaging* 38(2):195-198.

Corsjens PLA, Abrams WR, Malamud D. 2000. Saliva and viral infections *Periodontol 2000* 70(1):93-110.

Dang J, Feng Q. 2016. HPV16 infection in oral cavity cancer and oropharyngeal cancer patients. *J Oral Sci* 58(2):265-269.

D'Ascanio L, Cavuto C, Martinelli M, Salvinelli F. 2006. Radiological evaluation of major salivary gland agenesis. A case report. *Minerva Stomatol* 55(4):223-228.

Dutta M. 2017. The ectopic accessory parotid system with congenital cheek fistula: An overview and current update. *Laryngoscope* 127(6):1351-1360.

Enoz M, Suoglu Y. 2006. Salivary gland choristoma of the middle ear. *Laryngoscope* 116(6):1033-1034.

Entesarium M, Dalqvist J, Shashi V et al. 2007. FGF10 missense mutations in aplasia of major salivary gland agenesis. A case report. *Minerva Stomatol* 55(4):379-382.

Ezawa N, Katoh N, Oguchi K et al. 2018.Vizualization of multiple organ involvement in systemic amyloidosis using C-PiB PET imaging. *Eur J Nucl Med Imaging* 45(3):452-461.

Flaig MJ, Ihrier S. 2009. Sjögren-associated MALT-type lymphoma of labial salivary glands a rare constellation with amyloidosis and IgM-paraproteinemia. *Pathologe* 30(6):442-445.

Frydrych AM, Koong B. 2014. Hyposalivation in a 16-year-old girl: A case of salivary gland aplasia. *Aust Dent J* 59(1):125-128.

Fujita A, Sakai O, Chapman MN, Sugimoto H. 2012. IgG(4)-related disease of the head and neck; CT and MR imaging manifestations. *Radiographics* 32(7):1945-1958

Gabali A, Ross CW, Edwards PC et al. 2013. Pediatric extranodal marginal zone B-cell lymphoma presenting as amyloidosis in minor salivary glands: A case report and review of the literature. *J Pediatr Hematol Oncol* 35(3):E130-E133.

Garcia S, Martini F, Caces F et al. 1998. Polycystic disease of the salivary glands: Report of an attack on the submandibular glands (Article in French). *Ann Pathol* 18(1):58-60.

Gareb B, Perry M, Tadrous PJ. 2018. Isolated light chain amyloidosis involving the parotid gland: A case report. *J Oral Maxillofac Surg* 76(9):1917-1924.

Gertz MA. 2018. Immunoglobulin light chain amyloidosis: 2018 update on diagnosis, prognosis, and treatment. *Am J Hematol* 93:1169-1180.

Gever JT, Ferry JA, Harris NL et al. 2010. Chronic sclerosing sialadenitis (Küttner tumor) is an IgG(4)-associated disease. *Am J Surg Pathol* 34(2):202-210.

Giorgadze T, Baloch ZW, Thaler ER, Gupta PK. 2004. Unsuspected systemic amyloidosis diagnosed by fine needle aspiration of the salivary gland. *Diagn Cytopathol* 31(1):57-59.

Glynn F, O'Dwyer TP. 2007. Does the addition of sublingual gland excision to submandibular duct relocation give better overall results in drooling control? *Clin Otolaryngol* 32(2):103-107.

Godbehere J, Scotta GB, Tahir F, Sionis S. 2019. Küttner tumor of the parotid gland-A diagnostic rarity. *Ear Nose Throat J.* doi:10.1177/0145561319868450.

Goff C, Alfred C, Glade RS. 2012. Current management of congenital branchial cleft cysts, sinuses and fistulae. *Curr Opin Otolaryngol Head Neck Surg* 20(6):533-539.

Goldenberg D, Flax-Goldenberg R, Joachims HZ, Peled N. 2000. Misplaced parotid glands: Bilateral agenesis pf parotid glands associated with bilateral accessory parotid tissue. *J Laryngol Otol* 114:883-885.

Gonçalves AC, Marson FAL, Mendonça RMH et al. 2019. Chloride and Sodium ion concentrations in saliva and sweat as a method to diagnose cystic fibrosis. *J Pediatr (Rio J)* 95(4):443-450.

Greensmith AL, Johnstone BR, Reid SM et al. 2005. Prospective analysis of the outcome of surgical management of drooling in the pediatric population: A 10-year experience. *Plast Reconstr Surg* 116(5):1233-1242.

Gualtero DF, Castillo AS. 2016. Biomarkers in saliva for the detection of oral squamous cell carcinoma and their potential use for early diagnosis: A systematic review. *Acta Odontol Scand* 74(30;170-177.

Haen P, Slama B, Goudot P, Schouman T. 2017. Necrotizing sialometaplasia of the parotid gland associated with facial nerve paralysis. *J Stomatol Oral Maxillofac Surg* 118(1):63-65.

Hawkey NM, Zaorsky NG, Galloway TJ. 2016.The role of radiation therapy in the management of sialorrhea: A systematic review. *Laryngoscope* 126(1):80-85.

Heath N, McCleod I, Pearce R. 2006. Major salivary gland agenesis in a young child: Consequences for oral health. *Int J Pediatr Dent* 16(6):431-434.

Heptinstall L, Carroll C, Siddiqi J et al. 2017. Sclerosing mucoepidermoid carcinoma of the submandibular gland presenting as chronic sialadenitis: A case report and review of the literature. *Head Neck Pathol* 11(4):506-512.

Hernandez-Molina G, Faz-Munoz D, Astudillo-Angel M et al. 2018. Coexistence of amyloidosis and primary Sjögren's syndrome: An overview. *Curr Rheumatol Rev* 14(3):231-238.

Hinson D, Poteet P, Bower C. 2014. Duplicated facial nerve trunk with a first branchial cleft cyst. *Laryngoscope* 12(3):662-664.

Hoffrichter MS, Obeid G, Soliday JT. 2001. Bilateral submandibular duct atresia: Case report. *J Oral Maxillofac Surg* 59:445-447.

Hu F, Dai A-G, Zhu L-M. 2013. Sublingual gland amyloidosis causing obstructive sleep apnea syndrome: A case report and review of the literature. *Zhonghua Jie He He Hu Xi Za Zhi* 36(7):485-489.

Inan UU, Yilmaz MD, Demir Y et al. 2006. Characteristics of lacrimo-auriculo-dento-digital (LADD) syndrome: Case report of a family and literature review. *Int J Pediatr Otorhinolaryngol* 70(7):1307-1314.

Jaccard A, Desport E, Mohty D, Bridoux F. 2015. AL Amyloidosis (article in French) *Rev Med Interne* 36(2):89-97.

Jamet MP, Gnemmi V, Hachulla É et al. 2015. Distinctive patterns of Transthyretin amyloid in salivary tissue: A clinicopathologic study of 92 patients with amyloid-containing minor salivary gland biopsies. *Am J Surg Pathol* 39(8):1035-1044.

Jongerius PH, van Tiel P, van Limbeek J et al. 2003. A systematic review for evidence of efficacy of anticholinergic drugs to treat drooling. *Arch Dis Child* 88:911-914.

Jongerius PH, van den Hoogen FJ, van Limbeek J et al. 2004. Effect of botulinum toxin in the treatment of drooling: A controlled clinical trial. *Pediatrics* 114(3):620-627.

Kamisawa Y, Shimosegawa T, Okazaki K et al. 2009. Standard steroid treatment for autoimmune pancreatitis. *Gut* 58:1504-1507.

Kandula S, Manjuntha BS, Tayee P, Astehar M. 2016. Bilateral necrotizing sialometaplasia. *BMJ Case Rep* bcr2015211348. doi:10.1136/bcr-2015-211348.

Kaplan I, Alteman M, Kleiman S et al. 2012. The clinical, histological, and treatment spectrum. In necrotizing sialometaplasia. *Oral Surg Oral Med Oral Pathol Oral Radiol* 114;577-578.

Katz DA, Golden MR, Hughes JP et al. 2018. HIV self-testing increases HIV testing frequency in high-risk men who have sex with men: A randomized control trial. *J Acquir Immune Defic Syndr* 78(5):505-512.

Kojima M, Sugihara S, Lijima M et al. 2006. Marginal zone B-cell lymphoma of minor salivary gland representing tumor-forming amyloidosis of the oral cavity. A case report. *J Oral Pathol Med* 35950:314-316.

Kolokythas A, Karras M, Collins E et al. 2015. Salivary biomarkers associated with bone deterioration in patients with medication-related osteonecrosis of the jaws. *J Oral Maxillofac Surg* 73(9):1741-1747.

Koudounarakis E, Willems S, Karaullukcu B. 2016. Dysgenetic polycystic disease of the minor and submandibular glands. *Head Neck* 38(6):E2437-E2439.

Kulkami SS, Kulkami SS, Vastrad PP et al. 2011. Prevalence and distribution of high-risk human papillomavirus HPV Types 16 and 18 in carcinoma of cervix, saliva of patients with oral squamous cell carcinoma and in the general population in Karnataka India. *Asian Pac J Cancer Res* 12(3);645-648.

Lal D, Hotaling J. 2006. Drooling. *Curr Opin Otolaryngol Head Neck Surg* 14(6):381-386.

Law ST, Jafarzadeh SR, Govender P et al. 2019. Comparison of ultrasound features of major salivary glands in sarcoidosis amyloidosis and Sjögren syndrome. *Arthritis Care Res (Hoboken)* doi:10.1002/acr.24029 (Epub ahead of print).

Lecadet A, Bachmeyer C, Buob D et al. 2018. Minor salivary gland biopsy is more effective then normal appearing skin biopsy in the detection of systemic amyloidosis: A prospective monocentric study. *Eur J Intern Med* 57:e20-e21.

Leon ME, Santosh N, Agarwal A et al. 2016. Diagnostic challenges in the fine needle aspiration biopsy of chronic sclerosing sialadenitis (Küttner's tumor) in the context of head and neck malignancy: A series of 4 cases. *Head Neck Pathol* 10(3):389-393.

Li W, Xu H, Zhao L, Li X. 2018. Branchial anomalies in children: A report of 105 surgical cases. *Int J Pediatr Otorhinolaryngol* 104:14-18.

Lipp A, Trottenberg T, Schink T et al. 2003. A randomized trial of botulinum toxin A for treatment of drooling. *Neurology* 61(9):1279-1281.

Liu W, Chen M, Hao J et al. 2017. The treatment for first branchial cleft anomalies in children. *Eur Arch Otolaryngol* 274(9):3465-3470.

Lombaert L, Movahednia MM, Adine C, Ferreira JN. 2017. Concise review: Salivary gland regeneration: Therapeutic approaches from stem cells to tissue organoids. *Stem Cells* 35:97-105.

Lopes V, Murray P, Williams H et al. 2011. Squamous cell carcinoma of the oral cavity rarely harbours oncogenic human papilloma virus. *Oral Oncol* 47(8):698-701.

Machado de Sousa SO, Linares Ferrazzo LK, Mota lovola A, Dos Santos JN, de Araulo VC. 2008. Immunoprofile of Kütter tumor (chronic sclerosing sialadenitis). *Int J Surg Pathol* 16(2):143-149.

Maddy EA, Ashram YA. 2013. First branchial arch anomalies: Presentation, variability and safe surgical management. *Eur Arch Otorhinolaryngol* 270(6):1917-1925.

Maehara T, Moriyama M, Nakamura S. 2020. Review of a novel disease entity, immunoglobulin G4-related disease. *J Korean Assoc Oral Maxillofac Surg* 46(1):3-11.

Malek N, Swallow D, Grosset KA et al. 2014. Alpha-synuclein in peripheral tissues and body fluids as a biomarker for Parkinson's disease-A systematic Review. *Acta Nerol Scand* 130(2):59-72.

Mancini F, Zangaglia R, Cristina S et al. 2003. Double-blind, placebo-controlled study to evaluate the efficacy and safety of botulinum toxin type A in the treatment of drooling in Parkinsonism. *Mov Disord* 18(6):685-688.

Mandel L. 2006. An unusual pattern of dental damage with salivary gland aplasia. *J Am Dent Assoc* 137(7):984-989.

Manrique D, do Brasil Ode O, Ramos H. 2007. Drooling: Analysis and evaluation of 31 children who underwent bilateral submandibular gland excision and parotid duct ligation. *Rev Bras Otorhinolaryngol (Eng Ed)* 73(1):40-44.

Martinez DP, Majumdar S, Bateman N, Bull PD. 2007. Presentation of first branchial cleft anomalies: The Sheffield experience. *J Laryngol Otol* 121(5):455-459.

Masaki Y, Matsui S, Saeki T et al. 2017. A multicenter phase II prospective trial of glucocorticoid for patients with untreated IgG4-related disease *Mod Rheumatol* 27:849-845

Mateo Arias J, Molina Martinez M, Borrego A, Mayorga F. 2003.Amyloidosis of the submaxillary gland. *Med Oral*.8(1):66-70.

McInerney MS, Reddihough DS, Carding PN et al. 2019. Behavioural interventions to treat drooling in children with neurodisability: A systematic review. *Dev Med Child Neurol* 61(1):39-48.

Melo JC, Kitsko D, Reyes-Mugica M. 2012.Pediatric chronic sclerosing sialadenitis: Kütter tumor. *Pediatr Dev Pathol* 15(2):165-169.

Meningaud JP, Pitak-Arnnop P, Chikhani L, Bertrand JC. 2006. Drooling of saliva: A review of the etiology and management options. *Oral Surg Oral Med Oral Pathol Oral Radiol Endod* 101(1):48-57.

Mohan RP, Yerma S, Chawa VR, Tyaqi K. 2013. Non-syndromic, non-familial agenesis of major salivary glands: A report of two cases with review of literature. *J Clin Imaging Sci* 3:2.

Murube-Del-Castillo J. 1986. Transplantation of salivary gland to the lacrimal basin. *Scand J Rheumatol Suppl* 61:264-267.

Nandapalan V, Jones TM, Morar C et al. 1998. Localized amyloidosis of the parotid gland: A case report and review of localized amyloidosis in the head and neck. *Head Neck* 20(1):73-78.

Nienstedt JC, Buhman C, Bihler M et al. 2018. Drooling is no early sign of dysphagia in Parkinson's disease. *Neurogastroenterol Motil* 30(4):e13259.

Odeh M, Hershkovits M, Bornstein J, Loberant N, Blumenthal M, Ophir E. 2013. Congenital absence of salivary glands in Downs syndrome. *Arch Dis Child* 98(10):781-783.

Odell EW, Lombardi T, Shirlaw PJ, White CA. 1998. Minor salivary gland hyalinization and amyloidosis in low-grade lymphoma of MALT. *J Oral Pathol Med* 27(5):229-232.

Olsen KD, Maragos NE, Weiland LH. 1980. First branchial cleft anomalies. *Laryngoscope* 90:423-435.

Ormitti E, Ventura E, Bacciu A, Crisi G, Magnani C. 2013). Unilateral ectopic parotid gland in CHARGE syndrome. *Pediatr Radiol* 43(2):247-251.

Oshiro K, Rosenthal DI, Koomen JM et al. 2007. Pre-analytic saliva processing affects proteomic results and biomarker screening of head and neck squamous carcinoma. *Int J Oncol* 30(3):743-749.

Østerhus N, Skoogedal N, Akre H, Johnsen UL, Nordgarden H, Asten P. 2012. Salivary gland pathology as a new finding in Treacher Collins syndrome. *Am J Med Genet* 158A(6):1320-1325.

Paniello RC. 2007. Submandibular gland transfer for severe xerophthalmia. *Laryngoscope* 117(1):40-44.

Parker KH, Kemp TJ, Pan Y et al. 2018.) Evaluation of HPV-16 and HPV-18 specific antibody measurements in saliva collected in oral rinses and merocele sponges. *Vaccine* 36(19):2705-2711.

de Paula Eduardo F, de Mello Bezinelli L, de Carvalho DL et al. 2017. Minor salivary gland biopsy for the diagnosis of familial amyloid polyneuropathy. *Neurol Sci* 38(2):311-318.

Peixoto AP, Campos GS, Queiroz LB, Sardi SI. 2011. Asymptomatic oral human papillomavirus (HPV) infection in women with with a histopathologic diagnosis of genital HPV *J Oral Sci* 53(4):451-459.

Perera E, Revington P, Sheffield E. 2010. Low grade marginal zone B-cell lymphoma presenting as local amyloidosis in a submandibular salivary gland. *Int J Oral Maxillofac Surg* 39(11):1136-1138.

Pham Dang N, Picard M, Mondié JM, Barthélémy MD. 2010. Complete agenesis of all major salivary glands: A case report and review of the literature. *Oral Surg Oral Med Oral Pathol Oral Radiol Endod* 110:e23-e27.

Pickering V, Jordan RC, Schmidt BL. 2007. Elevated salivary endothelin levels in oral cancer patients-a pilot study. *Oral Oncol* 43(1):37-41.

Pradhu Y, Ingrams D. 2011. First branchial arch fistula: Diagnostic dilemma and improved surgical management. *Am J Otolaryngol* 32(6):617-619.

Qureishi A, Ali M, Fraser L et al. 2018. Saliva testing for human papilloma virus in oropharyngeal squamous cell carcinoma: A diagnostic accuracy study. *Clin Otolaryngol* 43(1):151-157.

Reid SM, McCutcheon J, Reddihough DS, Johnson H. 2012. Prevalence and predictors of drooling in 7-to-14-year-old children with cerebral palsy: A population study. *Dev Med Child Neurol* 54(11):1032-1036.

Reid SM, Westbury C, Chong C et al. 2019. Long-term impact of saliva control surgery in children with disability. *J Plast Reconstr Aesthet Surg* 72(7):1193-1197.

Reija MF, Gordilo DP, Palacio JC, Abascal LB. 2013. Bilateral submandibular gland aplasia with hypertrophy of the sublingual glands of a patient with cleft lip and palate: Case report. *J Craniofac Surg* 24(5)e532-e533.

Renker T, Haneke E, Röken C, Borradori L. 2014. Systemic light-chain amyloidosis revealed by progressive nail involvement, diffuse alopecia and Sicca Syndrome: Report of an unusual case with a review of the literature. *Dermatology* 228(2):97-102.

Reynolds H, Miller N, Walker R. 2018. Drooling in Parkinson's disease: Evidence of a role for divided attention. *Dysphagia* 33(6):809-817.

Russo N, Bellile E, Murdoch-Kinch CA et al. 2016. Cytokines in saliva increase in head and neck cancer patients after treatment. *Oral Surg Oral Med Oral Pathol Oral Radiol* 122(4):483-490.

Scafi M, Valleix S, Benyamine A et al. 2019. Lysozyme amyloidosis (article in French) *Rev Med Interne* 40(5):323-329.

Seifert G. 1992. Tumor-like lesions of the salivary glands. The new WHO classification. *Pathol Res Pracr* 188(7):836-846.

Seifert G, Donath K. 1977. On the pathogenesis of the Küttner tumor of the submandibular gland — Analysis of 349 cases with chronic sialadenitis of the submandibular (author's transl). *HNO* 25(3):81-92.

Seifert G, Thomsen ST, Donath K. 1981. Bilateral dysgenetic polycystic parotid glands. Morphological analysis and differential diagnosis of a rare disease of the salivary glands. *Virch Arch (Pathol Anat)* 390:273-288.

Shan XF, Lv L, Cai Z-G, Yu G-Y. 2019. Botulinum toxin A treatment of epiphora secondary to autologous submandibular gland transplantation. *Int J Oral Maxillofac Surg* 48(4):475-479.

Sheppard JP, Nguyen T, Alikhalid Y et al. 2018. Risk of brain tumor induction from pediatric head and neck CT procedures: A systematic literature review. *Brain Tumor Res Treat* 6(1):1-7.

Shimizu M, Okamura K, Kise Y et al. 2015. Effectiveness of imaging modalities for screening IgG4-related dacrocystitis and sialadenitis (Mikulicz's disease) and for differentiating it from Sjogren's syndrome (SS), with an emphasis on sonography. *Arthritis Res Ther* 17(1):223.

Shin YU, Oh YH, Lee YJ. 2012. Unusual involvement of igG(4)-related disease in lacrimal and submandibular and extraocular muscles. *Korean J Ophthalmol* 26(3):216-221.

Shpitzer T, Bahar G, Feinmesser R, Nagler RM. 2007. A comprehensive salivary analysis for oral cancer diagnosis. *J Cancer Res Clin Oncol* May 4 epub ahead of print.

Shree KH, Ranani P, Sherlin H et al. 2019. Saliva as a diagnostic tool in oral squamous cell carcinoma-A systematic review with meta-analysis. *Pathol Oncol Res* 25(2):447-453.

Singh P, Warnakulasuriya S. 2004. Aplasia of submandibular glands associated with ectodermal dysplasia. *J Oral Pathol Med* 33(10):634-636.

Smyth AG, Ward-Booth RP, High AS. 1993. Polycystic disease of the parotid glands: Two familial cases. *Br J Oral Maxillofac Surg* 31(1):38-40.

Solares CA, Chan J, Koltal PJ. 2003. Anatomical variations of the facial nerve in first branchial cleft anomalies. *Arch Otolaryngol Head Neck Surg* 129(3):351-355.

Sousa S, Rocha M, Patrão F et al. 2018. Submandibular duct transposition for drooling in children: A casuistic review and evaluation of grade of satisfaction. *Int J Pediatr Otolaryngol* 113:58-61.

Srikant N, Yellapurkar S, Poaz K et al. 2017. Dysgenetic polycystic disease of minor salivary gland: A rare case report and review of the literature. *Case Rep Pathol* .2017:5279025. doi:10.1155/2017/5279025.Epub 2017 Jan 19

Stulner C, Chambers PA, Telfer MR Corrigan AM. 2001. Management of first branchial cleft anomalies: Report of two cases. *Br J Oral Maxillofac Surg* 39(1):30-33.

Su J-Z, Liu X-J, Liu D-G et al. 2014. Sialography of the transplanted submandibular gland. *Ocul Surf* 12(3):215-220.

Sun L, Sun Z, Ma X. 2013. Partial duplication of the mandible, parotid aplasia and facial cleft: A rare developmental disorder. *Oral Surg Oral Med Oral Pathol Oral Radiol* 116(3):e202-e209.

Suzuki T, Kusumoto S, Yamashita T et al. 2016.Labial salivary gland biopsy for diagnosing immunoglobulin light chain amyloidosis retrospective analysis. *Ann Hematol* 95(2):279-285.

Takano K, Yamamoto M, Takahashi H, Shinomura Y, Imai K, Himi T. 2010.Clinopathologic similarities between Mikulicz disease and Küttner tumor. *Am J Otolaryngol* 16:429-434.

Teo NWY, Ibrahim SI, Tan KKH. 2015.Distribution of branchial anomalies in a pediatric Asian population. *Singapore Med J* 56(4):203-207/

Togni L, Mascitti M, Santarelli A et al. 2019. Unusual conditions impairing saliva secretion: Developmental anomalies of salivary glands. *Front Physiol* 10:855 eCollection 2019 https://doi.org/10.3389/fphys.2019.0085510:855.

Toros SZ, Egeli E, Kiliçarslan Y et al. 2010. Salivary gland choristoma of the middle ear in a child with sinus inversus totalis. *Auris Nasus Larynx* 37(3):356-358.

Triglia J-M, Nichollas R, Ducroz V et al. 1998. First branchial cleft anomalies: A study of 39 cases and a review of the literature. *Arch Otolaryngol Head Neck Surg* 124(3):291-295.

Tsai C-T, Robinson PV, de Cortez FJ et al. 2018. Antibody detection by agglutination -PCR (ADAP) enables early diagnosis of HIV infection by oral fluid analysis. *Proc Natl Acad Sci U S A* 115(6):1250-1255.

Turner DO, Williams-Cocks SJ, Bullen R et al. 2011. High-risk human papilloma virus (HPV) screening and detection in healthy patient saliva samples: A pilot study. *BMC Oral Health* 11;28.

Van der Burg JJ, Didden R, Jogerius PH, Rotteveel JJ. 2007. A descriptive analysis of studies on behavioral treatment of drooling (1975-2005). *Dev Med Child Neurol* 49(5): 390-394.

Vered M, Buchner A, Haimovici E et al. 2001. Focal lymphocytic infiltration in aging human palatal salivary glands: A comparative study with labial salivary glands. *J Oral Pathol Med* 30(1):7-11.

Wallace ZS, Zhang Y, Perugino CA et al. 2019. Clinical phenotypes of IgG4-related disease: An analysis of two international cross-sectional cohorts. *Ann Rheum Dis* 78:406-412.

Wasserman JK, Rourke R, Purgina B et al. 2017. HPV DNA in saliva from patients with SCC of the head and neck is specific for p16 -positive oropharyngeal tumors. *J Otolaryngol Head Neck Surg* 46(1):3.

Wilkie TF. 1967. The problem of drooling in cerebral palsy: A surgical approach. *Can J Surg* 10:60-67.

Williams HK, Connor R, Edmonson H. 2000. Chronic sclerosing sialadenitis of the submandibular and parotid glands; a report of a case and review of the literature. *Oral Surg Oral Med Oral Pathol Oral Radiol Endod* 89(6):720-723.

Wong DT. 2006. Salivary diagnostics powered by nanotechnologies proteomics and genomics. *J Am Dent Assoc* 137(3):313-321.

Work WP. 1972. Newer concepts of the first branchial cleft defects. *Laryngoscope* 106:137-143.

Yakob M, Fuentes L, Wang MB et al. 2014. Salivary biomarkers for detection of oral squamous cell carcinoma – current status and recent advances. *Curr Oral Health Rep* 1(2):133-141.

Yu GY, Zhu ZH, Mao C et al. 2004. Microvascular submandibular gland autologous transfer in severe cases of keratoconjunctivitis sicca. *Int J Oral Maxillofac Surg* 33(3):235-239.

Zhang L, Su J-Z, Cai Z-G et al. 2019. Factors influencing the long-term results of autologous microvascular submandibular gland transplantation for severe dry eyes disease. *Int J Oral Maxillofac Surg* 48(1):40-47.

Zimmerman BG, Park NJ, Wong DT. 2007. Genomic targets in saliva. *Ann N Y Acad Sci* 1098:184-191.

Chapter 18
Complications of Salivary Gland Surgery

Michael D. Turner DDS, MD
Division of Oral and Maxillofacial Surgery, Mount Sinai Hospital, Icahn Mount Sinai School of Medicine, New York, NY, USA

Outline

Introduction
General Considerations
Complications of Parotid Gland Surgery
　Facial Nerve Paralysis
　　Relationship of the Facial Nerve to the Parotid Gland
　　Approaches to the Parotid Gland
　　　Blair incision
　　　Retromandibular incision
　　Assessment of Facial Nerve Weakness
　The Auriculotemporal Nerve and Frey Syndrome
　　Diagnosis of Frey Syndrome
　　Management of Frey Syndrome
　　Surgical Prevention of Frey Syndrome and Facial Defects
　　　Temporoparietal fascia flap
　　　Sternocleidomastoid muscle flap
　　　Superficial musculoaponeurotic system flap
　　　Acellular dermal matrix
　　　Fat grafting
　Parotid Gland Salivary Leakage
　　Classification of Parotid Gland Salivary Leakage
　　Management of Parotid Salivary Leakage
　　　Conservative management of parotid gland salivary leakage
　　　Botulinum toxin for the management of parotid gland salivary leakage
　　　Scopolamine patch
　　　Sclerosing agents
　　　Surgical repair of parotid gland salivary leakage
　　　Tympanic neurectomy
　　　Radiotherapy
　　　Temporalis fascia and cyanoacrylate
　　Postoperative Infections
　Parotid Duct Leakage
　　Management of Parotid Duct Injuries
　　Endoscopic Management of Parotid Salivary Duct Injuries
　　　Surgical management of a parotid megaduct
　　Avulsion of the Parotid Duct
　　Stenosis of the Parotid Duct Orifice
Complications of Submandibular and Sublingual Gland Surgery
　Complications Associated with an Intraoral Approach to the Sublingual and Submandibular Glands
　　Ranulas (Mucous Extravasation Phenomenon)
　　　Complications associated with the management of ranulas
　　　Recurrence of ranulas
　　　Lingual nerve injury during sublingual gland removal
　　　Submandibular duct injury during sublingual gland removal
　　Complications Associated with Intraoral Surgery of the Submandibular Duct
　　　Stricture of the submandibular gland duct
　　　Lingual nerve injuries
　　　Extravasation of fluid and airway obstruction
　　　Ranula formation
　　　Submandibular duct avulsion
　Complications Associated with Transcervical Approaches to the Submandibular Gland
　　Marginal Mandibular Branch Injury during a Sialadenectomy
　　Lingual Nerve Injury during a Sialadenectomy
　　Hypoglossal Nerve Injury during a Sialadenectomy
　　Hematoma Formation
　　Hyposalivation
　Complications Associated with Removal of Minor Salivary Gland Mucoceles
　　Complications Associated with Removal of Mucoceles of the Lower Lip
　　Mucocele Recurrence
　　Neurosensory Change
　　Esthetic Defects of the Lip
Summary
Case Presentation – *Get It Right the First Time. That's the Main Thing*
References

Salivary Gland Pathology: Diagnosis and Management, Third Edition. Edited by Eric R. Carlson and Robert A. Ord.
© 2022 John Wiley & Sons, Inc. Published 2022 by John Wiley & Sons, Inc.
Companion website: www.wiley.com/go/carlson/salivary

Introduction

All surgical procedures have known associated complications, and salivary gland surgery is not an exception. The distinguishing feature, however, is that the term "salivary gland surgery" is a rather broad term that encompasses a wide range of procedures performed on organs that are intimately enmeshed in a variety of locations within the environs of the head and neck.

The complications of salivary gland surgery are for the most part site specific and result in a variety of problems. Some of these problems can be prevented with adjunctive procedures during the initial operation, and some can only be managed postoperatively. There are some complications of salivary gland surgery that cannot be treated at all.

This chapter reviews the most common complications that can occur during or after surgery to the parotid, submandibular, sublingual, and minor salivary glands. Like all complications, these complications have morbidities associated with them that can be worse than the primary diagnosis being addressed. A common theme in this subject is issues related to salivary function such as salivary fistulas, but also inadvertent complications associated with adjacent structures, like paralysis related to the facial nerve that can result in a significant decrease in the quality of life of the patient.

General Considerations

Complications inevitably occur following salivary gland surgery such that it is necessary that the surgeon understands the potential risks and complications associated with these surgical procedures with communication to the patient prior to the surgery. Patients are more accepting of complications when they occur with their informed consent.

A thorough history and physical examination can assist in the identification of patients who have predictive signs and/or symptoms of a possible complication that can that either be avoided or if it is not avoidable, attenuated in its severity. A good example of this opportunity is the inability to cannulate the submandibular duct. Evaluating the Wharton duct papilla prior to surgery with bimanual palpation of the submandibular gland will reveal if the orifice is visible or not (Figure 18.1). If it is not visible, the surgeon can be prepared to perform a dissection of the submandibular duct and entrance into the duct proper (Figure 18.2).

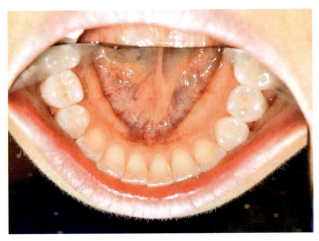

Figure 18.1. Bilateral submandibular duct orifices are not visible on examination on a 72-year-old woman with persistent bilateral submandibular sialadenitis.

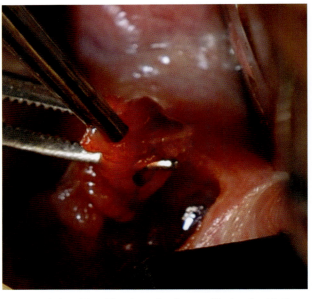

Figure 18.2. Identification of submandibular duct following papillotomy for the purpose of a lateral entry of a sialendoscope.

Complications of Parotid Gland Surgery

FACIAL NERVE PARALYSIS

The occurrence of facial nerve paralysis has been found to directly correlate with the violation of the capsule of the gland as well as nerve monitoring during the dissection (Eisele 1996; Eisele et al. 2010;

Guntinas-Lichius and Eisele 2016; Schapher et al. 2019). For management of parotid masses, extracapsular dissection was found in multiple studies to reduce the rate of temporary and permanent paralysis when compared with other approaches, particularly the superficial parotidectomy for the treatment of pleomorphic adenomas and other benign tumors (Bar et al. 2019; Bonavolontà 2019; Mantsopoulos et al. 2019). For superficial parotidectomies, the range for temporary facial nerve weakness has been reported as 9–20% and 9–41.7% for total parotidectomies (Aframian et al. 2004).

The range of permanent facial nerve paralysis varied, but is 0–1.8% for extracapsular dissections, 1.7–6.0% for superficial parotidectomies, and 7% for total or near total parotidectomies (Prichard et al. 1992; Bron and O'Brien 1997; Hancock 1999; Witt 2002; McGurk et al. 2003; Uyar et al. 2011; Albergotti et al. 2012). The incidence of permanent facial paralysis for total parotidectomies was difficult to determine since total parotidectomies are usually performed for the removal of malignant disease that occasionally necessitates sacrifice of the facial nerve.

Relationship of the Facial Nerve to the Parotid Gland

One of the major debilitating complications associated with parotid gland surgery is an injury to the facial nerve, cranial nerve VII. The main trunk of the facial nerve exits the temporal bone from the stylomastoid foramen. It then extends from the foramen to the parotid gland. The mean distance between the tip of the tragal cartilage to the main trunk is 6.37 mm on average and the distance between the main trunk and the tragal pointer 1 cm 91% of the time (Cannon et al. 2004). Once the nerve enters the parotid gland proper, it splits at the pes anserinus (see Figure 18.3) and divides into the upper temporofacial branch and the lower cervicofacial branch approximately 1–2 cm from the stylomastoid foramen (Wang and Eisele 2012). The temporofacial branch further divides into the temporal, zygomatic, and buccal branches, and the cervicofacial branch divides into the marginal mandibular and cervical branches. The facial nerve extends strands to the lingual nerve and other preganglionic fibers, a finding that will subsequently be discussed.

Approaches to the Parotid Gland

The approach to the parotid gland, the location of the pathologic process, and the specific disease

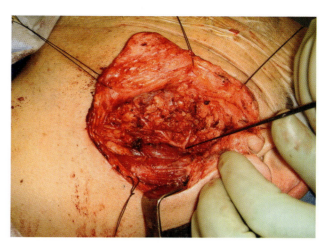

Figure 18.3. Following superficial parotidectomy, identification of the facial nerve is noted at the pes anserinus where it branches into the temporofacial and lower cervicofacial branches. Source: Photograph courtesy of David Eisele M.D.

process being treated (See Chapter 10) influence the decrease in postoperative facial animation and function. Two approaches include the Blair and retromandibular incisions.

Blair incision

The most common approach for access and management of parotid tumors is the modified Blair incision (See Chapter 10), although other approaches have been described (Terris et al. 1994; Hou et al. 2014; Casale et al. 2016). Regardless of the technique, a wide dissection provides for adequate visualization of the facial nerve to decrease the risk of an inadvertent injury (Figure 18.4).

Retromandibular incision

A common approach for the management of condylar fractures of the mandible is the retromandibular incision with a transparotid dissection to the condylar process. In short, a retromandibular incision is made starting approximately 1 cm inferior to the lobe of the ear, 2–3 cm posterior, and parallel to the posterior border of the mandibular ramus. The length of the incision is 3–5 cm in length as needed for exposure. Dissection toward the mandible is performed through the subcutaneous fat and platysma muscle to the parotid capsule. A small 3 mm incision is made through the capsule. Blunt dissection is performed through the parotid gland in an anterior posterior direction, and the marginal

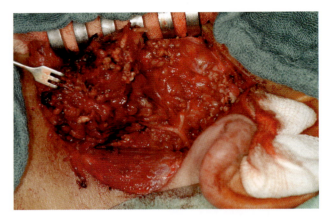

Figure 18.4. Forty-three-year-old man undergoing a superficial parotidectomy utilizing a Blair incision for removal of a pleomorphic adenoma. Note the wide dissection and identification of the facial nerve. Source: Photograph courtesy of Paul Covello DDS MD.

mandibular branch is identified and skeletonized to permit retraction. An incision is made through the pterygomandibular periosteum, and a subperiosteal reflection is performed. The majority of paralysis with this approach occurs in either the buccal branch (Hyde et al. 2002; Vesnaver et al. 2005; Bhutia et al. 2014; Shi et al. 2015) or the marginal mandibular branch (Ellis and Dean 1993; Manisali et al. 2003) (Figure 18.5).

Assessment of Facial Nerve Weakness

The House–Brackmann classification is a commonly utilized grading scale to evaluate and document facial paralysis as it relates to an injury to the facial nerve trunk (House and Brackmann 1985). The House–Brackmann scale is based upon the elevation of the eyebrow and the lateral movement of the labial commissure. The superior portion of the eyebrow is raised in gradients of 2.5 mm for a score of 1–4, with a similar score to lateral movement of the commissure (Table 18.1). Although this classification was designed for total trunk

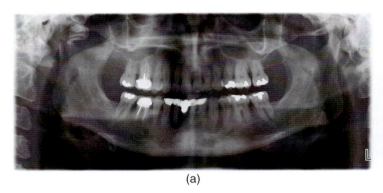
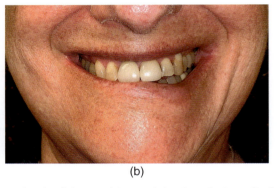

(a)   (b)

Figure 18.5. Panoramic radiograph (a) of a 56-year-old woman who sustained a right condylar neck fracture that resulted in a mechanical obstruction of the temporomandibular joint. Patient had a maximum incisal opening of 10 mm. Patient exhibiting weakness of the marginal mandibular nerve following a retromandibular incision (b). Patient regained full function three months postoperatively.

Table 18.1. House–Brackmann facial paralysis scale.

Grade	Description	Measurement	Function (%)	Estimated function (%)
I	Normal	8/8	100	100
II	Slight	7/8	76–99	80
III	Moderate	5/6–6/8	51–75	60
IV	Moderate-Severe	3/8–4/8	26–50	40
V	Severe	1/8–2/8	1–25	20
VI	Total	0/8	0	0

Complications of Salivary Gland Surgery **573**

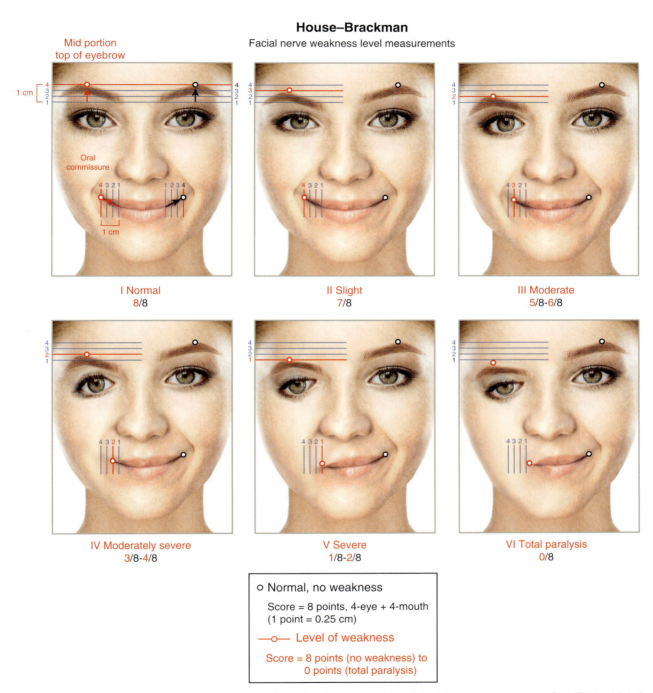

Figure 18.6. House–Brackmann grading scale for objective evaluation of facial nerve weakness. See Table 18.1 for explanation of scoring system. Source: Illustration by Joseph Chovan.

evaluation, it is also utilized for evaluation of upper and lower branches dysfunction (See Figure 18.6). Other grading systems have been developed but have not been widely adopted and are listed for completeness. They are the Terzis–Noah, Burres–Fisch, Nottingham, and Sunnybrook classifications (Burres 1986; Murty et al. 1994; Ross et al. 1996; Terzis and Noah 1997).

THE AURICULOTEMPORAL NERVE AND FREY SYNDROME

The auriculotemporal nerve is a branch of the third division of the trigeminal nerve. There are two major branches of the auriculotemporal nerve, and they divide at the juncture of the condylar neck and the sphenomandibular ligament. The superior, or somatosensory, branch provides sensation to the auricle, the external meatus, the tympanic membrane, and the general temporal region. The inferior, or parasympathetic, branch is comprised of postganglionic parasympathetic fibers from the glossopharyngeal nerve.

Injuries to the superior branch result in hypoesthesia or anesthesia of the overlying skin. The rate of occurrence of this complication following superficial parotidectomies ranges from 0 to 10.4% and 0–5% for complete parotidectomies. Unlike an injury to the facial nerve, this sensory change is well tolerated and does not decrease the quality of life index (Nahlieli 2017).

Frey syndrome can occur when the parasympathetic branch is damaged either from an injury or, more commonly, parotid gland surgery. This process is also referred to as gustatory sweating, but has also been termed auriculotemporal syndrome, Baillarger syndrome, or Frey–Baillarger syndrome (Dulguerov et al. 1999b). In a case series published in 1853, Baillarger first described two cases of auriculotemporal syndrome, but did not knowingly differentiate it from two other salivary gland fistulas (Baillarger 1853; Dulguerov et al. 1999a). Thereafter, multiple case reports and series described gustatory sweating following parotid surgery, infection, and trauma, but it wasn't until 1923 that the autonomic etiology of the phenomena was hypothesized by Lucie Frey (Brown-Sequard 1850; Rouyer 1859; New 1922; Frey 1923; Dulguerov et al. 1999a).

Frey syndrome occurs because of an abnormal connection during healing between the transected postganglionic parasympathetic fibers of the auriculotemporal nerve to the sympathetic subcutaneous nerves and vessels in the overlying region (Bonanno and Casson 1992) (See Figure 18.6). The acetylcholine released from the auriculotemporal nerve stimulates the postganglionic sympathetic cholinergic receptors of the sweat glands and the cutaneous vasculature, resulting in flushing, warmth, and sweating of the temporal and preauricular areas (de Bree et al. 2007) (See Figure 18.7).

The sequelae generally develop three to six months postsurgery or injury although there have been reports of it occurring years later (Baek et al. 2009).

The exact incidence of Frey syndrome is unclear since reports in the literature range from 1.7 to 97.6% (Neumann et al. 2011). The only significant predictor for the development of Frey syndrome has been found to be the size of the tumor. It has been suggested that larger tumors require a larger dissection and therefore result in a larger area of exposed parotid tissue (Lee et al. 2017), thereby predisposing patients to Frey syndrome.

Frey syndrome rarely progress in severity after onset and only needs to be managed in patients with subjective complaints, as opposed to objective findings. An outcome study of patients who underwent parotidectomies for benign salivary gland disease reported subjectively the presence of it 50.9% of the time (Baek et al. 2009).

Diagnosis of Frey Syndrome

A commonly used diagnostic evaluation for Frey syndrome is the Minor starch–iodine test (Minor 1927; O'Neill et al. 2008). Iodine solution comprised of 15.0 g iodine, 100.0 g castor oil, and 900.0 ml 70% alcohol is applied to the preauricular and temporal regions (see Chapter 10). A coat of starch is applied after the area dries (Jansen et al. 2017). A sialagogue is then administered. A positive response is noted when portions of the starch develop a purple color. The typical reaction time is approximately 30 seconds. The exact area of discoloration should be measured utilizing a 1 cm^2 grid and photographed to be able to evaluate for a change in intensity over time and the extent of the response (Linder et al. 1997).

Diagnosis can also be measured utilizing electrodes that detect the presence of l-lactate after stimulation, although a limited number of publications exist that describe this technique (Laccourreye et al. 1993).

Management of Frey Syndrome

The management of Frey syndrome includes utilizing different pharmacologic methods with varying success rates. Historically, treatment of these affected areas was topically with aluminum chloride, an antiperspirant, with generally poor results (Jansen et al. 2017). Botulinum toxin A is now the most frequent intervention and is considered the

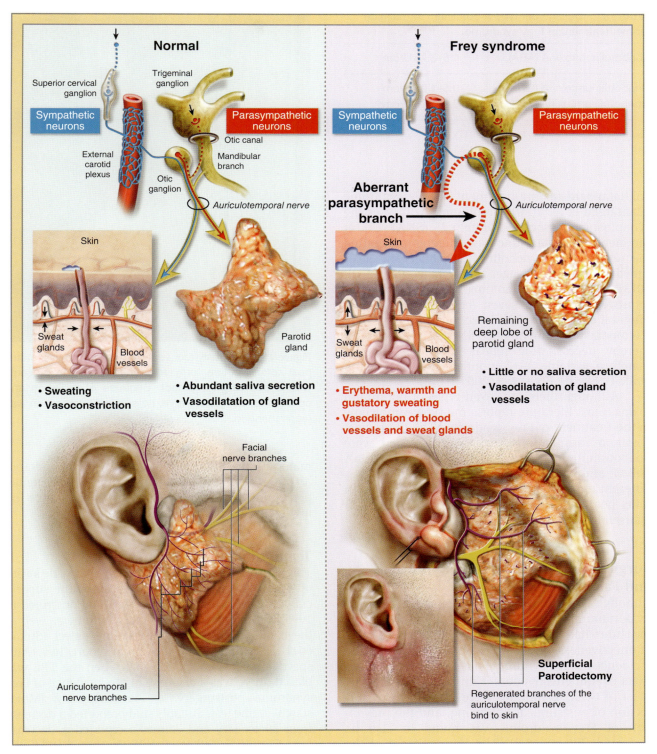

Figure 18.7. Illustration of abnormal neuromuscular junction between branches off the auricular-temporal nerve with a representative illustration of Frey Syndrome. Source: Illustration by Joseph Chovan.

Table 18.2. Dosage per type A botulinum formulation for the treatment of Frey syndrome.

AbobotulinumtoxinA (ABA)	1.5–3.75 U/cm^2
OnabotulinumtoxinA (ONA), IncobotulinumtoxinA (IBA)	0.5–1.25 U/cm^2 0.5–1.25 U/cm^2

Source: Based on Jansen S et. al., (2017).

gold standard for the treatment of Frey syndrome (Cantarella et al. 2010). Botulinum toxin lyses the synaptosomal-associated protein 25 (SNAP-25), at the neuromuscular junction, thereby preventing the release of acetylcholine (Tugnoli et al. 2002; Kreyden and Scheidegger 2004; Lawrence et al. 2013). Patients' symptoms are significantly improved in four to seven days after infiltration (Tugnoli et al. 2002). The injection of Botox is only a temporary treatment since SNAP-25 regenerates, thereby necessitating repeat injections approximately a variable 3–12 months later (Dulguerov et al. 1999a; de Bree et al. 2009).

Although there are seven types of botulinum toxins, most literature reports the type A molecule in the treatment of Frey syndrome. The three most common formulations that were reported were onabotulinumtoxinA (ONA), abobotulinumtoxinA (ABA), and incobotulinumtoxinA (IBA). The three different type A botulinum toxins are infiltrated in units per 1 cm^2 of the affected areas (Table 18.2) (Jansen et al. 2017).

Surgical Prevention of Frey Syndrome and Facial Defects

Although Frey syndrome can be effectively treated by botulinum toxin, a variety of surgical preventive measures has been developed with variable rates of effectiveness. As stated previously, the reported incidence of Frey syndrome has a wide range so an exact overall effectiveness is difficult to determine. Most of these techniques were developed for correction of postsurgical hollowing, and the prevention of Frey syndrome was found to also be indicated (Figure 18.8). The improvement of the cosmetic defect is somewhat variable and technique sensitive but there are four factors for consideration in selecting the appropriate procedure. These include the thickness of the interpositional material, the donor site morbidity, the predictability of the result and, most importantly, the patient's perception and acceptance of their appearance following surgery.

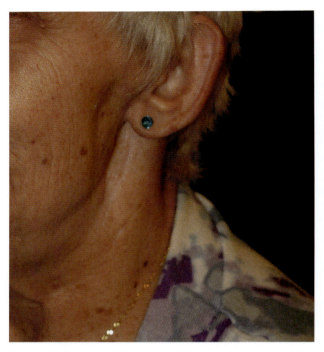

Figure 18.8. Seventy-four-year-old woman one-year status post total parotidectomy for adenocarcinoma presents with a postsurgical defect. Because of radiation and concern for the facial nerve, no surgical intervention was recommended.

Temporoparietal fascia flap

The temporoparietal fascia flap (TPF) is a wide swath of tissue that receives its vascularity by the superficial temporal artery. This flap was first described in 1995 for the prevention of Frey syndrome as well as the correction of the parotidectomy defect (Sultan et al. 1995). Following this initial report, two retrospective studies concluded that when the TPF was placed, there was a decrease in the incidence of Frey syndrome postsurgery, as determined by Minor starch–iodine test. Sultan's study reported a decrease from 39 to 4%, and Ahmed's reported a decrease from 57 to 17% (Sultan et al. 1995; Ahmed and Kolhe 1999). The TPF is esthetically effective in reducing the contour deficiency, although there is a risk of injury to the temporal branch of the facial nerve during the dissection (Motz and Kim 2016).

Sternocleidomastoid muscle flap

The sternocleidomastoid muscle flap (SCM) utilizes the sternocleidomastoid muscle as a barrier between the parotid gland surgical site and the overlying tissue. It was first described to prevent Frey syndrome in 1974 and has been regularly used since then (Kornblut et al. 1974). Although the flap is perfused by multiple arteries, the superiorly based flap is vascularized by the occipital artery. Unfortunately, the reported results varied in regards to its effectiveness in preventing Frey syndrome.

Some studies, including a meta-analysis, have shown the SCM flap to be effective in preventing Frey syndrome (Filho et al. 2004; Curry et al. 2009). In contrast, other studies have stated the exact opposite, reporting poor to no effect (Sanabria et al. 2012). Correction of the surgical defect has been found to be suboptimal, as well, because of the deficit of transferable bulk of soft tissue (Brennan et al. 2003). These two factors limit the effectiveness of the SCM flap for these indications.

Superficial musculoaponeurotic system flap

The superficial musculoaponeurotic system (SMAS) flap is a preventive barrier similar to the TPF. One of its advantages of this flap is it can be easily harvested directly through the Blair incision to preclude the necessity of a second incision or an unaesthetic extension (Figure 18.9). The SMAS flap has excellent cosmetic results, although its effectiveness in preventing Frey syndrome has mixed findings (Bonanno et al. 2000; Wille-Bischofberger et al. 2007; Motz and Kim 2016). One study reported that the affected area was decreased, although still present (Barbera et al. 2014). Because of this, the SMAS flap should be considered to be more useful in the correction of the surgical defect than as a preventative measure for Frey syndrome.

Acellular dermal matrix

Acellular dermal matrix is a tissue matrix harvested from cadaveric skin that has been processed to remove all cellular content. It is utilized as a scaffold for reconstruction and regeneration in many surgical procedures. When used in salivary gland surgery, particularly parotid gland surgery, the theory and practice is that it will serve as

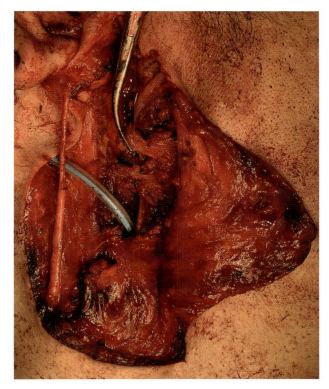

Figure 18.9. Superficial musculoaponeurotic system flap in a 66-year-old man undergoing a superficial parotidectomy for the excision of a pleomorphic adenoma. The SMAS flap is being developed and is being placed over the facial nerve and the remaining portion of the parotid gland. Because of the size of the tumor, portions of the SMAS are not present and an acellular dermal matrix will be placed over the remainder.

a physical barrier that will prevent the abnormal neural connection from occurring between the parotid gland and the overlying tissues (Figure 18.10). Its use for the prevention of Frey syndrome was first reported in 2001 as a case report, followed in the same year with a small prospective study that showed a 40% occurrence in the nontreated cohort and 0% in the subjects treated with an acellular matrix barrier (Clayman and Clayman 2001; Govindaraj et al. 2001). Thereafter, multiple studies, case series, and meta-analysis have been performed. All of these results had a decrease in Frey syndrome, but mixed findings were reported as with other interventional modalities. Regardless, in a 2010 meta-analysis, the subjective reduction of Frey syndrome was reported as 68%, with an objective measurement utilizing the Minor iodine–starch exam, by 85%

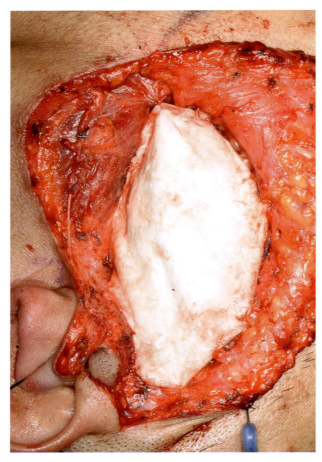

Figure 18.10. Forty-four-year-old man undergoing a superficial parotidectomy for a pleomorphic adenoma and placement of an interpositional membrane of acellular dermal matrix.

(Zhao-xuan 2010). As with any implanted, nonvascular substance, there is always a risk of infection. In the use of the acellular dermal matrix, it has been found that there is no significant increase in infection rates when compared to vascularized flaps. Cosmetically, because of the lack of bulk, a depression around the auricular lobule has been reported in comparative studies to fat grafting (Wang et al. 2016).

Fat grafting

Fat grafts are commonly utilized for the repair of surgical defects in many parts of the body. Although fat can be harvested from multiple locations, a predictable donor site is found in the periumbilical region. A half-circle incision is made along the inferior segment of the umbilicus and the fat is harvested as a segment, maintaining the interlobular architecture, that assists in stabilizing the graft (Conger and Gourin 2008). Unfortunately, fat has an unpredictable resorption rate, which is a particular problem when dealing with the correction of a parotidectomy surgical defect (Wang et al. 2016). The resorption rate of fat has been reported to range from 20 to 90% (Ersek 1991; Pinski and Roenigk 1992; Chandarana et al. 2009). Although there are anecdotal reports, there are no evidence-based studies regarding its utilization for the prevention of Frey syndrome.

A modification of the fat graft is the dermal-fat graft (DFG) in which the graft material is harvested with the overlying skin. Like the free fat graft, the periumbilical region is frequently utilized. Another donor site for the DFG is the upper quadrant in the gluteus region, close to the intergluteal crease. This region provides a substantial amount of tissue and can be easily closed because of the laxity of the skin at this site. After harvest, the overlying epidermis is removed, and the fat portion is trimmed to the desired depth. Like the free fat graft, the dermofat graft has an unpredictable reabsorption rate. If a free fat or DFG is being utilized to correct or prevent a surgical defect, 20–30% of extra volume should therefore be harvested.

When evaluating all available modalities for the prevention of Frey syndrome, it appears that all of the techniques reduce, but do not eliminate the symptoms of flushing and gustatory sweating. For surgical preventive measures, results suggest that the TPF flap has the best results in both the prevention of Frey syndrome and in the correction of the surgical defect. The SCM flap and acellular dermis had mixed results for the prevention of Frey syndrome and correction of the surgical defect. The SMAS flap had variable success in preventing Frey syndrome but is useful in correcting the surgical defect. Fat grafts are purely for correction of the surgical defect but have a variable resorption rate and therefore have unpredictable results.

PAROTID GLAND SALIVARY LEAKAGE

With violation of the parotid capsule, there is a risk of leakage and accumulation of salvia into either the overlying tissue or drainage through the skin. When the saliva collects in the overlying tissue, it is diagnosed as a sialocele, and when there is a passage to the skin, it is a fistula (Figures 18.11 and 18.12). Fistulas and sialoceles have a reported occurrence rate between 5 and 39% following partial resection

Complications of Salivary Gland Surgery   **579**

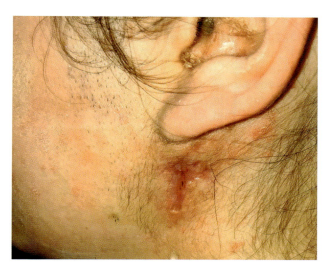

Figure 18.11. Thirty-one-year-old woman with an infected sialolith developed a salivary fistula following incision and drainage of an intra-parotid abscess. With no intervention, the fistula resolved in five weeks.

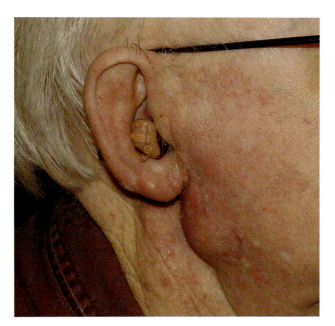

Figure 18.12. Seventy-seven-year-old man presented with a sialocele of the right parotid status post combined approach sialolithectomy. One week following surgery, patient developed sialocele which was treated with a pressure dressing and aspirations which was ineffective. The sialocele resolved after three weeks with no further intervention needed.

of the parotid gland and typically present within onse month following surgery.

The large range of the occurrence rate is most likely due to the subjective and objective diagnosis of these entities. Some authors rely on their clinical observations, which lend itself to nonstandardized diagnostic criteria, and others utilize objective findings, such as CT and ultrasound techniques for definitive diagnosis or as correlative tests to support their clinical diagnosis. Another confounding variable is that sialoceles progress to fistulas in 2–6% of cases and are therefore treated interchangeably (Lee et al. 2016). Both sialoceles and fistulas regularly resolve spontaneously by six months and are more common in the inferior and middle sections of the parotid gland (Witt 2009; Britt et al. 2017).

Classification of Parotid Gland Salivary Leakage

For the purpose of this chapter, salivary leakages are divided into three classes: minor, major, and sialoceles. Minor fistulae are the most commonly encountered. They are approximately 2–3 mm in diameter and regularly close on their own or with conservative management. Major fistulas are larger than 3 mm and are associated with dehiscence of the surgical wound. These also can also resolve spontaneously, although over a longer period of time.

Amylase testing of the fluid should show an amylase level of > 10 000 units/l to be considered positive for saliva (Darwish 2016).

Management of Parotid Salivary Leakage

As stated, minor fistulas and sialoceles generally resolve within the first postoperative month. When fistulas do develop, patients report expression of saliva through the wound during eating. For the patient's comfort and hygiene, the patients can place gauze overlying the area to absorb the leakage. Although tape can be used, it loses its adhesive property quickly following saturation. It is more effective to place a Barton bandage or pressure dressing around the head and jaws with the placement of interpositional gauze.

Conservative management of parotid gland salivary leakage

Initial management of parotid gland salivary leakage involves the placement of a pressure dressing with the intent that the overlying tissues scars to the remaining parotid tissue and create a seal (Witt 2009). The treatment of sialoceles also includes regular aspirations of the accumulated saliva. Not surprisingly, the sialoceles recur within 24 hours following aspiration and like fistulas, resolve within four to six weeks after onset, such that no intervention is needed.

Botulinum toxin for the management of parotid gland salivary leakage

For persistent parotid salivary leakage, injection of botulinum toxin has good results, with success rates ranging from 70 to 100% (Maharaj et al. 2020). After a complete superficial parotidectomy, injecting into the remaining deep lobe can be difficult because of the small target area. In partial superficial parotidectomies, there is still a large amount of parotid tissue present, so multiple injection sites are required to decrease the function throughout the remnant tissue.

A variety of doses has been suggested, with a range from 10 to 200 U of botulinum toxin A (Maharaj et al. 2020). Anecdotally, the author utilizes 50 U for patients with only the deep lobe remnant and 100 U in patients who underwent partial superficial parotidectomy or who developed sialoceles or fistulas following a traumatic injury to the gland.

Scopolamine patch

Scopolamine, an anticholinergic with an antimuscarinic effect, also decreases the incidence of the development of postsurgical leakage (Mantsopoulos et al. 2018). The theory is that the scopolamine decreases salivary flow, allowing area to close before fistula or sialocele occurs. One prospective study showed a reduction in the occurrence from 15 to 4% when the experimental cohort had a 2.5 cm^2 patch that contained 1.54 mg scopolamine that was released at a rate of approximately 1.0 mg/72 hours (Mantsopoulos et al. 2018). Patients reported the adverse effects of blurred vision, xerostomia, accommodation deficit, drowsiness, constipation, urinary retention, tachycardia, flushing, and dizziness.

Sclerosing agents

Another form of treatment for persistent sialoceles is the injection of sclerosing agents. Two agents, OK-432 and bleomycin, have been evaluated. OK-432, also named Picibanil, consists of lyophilized low-virulence group A Streptococcus pyogenes incubated with penicillin. This agent is used for sclerosis of a variety of lymphatic and other space forming lesions. Bleomycin is an antineoplastic drug that also functions as a sclerosing agent. A small cohort of subjects with postoperative sialoceles that persisted greater than four weeks were concurrently given an injection of both of these agents (Chen et al. 2013). All of the subjects had complete resolution of their sialoceles within three to five weeks, with no incidences of facial nerve injuries (Chen et al. 2013). Although of interest and included for completeness, this study had only nine subjects, without a comparative cohort, and utilized both agents together. It is impossible to determine which agent was responsible for the resolution of the leakages or even if the sialoceles would have resolved on their own given enough time.

Surgical repair of parotid gland salivary leakage

Chronic, untreated glandular sialoceles and fistulas are problematic and have a negative effect on the quality of life of the patient. In patients who underwent partial superficial parotidectomies, revision, and removal, the surgical site has been reported with mixed results (Powell and Clairmont 1983). The major concern of this intervention is that these sites have a significantly higher risk of postoperative facial nerve injuries (Motamed et al. 2003).

Tympanic neurectomy

The tympanic neurectomy procedure was first described by Golding-Wood in 1962 for the management of chronic parotitis (Golding-Wood 1962). The surgery consists of transecting the tympanic nerve, a branch of the glossopharyngeal nerve that carries the autonomic parasympathetic fibers to the parotid gland (See the Auriculotemporal Nerve and Frey Syndrome, for the description of this pathway).

To access this nerve, a tympanomeatal flap is raised and the nerve fibers are transected prior to synapsing within the otic ganglion. Historically, it was used for patients with hypersalivation and drooling, but the decrease in salivary function was found to be only temporary, having a duration for less than six months (Davis et al. 1977). The use of botulinum toxin has now replaced this technique because of the similar effect without the need for surgery.

Radiotherapy
An effective, although historical, management of intractable parotid leakage is the use of radiation. Doses between 6 and 20 Gy, with a mean of 12 Gy, are used to create atrophy of the gland, decreasing or even eliminating salivary flow (Ananthakrishnan and Parkash 1982; Powell and Clairmont 1983). Radiotherapy is no longer a treatment option because of the associated morbidity.

Temporalis fascia and cyanoacrylate
Transfer of temporalis fascia with skin closure using 2-octyl-cyanoacrylate has been used to close chronic fistulas. The cyanoacrylate stops the leakage from wound and allows for fibrosis of the fistula (Pesic et al. 2011). Although this management has only been reported as a case series, formation of abscesses from entrapment of the cyanoacrylate into the wound during healing is a known complication and should be taken into consideration. There is a report of a chronic fistula being injected with cyanoacrylate and lipiodol that caused a severe parotitis but ultimately resulted in resolution. Most likely, the injection of lipiodol, which causes exuberant inflammation, was responsible for sealing the fistula (Marcus and Nasser 1998).

Postoperative Infections
Reported postoperative infection of the parotid gland ranges from 0 to 1% (Nahlieli 2017). The reported infection rate is consistent with other head and neck surgical procedures.

Parotid Duct Leakage

Salivary duct fistulas and sialoceles should be considered different entities than what occurs in the gland parenchyma. Cutaneous fistulas occur from either transection of the duct or when there is an abscess that tracks superficially and erodes through the skin. Like glandular fistulas, cutaneous duct fistulas generally resolve within four weeks without the need for intervention. In patients that

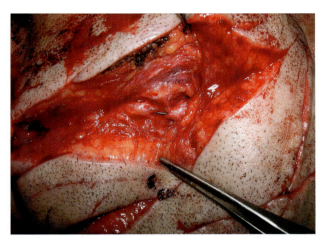

Figure 18.13. Twenty-three-year-old man presented following assault where he sustained a transection of the parotid duct. The distal and proximal segments were identified and anastomosed. Patency was confirmed by placement of 0.8 mm sialendoscope (Karl Storz, Tuttlingen, Germany), and a catheter was placed and sutured into position for four weeks.

present immediately following injury to the area, the duct can be repaired primarily, anastomosing the proximal and distal portion of the duct (Figure 18.13). If a sialendoscope is available, the patency of the duct can be verified and a surgical stent placed and secured for roughly four weeks to prevent adhesion and stricture formation.

Injury to the distal parotid duct can result in stricture of the duct or the orifice resulting in occlusion of the gland. This problem manifests as a gustatory swelling and can be repaired utilizing combined sialendoscopy techniques (See Chapter 19).

Iatrogenic injuries to the duct occur largely from lacrimal probes. When the probe is placed into the duct and advanced, if there is an obstruction from a sialolith or adhesion, the probe can be deflected thereby puncturing the duct wall (Figure 18.14). Different techniques are utilized to correct these injuries depending on their location.

MANAGEMENT OF PAROTID DUCT INJURIES

The most aggressive treatment for the management of a salivary duct injury is the superficial or complete parotidectomy. A complete parotidectomy will eliminate the problem but the benefit most likely outweighs the risks (See Complications of Parotid

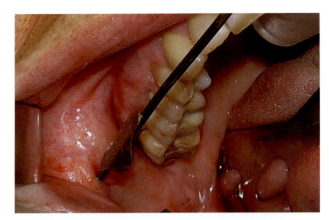

Figure 18.14. Placement of size eight lacrimal probe into right parotid orifice. Note that the full length of the probe is inserted into the gland. This should be done cautiously when there is a known or suspected obstruction. Transection or perforation can occur, particularly at the masseteric bend where the duct passes superficially. When bleeding occurs following removal of the probe, perforation is suspected and further probe placement should be discontinued.

symptoms. A less aggressive treatment is the elimination of salivary flow utilizing botulinum toxin. This is a temporary measure at best since it will not correct the underlying pathology.

Endoscopic Management of Parotid Salivary Duct Injuries

Surgical ductal procedures can be performed to decrease or eliminate the symptoms without removal of the gland tissue. If the major portion of the proximal and distal duct are still intact, but fully obstructed from scar tissue, a sialendoscope can be introduced to the obstruction, attempt to pass the scar tissue either with a micro drill, guide wire, or even a small sialendoscope can be used. Extreme caution and minimum force should be applied otherwise another perforation or complete transection of the duct can occur.

If the proximal stricture is not treated in a timely fashion, saliva accumulates within the proximal duct resulting in a megaduct or ductal aneurysm (Figure 18.15). A megaduct is diagnosed when the diameter of the duct exceeds 10 mm in diameter. This engorgement and dilation of the duct results in weakening of the duct wall and loss of elasticity. Once a megaduct is formed, it will not decrease in diameter, regardless of the intervention

Gland Surgery). A superficial parotidectomy can also be performed, and although this decreases salivary function, the issue of the continued function of the deep lobe of the parotid can result in continued

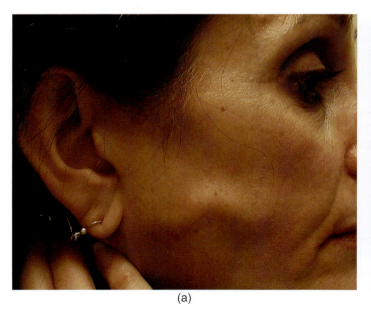

(a)

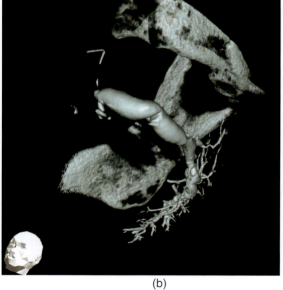

(b)

Figure 18.15. Forty-year-old woman who developed obstruction of the right parotid gland. She underwent multiple dilations with lacrimal probes multiple times over the course of six months. She developed a megaduct over the right cheek (a). The 3-D CBCT sialogram of the megaduct is noted (b).

and treatment of the etiology. Surgical intervention is therefore warranted. Megaducts create not only a functional issue but a cosmetic issue as well because of the bulge that is present on the patient's cheek (Koch et al. 2014).

Surgical management of a parotid megaduct

A pull-through sialodochoplasty is one of the techniques used to eliminate the megaduct. The orifice should first be identified and dilated if possible. A circular incision with a 5 mm cuff is made around the papilla. Utilizing blunt dissection, the duct is identified and skeletonized from the surrounding tissue to the stricture, if possible. Traction of the duct is applied, pulling as much of the megaduct and its associated stricture into the oral cavity. A longitude sectioning of the duct is performed, and the excess tissue is removed. The remaining duct is sutured primarily to the buccal mucosa, creating a neo-ostium (Figure 18.16). If available, verification of the patency can be performed by sialendoscopy. A cylindrical stent should be placed into the duct to prevent stricture of the neo-ostium (Gillespie 2018).

Avulsion of the Parotid Duct

Avulsion is a very rare complication of the parotid duct, with a reported occurrence of 0.5% (Nahlieli 2017). It occurs when either a fibrosed salivary gland stone or a large diameter stone (>5 mm) proximal to the masseteric bend is engaged with a retrieval basket. A complete transection of the duct can occur resulting in avulsion. There is no salvage surgery for this complication and either a superficial or complete parotidectomy becomes necessary to resolve this complication.

Stenosis of the Parotid Duct Orifice

The parotid duct orifice, when compared to the submandibular, is typically unforgiving when traumatized. In parotid gland sialendoscopy, aggressive dilatation, or trauma from insertion of the sialendoscope can induce scarring and direct occlusion of the salivary orifice occurs in 2–4% of cases (Iro et al. 2009; Nahlieli 2009). The management of this stenosis is regular dilation and stenting utilizing lacrimal probes, angiocatheters, and balloon dilators (Figure 18.17). Even with this treatment, it is not uncommon to require one to two years of weekly dilation to create a stable patency.

Complications of Submandibular and Sublingual Gland Surgery

The submandibular salivary gland can be approached utilizing intraoral and transcervical techniques. In terms of complications, the intraoral approach to the submandibular gland

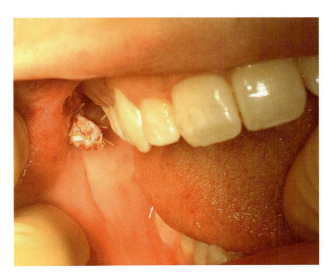

Figure 18.16. Completion of a pull through sialodochoplasty with the excess ductal tissue collar and surgical drain.

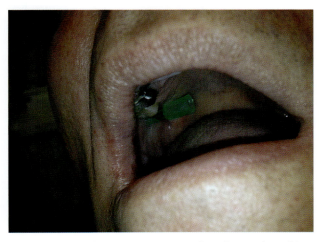

Figure 18.17. Eighteen-gauge angiocatheter placed into Stensen duct navigating around stricture without perforating the duct wall.

and sublingual gland are grouped together for the purpose of this discussion. The transcervical approaches to the submandibular gland are a separate and different entity and will presented as such.

COMPLICATIONS ASSOCIATED WITH AN INTRAORAL APPROACH TO THE SUBLINGUAL AND SUBMANDIBULAR GLANDS

The sublingual gland is frequently encountered when performing any procedure in the floor of the mouth. The sublingual gland is located anterior and superior to the submandibular gland and is covered by the mucosa of the floor of the mouth. The sublingual gland has two different duct systems. The minor ducts, which have been called the ducts of Rivinus, are small ducts, approximately 7–15 in number, and drain directly into the floor of the mouth. The larger, major duct is known as the Bartholin duct. In cadaveric studies, 36% had minor ducts without a major duct, 40% had the major sublingual gland duct draining into the submandibular gland, and 23% demonstrated the major sublingual gland draining directly into the mouth through the lingual caruncle, and there was only one major lingual duct in 1% of cases (Zhang et al. 2010) (Figure 18.18).

Ranulas (Mucous Extravasation Phenomenon)

Ranulas are formed from mucous extravasation when either the sublingual gland capsule is violated or when there is partial or full transection of the minor or major ducts of the gland. There are different types of ranulas that have been described. The first is the oral ranula or simple ranula, which is confined to the floor of the mouth. It appears as a bluish-grey, raised translucent lesion (Figure 18.19). In chronic lesions, patients report a cycle of rupture and drainage of mucous into the mouth, with apparent resolution. The lesion recurs approximately three to seven days later after epithelialization and closure of the perforated mucosa.

The other form of ranula is the cervical or plunging type. If the injury to the gland is further posterior or the mucous track posteriorly, it accumulates in the spaces of the neck with no oral findings (Figure 18.20).

A third type, called the mixed ranula, has been described with both oral and cervical findings.

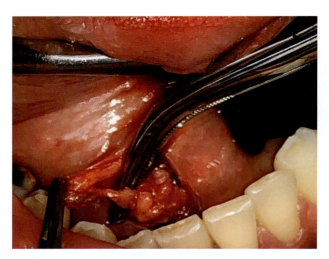

Figure 18.18. Bartholin duct entering into the Wharton duct during an intraoral dissection during a lingual gland removal.

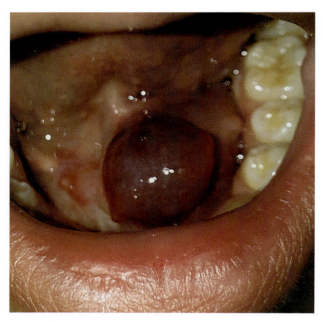

Figure 18.19. Twenty-five-year-old man presents with enlarged, translucent bluish hue lesion of the floor of the mouth. Patient relates history of this lesion draining and then recurring over a one-month period.

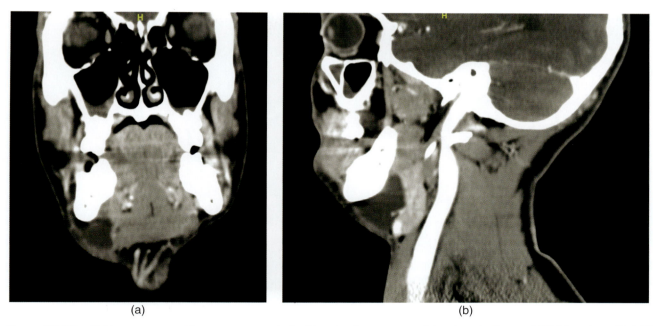

Figure 18.20. Thirty-one-year-old woman presented with enlarging mass on lateral neck. Coronal CT (a) and sagittal CT (b) obtained reveal a plunging ranula.

Complications associated with the management of ranulas

Regardless of the technique utilized, the major complications associated with the treatment of ranulas are recurrence, lingual nerve injury, and damage to the submandibular duct.

Recurrence of ranulas

When treating a ranula, the modality with the highest success rate is the excision of the sublingual gland that has been noted to have a cure rate of approximately 98% (Chung et al. 2019). When a recurrence occurs following resection, it is most likely from incomplete excision of all of the gland tissue. If the remnant of the gland is large enough, it can be removed with a secondary surgery. Small amounts of retained tissue can be difficult to treat with a secondary exploration, particularly in the posterior region, where visualization is limited. Consideration should be given to the use of sclerotherapy.

Similarly to the treatment of sialoceles, the most common agent used is OK-432. The most common reported adverse effect of this agent is pain and the onset of low-grade temperature of a short duration following the infiltration (Kim et al. 2008). It should be noted that OK-432, like most sclerosing agents, results in a robust inflammation. Close observation of the airway particularly, in larger plunging ranulas and pediatric patients, should therefore be considered (Kim et al. 2008; Zhi et al. 2014). Complete resolution of the ranula after utilizing OK-432 was found to be 79%, although 90% of patients did have some measurable decrease in size (Chung et al. 2019).

Lingual nerve injury during sublingual gland removal

Sensory change is the highest reported complication associated with removal of the sublingual gland, with an occurrence rate of 5% (Zhao et al. 2004). The lingual nerve is located anterior and medially to the sublingual gland and is encountered during gland removal (Figure 18.21). If the lingual nerve is transected during gland removal, the proximal and distal stumps should be identified and an immediate anastomosis of the two ends should be performed.

Submandibular duct injury during sublingual gland removal

The submandibular duct exits the submandibular hilum and, in most cases, is located above

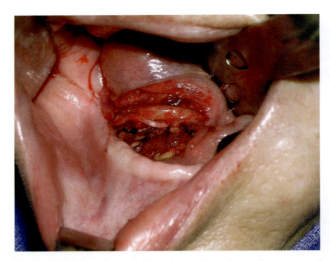

Figure 18.21. The relationship of the lingual nerve and the submandibular duct following sublingual gland removal. In the proximal region, the Wharton duct is superior and lateral to the lingual nerve.

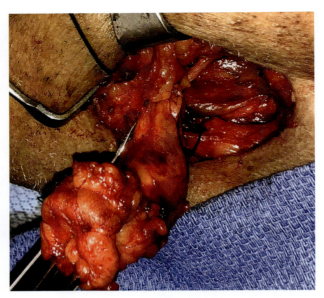

Figure 18.22. During sialadenectomy of right salivary gland through a transcervical approach secondary to large sialolith, the lingual nerve travels deep to the submandibular gland, enmeshed within the lingual gland tissues. Source: Photograph courtesy of Dr. Shahid Aziz.

(superficial from an intraoral perspective or deep from a transcervical perspective) to the lingual nerve and medial to the sublingual gland. It sharply turns at the posterior border of the mylohyoid and then courses medial to the insertion of the mylohyoid on the mylohyoid ridge. At the anterior hyoglossus, it once again is in contact with the lingual nerve, where this time, it crosses, with few exceptions, below the nerve (deep from an intraoral perspective or superficial from a transcervical perspective) (Figure 18.22).

Because of this close contact, the duct can easily be damaged, either during the dissection or by misidentification during the surgery. During removal of the sublingual glands, the incidence, like in most studies, varies, with a range between 1.93 and 14.67% (Zhao et al. 2005).

Complications Associated with Intraoral Surgery of Submandibular Ducts

Most surgeries of the submandibular duct are associated with sialendoscopic procedures. Sialendoscopy is a minimally invasive technique for the treatment of obstructive salivary gland disorders. Prior to its introduction, obstructive sialoliths and ductal strictures were managed by sialadenectomy (Nahlieli et al. 1994). For the most part, an injury to the salivary gland duct system is most likely related to insertion of a probe or endoscope. When placing a probe into a duct, if blood is expressed from the orifice on removal, a perforation has most likely occurred and further dilation should be discontinued. If unsure, and if available, a sialendoscopy or sialography should be performed to assess patency (Figure 18.23).

Sialendoscopy of the submandibular gland is divided into two different categories. The first is when the procedure is completely performed with the endoscope and no additional dissection is performed. For the most part, these surgeries are regulated to treatment of strictures, disruption of mucous plugs, and removal of sialoliths less than 5 mm in diameter. When a secondary approach, i.e. intraoral dissection to a sialolith > 5 mm, is performed, it is termed a combined or assisted approach (See Chapter 19).

Stricture of the submandibular gland duct

Stricture formation is the leading complication related to sialendoscopy. Strictures are created by injury to the duct wall from removal of an embedded sialolith or iatrogenic damage to the duct epithelium from instrumentation (Figure 18.24). The rate of stricture formation is roughly 2.5% (Nahlieli 2009).

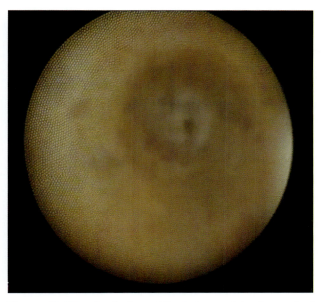

Figure 18.25. Occlusion of the left parotid salivary duct from stricture formation on a 58-year-old woman patient with advanced Sjögren syndrome.

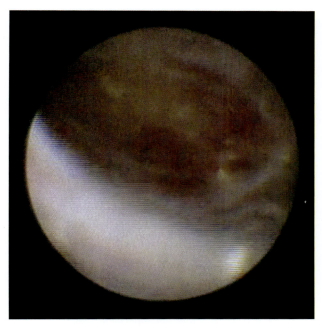

Figure 18.23. Perforation of the submandibular duct through a 1.1 mm sialendoscope (Karl Storz, Tuttlingen, Germany). The lingual gland tissue can be seen in the center of the image.

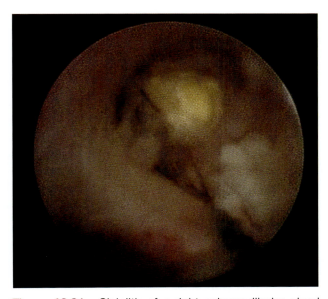

Figure 18.24. Sialolith of a right submandibular gland embedded into the duct wall. Chronic inflammation and reactive fibrotic tissue visualized surrounding the visible sialolith. Visualized through a 1.6 mm sialendoscope (Karl Storz, Tuttlingen Germany).

Stricture formation is identified by continued obstructive symptoms following surgery. If this occurs, a diagnostic sialendoscopy or sialogram should be performed to confirm the presence and location of the obstruction (Figure 18.25). These strictures should be dilated either by balloon dilation, microforcep stretching, or insertion of dilation probes. Attempting to dilate without ultrasound guidance or sialendoscopy visualization can result in perforation of the duct. Following successful dilation, drain placement for two to four weeks is recommended to maintain the patency of the duct.

Lingual nerve injuries

During a pure sialendoscopy with no extraductal surgical component, lingual nerve injuries have been reported as 0.7% when a perforation of the submandibular duct occurs where it contacts the lingual nerve. All of these cases were temporary and are reported for completeness (Iro et al. 2009; Nahlieli 2009). In a combined approach, particularly when the salivary duct is stretched and skeletonized away from the lingual nerve, it is not uncommon to have a transient altered sensation (Figure 18.26). Although most of these sensory changes are temporary, 0.4% of these patients have permanent residual hypoesthesia/anesthesia (Nahlieli 2009).

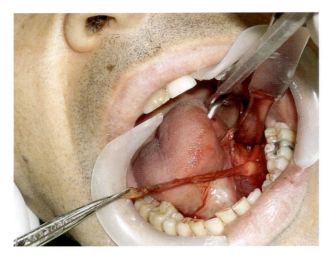

Figure 18.26. Twenty-six-year-old man with manipulation of the lingual nerve during a duct stretching procedure during a submandibular sialolithectomy. Source: Photograph courtesy of Dr. Oded Nahlieli.

Extravasation of fluid and airway obstruction

As stated previously, during a sialendoscopy, perforation of the submandibular duct can occur and the irrigation that is utilized to create the optical cavity extravasates into the floor of the mouth causing an obstruction of the airway. If this occurs in the operating room, the patient should remain intubated (Figure 18.27). This extravasated fluid is absorbed into the surrounding tissues within 24–48 hours.

Ranula formation

Although ranula formation has been discussed, sialendoscopy has an associated rate of formation between 1 and 2.5%, particularly if the sublingual duct enters into the submandibular duct and is inadvertently transected during a papillotomy procedure (Iro et al. 2009; Nahlieli 2017, 2009).

Submandibular duct avulsion

Avulsion of the submandibular duct during the performance of sialendoscopic sialolithectomy is a rare complication, and only a handful of cases have been reported in the literature (Walvekar et al. 2008). This complication occurs when a salivary gland stone is embedded into the duct wall. After the retrieval basket has engaged the sialolith, if excessive force is applied, the duct can be avulsed

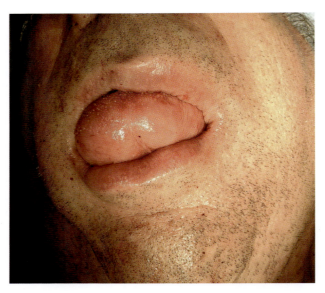

Figure 18.27. Seventy-five-year-old man following sialendoscopy with extravasation of saline into the floor of the mouth and tongue. Edema of the tongue resolved within 24 hours and patient was extubated without issue.

(Figure 18.28a). To salvage the procedure, a complex sialodochoplasty or sialadenectomy needs to be considered (Figure 18.28b). Similar to the parotid gland, the reported occurrence is 0.5% (Nahlieli 2017).

COMPLICATIONS ASSOCIATED WITH TRANSCERVICAL APPROACHES TO THE SUBMANDIBULAR GLAND

The complications associated with removal of the submandibular salivary glands are either injury to the marginal mandibular, lingual, and the hypoglossal nerves. The submandibular duct can also be injured, but since the gland is being removed, the results of this are of little consequence.

Marginal Mandibular Branch Injury During a Sialadenectomy

The marginal mandibular nerve is the most common nerve that is injured when performing the transcervical approach to the submandibular gland. Injury to this nerve results in partial or complete loss of animation to the lip and adjacent structures. The occurrence ranges from 1 to 7% (Springborg and Moller 2013; de Carvalho et al. 2015; Nocon et al. 2016) (Figure 18.5b).

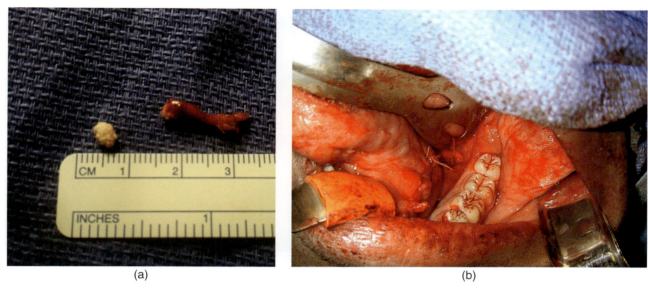

Figure 18.28. Sixty-two-year-old woman who had successful removal of a 4 mm distal sialolith of the left submandibular gland. When retrieval of the 3 mm proximal sialolith was attempted, duct was avulsed (a). Complex sialodochoplasty was performed (b).

Lingual Nerve Injury during a Sialadenectomy

Like in the transoral approach, injury of the lingual nerve is a known risk when performing submandibular gland excision. The most common cause is adhesion of the lingual nerve to the submandibular duct because of chronic inflammation. Another, less likely etiology, is the misidentification of the lingual nerve for the submandibular duct, resulting in a transection and removal. If this complication is identified during the surgery, immediate repair should be performed. The occurrence of lingual nerve injuries in total during this approach ranges from 0.5 to 4.4% (Springborg and Moller 2013; de Carvalho et al. 2015; Nocon et al. 2016; Nahlieli 2017).

Hypoglossal Nerve Injury during a Sialadenectomy

The hypoglossal nerve is located medial and deep to the submandibular gland. Except for an intraoral removal of a salivary gland, it is unlikely to be encountered during procedures performed in the mouth, and even if it is encountered, no injuries to this nerve have been reported (Capaccio et al. 2020). During the transcervical approach, injury to the hypoglossal nerve was reported with a range of 0–1.4% (Milton et al. 1986; Hald and Andreassen 1994; Preuss et al. 2007; Springborg and Moller 2013). This injury, although rare, is debilitating. On exam, the patient's tongue deviates to the affected side on extension (Figure 18.29). Over time, atrophy of the effected side occurs, leading to dysarthria and oral incompetence (Avitia and Osborne 2008).

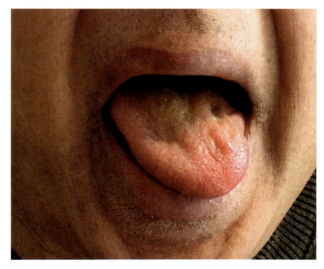

Figure 18.29. Seventy-one-year-old man status post removal of his left submandibular gland removal presented with hypoglossal nerve injury resulting in a deviation of the tongue during protrusion as well as atrophy of the left lateral surface. Source: Photograph courtesy Jack Kolenda MD, FRCS(C).

Hematoma Formation

Hematoma formation that occurs during any transcervical approach can result in an acute airway emergency. It is uncommon following sialadenectomy, with a range of occurrence from 0 to 14% (Hald and Andreassen 1994; Winkel et al. 2000; Springborg and Moller 2013). For the most part, hematomas are comprised of a collection of venous blood in into the dead space which self-tamponades. When the source is an artery, particularly the lingual artery, these complications necessitate a return to the operating room for surgical exploration and ligation of the bleeding vessel.

Hyposalivation

The submandibular glands each excrete 30% of the total whole saliva volume and have both a mucinous and serous component. The parotid glands excrete a predominantly serous saliva, supplying the remaining 20% each. This loss of salivary volume becomes more problematic in the geriatric population because of the increase of polypharmacy-induced hyposalivation. This results in an increase in the dental caries rate, candidiasis, erosion, and ulceration of the mucosal tissues, dysgeusia, dysphagia, gingivitis, and impaired use of removable prostheses (Turner et al. 2008). In these situations, patients should begin topical fluoride applications, saliva substitutes, and sialagogues.

Complications Associated with Removal of Minor Salivary Gland Mucocele

Extravasation mucoceles are caused by the disruption of minor salivary gland ducts, resulting in a submucosal accumulation of mucous. There is a disease entity of the mucous retention cyst, where the minor salivary gland duct is occluded, but for the purpose of this chapter, the extravasation and retention types will be grouped together and merely referred to as "mucoceles."

In the lower lip and the surrounding tissues, there are 800–1000 minor salivary glands with a large percentage of them located in the inferior–anterior labial vestibule. Because of this higher density, mucoceles of minor salivary glands present in this region (Sumi et al. 2007) (Figure 18.30).

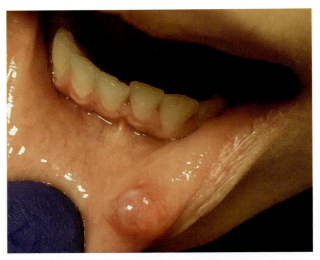

Figure 18.30. Twenty-six-year-old man with mucocele of the left lower lip.

The second region that are at risk for mucocele formation, although less frequently, is the ventral surface of the tongue. These types of mucoceles are difficult to manage because the causative minor salivary glands are found much deeper into the tissue than a labial mucocele and are much more difficult to identify and remove (Sugerman et al. 2000). This is supported in the current literature with mucoceles of the tongue having a recurrence rate of 8–50% (Oliveira et al. 1993; Choi et al. 2019) (Figure 18.31).

Mucoceles of the upper lip are very rare, and if there is a growth is in this region, the suspicion of a minor salivary gland tumor should be considered first (Choi et al. 2019).

COMPLICATIONS ASSOCIATED WITH REMOVAL OF MUCOCELE OF THE LOWER LIP

The three most common complications associated with removal of a mucocele of the lower lip are recurrence, neurosensory change to the lower lip, and soft tissue defects.

Mucocele Recurrence

A true recurrence occurs when just the mucocele is removed without the causative minor salivary gland,

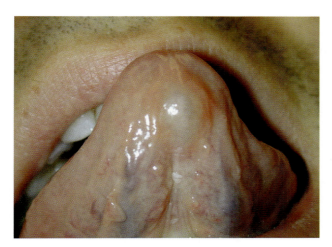

Figure 18.31. Twenty-three-year-old man with a mucocele of the tongue on the ventral surface.

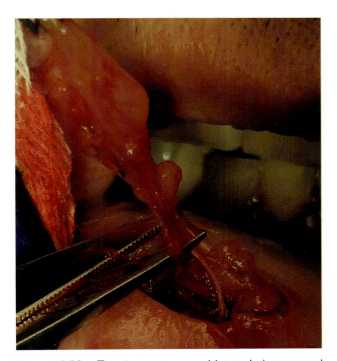

Figure 18.32. Twenty-seven-year-old man during removal of a mucocele with visualization of the adjacent minor salivary glands and their associated ducts.

as well. If the gland is removed and another mucocele occurs in the same area, it is likely that another minor salivary gland duct was injured during the dissection; thus, it should be considered a new occurrence (Figure 18.32) Regardless, the term recurrence will be utilized when referring to this phenomenon.

The incidence of recurrence can be decreased if all minor salivary glands that are visualized are removed during the excision of the mucocele. Reported recurrence rates are highly variable because of the different techniques utilized. These include excision with a scalpel, which is the most common, laser removal, cryotherapy, electrocautery, and sclerotherapy. Overall, the reported range was 2.8–18% (Yamasoba et al. 1990; Oliveira et al. 1993; Re Cecconi et al. 2010; Choi et al. 2019). The overall management of the recurrence is the same as the initial management, removal, or sclerosis of the causative minor salivary gland.

Neurosensory Change

Another complication of mucocele removal is injury to the nerve fibers that innervate the region where the mucocele is located. The lip is innervated by labial branches of the mental nerve (Figure 18.33). Like most nerves, they continue to branch as they move distally. This significance of this becomes important, because the mucoceles that are located more laterally on the lip have a higher incidence of sensory change when compared to the mucoceles located more medially. Of note, no prospective or retrospective evaluation of this complication has been reported.

Esthetic Defects of the Lip

Another significant complication is the postsurgical defect of the lip. Immediately after the surgery, there is an evident defect that typically resolves after one to two weeks, with final resolution in three to six months (Figure 18.34). Although rare, defects that persist after six months are treated with tissue fillers, like hyaluronic acid. Another type of cosmetic defect is the placement of a deep suture in close proximity to skin (Di Lauro et al. 2010). This causes a puckering defect in the adjacent skin, which becomes more pronounced when the surrounding edema resolves. If the defect is noticed during closure, the causative suture should be removed and placed closer to the labial mucosa. If the defect is observed postoperatively, massage of the region should release the entrapped tissue over time.

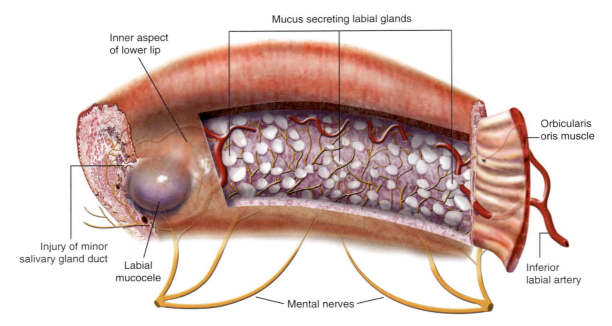

Figure 18.33. Illustration of the labial surface of the lip. The anatomy of the minor salivary glands and their position in the gland with an example of a transection of a duct and the formation of an extravasation mucocele. Small branches of the mental nerve branch and are present throughout the lip. Source: Illustration by Joseph Chovan.

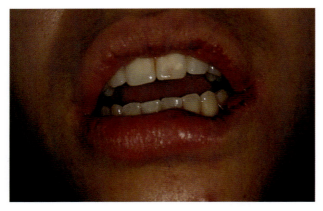

Figure 18.34. Twenty-five-year-old woman with a surgical defect immediately following the removal of a mucocele of the lower lip.

Summary

- Facial nerve paralysis can occur whenever the parotid capsule is violated.
- The House–Brackmann classification is a commonly used objective evaluation of facial nerve paralysis.
- Frey syndrome occurs following parotid gland tissue when an abnormal neural juncture occurs between the auricular temporal nerve and the overlying skin and sweat glands.
- Frey syndrome can be managed with infiltration of botulinum toxin, although it is only a temporary, palliative treatment.
- There are variety interpositional surgical techniques that decrease the incidence of Frey syndrome as well as correct the potential surgical defect. It is difficult to determine which is the most effective form of treatment because of the mixed results reported in the literature.
- Following parotid gland surgery, salivary gland leakage can occur. When it accumulates in the interstitial tissue, it is diagnosed as a sialocele. If there is a communication to the skin, it is diagnosed as a salivary fistula.
- Both salivary fistulas and sialoceles resolve without any intervention within four to six weeks of occurrence.
- Orifice to the parotid duct can be easily injured and result in stricture formation. These strictures are difficult to manage. This

can result in a robust dilation of the gland called a megaduct.
- When probing salivary gland ducts, passive pressure will prevent puncture or transection of the duct wall.
- When using a retrieval basket during sialolithectomy, excessive force can result in avulsion of the duct. If this occurs in the submandibular duct, a sialodochoplasty can be utilized as a salvage surgery. If it happens in the parotid gland, there is no salvage procedure and a superficial or total parotidectomy is necessary.
- Injury to the sublingual gland can result in extravasation of mucous into the surrounding tissues resulting in a ranula. When it is present in the floor of the mouth, it is an oral ranula, and when it drains past the mylohyoid muscle into the neck, it is a plunging ranula.
- Lingual gland removal is the most effective management of a ranula.
- The lingual nerve and the submandibular duct contact in two regions. These can be injured during intraoral and transcervical surgery on the sublingual and submandibular glands.
- During submandibular gland sialendoscopy, saline can extravasate into of floor of the mouth resulting in an airway obstruction.
- When removing a mucocele of the lower lip, damage to adjacent minor salivary glands can result in a new occurrence. Damage can also occur to the branches off the mental nerves causing a sensory deficit. An esthetic defect of the lip can be present following mucocele excision that resolves over time a majority of time.

Case Presentation – *Get It Right the First Time. That's the Main Thing*

A 72-year-old white woman was seen in August 1992 with a swelling of the left posterior hard palate extending into the soft palate. The lesion was asymptomatic. It was submucosal, firm to palpation 5 × 3 cm with overlying telangiectasia (Figure 18.35a) Biopsy was reported as showing pleomorphic adenoma with monomorphic features. In September 1992, she underwent excision with preservation of the underlying palatal bone using the periosteum as the deep margin. The final pathology confirmed pleomorphic adenoma with an atypical pattern.

Three months later she presented with a lump in the ipsilateral neck at the level of 2a. The mass was mobile and soft. CT scan was reported as a cystic lesion, possible branchial cyst. FNAB produced clear fluid and was reported as benign. In January, she had an excision of the mass, which was approximately 4 × 3 cm and appeared cystic in nature (Figure 18.35b). Initial report was of a metastatic node probably papillary thyroid. At this stage, we requested the pathologists to review the histopathology of the original palatal lesion. Following review, the original diagnosis was changed and the report was amended to show that the tumor was now diagnosed as polymorphous low-grade adenocarcinoma, papillary type. A CT of his facial bones showed recurrent/persistent disease at the base of the pterygoid plates (Figure 18.54c). In February 1993, she underwent a left hemi-maxillectomy via a Weber Fergusson incision and a left modified radical neck dissection to clear the neck (Figure 18.35d and e). Margins were negative, and no further nodes were seen. She underwent postoperative radiation therapy.

The patient did very well for almost five and a half years when she presented with local recurrence in the anterior maxilla in July 1998. Her CT scan showed a retropharyngeal node with a necrotic center (Figure 18.35f and g). In August 1998, she underwent surgery. An extra-oral vertical subsigmoid osteotomy via a cervical incision was used to access the retro pharyngeal nodes which were removed and an anterior maxillectomy was undertaken.

She recurred in the roof of the sinus in 2001 and refused further surgery. In August 2001, nine years following her original diagnosis she had clinical invasion of the orbit and involvement of the globe (Figure 18.35h–k). She wanted no further surgery at aged 81 years, and she died with disease six months later.

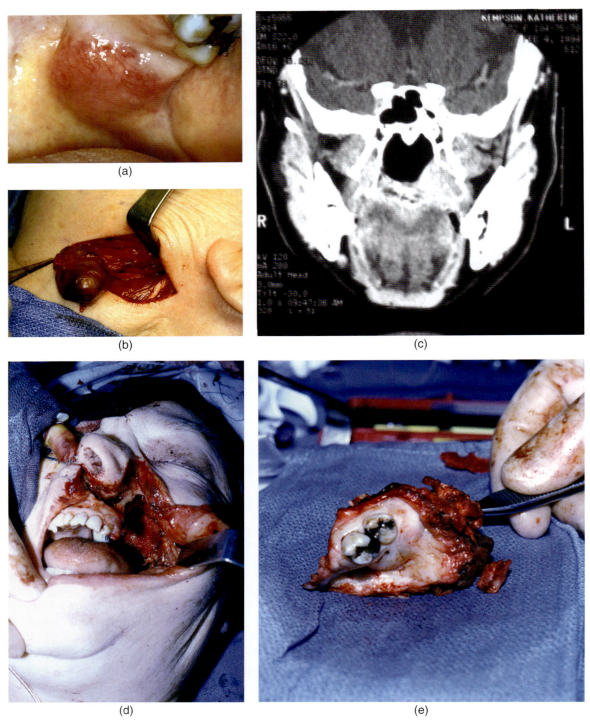

Figure 18.35. (a) Intraoral view shows of the left palate extending from the molar region into the soft palate. Note the overlying mucosal telangiectasia from tumor vessels. (b) Removal of the ipsilateral neck mass from level 2a. The mass lay partly in anterior to and partly deep to the sternocleidomastoid muscle. The mass is bluish soft and cystic in nature, with a thin wall. Note the greater auricular nerve crossing the muscle at the inferolateral aspect of the wound. (c) Coronal CT Scan following neck biopsy shows mass deep to left soft palate eroding the left pterygoid plates. The mass was not evident clinically. (d) Intraoperative view of left partial maxillectomy with excision of the overlying soft palate and pterygoid plates. (e) Surgical specimen left posterior maxilla. The scalpel handle is lifting the medial and lateral pterygoid muscles that form the posterior margin of the resection. (f) Axial CT scan. Note the large defect from the previous maxillectomy. Medial to the left mandibular ramus a 1.5cm lateral retropharyngeal node is seen with rim enhancement and a necrotic center. (g) Coronal CT shows the necrotic node medial to the left neck of condyle. (h) Intra oral view shows red-purple fleshy recurrence in the roof of the maxillectomy cavity abutting the orbital floor. (i) Patient now has orbital invasion with inability to open the left eye and redness and swelling of the periorbita. Note the hollowing of the left neck from the previous radical neck dissection. (j) Axial CT shows tumor destroying the lateral wall of the orbit and involving the globe. (k) Coronal CT bone window shows invasion of the orbit through the orbital floor.

Complications of Salivary Gland Surgery

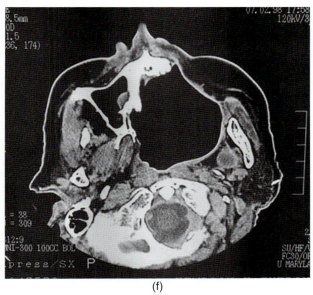

(f)

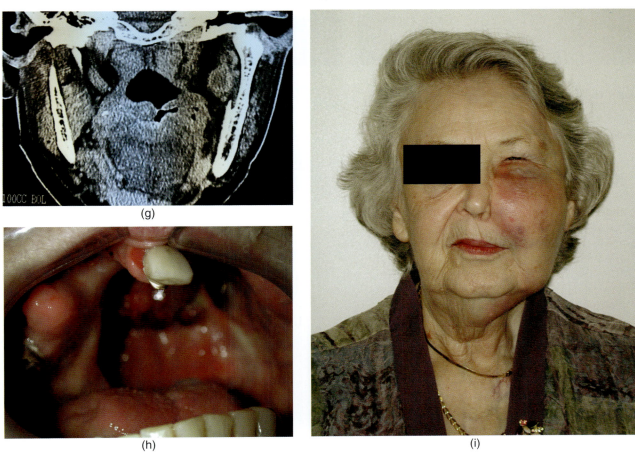

(g)

(h)

(i)

Figure 18.35. *(Continued).*

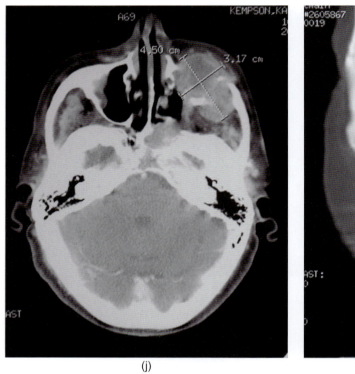
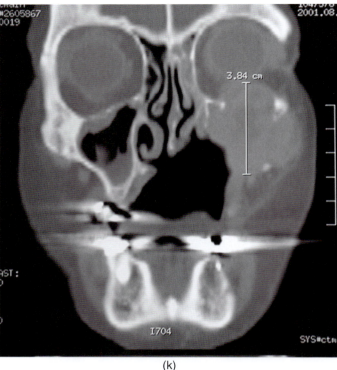

Figure 18.35. (Continued).

TAKE HOME POINTS

1. The initial histopathologic diagnosis both biopsy and final resection indicated the tumor to be benign. Unfortunately, this was a misdiagnosis as the lesion was malignant. The initial complication of the wrong diagnosis led to undertreatment of the primary tumor. Polymorphous adenocarcinoma (formerly PLGA) is a difficult diagnosis for the pathologist as its various patterns can mimic other salivary tumors such as pleomorphic adenoma and adenoid cystic carcinoma.

    It is a wise axiom in cancer surgery that the first chance is the best chance of cure. If the correct histopathologic diagnosis had been made, then the bone of the palate would not have been preserved and the patient would have had a partial maxillectomy as her primary treatment. This would have given an improved chance of cure. Whether she would have still developed a cervical node is debatable, but she would have had a neck dissection immediately and certainly not a biopsy of the neck node. The incorrect pathologic diagnosis led to an inadequate surgery with subsequent multiple recurrence and inability to control the disease locally.

2. Although the polymorphous adenocarcinoma was considered low grade in the 1990s, its name was changed in the 2017 World Health Organization classification of salivary gland cancers to reflect the fact that it can be more aggressive. There are certain sub types that are more likely to be aggressive in behavior and the papillary type as presented in this case is known to have a greater propensity for invasion and metastasis.

3. Obviously, a complication such as a misdiagnosis has legal consequences. In oncology, there are two possible disasters. First, a cancer may be called benign as in this case, and second, a benign tumor may be called malignant. The author has suffered both calamities. In the first, as in this case the patient is undertreated initially leading to recurrence and perhaps eventual death. In the second, the patient has surgery that is over-radical for the condition. The tumor is cured but at the expense of undue loss of normal tissue, a possible unnecessary neck dissection and resulting quality of like issues. When dealing with outside biopsy

diagnosis, the clinician should always have the slides reviewed by the pathology department within his institution. Even then as in the present case, mistakes can happen.

References

Aframian DJ, Palmon A, Nahlieli O. 2004. Future therapy strategies for salivary gland impairment. Refuat Hapeh Vehashinayim 21:43–50.

Ahmed OA, Kolhe PS. 1999. Prevention of Frey's syndrome and volume deficit after parotidectomy using the superficial temporal artery fascial flap. Br J Plast Surg 52:256–260.

Albergotti WG, Nguyen SA, Zenk J, Gillespie MB. 2012. Extracapsular dissection for benign parotid tumors: A meta-analysis. Laryngoscope 122:1954–1960.

Ananthakrishnan N, Parkash S. 1982. Parotid fistulas: A review. Br J Surg 69:641–643.

Avitia S, Osborne RF. 2008. Surgical management of iatrogenic hypoglossal nerve injury. Ear Nose Throat J 87:672–676.

Baek CH, Chung MK, Jeong HS et al. 2009. Questionnaire evaluation of sequelae over 5 years after parotidectomy for benign diseases. J Plast Reconstr Aesthet Surg 62:633–638.

Baillarger M. 1853. Memoire sur l'obliteration du canal de Stenon. Gazette Me'dicale de Paris 23:194–197.

Bar B, Mantsopoulos K, Iro H. 2019. Paradigm shift in surgery for benign parotid tumors: 19 years of experience with almost 3000 cases. Laryngoscope 130:1941–1946.

Barbera R, Castillo F, D'Oleo C, Benitez S, Cobeta I. 2014. Superficial musculoaponeurotic system flap in partial parotidectomy and clinical and subclinical Frey's syndrome. Cosmesis and quality of life. Head Neck 36:130–136.

Bhutia O, Kumar L, Jose A, Roychoudhury A, Trikha A. 2014. Evaluation of facial nerve following open reduction and internal fixation of subcondylar fracture through retromandibular transparotid approach. Br J Oral Maxillofac Surg 52:236–240.

Bonanno PC, Casson PR. 1992. Frey's syndrome: A preventable phenomenon. Plast Reconstr Surg 89:452–456, discussion 57-8.

Bonanno PC, Palaia D, Rosenberg M, Casson P. 2000. Prophylaxis against Frey's syndrome in parotid surgery. Ann Plast Surg 44:498–501.

Bonavolontà P. 2019. Postoperative complications after removal of pleomorphic adenoma from the parotid gland: A long-term follow up of 297 patients from 2002 to 2016 and a review of publications. Br J Oral Maxillofac Surg 57:998–1002.

de Bree R, van der Waal I, Leemans CR. 2007. Management of Frey syndrome. Head Neck 29:773–778.

de Bree R, Duyndam JE, Kuik DJ, Leemans CR. 2009. Repeated botulinum toxin type A injections to treat patients with Frey syndrome. Arch Otolaryngol Head Neck Surg 135:287–290.

Brennan PA, Kunjar J, Ramchandani P, Ilankovan V. 2003. Re: A prospective randomised trial of the benefits of a sternocleidomastoid flap after superficial parotidectomy. Br J Oral Maxillofac Surg 41:201–202.

Britt CJ, Stein AP, Gessert T, Pflum Z, Saha S, Hartig GK. 2017. Factors influencing sialocele or salivary fistula formation postparotidectomy. Head Neck 39:387–391.

Bron LP, O'Brien CJ. 1997. Facial nerve function after parotidectomy. Arch Otolaryngol Head Neck Surg 123:1091–1096.

Brown-Sequard CE. 1850. Production de sueur sous l'influence d'une excitation vive des nerfs du gofi. *Compte Reridu Socie'te' de Biologie* 1:104.

Burres SA. 1986. Objective grading of facial paralysis. Ann Otol Rhinol Laryngol 95:238–241.

Cannon CR, Replogle WH, Schenk MP. 2004. Facial nerve in parotidectomy: A topographical analysis. Laryngoscope 114:2034–2037.

Cantarella G, Berlusconi A, Mele V, Cogiamanian F, Barbieri S. 2010. Treatment of Frey's syndrome with botulinum toxin type B. Otolaryngol Head Neck Surg 143:214–218.

Capaccio P, Montevecchi F, Meccariello G et al. 2020. Transoral robotic submandibular sialadenectomy: How and when. Gland Surg 9:423–429.

de Carvalho AS, Dedivitis RA, de Castro MA, Nardi CE. 2015. Submandibular gland excision. Rev Col Bras Cir 42:14–17.

Casale M, Capuano F, Sabatino L et al. 2016. A safe transoral surgical approach to parapharyngeal tumor arising from deep lobe of parotid gland. SAGE Open Med Case Rep 4:2050313X16682131.

Chandarana S, Fung K, Franklin JH, Kotylak T, Matic DB, Yoo J. 2009. Effect of autologous platelet adhesives on dermal fat graft resorption following reconstruction of a superficial parotidectomy defect: A double-blinded prospective trial. Head Neck 31:521–530.

Chen WL, Zhang LP, Huang ZQ, Zhou B. 2013. Percutaneous sclerotherapy of sialoceles after parotidectomy with fibrin glue, OK-432, and bleomycin. Br J Oral Maxillofac Surg 51:786–788.

Choi YJ, Byun JS, Choi JK, Jung JK. 2019. Identification of predictive variables for the recurrence of oral mucocele. Med Oral Patol Oral Cir Bucal 24:e231–e235.

Chung YS, Cho Y, Kim BH. 2019. Comparison of outcomes of treatment for ranula: A proportion meta-analysis. Br J Oral Maxillofac Surg 57:620–626.

Clayman MA, Clayman LZ. 2001. Use of AlloDerm as a barrier to treat chronic Frey's syndrome. Otolaryngol Head Neck Surg 124:687.

Conger BT, Gourin CG. 2008. Free abdominal fat transfer for reconstruction of the total parotidectomy defect. Laryngoscope 118:1186–1190.

Curry JM, King N, Reiter D, Fisher K, Heffelfinger RN, Pribitkin EA. 2009. Meta-analysis of surgical techniques for preventing parotidectomy sequelae. Arch Facial Plast Surg 11:327–331.

Darwish HS, Satti KS. 2016. Post-traumatic right paroitd sialocele review of literature with report of a case. JSM Clin Med Imaging Cases Rev 1:1001.

Davis WE, Holt GR, Templer JW. 1977. Parotid fistula and tympanic neurectomy. Am J Surg 133:587–589.

Di Lauro AE, Abbate D, Dell'angelo B, Di Lauro F, Sammartino G. 2010. Treatment of a post surgery defect of the lower lip: A case report. Minerva Stomatol 59:663–669.

Dulguerov P, Marchal F, Gysin C. 1999a. Frey syndrome before Frey: The correct history. Laryngoscope 109:1471–1473.

Dulguerov P, Quinodoz D, Cosendai G, Piletta P, Marchal F, Lehmann W. 1999b. Prevention of Frey syndrome during parotidectomy. Arch Otolaryngol Head Neck Surg 125:833–839.

Eisele DW. 1996. Intraoperative electrophysiologic monitoring of the recurrent laryngeal nerve. Laryngoscope 106:443–449.

Eisele DW, Wang SJ, Orloff LA. 2010. Electrophysiologic facial nerve monitoring during parotidectomy. Head Neck 32:399–405.

Ellis E, 3rd, Dean J. 1993. Rigid fixation of mandibular condyle fractures. Oral Surg Oral Med Oral Pathol 76:6–15.

Ersek RA. 1991. Transplantation of purified autologous fat: A 3-year follow-up is disappointing. Plast Reconstr Surg 87:219–227, discussion 28.

Filho WQ, Dedivitis RA, Rapoport A, Guimaraes AV. 2004. Sternocleidomastoid muscle flap preventing Frey syndrome following parotidectomy. World J Surg 28:361–364.

Frey L. 1923. Le syndrome du nerf auriculo-temporal. Rev Neurol 2:97–104.

Gillespie MB. 2018. Combined Parotid Techniques. Atlas Oral Maxillofac Surg Clin North Am 26:133–143.

Golding-Wood PH. 1962. Tympanic neurectomy. J Laryngol Otol 76:683–693.

Govindaraj S, Cohen M, Genden EM, Costantino PD, Urken ML. 2001. The use of acellular dermis in the prevention of Frey's syndrome. Laryngoscope 111:1993–1998.

Guntinas-Lichius O, Eisele DW. 2016. Facial nerve monitoring. Adv Otorhinolaryngol 78:46–52.

Hald J, Andreassen UK. 1994. Submandibular gland excision: Short- and long-term complications. ORL J Otorhinolaryngol Relat Spec 56:87–91.

Hancock BD. 1999. Clinically benign parotid tumours: Local dissection as an alternative to superficial parotidectomy in selected cases. Ann R Coll Surg Engl 81:299–301.

Hou J, Chen L, Wang T et al. 2014. A new surgical approach to treat medial or low condylar fractures: The minor parotid anterior approach. Oral Surg Oral Med Oral Pathol Oral Radiol 117:283–288.

House JW, Brackmann DE. 1985. Facial nerve grading system. Otolaryngol Head Neck Surg 93:146–147.

Hyde N, Manisali M, Aghabeigi B, Sneddon K, Newman L. 2002. The role of open reduction and internal fixation in unilateral fractures of the mandibular condyle: A prospective study. Br J Oral Maxillofac Surg 40:19–22.

Iro H, Zenk J, Escudier MP et al. 2009. Outcome of minimally invasive management of salivary calculi in 4,691 patients. Laryngoscope 119:263–268.

Jansen S, Jerowski M, Ludwig L, Fischer-Krall E, Beutner D, Grosheva M. 2017. Botulinum toxin therapy in Frey's syndrome: A retrospective study of 440 treatments in 100 patients. Clin Otolaryngol 42:295–300.

Kim MG, Kim SG, Lee JH, Eun YG, Yeo SG. 2008. The therapeutic effect of OK-432 (picibanil) sclerotherapy for benign neck cysts. Laryngoscope 118:2177–2181.

Koch M, Kunzel J, Iro H, Psychogios G, Zenk J. 2014. Long-term results and subjective outcome after gland-preserving treatment in parotid duct stenosis. Laryngoscope 124:1813–1818.

Kornblut AD, Westphal P, Miehlke A. 1974. The effectiveness of a sternomastoid muscle flap in preventing post-parotidectomy occurrence of the Frey syndrome. Acta Otolaryngol 77:368–373.

Kreyden OP, Scheidegger EP. 2004. Anatomy of the sweat glands, pharmacology of botulinum toxin, and distinctive syndromes associated with hyperhidrosis. Clin Dermatol 22:40–44.

Laccourreye O, Bernard D, de Lacharriere O, Bazin R, Brasnu D. 1993. Frey's syndrome analysis with biosensor. A preliminary study. Arch Otolaryngol Head Neck Surg 119:940–944.

Lawrence GW, Ovsepian SV, Wang J, Aoki KR, Dolly JO. 2013. Therapeutic effectiveness of botulinum neurotoxin A: Potent blockade of autonomic transmission by targeted cleavage of only the pertinent SNAP-25. Neuropharmacology 70:287–295.

Lee YC, Park GC, Lee JW, Eun YG, Kim SW. 2016. Prevalence and risk factors of sialocele formation after partial superficial parotidectomy: A multi-institutional analysis of 357 consecutive patients. Head Neck 38(Suppl 1):E941–E944.

Lee CC, Chan RC, Chan JY. 2017. Predictors for Frey syndrome development after parotidectomy. Ann Plast Surg 79:39–41.

Linder TE, Huber A, Schmid S. 1997. Frey's syndrome after parotidectomy: A retrospective and prospective analysis. Laryngoscope 107:1496–1501.

Maharaj S, Mungul S, Laher A. 2020. Botulinum toxin A is an effective therapeutic tool for the management of parotid sialocele and fistula: A systematic review. Laryngoscope Investig Otolaryngol 5:37–45.

Manisali M, Amin M, Aghabeigi B, Newman L. 2003. Retromandibular approach to the mandibular condyle: A clinical and cadaveric study. Int J Oral Maxillofac Surg 32:253–256.

Mantsopoulos K, Goncalves M, Iro H. 2018. Transdermal scopolamine for the prevention of a salivary fistula after parotidectomy. Br J Oral Maxillofac Surg 56:212–215.

Mantsopoulos K, Goncalves M, Koch M, Traxdorf M, Schapher M, Iro H. 2019. Going beyond extracapsular dissection in cystadenolymphomas of the parotid gland. Oral Oncol 88:168–171.

Marcus AJ, Nasser NA. 1998. Case report: The treatment of a chronic parotid cutaneous fistula by the injection of a solution of lipiodol with cyanoacrylate. Clin Radiol 53:616–618.

McGurk M, Thomas BL, Renehan AG. 2003. Extracapsular dissection for clinically benign parotid lumps: Reduced morbidity without oncological compromise. Br J Cancer 89:1610–1613.

Milton CM, Thomas BM, Bickerton RC. 1986. Morbidity study of submandibular gland excision. Ann R Coll Surg Engl 68:148–150.

Minor V. 1927. Ein neues Verfahren zu der klinischen Unter schung der Schweissabsonderung. Dtsch Z Nervenheilkd 101:302.

Motamed M, Laugharne D, Bradley PJ. 2003. Management of chronic parotitis: A review. J Laryngol Otol 117:521–526.

Motz KM, Kim YJ. 2016. Auriculotemporal syndrome (Frey Syndrome). Otolaryngol Clin North Am 49:501–509.

Murty GE, Diver JP, Kelly PJ, O'Donoghue GM, Bradley PJ. 1994. The Nottingham system: Objective assessment of facial nerve function in the clinic. Otolaryngol Head Neck Surg 110:156–161.

Nahlieli O. 2009. Advanced sialoendoscopy techniques, rare findings, and complications. Otolaryngol Clin North Am 42:1053–1072, Table of Contents.

Nahlieli O. 2017. Complications of traditional and modern therapeutic salivary approaches. Acta Otorhinolaryngol Ital 37:142–147.

Nahlieli O, Neder A, Baruchin AM. 1994. Salivary gland endoscopy: A new technique for diagnosis and treatment of sialolithiasis. J Oral Maxillofac Surg 52:1240–1242.

Neumann A, Rosenberger D, Vorsprach O, Dazert S. 2011. The incidence of Frey syndrome following parotidectomy: Results of a survey and follow-up. HNO 59:173–178.

New GB, Bozer HE. 1922. Hyperhydrosis of the cheek associated with the parotid region. Minn Med 5:652–657.

Nocon CC, Cohen MA, Langerman AJ. 2016. Quality of neck dissection operative reports. Am J Otolaryngol 37:330–333.

Oliveira DT, Consolaro A, Freitas FJ. 1993. Histopathological spectrum of 112 cases of mucocele. Braz Dent J 4:29–36.

O'Neill JP, Condron C, Curran A, Walsh A. 2008. Lucja Frey--historical relevance and syndrome review. Surgeon 6:178–181.

Pesic Z, Buric N, Vuckovic I et al. 2011. Use of 2-Octyl-Cyanoacrylate in surgical closing of Postparotidectomy salivary fistulas. Eur Arch Otorhinolaryngol 268:1691–1694.

Pinski KS, Roenigk Jr, HH. 1992. Autologous fat transplantation. Long-term follow-up. J Dermatol Surg Oncol 18:179–184.

Powell ME, Clairmont AA. 1983. Complications of parotidectomy. South Med J 76:1109–1112.

Preuss SF, Klussmann JP, Wittekindt C, Drebber U, Beutner D, Guntinas-Lichius O. 2007. Submandibular gland excision: 15 years of experience. J Oral Maxillofac Surg 65:953–957.

Prichard AJ, Barton RP, Narula AA. 1992. Complications of superficial parotidectomy versus extracapsular lumpectomy in the treatment of benign parotid lesions. J R Coll Surg Edinb 37:155–158.

Re Cecconi D, Achilli A, Tarozzi M et al. 2010. Mucoceles of the oral cavity: A large case series (1994-2008) and a literature review. Med Oral Patol Oral Cir Bucal 15:e551–e556.

Ross BG, Fradet G, Nedzelski JM. 1996. Development of a sensitive clinical facial grading system. Otolaryngol Head Neck Surg 114:380–386.

Rouyer J. 1859. Note sur l'ephidrose parotidienne. Journal de la Physiologie de l'homme et des animaux 2:447–449.

Sanabria A, Kowalski LP, Bradley PJ et al. 2012. Sternocleidomastoid muscle flap in preventing Frey's syndrome after parotidectomy: A systematic review. Head Neck 34:589–598.

Schapher M, Koch M, Agaimy A, Goncalves M, Mantsopoulos K, Iro H. 2019. Parotid pleomorphic adenomas: Factors influencing surgical techniques, morbidity, and long-term outcome relative to the new ESGS classification in a retrospective study. J Craniomaxillofac Surg 47:1356–1362.

Shi D, Patil PM, Gupta R. 2015. Facial nerve injuries associated with the retromandibular transparotid approach for reduction and fixation of mandibular condyle fractures. J Craniomaxillofac Surg 43:402–407.

Springborg LK, Moller MN. 2013. Submandibular gland excision: Long-term clinical outcome in 139 patients operated in a single institution. Eur Arch Otorhinolaryngol 270:1441–1446.

Sugerman PB, Savage NW, Young WG. 2000. Mucocele of the anterior lingual salivary glands (glands of Blandin and Nuhn): Report of 5 cases. Oral Surg Oral Med Oral Pathol Oral Radiol Endod 90:478–482.

Sultan MR, Wider TM, Hugo NE. 1995. Frey's syndrome: Prevention with temporoparietal fascial flap interposition. Ann Plast Surg 34:292–296, discussion 96-7.

Sumi M, Yamada T, Takagi Y, Nakamura T. 2007. MR imaging of labial glands. AJNR Am J Neuroradiol 28:1552–1556.

Terris DJ, Tuffo KM, Fee Jr, WE. 1994. Modified facelift incision for parotidectomy. J Laryngol Otol 108:574–578.

Terzis JK, Noah ME. 1997. Analysis of 100 cases of free-muscle transplantation for facial paralysis. Plast Reconstr Surg 99:1905–1921.

Tugnoli V, Marchese Ragona R, Eleopra R et al. 2002. The role of gustatory flushing in Frey's syndrome and its treatment with botulinum toxin type A. Clin Auton Res 12:174–178.

Turner M, Jahangiri L, Ship JA. 2008. Hyposalivation, xerostomia and the complete denture: A systematic review. J Am Dent Assoc 139:146–150.

Uyar Y, Caglak F, Keles B, Yildirim G, Salturk Z. 2011. Extracapsular dissection versus superficial parotidectomy in pleomorphic adenomas of the parotid gland. Kulak Burun Bogaz Ihtis Derg 21:76–79.

Vesnaver A, Gorjanc M, Eberlinc A, Dovsak DA, Kansky AA. 2005. The periauricular transparotid approach for open reduction and internal fixation of condylar fractures. J Craniomaxillofac Surg 33:169–179.

Walvekar RR, Razfar A, Carrau RL, Schaitkin B. 2008. Sialendoscopy and associated complications: A preliminary experience. Laryngoscope 118:776–779.

Wang SJ, Eisele DW. 2012. Parotidectomy--Anatomical considerations. Clin Anat 25:12–18.

Wang S, Li L, Chen J et al. 2016. Effects of free fat grafting on the prevention of Frey's syndrome and facial depression after parotidectomy: A prospective randomized trial. Laryngoscope 126:815–819.

Wille-Bischofberger A, Rajan GP, Linder TE, Schmid S. 2007. Impact of the SMAS on Frey's syndrome after parotid surgery: A prospective, long-term study. Plast Reconstr Surg 120:1519–1523.

Winkel R, Overgaard TI, Balle VH, Charabi S. 2000. Surgical results of submandibular gland excision. Ugeskr Laeger 162:5354–5357.

Witt RL. 2002. The significance of the margin in parotid surgery for pleomorphic adenoma. Laryngoscope 112:2141–2154.

Witt RL. 2009. The incidence and management of siaolocele after parotidectomy. Otolaryngol Head Neck Surg 140:871–874.

Yamasoba T, Tayama N, Syoji M, Fukuta M. 1990. Clinicostatistical study of lower lip mucoceles. Head Neck 12:316–320.

Zhang L, Xu H, Cai ZG et al. 2010. Clinical and anatomic study on the ducts of the submandibular and sublingual glands. J Oral Maxillofac Surg 68:606–610.

Zhao YF, Jia Y, Chen XM, Zhang WF. 2004. Clinical review of 580 ranulas. Oral Surg Oral Med Oral Pathol Oral Radiol Endod 98:281–287.

Zhao YF, Jia J, Jia Y. 2005. Complications associated with surgical management of ranulas. J Oral Maxillofac Surg 63:51–54.

Zhao-xuan Z. 2010. Department of Oral and Maxillofacial Surgery, The Second Hospital of Fuzhou, Fujian Fuzhou 350007, China.; The clinical value of parotid masseter fascia and acellular dermal matrix in prevention of Frey's syndrome after parotidectomy. J Clin Stomatol 1:40–42.

Zhi K, Gao L, Ren W. 2014. What is new in management of pediatric ranula? Curr Opin Otolaryngol Head Neck Surg 22:525–529.

Chapter 19
Innovations in Salivary Gland Surgery

Mark McGurk[1] and Katherine George[2]

[1]Head and Neck Academic Center, Department of Head and Neck Surgery, University College London Hospital, London, UK

[2]Department of Oral and Maxillofacial Surgery, Kings College Hospital NHS Foundation Trust, London, UK

Outline

Minimally Invasive Parotid Gland Surgery
  History of Parotid Surgery
  Minimally Invasive Surgical Approaches to the Parotid Gland
    Partial Superficial Parotidectomy
    Extracapsular Dissection with Extended Option
      ECD Performed for Malignant Parotid Tumors
    Extended ECD
Minimally Invasive Sublingual Gland Surgery
  Sublingual Gland Anatomy
  Diagnosis of Mucocele, Ranula, and Plunging Ranula
  Treatment of Mucocele, Ranula, and Plunging Ranula
    Mucocele
    Simple Ranula in Floor of Mouth
    Plunging Ranula
Minimally Invasive Salivary Gland Surgery with Sialendoscopy
  Imaging Modalities in the Management of Sialolithiasis
    Sialography
    Other Imaging Modalities
  Sialendoscopy
    Basket Retrieval of Stones
    Fragmentation of Stones
      Microforceps
      Laser Lithotripsy
      Intracorporeal Shock Wave Lithotripsy
      Extracorporeal Shock Wave Lithotripsy
    Intraoral Stone Release of Submandibular Gland Hilar Stones
    Combined Open and Endoscopic Removal of Parotid Stones
  Robotic-Assisted Procedures
  Salivary Duct Strictures
    Investigation of Salivary Duct Strictures
    Classification of Salivary Duct Strictures
    Treatment of Salivary Duct Strictures
      Sialendoscopy-Guided Duct Dilatation
      Balloon Dilatation
      Treatment Adjuncts
      Treatment Outcomes of Salivary Duct Dilatation
      Other Treatment Options for Stenoses
Summary
References

Surgery has historically gone through a number of recognizable evolutionary and transformational cycles. Prior to the availability of general anesthesia, surgery had limited application and most hospitals had an operating list running only once a week. Surgery gained more utility as an acceptable treatment modality following the introduction of general anesthesia. This notwithstanding, endotracheal intubation was not introduced until after the second world war, and prior to this, many operations were still performed under spinal or local anesthesia. In the 1950s, the scope of surgery was transformed by the combination of endotracheal intubation, blood replacement, and antibiotics. Surgery was released and the magnitude of operations expanded while surgeons sought the limits of what the patient and public could withstand. In the last three decades, the cycle has changed again with the introduction of specialist practice leading to retrenchment and the development of minimally invasive surgery that maintain and extend standards of surgery. This has had a huge impact in surgery overall but has largely

---

Salivary Gland Pathology: Diagnosis and Management, Third Edition. Edited by Eric R. Carlson and Robert A. Ord.
© 2022 John Wiley & Sons, Inc. Published 2022 by John Wiley & Sons, Inc.
Companion website: www.wiley.com/go/carlson/salivary

passed by the head and neck. This chapter describes innovations in salivary gland surgery with an emphasis on minimally invasive approaches to salivary gland disease.

Minimally Invasive Parotid Gland Surgery

HISTORY OF PAROTID SURGERY

A history of parotid gland surgery helps to explain the general reluctance to embrace minimally invasive procedures. A recognizable form of parotid gland surgery was practiced in the 1920s and 1930s mainly under local anesthesia and by general surgeons. These individuals were true general surgeons with operating lists consisting of amputations, abdominal procedures, and craniotomies. A lump in the parotid gland was of little significance to this generation of surgeons. To compound matters, no classification of parotid gland pathology had been devised. The parotid gland lumps were pleomorphic in consistency and thought to be hamartomas rather than neoplasms. Consequently, wide excision was not contemplated. Rather an incision was made directly over the surface of the lump that was then enucleated and frequently ruptured. Parotid tumors have a mean time to recurrence of approximately 10 years so it took time for the recurrence to be appreciated. It was only in 1933 when McFarland recognized this phenomenon. By the 1940–1950s, parotid gland surgery was becoming a niche subject and a small coterie of surgeons, Janes in Canada, Hamilton Bailey in London, and Redon in Paris, took up the challenge to contrive a new surgical approach to the parotid gland. They used the facial nerve as a plane of dissection (Janes 1940; Bailey 1947). This nerve divided the parotid gland into a superficial and deep lobe and so the superficial and total parotidectomy procedures were born. The adoption of the surgical technique was slow but received added momentum by the work of Patey and Thackray (1957) who reported tumors in the parotid gland to have an incomplete capsule. This was a ready explanation for the high rate of recurrence prevalent at the time. The superficial and total parotidectomies gave the tumor a wide berth and the adoption of this technique coincided with a reduced incidence of recurrent disease. Superficial parotidectomy was adopted universally and became the standard of care internationally. This situation would still pertain but for one surgeon in Mr. Nicholson of the Christie Hospital in Manchester (Gleave et al. 1979). He was practicing in the 1940s and 1950s and held the opinion that the high risk of recurrence was not due to the incomplete tumor capsule but rather to the lack of access available with the incision made directly over the lump. By contrast, he used a different surgical approach that consisted of first exposing the parotid gland followed by making a cruciate incision over the lump. The lump was then removed carefully with a thin cuff of surrounding normal parotid tissue. Nicholson believed that wide exposure with improved access was the defining factor limiting recurrence. Stated differently, one needed wide exposure of the gland in order to perform a successful superficial parotidectomy. He had maintained meticulous records and had very few recurrent tumors. Consequently, he did not switch to the now accepted nerve dissection procedure but continued with extracapsular dissection (ECD). The analysis of over 600 cases showed conclusively that extracapsular dissection was a safe procedure with recurrence rates similar to superficial parotidectomy but with much less morbidity (McGurk et al. 1996). Four meta-analyses now confirm Nicholson's impression (Albergotti et al. 2012; Foresta et al. 2014; Xie et al. 2015; Martin et al. 2020). The cause of recurrence was not the biological nature of the tumor, for example incomplete capsule, but rather an inappropriate surgical approach. The argument for persisting with superficial parotidectomy versus ECD cannot be based on reducing the risk of recurrent disease.

MINIMALLY INVASIVE SURGICAL APPROACHES TO THE PAROTID GLAND

Partial superficial parotidectomy and extracapsular dissection are based on fundamentally different principles. Superficial parotidectomy is essentially a nerve dissection technique; the parotid gland is exposed in its entirety, the facial nerve trunk is identified and the dissection proceeds along the epineurial surface of the nerve, filleting the superficial lobe of the parotid from the underlying nerve structures. It is not widely appreciated that the facial nerve and its branches are supported by a dense network of interlacing tiny fibers that are lost in this dissection. The exposure of the nerve consequently carries a degree of morbidity in terms of nerve injury (permanent 1%; temporary 25–30%), and a significant incidence of Frey syndrome (Bron and O'Brien 1997; Koch et al. 2010; Stathopoulos et al. 2018; Zheng et al. 2019). In contrast, extracapsular dissection focuses attention on the tumor rather than the facial nerve, the latter being assessed by continuous facial nerve monitoring. The philosophy of these procedures differs significantly, and surgeons find it difficult to shift between the two and hence align with one procedure or the other. Regardless of the exact minimally invasive parotid surgery being performed, attention to holograms is useful to visualize the relationship of the tumor to the facial nerve (Videos 19.1 and 19.2).

Video 19.1. Hologram demonstrating the relationship of a tumor of the parotid gland and the facial nerve.

Video 19.2. Hologram demonstrating the relationship of a tumor of the parotid gland and the facial nerve.

Partial Superficial Parotidectomy

This procedure is an adaption to the superficial parotidectomy. It became apparent to surgeons who regularly performed superficial parotidectomies that at times a lump was in a position where not all of the superficial lobe of the parotid had to be sacrificed, but only a portion of the superficial lobe (Poncet et al. 1991). This is typically the case for lumps 2–3 cm in the tail of the parotid or those in the superficial aspect of the gland. The approach is identical to that for a superficial parotidectomy. A preauricular incision leads to exposure of the parotid gland and dissection then proceeds in the pre-tragal area to identify the main trunk of the facial nerve. The technique is reviewed in Chapter 10. Once the main trunk is identified, it is traced forward to the pes anserinus where the upper and lower divisions of the facial nerve are identified. The lower branch coursing toward the tail of the parotid is then followed, releasing a smaller V-shaped portion of parotid tissue that encompasses the lump rather than the whole superficial lobe. As in the case of superficial parotidectomy, a skirt of normal tissue can remain attached to the tumor but not always on its deep surface. In approximately 60% of cases, the lump sits on a branch of the facial nerve that has to be dissected from the tumor capsule (the bare area). In the tail of parotid, once the triangle of parotid tissue is removed, the ideal situation is to suture the remaining parotid fascia to the sternocleidomastoid muscle producing a seal that minimizes the risk of Frey syndrome and also retains normal facial contour. This is not easy to accomplish if segments are taken from the middle of the parotid gland. The parotid fascia is fixed to the underlying parotid tissue and is difficult to approximate the two edges of the resection to form a seal. The procedure is not as versatile as ECD, but in selected cases, it produces results comparable to extracapsular dissection. As long as the parotid fascia can be closed, there is only a limited risk of Frey syndrome and minimal change in facial contour, and because most of the facial nerve is not exposed, there is a reduced risk of temporary nerve injury (Roh et al. 2007; Li et al. 2020). In these circumstances, partial superficial parotidectomy is a reasonable alternative to extracapsular dissection.

Extracapsular Dissection with Extended Option

As with partial superficial parotidectomy, every opportunity should be taken to establish that the lump in question is in fact a benign tumor. Clinical examination and history are important and can tease out the majority of malignant lumps. The addition of ultrasound and fine needle aspiration reduces the risk of encountering a low-grade malignant tumor to less than 1%. Low-grade malignant tumors, however, do masquerade as benign lumps. This is particularly the case with small lumps (<1cm) that have not had time to express their clinical features (surgeons by reflex choose a small simple lump when starting a new technique). It is always an embarrassment to have a lump reported unexpectedly as a low-grade mucoepidermoid or acinic cell carcinoma rather than a pleomorphic adenoma. It is recommended that these small lumps be routinely removed with a margin of approximately 1cm of normal parotid tissue to avoid this situation (see Video 19.3). The ECD technique can be used but with blunt dissection taking place peripheral to the tumor. This approach leaves a soft tissue deficit, which in the tail of the parotid can be masked by suturing the platysma and sternocleidomastoid muscles to the remaining tail of the parotid. The defect is more apparent in the preauricular area. This defect can be closed by mobilizing the parotid gland ("Extended ECD") and suspending the tail of the parotid gland superiorly. An alternative is to rotate a small sternocleidomastoid muscle flap into the defect to retain a normal facial contour.

Video 19.3. Extracapsular dissection for treatment of a small parotid tumor.

The technique of extracapsular dissection has been reported previously (Chapter 10). In principle, this procedure consists of a preauricular incision that is normally much less than that required for a superficial parotidectomy as only the area around the lump needs to be exposed. The skin flap is raised to expose an area of parotid gland at least 1 cm peripheral to the lump. Tumors in the superficial lobe that are easily palpable and just below the fascia can then be approached through a cruciate incision where the intersection is gripped by four artery clips that elevate the fascia off the lump and allows the incision to be safely made (Figures 19.1a and b). It is emphasized that this relieving incision must extend at least 1 cm past the periphery of the lump. The basic technique is one of blunt dissection. This procedure, familiar to all parotid surgeons, is frequently used in the superficial parotidectomy when identifying the main trunk of the facial nerve. A rule that ensures safety is that parotid tissue cannot be divided unless one can see through the tissues lying between the blades of the scissors. Careful hemostasis is maintained at all times. As indicated above, continuous facial nerve monitoring is used to warn of the presence of the facial nerve although the nerve is usually easily identified by visual inspection. As the leaves of the cruciate are lifted upwards and backwards on the artery clips, the periphery of the tumor is dissected in normal parotid tissue 1 or 2 mm peripheral to the lump. The mass slowly rises out of the parotid gland. Dissection should proceed around the lump picking the easiest areas to dissect at any one time. Branches of the facial nerve running under the lump are preserved, those running over the lump are freed and laid to the side while the dissection proceeds as normal (see Video 19.4).

Video 19.4. Extracapsular dissection for treatment of a large parotid tumor. Source: Directed by Mark McGurk.

ECD Performed for Malignant Parotid Tumors

McGurk et al. (2003) investigated the utility and outcomes of performing ECD for clinically benign tumors of the parotid gland that later proved to be malignant based on final histopathology of the specimen. In doing so, these authors reviewed 821 parotid specimens where the surgical strategy was established on clinical grounds rather than fine aspiration cytology of the parotid lump. ECD was executed for simple lumps, defined clinically as lumps that were discrete, mobile, and smaller than

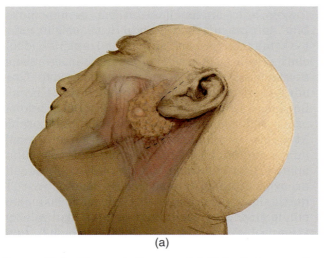
(a)

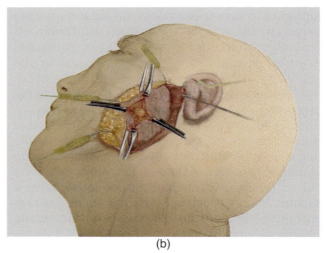
(b)

Figure 19.1. Tumors in the superficial lobe that are easily palpable and just below the fascia (a) can then be approached through a cruciate incision where the intersection is gripped by four artery clips that elevate the fascia off the lump and allows the incision to be safely made (b).

4 cm in diameter, and therefore classified as clinically benign. The authors identified 662 simple lumps, of which 503 were operated with ECD and 159 were operated with superficial parotidectomy. Thirty-two (5%) of the 503 simple lumps proved to be malignant tumors on final histopathology, with seven mucoepidermoid carcinomas, 1 acinic cell carcinoma, 1 adenoid cystic carcinoma, and 3 other carcinomas diagnosed. Twelve of these 32 malignant tumor patients had undergone ECD and 20 of these 32 malignant tumor patients had undergone superficial parotidectomy. Two patients undergoing ECD for malignant tumors realized a positive margin on final histopathology while no patients realized a positive margin following superficial parotidectomy for malignant tumors. Seven of 12 ECD patients and 12 of 20 superficial parotidectomy patients underwent postoperative radiation therapy. The 5-year and 10-year cancer-specific survival rates were 100% for ECD and 98% for superficial parotidectomy. Local recurrences developed in one patient who underwent ECD and five patients who underwent superficial parotidectomy. The authors concluded that ECD is a scientifically valid and oncologically safe approach to the management of the clinically benign parotid lump. Additional studies with larger numbers of patients are required to validate the conclusion of this study.

Extended ECD

It is inappropriately suggested that the basic ECD procedure is not compatible with large tumors or those that lie in the deep lobe or are wedged between the mastoid process and the mandible (Quer et al. 2016, 2017). It is not widely appreciated that the parotid gland is a mobile structure. Once the skin flap has been raised to expose the tumor, the parotid gland can be released from its attachments that include the pre-tragal tissues, the mastoid process and along its attachment to the sternocleidomastoid muscle. The plane of the deep cervical fascia is very apparent on the muscle surface and can be followed over the edge of the sternocleidomastoid and down its deep surface until the accessory nerve is encountered. This defines the depth of the dissection. Every head and neck surgeon will be familiar with this procedure as it is routine in neck dissection. The freeing of the fascia from the mastoid process and sternocleidomastoid muscle allows the parotid tail to be lifted so the posterior belly of the digastric can be exposed and the parotid must be released off its surface. The final point of attachment is the tail of the parotid to the platysma muscle that is subsequently divided. At this point, the parotid gland can be rotated anteriorly which lifts the parotid tissue that is wedged between the mastoid and the mandible into view. The tumor is now superficial and can be approached by a cruciate incision across its surface (Figure 19.2a and b). Similarly, lumps on the deep aspect of the parotid gland and sitting on the digastric muscle may be approached by lifting the tail up and a cruciate incision is then made on the deep surface of the parotid gland over the lump (see Video 19.5). In many instances, the lump then falls out without the facial nerve being seen. Using the two

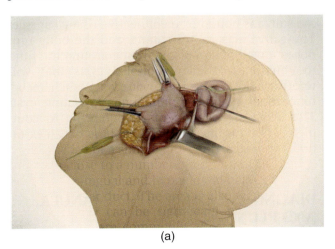
(a)

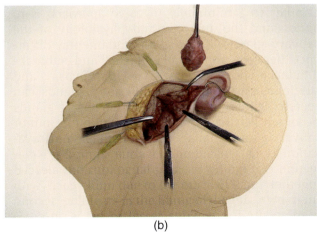
(b)

Figure 19.2. Depiction of the approach to deep parotid tumors where the gland is first released (a) then it is rotated into a position that gives the easiest access to the tumor by splitting the gland over its surface and release it by ECD (b).

approaches (ECD and the extended procedure), all parotid lumps can be safely delivered while retaining the parotid gland and with minimal risk of temporary injury to the facial nerve. The author has practiced extracapsular dissection exclusively for the last two decades. The results of the last 100 consecutive parotid tumors have been analyzed recently with a temporary nerve injury rate for benign disease of 4%, no recorded Frey syndrome, and no permanent injury in these 100 cases. The extended approach is best explained in Video demonstrations made available in this chapter.

Video 19.5. Extended extracapsular dissection of deep lobe tumor of the parotid gland.

Minimally Invasive Sublingual Gland Surgery

Following the theme of minimally invasive treatment, it is possible for this approach to be applied to the salivary ranula. The pathogenesis of the ranula has not been clearly elucidated or understood which has possibly led to more invasive surgical approaches than are required. The oral extravasation cyst (mucocele, simple, and plunging ranula) can be successfully treated when approached through the oral cavity and without an external incision. This is a real consolation to the patients who are usually affected by this disorder namely children and young adults.

SUBLINGUAL GLAND ANATOMY

The key to a minimally invasive approach is to understand the anatomy and physiology of the salivary glands. There is a fundamental difference between the major (parotid and submandibular) and the minor (submucosa and sublingual gland) in that the minor glands can secrete against pressure while the major glands become obstructed and atrophy. It is the minor salivary glands that are the root cause of extravasation cysts. The sublingual gland is simply a collection of 15–30 minor salivary glands coalesced together into a discernible structure, each with their own duct (ducts of Ranvier). The second prerequisite for an extravasation cyst is an environment of loose connective tissue into which the saliva can flow. Extravasation cysts do not develop in the hard palate.

The sublingual gland has been anatomically described in detail by Leppi (1967). It consists of two portions, the greater (tail) and the lesser (head) of the sublingual gland. The head is visible in the anterior mouth and contains the ducts of Ranvier. This portion of the gland is the origin of the simple ranula, and the trigger is probably trauma to a duct of Ranvier. The tail passes along the floor of the mouth and descends toward the submandibular gland. It is not present in approximately 20% of cases. The tail has no connection with the overlying mucosa that can be easily stripped off its surface during a sublingual gland removal. The contrary applies to the lesser portion of the sublingual gland (head). The tail is not usually the cause of simple ranulas.

The trigger for the plunging ranula is unclear. For one reason or another, a leak of saliva develops on the under-surface of the sublingual gland and either collects between it and the mylohyoid muscle or passes through to collect in the submandibular triangle. In the former, there is no swelling or evidence of leak until the patient presses their tongue down into the floor of their mouth when a surprisingly large submental (not submandibular) swelling may appear. The fluid is confined in the compartment between the sublingual gland above and the mylohyoid below, but eventually it will dissect through the fibers of the mylohyoid muscle to track into the submandibular space. On occasion, a dehiscence is evident in the mylohyoid muscle with herniation of the sublingual gland. It is possible that trauma from the muscle could trigger a leak. An important point to appreciate with all the extravasation cysts is that the saliva is bound by a connective tissue capsule. The saliva acts as an irritant, and the body produces a wall of connective tissue around the fluid to contain it. Unlike epithelial cysts that will reform if the lining is not removed, such recurrence does not apply to the extravasation cyst. This releases the surgeon from having to completely remove the sac that would dictate an extra-oral approach.

DIAGNOSIS OF MUCOCELE, RANULA, AND PLUNGING RANULA

The appearance of the mucocele on the lip and a ranula in the floor of the mouth is self-evident. They present as a thin-walled bluish cyst. The saliva produces this blue color. The plunging ranula poses the diagnostic problem. It presents as a diffuse swelling in the submandibular triangle and can be mistaken for a lymphangioma. An ultrasound or MRI scan should show the cyst passing through the mylohyoid muscle, but the diagnosis is confirmed by aspirating a collection of yellow sticking fluid from the cyst cavity (Hills et al. 2016).

TREATMENT OF MUCOCELE, RANULA, AND PLUNGING RANULA

Mucocele

A mucocele on the lower lip does not pose a therapeutic problem. It can be excised under local anesthetic on an ambulatory basis. This is accomplished with an elliptical incision around the cyst followed by careful blunt dissection to remove the sac and attached minor salivary glands. A minor complication is that tiny fibers of the mental nerve run in the submucosal plane. Injury to these fibers, which is common, leaves a small area of altered sensation on the vermilion of the lip. Patients should be warned of these possible sequelae during preoperative informed consent discussions as this complication is difficult to avoid.

Simple Ranula in Floor of Mouth

Simple ranulas can be small and discrete, but if left to persist, they can extend along the floor of mouth toward the posterior margin of the mylohyoid muscle. It has been established that each is developed from a leak of saliva from an associated minor salivary gland (McGurk et al. 2008). Unfortunately, the tract is miniscule and invisible to the naked eye. The literature is replete with suggestions on how to treat these lesions, most based on experience of just a few successful cases. The most predictable way of eliminating a simple ranula in the floor of the mouth is to remove the sublingual gland (Zhao et al. 2005). However, the removal of this gland is not a simple procedure and the dissection runs close to a number of important structures such as the lingual and hypoglossal nerves and the submandibular duct. The area is also well perfused and morbidity can be significant particularly in children who are commonly affected. Sublingual gland removal is the safe salvage procedure, but there are two relatively reliable minimally invasive alternatives to adopt first.

One approach is to identify the site of the leak on the sublingual gland and then seal it (Goodson et al. 2015). This can be accomplished by first aspirating the ranula and then re-evaluating the patient the following day. The cyst starts to reform, and a small blue patch signals the origin of the leak. A suture is placed to suspend the site in question then two or three black silk sutures can be placed through the base to seal the leak. The procedure is acceptable to children of eight and nine years old under local anesthetic (see Video 19.6). The success rate of this technique is approximately 85% and can be repeated if the first attempt fails. This technique is not a reproduction of the historical suture method. The latter simply involves placing black silk suture through the dome of the cyst hoping that a new tract will form. The latter is not very effective. The second approach consists of making two parallel incisions at each end of the cyst then suturing the dome to the floor of the cavity. This in principle forms a permanent conduit for saliva to enter the floor of mouth. There have been initial reports of success with this method (Wang et al. 2016).

Video 19.6. Main suture technique for treatment of a ranula.

Plunging Ranula

The principal impact of the minimally invasive approach to salivary extravasation cysts lies with the plunging ranula. Historically, these lesions have caused confusion as the swelling lies adjacent to the submandibular gland and so it was unclear if the salivary leak arose from the submandibular or the sublingual gland. Some unfortunate patients have had both glands removed. The origin of the salivary leak is the sublingual gland. The key to the plunging ranula, therefore, is the removal of the sublingual gland (see Chapter 4). The surgical procedure is well described in Chapter 4 and need not be repeated in detail. The key is to release the sublingual gland initially by rotating it laterally toward the mandible, then release the tail and free the oral mucosa from its surface. The mucosa covering the head of the sublingual gland is bound tenaciously to the epithelium due to the ducts of Ranvier that in turn leads to tears in the lining of the floor of mouth. Once the head or lesser sublingual component is released, the gland can be lifted free of the floor of mouth and the salivary sac is pulled up into view through the dehiscence in the mylohyoid. A small suction drain is placed into the sac via the oral cavity emerging in the submental region. Only then should the saliva be aspirated from the sac. Once deflated, a suture or clip is placed across its neck of the empty sac. It is then allowed to fall back into the submandibular triangle. Due to perforations in the mucosa, an oral seal is never achieved. If the neck of the sac is not sealed adequately, saliva will trickle from the mouth into the sac and cause a transient but troublesome infection. The result is otherwise very reliable[5] and avoids an extra oral incision in the neck.

Minimally Invasive Salivary Gland Surgery with Sialendoscopy

Salivary gland stones and strictures are the commonest cause of benign obstructive salivary gland disease, which in turn is the commonest reason for salivary gland complaints (Ngu et al. 2007). Other causes include mucus plugs, polyps, foreign bodies, external compression, and anatomical duct anomalies. The submandibular gland is most often affected, representing 80–90% of cases with the remaining 5–10% in the parotid gland. The sublingual gland is affected in less than 1% of cases (Strychowsky et al. 2012).

Approximately 70% of benign obstructive salivary gland disease is caused by stones and characteristic symptoms are meal time syndrome, manifesting as pain and swelling over the affected gland on eating and sometimes accompanied by a salty and unpleasant tasting discharge in the mouth. Typically, sialadenitis follows many months or years of intermittent and recurrent meal time syndrome. The submandibular glands are more commonly affected, with approximately 80% of sialolithiasis occurring in the submandibular glands and 20% in the parotid glands (Bodner 1999; McGurk et al. 2004). It is rare for sialolithiasis to present in the sublingual glands. Salivary calculi tend to be unilateral and although they can occur at any age, they are more common in midlife (Lustmann et al. 1990).

The incidence of symptomatic salivary calculi is estimated to be 59 per million population per annum in the United Kingdom and the prevalence is estimated to be 0.45% (Escudier and McGurk 1999). The cause of sialolithiasis is, as yet unclear but is thought to be related to differences in salivary gland duct anatomy which lead to increased saliva stasis and an altered biochemical composition of saliva, both of which could contribute to the precipitation of calcium and other minerals. It is well documented that stones are more common in the submandibular gland that secretes saliva with a high mucin content and high calcium concentration with flow against gravity. The course of the submandibular duct is long and has an anatomical bend around the free edge of the mylohyoid muscle with saliva stasis being more likely at this site. It is therefore unlikely to be a coincidence that stones are most common in the proximal duct and hilum of the submandibular gland. Harrison et al. (1997) provided evidence of spontaneous micro calculi formation in the salivary gland ducts through calcification of cellular debris and this may also play a role. Marchal et al. (2001) proposed retrograde migration of food, bacteria, or foreign bodies provided a nidus for further calcification. Stones grow in layers with a mineralized central nucleus, surrounded by layers of organic and inorganic matter and bacterial DNA can occasionally be found between them; however, the presence of foreign bodies within stones is uncommon (Teymoortash et al. 2002).

Eighty percent of asymptomatic stones arise in the submandibular gland and the traditional approach to remove those in the proximal duct or hilum of the gland is by sialoadenectomy (McGurk et al. 2004). The risks of submandibular gland removal include permanent marginal mandibular nerve injury (1–8%), hypoglossal nerve injury (3%), and lingual nerve injury (2%) (Strychowsky et al. 2012). Parotid stones are less common but risks of parotidectomy include permanent facial nerve injury (1–3%), sensory loss in the greater auricular nerve distribution (2–100%), and Frey Syndrome (8–33%) (Strychowsky et al. 2012). The advent of micro-endoscopes allowed the examination and instrumentation of the salivary gland ducts and stone removal with techniques adapted from urology was soon to follow (Katz 1991). This enabled more minimally invasive, gland preserving surgery often amenable to treatment in the outpatient department with reduced risk of complications and less time for nonproductive patient recovery. Sialendoscopic management of obstructive salivary gland pathology has been so successful that the incidence of sialadenectomy has reduced to 0–11% (Strychowsky et al. 2012). When sialendoscopy is combined with other minimally invasive therapy, such as lithotripsy or a combined surgical approach, rates of sialadenectomy are reduced to approximately 3% (McGurk et al. 2004; Strychowsky et al. 2012). Furthermore, studies have demonstrated that the secretory function of the gland can recover following removal of the obstruction (Makdissi et al. 2004; Su et al. 2009).

Sialendoscopy has been shown to be an efficacious, safe, and gland preserving option for patients with benign obstructive salivary gland disease on a systematic review and meta-analysis and it is well received by patients (Overton et, al. 2012; Strychowsky et al. 2012; Kroll et al. 2013; Ianovski et al. 2014).

IMAGING MODALITIES IN THE MANAGEMENT OF SIALOLITHIASIS

Ultrasound

Ultrasound provides a quick, simple, and safe method to evaluate the salivary glands in patients with suspected obstructive salivary gland disease and is the most common imaging modality used (Figure 19.3). Sensitivity approaches 100% in series where stones are 3 mm or larger in size, however, sensitivity decreases for stones less than 3 mm in size to 78%. Specificity of ultrasound is in the region of 95%. Fibrotic duct stenosis, phleboliths, arterial vascular calcifications, and calcified lymph nodes may give false positive results (Terraz et al. 2013). When a patient has symptoms of sialolithiasis but the ultrasound is negative for a stone, further imaging should be considered.

Sialography

Sialography is an invasive imaging modality relying on the injection of an iodized contrast agent into the duct. A calculus appears as a filling defect within the duct system and further information relating to duct caliber and stone mobility within the duct can be obtained. A drawback of this technique is that ionizing radiation is required and intraparenchymal stones will not be identified by sialography. Figure 19.4 demonstrates a left submandibular sialogram with filling defect/stone at the proximal end of the main duct.

Other Imaging Modalities

There is less of a role for MR sialography and CT imaging in the diagnosis of sialolithiasis. MR sialography is a noninvasive imaging modality that relies

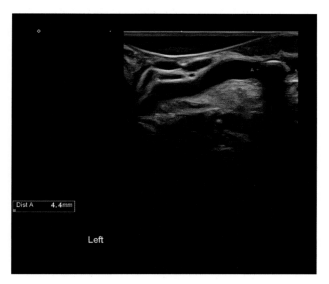

Figure 19.3. Intra-oral ultrasound showing a stone in the distal third of the left submandibular duct, with associated duct dilatation.

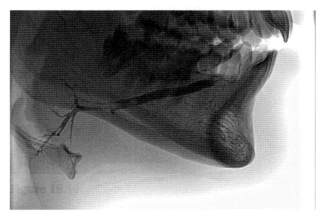

Figure 19.4. Left submandibular sialogram with filling defect/stone at the proximal end of the main duct.

on adequate gland function as the patient's own saliva is used as a natural contrast agent. If gland function is poor, this can compromise images and small stones can be missed (Ibrahim and Badry el 2013). Salivary calculi can also be diagnosed by use of CT; however, the slices must be very fine in order to identify small stones (Figure 19.5).

SIALENDOSCOPY

Sialendoscopy, introduced into clinical practice in the 1990s, allows exploration of almost the entire ductal system by the use of micro-endoscopes

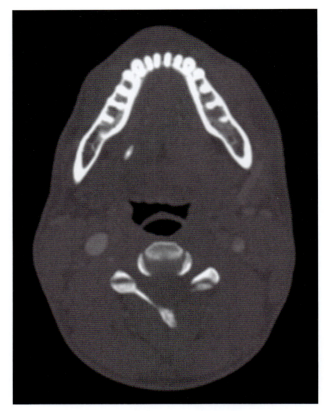

Figure 19.5. CT scan showing a stone just anterior to the right submandibular gland hilum on an axial image.

areas with site-specific sheath designs. Karl Storz salivary endoscopes (El Segundo, California) range in size from 0.8 to 1.6 mm and are autoclavable with the optical fibers fixed within a fine hollow tube containing an irrigation channel. The 1.1, 1.3, and 1.6 mm Karl Storz endoscopes also have a working channel through which baskets or other micro-instruments can be inserted. The advantage of using the smallest sialendoscope is that it is easier to introduce into and manipulate the kinks and bends of the duct and to pass deeper into the duct system. However, micro-endoscope choice is a balance between ease of duct cannulation and the need for a working channel (Figures 19.6–19.8).

Basket Retrieval of Stones

Stones that are smaller than 4–5 mm and that are mobile within the duct can usually be removed by sialendoscopic-assisted basket retrieval as a

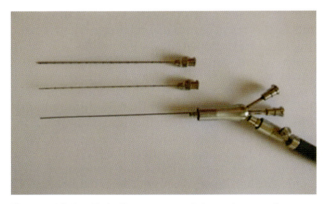

Figure 19.6. Polydiagnost modular micro-endoscope with sheaths of two different sizes.

(Katz 1991). It can be used as a diagnostic for obstructive salivary gland disease, but it is also an effective and safe therapeutic modality which has fundamentally changed the way in which obstructive salivary gland disease is managed by enabling gland preserving treatments (Strychowsky et al. 2012). Sialendoscopy is well suited to the outpatient department and usually carried out under a local anesthetic. Semirigid 0° micro-endoscopes are recommended as they can pass through the kinks and turns in the duct but are easier to handle than flexible endoscopes and have better resolution. Modular systems are available, such as those produced by Polydiagnost (Pfaffenhofen, Germany), where the optical fibers are contained within a single probe that can be sterilized and reused and a disposable front sheath is then applied over the probe to create an irrigation channel. A larger sheath can be selected if a working channel is required. This system has the advantage that the sheath size can be changed during a procedure within seconds, without the need to open a second micro-endoscope. It is a versatile system in that the micro-endoscope can be used in different anatomical

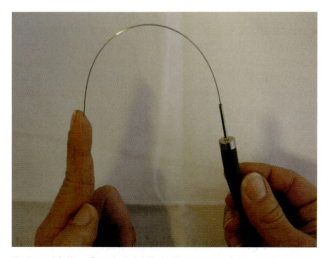

Figure 19.7. Semi-rigid Polydiagnost micro-endoscope.

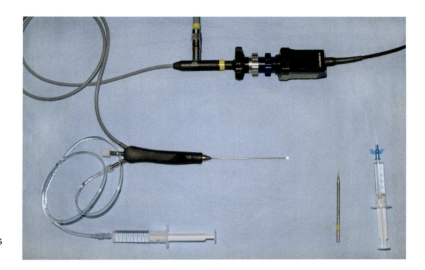

Figure 19.8. Karl Storz micro-endoscopes with working channel.

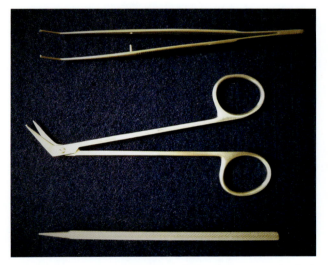

Figure 19.9. Instruments for salivary duct access including Nettleship dilator.

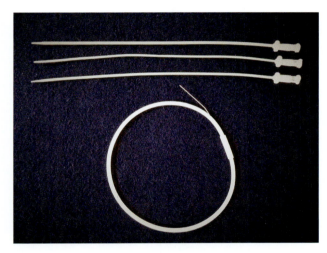

Figure 19.10. Cook Medical salivary duct dilators.

single modality treatment or by radiologically guided techniques with equal success. The size of the stone can be assessed by a preoperative ultrasound scan and the mobility within the duct is evident at sialendoscopy or on sialogram imaging. The procedure is well suited to local anesthetic in the outpatient department. For submandibular duct sialoliths, a lingual nerve block and infiltration of 2% lidocaine with 1:80000 epinephrine at the submandibular duct papilla is administered. For the parotid gland, local anesthetic is injected around the parotid duct papilla. Where stone retrieval is endoscopically assisted, 2% plain lidocaine is flushed through the endoscope during the sialendoscopy to ensure pain control.

The duct is dilated by way of salivary gland dilators in order to facilitate the introduction of the micro-endoscope. There are several dedicated salivary gland dilators available and include salivary probes of increasing size and rigidity, hollow bougies of increasing size which allow duct dilatation via a Seldinger technique or the use of a Nettleship dilator (Katena Products, Inc., Parsippany, New Jersey) to widen the duct orifice. If a Nettleship dilator is used care needs to be taken not to create a false passage that is more likely if the tip of the Nettleship is very sharp (Figure 19.9). Cook Medical (Bloomington, Indiana) have produced a single use salivary dilator system which uses a Seldinger technique; accessing the duct with a wire and then introducing flexible serial dilators, less likely to traumatize the duct, over the wire to gradually dilate the duct (Figure 19.10). Whichever method is selected, once duct access is achieved, the micro-endoscope can then be introduced. In order to maintain duct access a Kolenda introducer sheath (Cook Medical, Bloomington, Indiana) can be used to maintain access to the salivary gland duct for the duration of the procedure (Figure 19.11 and Video 19.7). This is particularly helpful when the micro-endoscope needs to be inserted and removed repeatedly during the procedure, for example, when more than one stone is present or intracorporeal stone fragmentation techniques are used.

Video 19.7. Kolenda introducer used to maintain access to the salivary duct as part of sialendoscopy.

Once the sialendoscope has been introduced into the duct, irrigation is required in order to inflate and examine the duct lumen. Isotonic saline is used throughout the procedure once the duct has been anesthetized. It is important to note that the size of a salivary calculus cannot be accurately determined through the micro-endoscope because of optical distortion. The size of the stone must be determined by the preoperative ultrasound scan. Stones smaller than 4 mm can be retrieved by basket in most cases as the submandibular duct will usually stretch by up to 50% to accommodate passage of the stone and the basket (Figure 19.12). There are a variety of baskets that have been designed for salivary stone retrieval that may be selected for use (Figure 19.13). Some baskets have the ability to open and release the stone once it has been captured (Figure 19.14). This is an advantage where a distal stricture is present or the stone is larger than the duct as there is a risk of impaction of the stone and the basket in these cases. Where nonreleasing baskets are selected, an open approach is usually required to release a basket and stone trapped together in the duct.

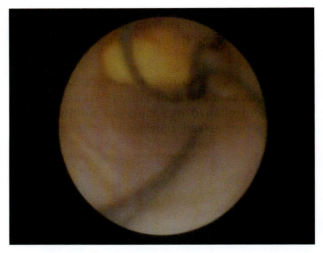

Figure 19.12. Sialendoscopy guided basket retrieval of a stone.

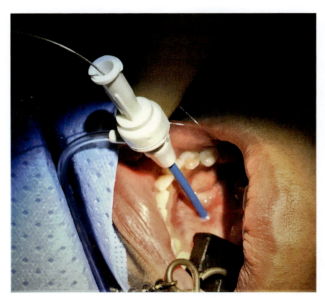

Figure 19.11. Kolenda introducer sheath (Cook Medical) in situ.

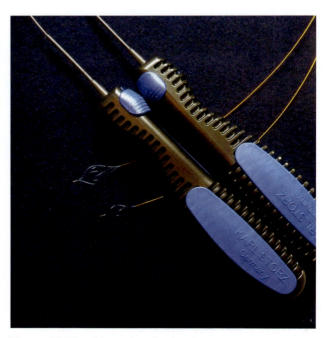

Figure 19.13. Non-releasing baskets.

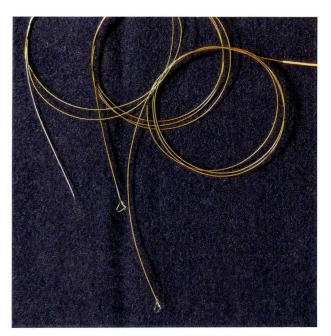

Figure 19.14. Releasing baskets.

Bacteria are often found on the surface of a stone and when manipulated there is an increased risk of sialadenitis. For this reason, a course of antibiotics is prescribed postoperatively for five days. Patients are also advised to keep well hydrated and to stimulate saliva flow by chewing sugar free gum or similar for several weeks following the procedure. Gland massage is also advised.

Radiologically guided techniques to removal stones rely on the use of x-ray fluoroscopy and digital subtraction imaging to demonstrate the position of the stone within the duct and measure its size. The basket is introduced into the duct orifice and advanced toward the stone. This can be visualized on the dynamic radiographic images and once the basket is in position it can be opened and the stone captured. The technique is similar to the sialendoscopy-guided procedure except in the technique used to visualize the stone. Acute sialadenitis is a contraindication for both techniques. An added contraindication for radiologically guided stone retrieval is an allergy to iodine as iodine-based contrast media is commonly utilized, although alternatives are available (Brown et al. 2002).

In a review of 1522 cases of basket or microforceps retrieval of stones, 91.6% were successfully as a sole procedure. Other minimally invasive techniques were employed in those cases that were not successful, achieving a cure of 95.9% of cases (Iro et al. 2009). Complications following basket retrieval of a stone, regardless of the technique used are uncommon. Duct avulsion can occur if a stone is captured in the basket and excessive force is used in the attempt to remove it from the duct; however, this is rare. Secondary strictures are more common and are reported to be in the region of 2–2.45% (Marchal et al. 2000; Nahlieli 2017). Duct perforation can occur if a false passage is created by the endoscope or other instruments used to cannulate or dilate a duct. If this occurs, it is usually best to abort the procedure and allow time for the duct to heal before reattempting the procedure. Postoperative gland swelling is common and usually resolves over 24–48 hours. Ranula formation results from injury to the sublingual gland during the procedure and lies in the region of 1–2.45% (Nahlieli 2017). Lingual nerve paresthesia is rare following sialendoscopy of the submandibular gland and is reported to be between 0.7 and 0.4% (Strychowsky et al. 2012).

Fragmentation of Stones

Intraductal fragmentation is a treatment option for stones that are accessible by sialendoscopy but are larger than 4–5 mm and so cannot be removed by basket alone. Various methods are available and include mechanical fragmentation with microdrills or microforceps and may be guided by ultrasound or sialendoscopy. Extracorporeal shock wave lithotripsy is a method of extra-ductal stone fragmentation and is suitable for large stones that are easily identifiable on ultrasound scan, that cannot be removed by basket and cannot be easily accessed by sialendoscopy.

Microforceps

Microforceps with a diameter of 2 mm can be introduced into the salivary ducts and stones crushed intraductally by ultrasound guidance or sialendoscopy guided. This is a simple and inexpensive technique; however, the duct caliber must be sufficiently wide for passage of the microforceps and this technique is not suitable for stones deep in the gland (Geisthoff and Maune 2010). Smaller forceps measuring 0.8 mm with serrated jaws have been designed for sialendoscopy-guided stone fragmentation.

Laser Lithotripsy

Laser lithotripsy is a method of sialendoscopy-assisted intraductal stone fragmentation. Holmium:

YAG and pulsed dye lasers have both been used. There is a high risk, however of thermal damage to the duct wall and surrounding tissue with the Holmium:YAG laser and copious irrigation with saline is required (McGurk et al. 1994). Success rates with the pulsed dye laser are such that multiple treatment sessions are often necessary which makes it a labor-intensive option (Ito and Baba 1996). Lasers are also very expensive and for these reasons have not gained popularity.

Intracorporeal Shock Wave Lithotripsy

Intracorporeal shock wave lithotripsy is the use of electrohydraulic or pneumatic devices introduced intraductally to fragment stones. Until recently, results were variable and the technique was largely abandoned due to local tissue damage. However, a pneumatic lithotripter (StoneBreaker™, Cook Medical, Bloomington, Indiana) designed specifically for the salivary glands has been developed by adaptation of a pneumatic lithotripter used for fragmentation of renal calculi, with successful fragmentation in 97.7% (Figure 19.15) (Koch et al. 2016). The device is powered by carbon dioxide cartridges, producing a mechanical shock that is transferred as kinetic energy through a salivary probe measuring 0.56 mm in diameter onto the surface of the stone that is accessed through a sialendoscope. Stone fragments pass out of the duct spontaneously, facilitated by gland massage and stimulation of salivary flow with sialagogues or they can be removed by basket (Figure 19.16 and Video 19.8). This technique is suitable for stones that are too large for basket retrieval, but are accessible endoscopically using a sialendoscope with an appropriately sized working channel through which the salivary probe of the lithotripter can be passed. There is a risk of retropulsion of stone fragments and the duct wall can become macerated following fragmentation of immobile stones, tethered to the duct wall. Postoperative follow-up is therefore required with the potential need for further interventional therapy.

Video 19.8. Fragmentation of sialoliths with the pneumatic lithotripter.

Extracorporeal Shock Wave Lithotripsy

Extracorporeal shock wave lithotripsy (ECSWL) for salivary gland stones is another minimally invasive technique adapted from the treatment of renal calculi. Its use for the fragmentation of salivary stones was reported in 1989 by Iro et al. It is a noninvasive method of stone fragmentation and usually no analgesia is required. Multiple treatment sessions are usually required. Pressure waveforms are generated by piezoelectric or electromagnetic techniques depending upon the design of the lithotripter. The shock wave produced passes through a water filled cushion that sits against the skin centered over the target stone. Fragmentation of the stone arises due to the propagation of microcracks inside the stone that arise during stone formation or by the collapse of cavitation bubbles near the stone surface, a process known as erosion (Zhu et al. 2002). Suitable stones are those that are readily identifiable by ultrasound scan and salivary duct strictures that could impede passage of stone fragments must be excluded prior to treatment. Success rates are lower for submandibular gland stones because of the position of the mandible relative the

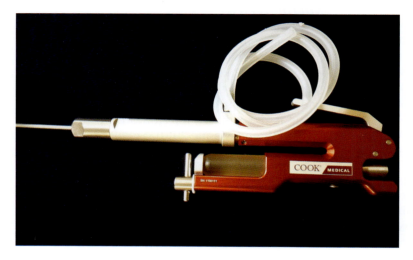

Figure 19.15. Stonebreaker™ (Cook Medical, Bloomington, USA). Source: Cook Medical, Bloomington, USA.

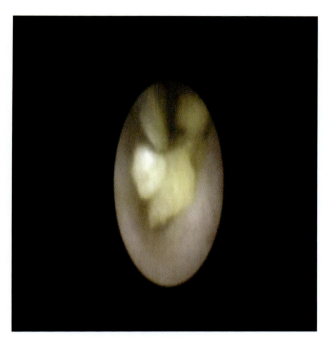

Figure 19.16. Stone fragmentation with Stonebreaker. Source: Cook Medical, Bloomington, USA.

gland and the resultant difficulty in the placement of the water-filled cushion of the lithotripsy device. Approximately, one-third of submandibular gland stones can be successfully treated by ECSWL compared with two-thirds of parotid stones (Iro et al. 1989; Escudier et al. 2003; Zenk et al. 2004).

Intraoral Stone Release of Submandibular Gland Hilar Stones

Most submandibular salivary stones are positioned in the hilum of the gland and sialadenectomy was the treatment of choice for proximal and hiloparenchymal stones before the advent of minimally invasive gland sparing treatment. Complications of sialadenectomy include temporary (23%) or permanent (8%) weakness of the marginal mandibular branch of the facial nerve; temporary (1–2%) or permanent (3%) hypoglossal nerve palsy, temporary (2–6%) or permanent (2%) anesthesia or paresthesia of the lingual nerve. Other complications include hematoma (2–4%), salivary fistulas (1%), sialoceles (1–3%), wound infections (3–8%), hypertrophic scars (2–5%), inflammation caused by residual stones in the Wharton duct (2–8%) (Capaccio et al. 2009).

Transoral stone release is a technique designed for removal of large proximal and hiloparenchymal stones that are not suitable for endoscopic basket retrieval or fragmentation. Ideally, the stone should be palpable intraorally on bimanual palpation of the gland. There is an increased risk of treatment failure when the stone is purely parenchymal and not palpable clinically. The procedure is usually performed under general anesthetic as a day case unless comorbidities prevent such an approach. The patient is positioned supine with the head secured in a head ring. A mouth gag placed on the ipsilateral side and headlight illumination aid surgical access. Local anesthetic (2% lidocaine with 1:80000 epinephrine) is infiltrated along the floor of the mouth, just beneath the oral mucosa and medial to the sublingual gland that can usually be easily identified on retraction of the tongue. A longitudinal incision is made along the floor of the mouth just through the mucosa and then the loose areolar tissue is dissected with sharp scissors. Hemostasis is essential throughout the procedure to aid identification of the lingual nerve and the submandibular duct. The sublingual gland is rotated laterally with the aid of a 3–0 silk suture and the submandibular duct comes into view. The lingual nerve can be seen to pass beneath the Wharton duct as it runs from lateral to medial towards the tongue. The duct is traced proximally as an assistant pushes up on the submandibular gland from an external approach, facilitating palpation of the calculus. Care must be taken to prevent damage to the lingual nerve as it travels medial to the duct and then crosses it superiorly on its pathway to the infratemporal fossa (Figure 19.17). Once the calculus can be easily palpated and, in some cases, seen through the duct wall, an incision is

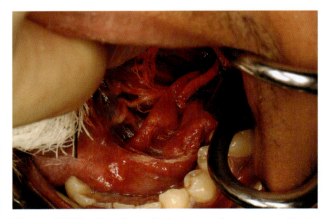

Figure 19.17. Relationship between the submandibular duct and nerve as seen during intra oral stone release procedure for large submandibular hilar-parenchymal stones.

made directly over the duct and the stone is removed. A sialendoscope is then introduced into the hilar opening to wash out the cavity and to examine for residual stone fragments. The distal duct can then be examined endoscopically through the duct ostium. The hilar opening can be closed with resorbable sutures such as a 6–0 Vicryl Rapide (Ethicon, Somerville, New Jersey), left to heal by secondary intention or marsupialized to the floor of the mouth by a duct slitting procedure, thus creating a new gland opening (Zenk et al. 2001; Combes et al. 2009; Witt et al. 2012). Results for this technique are very good with 0.8–4% of patients requiring further treatment with gland removal and a low risk of lingual nerve injury (0–6% permanent paresthesia) (Nahlieli et al. 2007; Combes et al. 2009; Iro et al. 2009; Zhang et al. 2010).

Combined Open and Endoscopic Removal of Parotid Stones

Parotid stones that are not amenable or have been resistant to basket retrieval or stone fragmentation can be removed by a combined endoscopic and open approach, thus avoiding a superficial parotidectomy and its attendant risks (Nahlieli et al. 2002; McGurk et al. 2006; Marchal 2015). In essence, stones treated by this approach are large (greater than 5 mm), fixed to the duct wall or complicated by a distal stricture making an endoscopic approach more difficult. Intraparenchymal stones may also be approached in this fashion.

The procedure is performed under a general anesthetic without muscle relaxants and with continuous facial nerve monitoring. Augmentin antibiotic is given on induction and a five-day postoperative course is prescribed. A sialendoscopic is introduced into the parotid duct ostia following duct dilatation. Once the stone is located the light source on the sialendoscope is turned up to the maximum intensity, and a red light is seen illuminating the skin surface at the sight of the stone. This location is marked on the skin with a surgical marker and the sialendoscope is withdrawn. An alternative is to locate the stone with an ultrasound scan and mark the position on the skin in the same way. Once the location of the stone has been identified, a pre-auricular incision is made, extended behind the ear and then into a skin crease in the neck for a short distance. A flap is then raised on the parotid fascia for approximately 1 cm beyond the position of the stone. The sialendoscope is then reintroduced into the duct and used to identify the position of the stone. Once again, the light on the endoscope stack is intensified and transillumination through the parotid tissue at the site of the stone can be seen (Figure 19.18). This directs dissection through the parotid fascia, followed by blunt dissection through the parotid gland tissue to the level of the parotid duct. The buccal branch of the facial nerve is closely related to the duct and dissection continues on a broad front, to both define the duct and prevent traumatic injury to the nerve. It is not necessary to identify the nerve but it is usually seen at this point in the operation. Once the duct has been adequately defined, it is opened longitudinally with a blade onto the stone which is retrieved by a fine dental excavator. Once removed, the sialendoscope is advanced to examine the rest of the duct system and identify any residual stone fragments. Once the endoscopic examination is complete, a sialodrain can be inserted along the duct to the hilum, secured to the oral buccal mucosa and removed at four weeks. The duct wall is closed over the drain with 6–0 Vicryl sutures. The parotid fascia is then closed as is the subcutaneous tissue and the skin and a pressure dressing applied for 24–48 hours.

In a series of 57 glands, patients were either symptom free or had minimal symptoms that did not require further treatment in 97.5% of cases and there were no documented cases of permanent facial nerve weakness (Overton et al. 2012). Sialoceles occurred in 10% of patients post operatively and were managed by serial aspiration and pressure dressings.

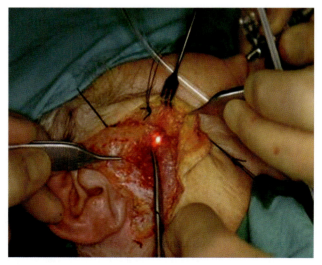

Figure 19.18. Combined endoscopic and open approach for removal of a parotid stone.

Most salivary gland stones (80%) can now be successfully removed by minimally invasive gland preserving surgery leaving a functioning gland intact. These procedures have reduced the need for submandibular gland removal to approximately 3% of cases, and there is never a need to remove a parotid gland for sialolithiasis.

ROBOTIC-ASSISTED PROCEDURES

Robotic-assisted procedures to remove salivary stones are the next advance in the management of benign obstructive salivary gland disease, and reports of the technique have been published for the removal of large submandibular stones in the hilum of the gland (Walvekar et al. 2011; Capaccio et al. 2019). Transoral robotic submandibular sialoadenectomy has also been reported for patients who require submandibular gland removal but will not tolerate a cervical scar or risk of facial nerve paralysis (Capaccio et al. 2020).

SALIVARY DUCT STRICTURES

A salivary duct stricture or stenosis is a narrowing of the salivary duct that impedes the out-flow of saliva. The obstructive symptoms of a stricture are slightly different to that of the obstructive symptoms of sialolithiasis. Most patients with a stricture report intermittent salivary gland swelling present on waking or developing at breakfast. The hypothesis is that as saliva flow decreases at night time, the saliva stagnates behind the stricture and thickens to form a mucus plug, thus obstructing saliva flow. The swelling resolves once saliva flow is stimulated, and the mucus plug is flushed through the stricture. A complaint of an associated "bad taste" in the mouth with a sudden rush of saliva is not uncommon.

Approximately 25% of benign obstructive salivary gland cases are caused by duct strictures, 75% of which arise in the parotid gland (Ngu et al. 2007). Strictures are more common in women but symptoms usually arise in middle age regardless of gender (Ngu et al. 2007). The cause of a stricture is unknown but 40% of cases are associated with other conditions such as salivary stones, allergic reactions within the gland, autoimmune disease, bruxism, previous parotid surgery, and radiotherapy (Koch et al. 2008, 2009). The parotid duct may be more often affected as it is anatomically smaller than the submandibular gland duct and so may be more likely to obstruct even in the case of mild fibrosis.

Minimally invasive salivary therapies have changed the landscape of benign obstructive salivary gland disease management over the last 20 years. Previously, if conservative management failed, as it did in approximately 50% of cases of salivary duct stenoses, gland resection, with all of its attendant risks, was the next step (Moody et al. 2000; Amin et al. 2001). The development of sialendoscopy and minimally invasive salivary gland surgical techniques has made gland preservation possible in over 95% of cases (Koch and Iro 2017a).

Investigation of Salivary Duct Strictures

Ultrasound is the first-line investigation for strictures, although it is the associated duct dilatation that is evident on ultrasound, and not the stricture itself. Stimulation of saliva flow by use of sialogogues, such as vitamin C drops, assists detection of a stricture by enhancing duct dilatation (Bozzato et al. 2009). If further imaging is required other options include conventional sialography, MR sialography, CT or cone-beam CT sialography, or sialendoscopy.

Conventional sialography relies on the injection of water-soluble contrast media into the salivary duct that is imaged by use of serial radiographs with or without digital subtraction. Imaged in this way, strictures are evidenced by filling defects within the ductal system and are diagnosed with a high sensitivity (Ngu et al. 2007). Care must be taken to avoid infiltration of air into the duct as air bubbles appear as signal voids that can be confused with sialoliths on the resultant images. Sialography can also be coupled with MRI, CT or cone-beam CT images thus offering three-dimensional views of the duct anatomy.

A disadvantage of conventional sialography as well as CT and cone beam CT (CBCT) sialography is the need for radiation exposure. This is not the case for sialography coupled with MRI. In addition, saliva acts as a natural contrast agent in MR sialography, allowing the duct anatomy to be easily evaluated on heavily T2-weighted images thus avoiding the need for duct cannulation. MR sialography can also be carried out in the presence of acute sialadenitis which is not the case for sialography requiring contrast or sialendoscopy. Citric acid can also be used to stimulate salivary flow, enhancing the image and giving an indication of gland function (Capaccio et al. 2008). The limitations of MRI sialography include cost and accessibility.

Sialendoscopy has the advantage of being both a diagnostic and therapeutic tool and allows treatment of inflammatory strictures by endoscopic irrigation with sterile saline and infiltration of intraductal steroids. Fibrous strictures can be also be managed by sialendoscopic duct dilatation using balloons, baskets, or microdrills.

Classification of Salivary Duct Strictures

Strictures have been classified by their appearance on sialography or sialendoscopy. Ngu et al. (2007) retrospectively reviewed over 1300 sialograms taken over a 10-year period for patients with symptoms of salivary obstruction. A stricture was diagnosed as the cause of obstruction in approximately 200 cases, 2/3 of which were point strictures, 1/3 multiple and 7% were bilateral. Most strictures occurring in the parotid duct were in the middle third of the main duct (41%) and most submandibular strictures were in the proximal-hilar region (70%) (Ngu et al. 2007). The findings were in contrast to a case series of 153 submandibular duct stenoses examined by sialendoscopy and published by Koch et al. (2012b). In this series, most Wharton duct stenoses were fibrous (87.3%) and at the papilla or distal duct (62.7%) (Koch et al. 2012a).

A sialendoscopy-based classification system of parotid stenoses has been published by Koch and Iro (2017b) initially describing the sialendoscopic appearance in 111 stenoses and subsequently 550 stenoses, they describe 3 types of stenosis (Koch et al. 2009; Koch and Iro 2017b). Type 1 is characterized by the appearance of inflammatory changes at the site of the stenosis (8.9%), type 2 have an abnormal duct system with web-like changes and megaduct (19.5%), and type 3 are fibrotic with diffuse duct wall involvement that result in high-grade luminal narrowing (71.6%). Multiple stenoses were found in 2.8% and bilaterally in 11.9%. Most were located in the distal or middle duct and approximately 80% were short segments (Koch and Iro 2017b). Kopeć et al. (2013) divided stenoses of Stensen duct into 3 segments: the papilla and distal part of the duct; the middle and the hilum. They used the measurements on the shaft of the sialendoscope to measure the exact position of the stricture and also found that stenoses of the distal and middle duct were more common (Kopeć, et al. 2013). Marchal et al. (2008) introduced a classification system of salivary stones and stenosis based on the presence of lithiasis, stenosis, or dilatation (LSD classification) also taking into account the site, number, and severity of the stenosis but patient numbers were not published.

Treatment of Salivary Duct Strictures

Conservative treatment by way of gland massage, good hydration, and stimulation of salivation with sialagogues may be all that is required for a patient who has minimal symptoms and no treatment is an option if the patient is asymptomatic with or without signs of gland atrophy. However, minimally invasive treatments are available and effective at managing symptomatic cases of duct stenoses with gland preservation possible in over 95% of cases (Nahlieli et al. 2001; Papadaki et al. 2008; Koch et al. 2012b; Kopeć et al. 2013).

Sialendoscopy-Guided Duct Dilatation

Sialendoscopically guided duct dilatation is routinely carried out under local anesthetic in the outpatient department in a similar way to basket retrieval of a stone. Local infiltration of 2% lidocaine with epinephrine 1:80000 close to the salivary gland papilla is performed and in the case of the submandibular gland, a lingual nerve block can also be considered. The duct orifice is then dilated to allow the introduction of the sialendoscope, and this can be achieved by the use of a Nettleship dilator (Katena Products, Inc., Parsippany, New Jersey) or lacrimal probe. An alternative option is the use serial salivary duct dilators introduced via a Seldinger technique. A guide wire is inserted into the duct, and salivary duct dilators of increasing size are passed over the wire until the sialendoscope can be easily passed into the duct. Using these dilator sets to blindly dilate, a duct stricture is not recommended as this approach could easily lead to a duct perforation. If a perforation of the duct occurs, there is little risk of permanent harm. However, it is best to abort the procedure and wait until the duct has healed before repeating the procedure. Once, the sialendoscope has been successfully inserted the duct system can be explored and the stricture examined with the aid of duct irrigation with sterile saline or local anesthetic.

The act of irrigation alone can be an effective way of dilating the duct. This is particularly true if the stenosis is inflammatory in nature and in this case infiltration of steroid is recommended. Dexamethasone, 3.3 mg is used and infiltrated through the endoscope directly into the duct. If the stricture is fibrotic; as in type 2 and type 3 strictures; baskets, microdrills and balloons can be used (Nahlieli et al. 2001; Koch et al. 2008). When a basket is selected, it is inserted into the fibrotic stricture and opened in order to distend the wall. A microdrill is a handheld device of two different sizes. The smallest size is usually the best for strictures, and the largest for stone fragmentation. The tip of the microdrill is inserted into the stricture and gently turned in order to cut the fibrotic tissue and open the stenosis. Point strictures tend to spring open suddenly when dilated in this way.

Balloon Dilatation

Balloon dilatation of salivary strictures was first reported in 1992 by use of an angioplasty balloon under sialographic guidance (Buckenham et al. 1992). Angioplasty balloons are still commonly used for balloon dilatation of salivary gland strictures; however, dedicated high pressure balloons designed specifically for the treatment of salivary duct stenosis have been developed. Cutting balloons can also be used, which have small microtomes on the surface which cut the fibrous tissue of a noninflammatory stricture as it inflates, thus encouraging dilatation. High-pressure balloons are favored over low-pressure ones as they are less likely to burst and sterile saline is the inflation medium of choice as it is harmless should it come into contact with the tissues. Balloon choice is also influenced by the gland being treated and balloons of a smaller diameter are chosen for dilatation of a parotid stricture and balloons larger in diameter for dilatation of a submandibular stricture. Once correctly positioned within the stricture the balloon is inflated to pressures of 10 bar for 1–3 minutes (Figures 19.19–19.21). Balloons can be used under ultrasound guidance, sialography, or sialendoscopy, but in all cases, care needs to be taken to ensure that the balloon does not displace during the procedure. The disadvantage of sialography-guided duct dilatation is the need for radiation exposure. In addition, the stricture can only be examined by indirect visualization and so diagnostic information is lost when compared to sialendoscopy guided duct dilatation.

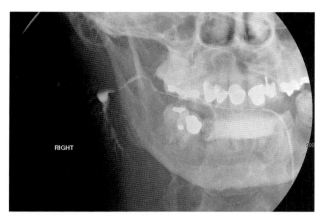

Figure 19.19. Right parotid sialogram showing a stricture at the mid-distal part of the main duct.

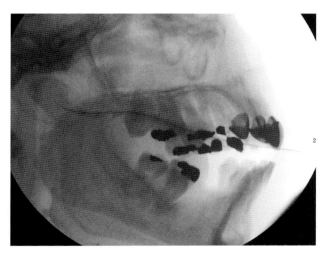

Figure 19.20. Right parotid sialogram with guide wire and inflated balloon in situ during sialography guided duct dilatation.

Treatment Adjuncts

Once dilatation is complete, a polyurethane stent may be placed. These stents are available in a variety of lengths and diameters and can be guided into place with a sialendoscope or under ultrasound guidance. They have a tendency to fall out, unless secured to the oral mucosa with sutures. If used, they are usually left in situ for several weeks as healing progresses and they are normally well-tolerated by the patient.

Many centers advocate the use of intraductal steroids as part of sialendoscopy-guided duct dilatation (Nahlieli et al. 2001; Kopeć et al. 2013; Koch et al. 2008, 2014). This has been supported by a prospective study comparing the outcomes of

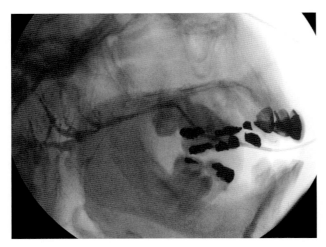

Figure 19.21. Sialogram following sialography guided duct dilatation for a right parotid stricture.

patients who received intraductal steroids as part of sialendoscopy-guided treatment with those that did not. Improved outcomes were reported when steroids had been given (Capaccio et al. 2017).

Regardless of the technique, postoperative inflammation of the tissues and local swelling can be sufficient to occlude the duct temporarily and it is not uncommon for patients to complain of obstructive symptoms during this time. Encouragement of oral fluid intake, a soft diet, and anti-inflammatory medications are helpful during the healing process. Once healing has progressed, patients are encouraged to maintain good hydration and stimulate salivary flow with sialogogues. Antibiotics are not usually prescribed following minimally invasive duct dilatation procedures.

Treatment Outcomes of Salivary Duct Dilatation

When sialendoscopy-guided, stricture dilatation is considered successful when a 1.1 mm sialendoscope can pass along the duct with ease. If the procedure has been carried out under radiographic control success is gauged by a postoperative sialogram taken to assess the degree of dilatation obtained. Results of sialography-guided balloon duct dilatation published in the literature are good, with success characterized by partial or complete opening of the stricture reported in over 80% of cases (Drage et al. 2002; Brown 2006). Success rates for sialendoscopy-guided duct dilatation are consistently 80% or greater, with some studies quoting 100% success for dilatation of parotid duct stenosis (Koch et al. 2008, 2012a, Papadaki et al. 2008; Kopeć et al. 2013). Furthermore, greater than 95% of patients avoid the need for gland removal (Nahlieli et al. 2001; Kopeć et al. 2013; Koch et al. 2014, 2012a).

Successful dilatation is more likely in younger patients with a shorter history of obstructive symptoms presenting with a point strictures without significant associated ductal dilatation (Brown 2002). This seems to support the hypothesis that type 1 inflammatory strictures may be a precursor to type 3 and more responsive to treatment with more conservative treatments such as steroid infiltration before development of a fibrotic type 3 stenosis. Type 2, low-grade, short stenoses associated with an abnormal duct system may also respond to more conservative methods of management such as irrigation and gland massage (Koch and Iro 2017b). Stricture recurrence has been reported in between 10 and 47% of cases, the reason for which is unknown, although it may be related to postoperative inflammation (Brown 2006; Drage et al. 2002; Koch et al. 2014). However, they usually respond to repeat duct dilatation (Koch et al. 2014). Despite this symptomatic improvement is the norm in the majority of cases and unrelated to the type of stenosis present (Koch et al. 2014). It is presumed that this is because the gland becomes nonfunctional over time as a result of chronic obstruction (Drage et al. 2002; Koch et al. 2014).

Other Treatment Options for Stenoses

Duct dilatation procedures are not the only option for management of symptomatic duct stenosis. In the case of the submandibular gland, a stricture of the distal Wharton duct may be better managed by a papillotomy or duct slitting. Koch et al. (2012b) published a series of 153 stenoses of the submandibular duct, most affecting the distal third and bilateral involvement documented in 8.6% of cases. They recommended papillotomy or duct incision procedures for distal stenoses and interventional sialendoscopy for more centrally located stenoses. Submandibular gland preservation rates were reported to be 97.8%. This is not the case in the parotid as papillotomy characteristically leads to stricture formation resistant to treatment (Cohen 2003; Koch et al. 2008). A megaduct can also result as a complication of a distal parotid stricture and is the result of proximal duct dilatation as a response to the increase in pressure caused by the obstruction. They are a very uncommon but troublesome sequelae of a stricture at the parotid papilla as the duct dilatation is visible, looking like a sausage lying in the cheek, just under the skin. Treatment options include duct dilatation and long-term stent placement, botulinum toxin injections into the gland to reduce salivation or surgery to over-sew the duct.

In cases of treatment failure, botulinum toxin injections into the affected gland have been successful in achieving symptomatic relief by inhibiting salivation (Ellies et al. 2004). Duct ligation can be considered where other treatments have failed; however, success rates of only 50% have been reported (Baurmash 2004). Alpha blockers are used successfully in urology for the management of stenoses and one study has shown good results, with 80% of patients noting significant improvement in symptoms, when used for salivary gland stenoses resistant to treatment (Guerre et al. 2010). However, in the absence of duct dilatation the usual course of events is for glandular function to reduce in the presence of a stricture and as this occurs the symptoms reduce.

Summary

- Head and neck surgery has been slow to embrace the introduction of minimally invasive and other innovative procedures.
- Both the partial superficial parotidectomy and extracapsular dissection are a contribution in this respect. They have similar outcomes with respect to reduced risk of complications and morbidity.
- Extracapsular dissection is a very versatile surgical technique. New impetus has been given to the choice of surgical technique by our recent breakthroughs in the imaging of the facial nerve with holograms.
- Holograms permit tracing the facial nerve through the parotid tissue while observing its relationship to the tumor. Without this modality, the surgeon has to adapt blindly to situations evolving during surgery, whereas now the operator can identify the most appropriate direction to approach the tumor and deliver it down a path that does not encompass or may only minimally approach branches of the facial nerve. The information produced by the new imaging modalities and the ability to project them in 3D in a hologram gives the surgeon the opportunity to move away from a standard approach to facial nerve dissection.
- It is now accepted that these parotid tumors can be dissected safely in a plane of normal parotid tissue close to the periphery of the tumor (1 or 2 mm) and surgery can be designed around the tumor and not the facial nerve.
- Minimally invasive salivary therapies, centered on sialendoscopy, have changed the management of benign obstructive salivary gland disease.
- Gland preservation is now possible in the majority of cases of benign obstructive salivary gland disease treated with sialendoscopy with the need for sialadenectomy reduced to 4.6% (Atienza and López-Cedrún 2015).
- The specific technique employed for salivary gland stone retrieval is dictated by the site and size of the stone within the intra- or extra-glandular ducts with more than one approach often being required based on established treatment algorithms (Koch et al. 2009).
- A combination of minimally invasive therapies might be required to best manage individual cases of salivary obstructive disease and treatment algorithms have been developed to aid clinicians in treatment planning (Koch et al. 2009).

References

Albergotti WG, Nguyen SA, Zenk J, Gillespie MB. 2012. Extracapsular dissection for benign parotid tumours: A meta-analysis. *Laryngoscope* 122:1954–1960.

Amin MA, Bailey BMW, Patel SR. 2001. Clinical and radiological evidence to support superficial parotidectomy as the treatment of choice for chronic parotid sialadenitis: A retrospective study. *Br J Oral Maxillofac Surg* 39(5):348–352.

Atienza G, López-Cedrún JL. 2015. Management of obstructive salivary disorders by sialendoscopy: A systematic review. *Br J Oral Maxillofac Surg* 53(6):507–519.

Bailey H. 1947. Parotidectomy: Indications and results. *Br Med J* 1(4499):404–407.

Baurmash HD. 2004. Chronic recurrent parotitis: A closer look at its origin, diagnosis, and management. *J Oral Maxillofac Surg* 62(8):1010–1018.

Bodner L. 1999. Parotid sialolithiasis. *J Laryngol Otol* 113(3):266–267.

Bozzato A, Hertel V, Bumm K, et al. 2009. Salivary simulation with ascorbic acid enhances sonographic diagnosis of obstructive sialadenitis. *J Clin Ultrasound* 37(6):329–332.

Bron LP. O'Brien CJ. 1997. Facial nerve function after parotidectomy. *Arch Otolaryngol Head Neck Surg* 123:1091–1096.

Brown JE. 2002. Minimally invasive techniques for the treatment of benign salivary gland obstruction: A review. *Cardiovasc Intervent Radiol* 25(5):345–351.

Brown JE. 2006. Interventional Sialography and minimally invasive techniques in benign salivary gland obstruction. *Semin Ultrasound CT MR* 27(6):465–475.

Brown JE, Drage NA, Escudier MP, et al. 2002. Minimally invasive radiologically guided intervention for the treatment of salivary calculi. *Cardiovasc Intervent Radiol* 25(5):352–355.

Buckenham TM, Page JE, Jeddy T. 1992. Technical report: interventional sialography – Balloon dilatation of a Stensen's duct stricture using digital subtraction sialography. *Clin Radiol* 45(1):34.

Capaccio P, Cuccarini V, Ottaviani F, et al. 2008. Comparative Ultrasonographic, magnetic resonance Sialographic, and Videoendoscopic assessment of salivary duct disorders. *Ann Otol Rhinol Laryngol* 117(4):245–252.

Capaccio P, Torretta S, Pignataro L. 2009. The role of Adenectomy for salivary gland obstructions in the era of Sialendoscopy and lithotripsy. *Otolaryngol Clin N Am* 42(6):1161–1171.

Capaccio P, Torretta S, di Pasquale D, et al. 2017. The role of interventional sialendoscopy and intraductal steroid therapy in patients with recurrent *sine causa* sialadenitis: A prospective cross-sectional study. *Clin Otolaryngol* 42(1):148–155.

Capaccio P, Montevecchi F, Meccariello G, et al. 2019. Transoral robotic surgery for Hilo-parenchymal submandibular stones: Step-by-step description and reasoned approach. *Int J Oral Maxillofac Surg* 48(12):1520–1524.

Capaccio P, Montevecchi F, Meccariello G, et al. 2020. Transoral robotic submandibular sialadenectomy: How and when. *Gland Surgery* 9(2):423–429.

Cohen D. 2003. Surgery for prolonged parotid duct obstruction: A case report. *Otolaryngol Head Neck Surg* 128(5):753–754.

Combes J, Karavidas K, McGurk M. 2009. Intraoral removal of proximal submandibular stones – An alternative to sialadenectomy? *Int J Oral Maxillofac Surg* 38(8):813–816.

Drage NA, Brown JE, Escudier MP, et al. 2002. Balloon dilatation of salivary duct strictures: Report on 36 treated glands. *Cardiovasc Intervent Radiol* 25(5):356–359.

Ellies M, Gottstein U, Rohrbach-Volland S, et al. 2004. Reduction of salivary flow with botulinum toxin: Extended report on 33 patients with drooling, salivary fistulas, and Sialadenitis. *Laryngoscope* 114(10):1856–1860.

Escudier MP, McGurk M. 1999. Symptomatic sialoadenitis and sialolithiasis in the English population, an estimate of the cost of hospital treatment. *Br Dent J* 186(9):463–466.

Escudier MP, Brown JE, Drage NA, McGurk M. 2003. Extracorporeal shockwave lithotripsy in the management of salivary calculi. *Br J Surg* 90(4):482–485.

Foresta E, Torroni A, Di Nardo F, et al. 2014. Pleomorphic adenoma and benign parotid tumors: Extracapsular dissection vs superficial parotidectomy – Review of literature and meta-analysis. *Oral Surg Oral Med Oral Pathol Oral Radiol* 117:663–676.

Geisthoff UW, Maune S. 2010. Ultrasound-guided mechanical fragmentation of sialoliths (sonoguide forceps). *Head Neck* 32(12):1641–1647.

Gleave EN, Whittaker JS, Nicholson A. 1979. Salivary tumours – Experience over thirty years. *Clin Otolaryngol* 4:247–257.

Goodson AM, Payne KF, George K, McGurk M. 2015. Minimally invasive treatment of oral ranulae: Adaption to an old technique. *Br J Oral Maxillofac Surg* 53(4):332–335.

Guerre A, Hartl D-M, Katz P. 2010. Les Alpha-1-Bloquants (alfuzosine) en pathologie salivaire obstructive. *Rev Stomatol Chir Maxillofac* 111(3):135–139.

Harrison JD, Epivatianos A, Bhatia SN. 1997. Role of microliths in the aetiology of chronic submandibular sialadenitis: A clinicopathological investigation of 154 cases. *Histopathology* 31(3):237–251.

Hills A, Holden A, McGurk M. 2016. Evolution of the management of ranulas: Change in a single surgeon's practice 2001–2014. *Br J Oral Maxillofac Surg* 54(9):992–996.

Ianovski I, Morton RP, Ahmad Z. 2014. Patient-perceived outcome after sialendoscopy using the Glasgow benefit inventory. *Laryngoscope* 124(4):869–874.

Ibrahim NMA, Badry A. 2013. Diagnostic accuracy of MR sialography in sialolithiasis and salivary ductal stenosis. *Egypt J Radiol Nucl Med* 44(1):45–50.

Iro H, Nitsche N, Schneider HT, Ell C. 1989. Extracorporeal shockwave lithotripsy of salivary gland stones. *Lancet* 334(8654):115.

Iro H, Zenk J, Escudier MP, et al. 2009. Outcome of minimally invasive management of salivary calculi in 4,691 patients. *Laryngoscope* 119(2):263–268.

Ito H, Baba S. 1996. Pulsed dye laser lithotripsy of submandibular gland salivary calculus. *J Laryngol Otol* 110(10):942–6.

Janes RM. 1940. Treatment of tumours of the salivary glands by radical excision. *Can Med Assoc J* 43(6): 554–559.

Katz P. 1991. Endoscopy of the salivary glands. *Ann Radiol (Paris)* 34:110–113.

Koch M, Iro H. 2017a. Salivary duct stenosis: Diagnosis and treatment. *Acta Otorhinolaryngol Ital* 37:132–141.

Koch M, Iro H. 2017b. Extended and treatment-oriented classification of parotid duct stenosis. *Laryngoscope* 127(2):366–371.

Koch M, Iro H, Zenk J. 2008. Role of Sialoscopy in the treatment of Stensen's duct strictures. *Ann Otol Rhinol Laryngol* 117(4):271–278.

Koch M, Zenk J, Iro H. 2009. Algorithms for treatment of salivary gland obstructions. *Otolaryngol Clin N Am* 42(6):1173–1192.

Koch M, Iro H, Zenk J. 2009. Sialendoscopy-based diagnosis and classification of parotid duct stenoses. *Laryngoscope* 119(9):1696–1703.

Koch M, Zenk J. Iro H. 2010. Long-term results of morbidity after parotid gland surgery in benign disease. *Laryngoscope* 120:724–730.

Koch M, Iro H, Klintworth N, et al. 2012a. Results of minimally invasive gland-preserving treatment in different types of parotid duct stenosis. *Arch Otolaryngol Head Neck Surg* 138(9):804.

Koch M, Iro H, Künzel J, et al. 2012b. Diagnosis and gland-preserving minimally invasive therapy for Wharton's duct stenoses. *Laryngoscope* 122(3):552–558.

Koch M, Künzel J, Iro H, et al. 2014. Long-term results and subjective outcome after gland-preserving treatment in parotid duct stenosis. *Laryngoscope* 124(8):1813–1818.

Koch M, Mantsopoulos K, Schapher M, et al. 2016. Intraductal pneumatic lithotripsy for salivary stones with the StoneBreaker: Preliminary experience. *Laryngoscope* 126(7):1545–1550.

Kopeć T, Szyfter W, Wierzbicka M, Nealis J. 2013. Stenoses of the salivary ducts-sialendoscopy based diagnosis and treatment. *Br J Oral Maxillofac Surg* 51(7):e174–e177.

Kroll T, Finkensieper M, Sharma SJ, et al. 2013. Short-term outcome and patient satisfaction after sialendoscopy. *Eur Arch Otorhinolaryngol* 270(11):2939–2945.

Leppi TJ. 1967. Gross anatomical relationships between primate submandibular and sublingual salivary glands. *J Dent Res* 46:359–365.

Li C, Matthies L, Hou X, et al. 2020. A meta-analysis of the pros and cons of partial superficial parotidectomy versus superficial parotidectomy for the treatment of benign parotid neoplasms. *J Craniomaxillofac Surg*, 48 (2929) 590–598.

Lustmann J, Regev E, Melamed Y. 1990. Sialolithiasis. *Int J Oral Maxillofac Surg* 19: 135–318.

Makdissi J, Escudier MP, Brown JE, et al. 2004. Glandular function after intraoral removal of salivary calculi from the hilum of the submandibular gland. *Br J Oral Maxillofac Surg* 42(6):538–541.

Marchal F. 2015. A combined endoscopic and external approach for extraction of large stones with preservation of parotid and submandibular glands. *Laryngoscope* 125(11):2430–2430.

Marchal F, Becker M, Dulguerov P, Lehmann W. 2000. Interventional Sialendoscopy. *Laryngoscope* 110(2):318.

Marchal F, Kurt A-M, Dulguerov P, Lehmann W. 2001. Retrograde theory in sialolithiasis formation. *Arch Otolaryngol Head Neck Surg* 127(1):66.

Marchal F, Chossegros C, Faure F, et al. 2008. Salivary stones and stenosis. A comprehensive classification. *Rev Stomatol Chir Maxillofac* 109(4):233–236.

Martin, H. Jayasinghe, J. Lowe, T. 2020. Superficial parotidectomy versus extracapsular dissection: Literature review and search for a gold standard technique. *Int J Oral Maxillofac Surg* 49:192–199.

McFarland, J. 1933. Three hundred mixed tumours of the salivary gland of which 69 recurred. *Surg Gynecol Obstet* 63: 457.

McGurk M, Prince MJ, Jiang ZX, King TA. 1994. Laser lithotripsy: A preliminary study on its application for sialolithiasis. *Br J Oral Maxillofac Surg* 32(4):218–221.

McGurk M, Renehan A, Gleave EN, Hancock BD. 1996. Clinical significance of the tumour capsule in the treatment of parotid pleomorphic adenomas. *Br J Surg* 83:1747–1749.

McGurk M, Thomas BL, Renehan AG. 2003. Extracapsular dissection for clinically benign parotid lumps: Reduced morbidity without oncological compromise. *Br J Cancer* 89:1610–1613.

McGurk M, Makdissi J, Brown JE. 2004. Intra-oral removal of stones from the hilum of the submandibular gland: Report of technique and morbidity. *Int J Oral Maxillofac Surg* 33(7):683–686.

McGurk M, MacBean AD, Fan KFM, et al. 2006. Endoscopically assisted operative retrieval of parotid stones. *Br J Oral Maxillofac Surg* 44(2):157–160.

McGurk M, Eyeson J, Thomas B, Harrison JD. 2008. Conservative treatment of oral ranula by excision with minimal excision of the sublingual gland: Histological support for a traumatic aetiology. *J Oral Maxillofac Surg* 66:2050–2057.

Moody AB, Avery CME, Walsh S, et al. 2000. Surgical management of chronic parotid disease. *Br J Oral Maxillofac Surg* 38(6):620–622.

Nahlieli, O. 2017. Complications of traditional and modern therapeutic salivary approaches. *Acta Otorhinolaryngol Ital* 37(2):142–147.

Nahlieli O, Shacham R, Yoffe B, Eliav E. 2001. Diagnosis and treatment of strictures and kinks in salivary gland ducts. *J Oral Maxillofac Surg* 59(5):484–490.

Nahlieli O, London D, Zagury A, Eliav E. 2002. Combined approach to impacted parotid stones. *J Oral Maxillofac Surg* 60(12):1418–1423.

Nahlieli O, Shacham R, Zagury A, et al. 2007. The ductal stretching technique: An endoscopic-assisted technique for removal of submandibular stones. *Laryngoscope* 117(6):1031–1035.

Ngu R, Brown J, Whaites E, et al. 2007. Salivary duct strictures: Nature and incidence in benign salivary obstruction. *Dentomaxillofacial Radiology* 36(2):63–67.

Overton A, Combes J, McGurk M. 2012. Outcome after endoscopically assisted surgical retrieval of symptomatic parotid stones. *Int J Oral Maxillofac Surg* 41(2):248–251.

Papadaki ME, McCain JP, Kim K, et al. 2008. Interventional Sialoendoscopy: Early clinical results. *J Oral Maxillofac Surg* 66(5):954–962.

Patey DH, Thackray AC. 1957. The treatment of parotid tumours in the light of a pathological study of parotidectomy material. *Br J Surg* 45:477–487.

Poncet J, Rondet P, Kossowski M, et al. 1991. Surgery of the parotid gland. Indications. Review of the anatomy. *Ann Radiol* 34(1–2):122–129.

Quer M, Guntinas-Lichius O, Marchal F, et al. 2016. Classification of parotidectomies: A proposal of the European salivary gland society. *Eur Arch Otorhinolaryngol* 273: 3307–3312.

Quer M, Vander Poorten V, Takes RP, et al. 2017. Surgical options in benign parotid tumors: A proposal for classification. *Eur Arch Otorhinolaryngol* 274(11): 3825–3836.

Roh J-L, Kim HS and Park CI. 2007. Randomized clinical trial comparing partial parotidectomy versus superficial or total parotidectomy. *Br J Surg* 94: 1081–1087.

Stathopoulos P. Igoumenakis D. Smith WP. 2018. Partial superficial, superficial and Total parotidectomy in the management of benign parotid gland tumours: A 10-year prospective study of 205 patients. *J Oral Maxillofac Surg* 76:455–459.

Strychowsky JE, Sommer DD, Gupta MK, et al. 2012. Sialendoscopy for the management of obstructive salivary gland disease. *Arch Otolaryngol Head Neck Surg* 138(6):541.

Su Y-X, Xu J-H, Liao G-Q, et al. 2009. Salivary gland functional recovery after sialendoscopy. *Laryngoscope* 119(4):646–652.

Terraz S, Poletti PA, Dulguerov P, et al. 2013. How reliable is sonography in the assessment of Sialolithiasis? *Am J Roentgenol* 201(1):W104–W109.

Teymoortash A, Wollstein AC, Lippert BM, et al. 2002. Bacteria and pathogenesis of human salivary calculus. *Acta Otolaryngol* 122(2):210–214.

Walvekar RR, Tyler PD, Tammareddi N, Peters G. 2011. Robotic-assisted transoral removal of a submandibular megalith. *Laryngoscope* 121(3):534–537.

Wang S, Zhang Z, Yang C. 2016. Clinical evaluation of a two-incision fistula technique for the treatment of oral ranulas. *Br J Oral Maxillofac Surg* 54(1):22–24.

Witt RL, Iro H, Koch M, et al. 2012. Minimally invasive options for salivary calculi. *Laryngoscope* 122(6):1306–1311.

Xie S, Wang K, Xu H, et al. 2015. PRISMA-extracapsular dissection versus superficial parotidectomy in treatment of benign parotid tumors: Evidence from 3194 patients. *Medicine (Baltimore)* 94(34):e1237.

Zenk J, Constantinidis J, Al-Kadah B, Iro H. 2001. Transoral removal of submandibular stones. *Arch Otolaryngol Head Neck Surg* 127(4):432.

Zenk J, Bozzato A, Gottwald F, et al. 2004. Extracorporeal shock wave lithotripsy of submandibular stones: Evaluation after 10 years. *Ann Otol Rhinol Laryngol* 113(5):378–383.

Zhang L, Escudier M, Brown J, et al. 2010. Long-term outcome after intraoral removal of large submandibular gland calculi. *Laryngoscope* 120(5):964–966.

Zhao YF, Jia J, Jia Y. 2005. Complications associated with surgical management of ranulas. *J Oral Maxillofac Surg* 63(1):51–54.

Zheng CY, Cao R, Gao MH, et al. 2019. Comparison of surgical techniques for benign parotid tumours: A multicentre retrospective study. *Int J Oral Maxillofac Surg* 48:187–192.

Zhu S, Cocks FH, Preminger GM, Zhong P. 2002. The role of stress waves and cavitation in stone comminution in shock wave lithotripsy. *Ultrasound Med Biol* 28(5):661–671.

Index

Page locators in **bold** indicate tables. Page locators in *italics* indicate figures. This index uses letter-by-letter alphabetization.

3D-CRT *see* three-dimensional conformal radiation therapy
aberrant glands, 544–545
ABP *see* acute bacterial parotitis
absolute effect measures, 226
ABSS *see* acute bacterial submandibular sialadenitis
ACC *see* adenoid cystic carcinoma
accessory parotid gland (APG)
    hereditary and congenital conditions, 544–545
    tumors of the parotid gland, 304, 314–315
access parasymphyseal mandibulotomy, *316*
acellular dermal matrix, 577–578, *578*
achalasia, 192, *193*
acini
    acinar atrophy, 557
    acinar degeneration, 177, 179
    acinar hyperplasia, 179, 193
    histology of the salivary glands, 14
acinic cell carcinoma
    classification systems for salivary gland tumors, 237, *237*
    molecular biology of salivary gland tumors, 282, 285–287
    radiation therapy for malignant tumors, 436–438, 446–447
    tumors of the minor salivary glands, 414–417, *418*
    tumors of the parotid gland, 302–303, 325, *328*, 330–334
acute bacterial parotitis (ABP), 85–89
    case presentation, 111–114, *112–113*
    diagnosis, 86–87, *87*
    historical context and epidemiology, 85
    treatment, 87–89, *88*, *90–91*
    variants and their etiology, 82, *83–84*, 86
acute bacterial submandibular sialadenitis (ABSS), 98–99
    children and adolescents, 203–206, *205–207*
    etiology and pathophysiology, 98, *98*
    treatment, 99, *99*
acute suppurative parotitis, 206, *206*
adamantinoma-like Ewing sarcoma (ALES), 479
ADC *see* apparent diffusion coefficient
adenocarcinoma
    children and adolescents, 214
    classification systems for salivary gland tumors, 239, *239*
    molecular biology of salivary gland tumors, 283
    radiation therapy for malignant tumors, 436, 440–441
    systemic therapy for salivary gland cancer, 457, 462, *465*
    tumors of the minor salivary glands, 423
    tumors of the parotid gland, 325, 330–333
    tumors of the submandibular and sublingual glands, *351*
adenoid cystic carcinoma (ACC)
    classification systems for salivary gland tumors, 235–236, *236–237*
    diagnostic imaging, 60, *61–62*
    grading and staging of salivary gland tumors, 253
    molecular biology of salivary gland tumors, 277, *278*, 280–283, 285–288
    radiation therapy for malignant tumors, 435–436, 441, 447–449, *449*, 451
    systemic therapy for salivary gland cancer, 456–458, 460
    tumors of the minor salivary glands, 388–389, 400, *401–408*
    tumors of the parotid gland, 302–303, 325, 330–333, *331*

Salivary Gland Pathology: Diagnosis and Management, Third Edition. Edited by Eric R. Carlson and Robert A. Ord.
© 2022 John Wiley & Sons, Inc. Published 2022 by John Wiley & Sons, Inc.
Companion website: www.wiley.com/go/carlson/salivary

adenoid cystic carcinoma (ACC) (*Cont'd*)
　tumors of the submandibular and sublingual
　　glands, 345–346, *348*, 355–370, *360–361*,
　　366–368
adenosquamous carcinoma (ASC), 250
adolescents *see* children and adolescents
adrenergic axons, 15–16
ADT *see* androgen deprivation therapy
airway obstruction, 588, *588*
AJCC *see* American Joint Committee on Cancer
aldosterone, 16
ALES *see* adamantinoma-like Ewing sarcoma
ALS *see* amyotrophic lateral sclerosis
alveolar nerve graft, 519, *522*
American Joint Committee on Cancer (AJCC),
　255–256, **257–259**
amifostine, 532
amyloidosis
　hereditary amyloidosis, 558–559
　primary (AL) amyloidosis, 559
　salivary gland biopsy, 558–560, *559*
　secondary (AA) amyloidosis, 559–560
amyotrophic lateral sclerosis (ALS), 555
anaplastic fibrosarcoma, 389
anaplastic osteosarcoma, 389
anastomosis, 515–520, *517–522*
anatomy, embryology, and physiology, 1–18
　case presentation, 16–17, *17*
　control of salivation, 14–16
　diagnostic imaging, 42–49
　histology of the salivary glands, 14, *15*
　minor salivary glands, 13
　parotid gland, 2–9, *2–9*
　sublingual gland, 13, 606
　submandibular gland, 9–13, *10–12*
　tubarial salivary glands, 13–14
androgen deprivation therapy (ADT), 461
androgen receptor (AR) inhibition, 460–461
angiosarcoma, 479
antibiotics
　acute bacterial parotitis, 87–89, 111–114, *112–113*
　acute bacterial submandibular sialadenitis, 99
　bacterial sialadenitis in pregnancy, 110
　cat-scratch disease, 102
　chronic recurrent submandibular sialadenitis, 99
　sialolithiasis, 150–152
APG *see* accessory parotid gland
aplasia, 543–544

apoptosis, 277–279
apparent diffusion coefficient (ADC), 28–29, *29*
AR *see* androgen receptor
ASC *see* adenosquamous carcinoma
auriculotemporal nerve
　anatomy, embryology, and physiology, 5–6
　complications of salivary gland surgery, 574–578,
　　575–578, **576**
autoimmune parotitis, 148
autoimmune sialadenitis, 110–111
avulsive injury, 510, *511*
　see also duct avulsion

BAFF *see* B-cell activating factor
balloon dilatation, 619, *619–620*
barotrauma, 534–535
Bartholin duct, *584*
Bartonella henselae, 99–102, *103–104*
basal cell adenocarcinoma, 239–240, *239*
basal cell adenoma, 230–231, *230*, 271
basal cell carcinoma, 253
basaloid salivary carcinoma, 479
BAT *see* brown adipose tissue
B-cell activating factor (BAFF), 176, 178
benign lymphoepithelial lesion (BLL)
　classification systems for salivary gland tumors,
　　251–252, *251–252*
　cysts and cyst-like lesions, 130, *131*
　Sjögren syndrome, 177, *177*, 179–180, *179*,
　　181–182
benign mixed tumor *see* pleomorphic adenoma
benign neoplasms
　children and adolescents, 201–202, 208–209
　classification systems for salivary gland tumors,
　　225–234, **227**, *229–233*, 251–253, *251–252*
　complications of salivary gland surgery, 593–596,
　　594–596
　diagnostic imaging, 57–60, *58–59*, 61–64, *62–64*,
　　68, *68–74*
　molecular biology of salivary gland tumors,
　　269–299
　non-salivary tumors of the salivary glands,
　　471–478, *472–478*
　radiation therapy for malignant tumors, 436–438
　tumors of the minor salivary glands, 373–386,
　　375, **377–378**, *380–388*
　tumors of the parotid gland, 301–304, *307*, 308,
　　309–313, 315–325, *316*, *322–324*, *326–327*

tumors of the submandibular and sublingual glands, 345–372
see also individual neoplasms
biofilm, 146
biomarkers
    cellular classification of salivary gland tumors, 226–227
    molecular biology of salivary gland tumors, 285–288, *286*
    non-salivary tumors of the salivary glands, 484
    saliva, 548–554, 560
biopsy/histopathology
    amyloidosis, 558–560, *559*
    children and adolescents, *205*, 214, *215–218*, 219–223, *221–222*
    classification systems for salivary gland tumors, 229–244, 246–253, 259–261, *260–262*
    complications of salivary gland surgery, 593, 596
    hereditary and congenital conditions, *553*
    image-guided biopsies, 35–36, *37*
    IgG4-related disease, 194–195, *197–198*
    Küttner tumor, 561, *563*
    molecular biology of salivary gland tumors, 284–285
    non-salivary tumors of the salivary glands, *477*, 485, *495, 497, 503–504*
    Parkinson disease, 560
    sarcoidosis, 187–192, *191–192*
    sialadenitis, 102–104, *103–104, 106*
    sialolithiasis, *151, 153, 171–172*
    sialosis, 193–194, *194*
    Sjögren syndrome, *179*, 180–185, *183–185*
    systemic therapy for salivary gland cancer, 462, *464–465*
    tumors of the minor salivary glands
        benign tumors, 376–377, *380–382, 384–386*, 388
        malignant tumors, 390–393, *391*, 394–395, *401–402, 405–408*, 410–416, 420, 429–430
    tumors of the parotid gland, 303–308, *305, 307*, 325, *326–329, 331, 336*
    tumors of the submandibular and sublingual glands, *348*, 349, *350*, 351, *352, 356, 362, 367–368*, 369
Blair incision, 571, *572*
Blandin and Nuhn's gland, 127, *127*
BLL *see* benign lymphoepithelial lesion
blunt trauma, *535*
botulinum toxin
    complications of salivary gland surgery, 574–576, **576**, 580
    saliva, 555–556
    traumatic injury to the salivary glands, 512, 515, 523, 528
branchial cleft
    cysts and cyst-like lesions, 130, 348
    hereditary and congenital conditions, 545–548, *547, 549–553*
    tumors of the submandibular and sublingual glands, 348
breast cancer, 302, 375–376
brown adipose tissue (BAT), 38–39, *40*
buccal mucosal tumors, 378–380, **378**, 394–395, *397–398*, 409, *415–416*
bulimia nervosa, 192

cadherins, 280, 287
calcified lymph nodes, 150, *151–152*
cAMP *see* cyclic adenosine monophosphate
cAMP response element binding protein (CREB), 456
CAMSG *see* cribriform adenocarcinoma of minor salivary glands
canalicular adenoma
    classification systems for salivary gland tumors, *230*, 231
    tumors of the minor salivary glands, 386, *386–388*
    tumors of the parotid gland, 302–303
capillary hemangioma, 202
carbon ion therapy, 451
carcinoma ex-pleomorphic adenoma, 219–220
    classification systems for salivary gland tumors, 244–245, *244*
    molecular biology of salivary gland tumors, 283, 285–287
    non-salivary tumors of the salivary glands, *480–481*
    radiation therapy for malignant tumors, 439
    tumors of the minor salivary glands, 379, 385
    tumors of the parotid gland, 308, 334
carcinosarcoma, 385
carotid space (CS), 45
Castleman's disease, 497
cat-scratch disease (CSD), 99–102, *103–104*
CBCT *see* cone beam computerized tomography
CCC *see* clear cell carcinoma
CCOC *see* clear cell odontogenic carcinoma

CD30-positive T-cell lymphoproliferative disorders, 479
cell phones, 302
central mucoepidermoid carcinoma, 397–399, *399*
cerebrospinal fluid (CSF), 25
cerebrovascular accident (CVA), *518*
cervical lymphadenopathy, 196
cevimeline, 532–533
CF *see* cystic fibrosis
CHARGE syndrome, 545, 555
chemotherapy, 455–469
    adjuvant treatment, 457
    androgen receptor inhibition, 460–461
    case presentation, 461–466, *463–465*
    C-Kit inhibition, 458
    clinical presentation, 456–457
    diagnostic imaging, 39–41
    EFGR inhibition, 459
    epidemiology and risk factors, 455–456
    Her2 inhibition, 459–460, 462, 466
    immune checkpoint inhibition, 461
    metastatic disease, 457–458, **458, 460**, *465*
    molecular biology of salivary gland tumors, 274, 456
    multi kinase inhibition, 460
    non-salivary tumors of the salivary glands, 479, 485
    NTRK inhibition, 461
    proteasome inhibition, 460
    radiation therapy for malignant tumors, 441, 449
    Sjögren syndrome, 178
    targeted therapy, 458–461, *459*, **460**
    tumors of the minor salivary glands, 424
    tumors of the parotid gland, 301, 330
children and adolescents, 201–224
    acute submandibular sialadenitis, 203–206, *205–207*
    acute suppurative parotitis, 206, *206*
    bacterial sialadenitis, 203–207
    case presentation, 218–223, *221–222*
    chronic juvenile recurrent parotitis, 206–207, *207*
    epidemiology, 201–202
    epithelial tumors, 208–210
    lymphatic malformations, 211, *213*
    mesenchymal tumors, 201, 210–214, *210–213*
    minor salivary gland tumors, 214–218
    mucous escape reaction, 203
    neoplastic salivary gland disease, 207–218, **208**, *210–213, 215–218*
    neural tumors, 214, *215–216*
    nonneoplastic salivary gland lesions, 202–207, **202**, *204–207*
    parotid tumors, 214
    submandibular tumors, 214
cholelithiasis, 147, 166–168
cholinergic axons, 15–16
chondrosarcoma, 389
chromosomal DNA alterations, 281–283, *282*, 285–287
chronic alcoholism, 192–194
chronic bacterial parotitis, 89–97
    etiology and pathophysiology, 89
    parotidectomy, 89–90, 95–96, 97
    sialendoscopy, 89, *92–94*
    treatment algorithm, *91*
chronic recurrent juvenile parotitis
    etiology and pathophysiology, 97, 206–207, *207*
    treatment, 97–98, 206–207
chronic recurrent submandibular sialadenitis, 99, *100–102*
chronic sialadenitis, 52–53
C-Kit inhibition, 458
clear cell adenocarcinoma, 495–497
clear cell carcinoma (CCC)
    classification systems for salivary gland tumors, 240–241, *240*
    grading and staging of salivary gland tumors, 254–255
    molecular biology of salivary gland tumors, 274
    non-salivary tumors of the salivary glands, 495–497
    tumors of the minor salivary glands, 389
clear cell odontogenic carcinoma (CCOC), 255
clinical treatment volume (CTV), 442, *442*, 447
Clostridium difficile, 83
CNB *see* core needle biopsy
community acquired parotitis, *84, 86*, 88–89
complications of salivary gland surgery, 569–600
    case presentation, 593–596, *594–596*
    concepts and definitions, 570, *570*
    minor salivary gland mucocele removal, 590–591, *590–592*
    parotid gland surgery, 570–583
        auriculotemporal nerve and Frey syndrome, 574–578, *575–578*, **576**
        facial nerve paralysis, 570–573, *571–573*, **572**
        parotid duct leakage, 581–583, *581–583*
        parotid gland salivary leakage, 578–581, *579*

submandibular and sublingual gland surgery, 583–590
  intraoral approach, 584–588, *584–589*
  transcervical approach, 588–590, *589*
computerized tomography angiography (CTA)
  case presentation, 16–17, *17*
  technique, 23
  vascular lesions, 52
computerized tomography (CT)
  acute bacterial parotitis, 83, 87, 89, 90, 111, *112*
  acute bacterial submandibular sialadenitis, 98, *98*
  acute/chronic sialadenitis, 52, *52–53*
  advanced techniques, 24, 42
  artifacts, 23–24
  bacterial sialadenitis in pregnancy, 108, *109*
  benign neoplasms, 57–60, *58–59*, 61–64, *62–63*, 68, *69–70*, 73
  cat-scratch disease, *103*
  children and adolescents, *204, 213, 215, 217*
  chronic bacterial parotitis, *93, 95*
  classification systems for salivary gland tumors, 260–261
  complications of salivary gland surgery, *585*, 594–596
  concepts and definitions, 20
  cysts and cyst-like lesions, *121, 126, 128, 131, 135, 137, 140*
  first branchial cleft cyst, 56–57, *57–58*
  hereditary and congenital conditions, *544, 550*
  HIV-associated lymphoepithelial lesions, 54, *54*
  Hounsfield units, 21–23, **23**
  image-guided biopsies, 35–36, *37*
  IgG4-related disease, *197–198*
  innovations in salivary gland surgery, 609, *610*, 617–618
  malignancies, 60, *60–62*, 64–67, *65–66*
  mucous escape reaction, 54
  mumps, *107*
  non-salivary tumors of the salivary glands, 475–478, *476–477, 480, 486, 489, 491, 494–495, 499, 501–502*
  parotid gland, 42–45, *43–44*
  radiation therapy for malignant tumors, 442, *442*
  sarcoidosis, 56
  sialadenosis/sialosis, 54–55
  sialography, 35
  sialolithiasis, 55, *55–56*, 149, 162, *162, 164–165, 169–170*
  Sjögren syndrome, 55–56, *180–181*
  sublingual gland, 48–49, *48*
  submandibular gland, 45–48, *46–47*
  systemic therapy for salivary gland cancer, *463*
  technique, 20–24, *21–23*
  traumatic injury to the salivary glands, 513, *513*
  tubarial salivary glands, 13
  tumors of the minor salivary glands
    benign tumors, *380–381, 383, 387*
    malignant tumors, 390–393, *391–393, 395, 397–398, 401–408, 409, 413, 419, 426–427*
  tumors of the parotid gland, 304, *305, 309, 317, 319, 325, 326*
  tumors of the submandibular and sublingual glands, 349, *349*, 351, *351, 354, 356–357, 361, 364, 366*
  vascular lesions, 50–52, *50–51*
cone beam computerized tomography (CBCT), 617–618
congenital conditions *see* hereditary and congenital conditions
connective tissue disorders, 29
core needle biopsy (CNB)
  diagnostic imaging, 35–36, *37*
  non-salivary tumors of the salivary glands, 485
  Parkinson disease, 560
  tumors of the parotid gland, 308
  tumors of the submandibular and sublingual glands, 349
corticosteroids, 211, 473
CREB *see* cAMP response element binding protein
cribriform adenocarcinoma of minor salivary glands (CAMSG), 238–239, 255, 409, 503, *504*
cross-validation, 226
CS *see* carotid space
CSD *see* cat-scratch disease
CSF *see* cerebrospinal fluid
CT *see* computerized tomography
CTA *see* computerized tomography angiography
CTV *see* clinical treatment volume
CVA *see* cerebrovascular accident
cyanoacrylate, 581
cyclic adenosine monophosphate (cAMP), 16
cystadenocarcinoma, 241–242, *241*
cystadenoma, 232–233, *232*
cystic fibrosis (CF), 548
cystic hygroma, 475

cysts and cyst-like lesions, 117–143
  branchial cleft cysts, 130
  case presentation, 139–142, *139–142*
  children and adolescents, 203
  hereditary and congenital conditions, 545–548, *546–547, 549–553*
  mucous escape reaction, 117–127, *119–121, 123–127*
  mucous retention cyst, 127, *128–129*
  nomenclature and classification, 117, **118**
  parotid cysts associated with HIV/AIDS, 127–130, *131–135*
  parotid neoplasms masquerading as cysts, 130–138, *136–138*, **136**
  traumatic injury to the salivary glands, 513, *513*
  tumors of the minor salivary glands, 399
  tumors of the parotid gland, 304
  tumors of the submandibular and sublingual glands, 348

dedifferentiated tumors, 389
deep lobe
  anatomy, embryology, and physiology, 11, *12*
  tumors of the parotid gland, 304, 314, *317–318*, 321
demethylation, 283–284
dermal-fat graft (DFG), 578
desmoid melanoma, *482*
DFG *see* dermal-fat graft
diabetes mellitus, 88
diffuse infiltrative lymphocytosis syndrome (DILS), 107, *108*
diffuse large B-cell lymphoma (DLBCL), 178, 483–486
diffusion weighted imaging (DWI), 28–29, *29*
DILS *see* diffuse infiltrative lymphocytosis syndrome
DLBCL *see* diffuse large B-cell lymphoma
Down syndrome, 544
doxycycline, 475
drooling, 554–556
ductal aneurysm, 582–583, *582*, 620–621
ductal papilloma, 233, *233*
duct atresia, 544, *545*
duct avulsion
  complications of salivary gland surgery, 583, 588, *589*
  innovations in salivary gland surgery, 613
ducts of Ranvier, 606
ducts of Rivinus, 122

DWI *see* diffusion weighted imaging
dynamic contrast-enhanced MRI, 30
dysphagia, 446

EAPS *see* ectopic accessory parotid gland system
EBV *see* Epstein-Barr virus
ECA *see* external carotid artery
ECD *see* extracapsular dissection
ectopic accessory parotid gland system (EAPS), 544–545
EDX *see* X-ray diffraction analysis
EGFR *see* epidemal growth factor receptor
EIA *see* enzyme immunoassay
elective nodal irradiation (ENI)
  radiation therapy for malignant tumors, 439, *440*, 441
  tumors of the parotid gland, 333
EMC *see* epithelial-myoepithelial carcinoma
ENE *see* extranodal extension
enhanced cellular proliferation, 276–277, *278*
ENI *see* elective nodal irradiation
environmental carcinogens, 456
enzyme immunoassay (EIA), 102
EPE *see* extraparenchymal extension
epidermal growth factor receptor (EGFR)
  molecular biology of salivary gland tumors, 277, *278*, 287–288, *289*
  systemic therapy for salivary gland cancer, 456, 459
epigenetic alteration of gene expression, 283–284, 287
epithelial-myoepithelial carcinoma (EMC)
  classification systems for salivary gland tumors, 246–247, *247*
  molecular biology of salivary gland tumors, 271
  tumors of the minor salivary glands, 389, 417, *419–422*
epithelial tumors
  children and adolescents, 208–210
  non-salivary tumors of the salivary glands, 479, *482*
Epstein-Barr virus (EBV)
  non-salivary tumors of the salivary glands, 488
  systemic therapy for salivary gland cancer, 455
  tumors of the parotid gland, 302
erythema nodosum, 186
Escherichia coli, 86
external carotid artery (ECA), 8, 45

extracapsular dissection (ECD), 602–606
   extended ECD, 605–606, *605*
   malignant parotid tumors, 604–605, *605*
   tumors of the parotid gland, 320–321
   with extended option, 603–604, *604*
extracorporeal shock wave lithotripsy, 154–158, 160–162, 206, 614–615
extranodal extension (ENE), 255
extraparenchymal extension (EPE), 255–256
extravasation of fluid, 588, *588*

facial hemangioma, 150
facial nerve
   anatomy, embryology, and physiology, 4–5, *5–6*
   complications of salivary gland surgery, 570–573, *571–573*, **572**
   traumatic injury to the salivary glands, 515–522, *516–522*
   tumors of the parotid gland, 312–314, *314–315*, 320–324
facial transplantation surgery, 522
familial amyloid polyneuropathy (FAP), 558–559
fast neutron therapy, 330
fat grafting, 578
fibrous histiocytoma, 478–479
fine needle aspiration (FNA)
   diagnostic imaging, 35–36, *37*
   Küttner tumor, 561, *563*
   molecular biology of salivary gland tumors, 284–285
   non-salivary tumors of the salivary glands, 485, *497*
   sialadenitis, 104
   systemic therapy for salivary gland cancer, 462
   tumors of the minor salivary glands, 376
   tumors of the parotid gland, 303–308, *305*, *307*, 325, *326–327*, 331
   tumors of the submandibular and sublingual glands, *348*, *349*, *351*, *356*
first branchial cleft cyst, 56–57, *57–58*
fistulae
   complications of salivary gland surgery, 578–579, *579*
   hereditary and congenital conditions, 544–548, *547*, *549–553*
   traumatic injury to the salivary glands, 509–512, *510–511*
fluid attenuation inversion recovery (FLAIR), 28, *29*

fluoroscopy, *526*
fMRI *see* functional magnetic resonance imaging
FNA *see* fine needle aspiration
focal lymphocytic infiltration, 557
Frey syndrome
   complications of salivary gland surgery, 574–578, *575–578*, **576**
   diagnosis, 574
   management, 574–576, **576**
   surgical prevention, 576–578, *576–578*
   traumatic injury to the salivary glands, 522–524, *524*
functional magnetic resonance imaging (fMRI), 30

gadolinium contrast MRI, 28, *28*
Gardner's syndrome, 150, *153*
gene fusion proteins
   grading and staging of salivary gland tumors, 253–255
   molecular biology of salivary gland tumors, 281–282, *282*, 285–286, 288–290
   systemic therapy for salivary gland cancer, 456
   tumors of the parotid gland, 302, 334
generalized acinar atrophy, 557
genomics, 226, 548–550
glucose metabolism, 38, *39*
gout, 147, 166–168
gradient recalled echo (GRE) imaging, 26, *27*
gunshot wounds, *514–515*, *517–518*, *528*
gustatory sweating, 522–524, *524*, 574

H3N2 influenza, 107–108
HAART *see* highly active antiretroviral therapy
Haemophilus influenza, 97
hazard ratios, 226
HCCC *see* hyalinizing clear cell carcinoma
HCV *see* hepatitis C virus
Heerfordt syndrome, 186
hemangioendothelioma
   children and adolescents, 210–211, *210–211*
   non-salivary tumors of the salivary glands, 471–473, *472–474*
hemangioma
   children and adolescents, 210–211, *212*
   diagnostic imaging, 51–52, *51*
   non-salivary tumors of the salivary glands, 471–473, *472–474*
   sialolithiasis, 150

hematoma formation, 590
hepatitis C virus (HCV), 484
Her2 inhibition, 459–460, 462, 466
hereditary and congenital conditions, 543–548
   aberrant glands, 544–545
   amyloidosis, 558–559
   aplasia, 543–544
   children and adolescents, 201–202
   cystic fibrosis, 548
   diagnostic imaging, 56–57, *57–58*
   duct atresia, 544, *545*
   first branchial cleft cysts, fistulae, and sinuses, 545–548, *547, 549–553*
   polycystic disease of the salivary glands, 545, *546–547*
herpes labialis, 543
HGT *see* high-grade transformation
high-grade transformation (HGT), 389
highly active antiretroviral therapy (HAART), 130, *131–135*
hilar lymphadenopathy, 186
hilar stones, 615–616, *615*
histogenetic tumor classification, 271–274, *272–273*
HIV/AIDS
   cysts and cyst-like lesions, 127–130, *131–135*
   diagnostic imaging of HIV-associated lymphoepithelial lesions, 54, *54*
   non-salivary tumors of the salivary glands, 479, 484, *484*
   saliva, 554
   sialadenitis, 82, 105–107, *108*
   sialolithiasis, 148
   Sjögren syndrome, 180
   systemic therapy for salivary gland cancer, 455–456
Hodgkin lymphoma (HL)
   classification systems for salivary gland tumors, 252, *252*
   non-salivary tumors of the salivary glands, 479–483
   tumors of the parotid gland, 324–325
hollowing, 524, 576
hospital acquired parotitis, *84, 86,* 89
House–Brackmann scale, 466, 516, 521–522, 572–573, **572**, *573*
human papillomavirus (HPV), 456, 552–554
hyalinizing clear cell carcinoma (HCCC)
   classification systems for salivary gland tumors, 241
   grading and staging of salivary gland tumors, 254–255
   non-salivary tumors of the salivary glands, 495
   tumors of the minor salivary glands, 389
   tumors of the submandibular and sublingual glands, 345
hydroxyapatite, 146
hypermethylation, 283–284, 287
hyperparathyroidism, 147, 166–168
hypersalivation, 554–556
hypoglossal nerve injury, 589, *589*
hyposalivation, 590
   see also xerostomia

IFA *see* indirect fluorescent antibody
IFN *see* interferons
Ig *see* immunoglobulin
IHC *see* immunohistochemistry
immortalization, 279
immune checkpoint inhibition, 461
IgG4-related disease, 194–196
   case presentation, 196–199, *197–198*
   diagnosis with salivary gland biopsy, 194–195, *197–198*
   epidemiology and pathophysiology, 110–111, 195–196
   etiology and classification, 194–195, *195*
   Küttner tumor, 557–558
immunohistochemistry (IHC)
   classification systems for salivary gland tumors, 227, *249*
   molecular biology of salivary gland tumors, 274, 284–287
   non-salivary tumors of the salivary glands, 495–497, *497*
   tumors of the minor salivary glands, 423
IMRT *see* intensity-modulated radiation therapy
independent validation, 226
indirect fluorescent antibody (IFA), 102
infections of the salivary glands *see* sialadenitis
infiltrating lipoma, 478, *478*
influenza A, 107–108
innovations in salivary gland surgery, 601–624
   minimally invasive parotid gland surgery, 602–606, *604–605*
   minimally invasive sublingual gland surgery, 606–608
   minimally invasive surgery with sialendoscopy, 608–617, *609–616*

robotic-assisted procedures, 617
salivary duct strictures, 617–621, *619–620*
intensity-modulated radiation therapy (IMRT)
   advanced techniques, 449–451, *450*
   complications of radiation therapy, 445–446, *445*
   evolution of radiation techniques, 436, 442–444, *444*
   high-risk salivary gland malignancies, 441, *449*
   low- and moderate-risk salivary gland malignancies, 446–447
   non-salivary tumors of the salivary glands, 488
   saliva, 552
   traumatic injury to the salivary glands, 532
intercalated duct cells, 14
interferons (IFN), 176, 473
interventional sialendoscopy, 146, 149, 157–158, *158*
intracorporeal shock wave lithotripsy, 154, 157–158, 614, *614–615*
invasion, 280
ischemic/degenerative disease, 556–557, *557*

keratoconjunctivitis sicca, 175, 177
Küttner tumor, 557–558
   case presentations, 196–199, *197–198*, 561, *562–563*

laceration injury, 515, *516*, *520*, *526–527*
lacrimal glands
   hereditary and congenital conditions, 544
   Sjögren syndrome, 177
   tumors of the submandibular and sublingual glands, 369
lacrimal probes, 84–85, *84*
lacrimo-auriculo-dento-digital (LADD) syndrome, 544
large B-cell lymphoma, 483–486
large cell neuroendocrine carcinoma (LCNEC), 248–249, *248–249*
large T3/T4 tumors, 436, 438–439
laser lithotripsy, 613–614
LCNEC *see* large cell neuroendocrine carcinoma
leukemia, 202
Lewy type α-synucleinopathy (LTS), 560
LGCCC *see* low-grade cribriform cystadenocarcinoma
likelihood ratios, 226
lingual nerve injury, 585, *586*, 587, *588*, 589
Linnaean taxonomy, 226
lipoma

   diagnostic imaging, 61–62, *62*
   non-salivary tumors of the salivary glands, 476–478, *477–478*
lip tumors, 378–380, **378**, *397–398*, 409
Lofgren syndrome, 186
low-grade cribriform cystadenocarcinoma (LGCCC), 241–242, *241*, 254
LTS *see* Lewy type α-synucleinopathy
lymphadenopathy
   diagnostic imaging, 39, *40–41*
   non-salivary tumors of the salivary glands, 484
   tumors of the submandibular and sublingual glands, 347–348, *364*
lymphangioma
   children and adolescents, 211, *213*
   diagnostic imaging, 50–51, *50*
   non-salivary tumors of the salivary glands, 473–475, *475*
lymphatic malformations, 475
lymph nodes
   non-salivary tumors of the salivary glands, 479–497, *483–486*, *488–492*, *494–497*
   parotid gland, 8
   see also metastatic disease
lymphoepithelial carcinoma
   classification systems for salivary gland tumors, 249, *249*
   systemic therapy for salivary gland cancer, 455
   tumors of the parotid gland, 302
lymphoma
   classification systems for salivary gland tumors, 251–252, *251–252*
   diagnostic imaging, 64–65, *65–66*
   non-salivary tumors of the salivary glands, 479–486, *483–486*
   Sjögren syndrome, 177–180, *177–178*, 184–185
lympho-vascular space invasion, 437, 438–439
lysozyme amyloidosis, 559

magnetic resonance angiography (MRA), 52
magnetic resonance imaging (MRI)
   acute/chronic sialadenitis, 52, *53*
   bacterial sialadenitis in pregnancy, 108–110
   benign neoplasms, 57–60, 61–64, *63–64*
   children and adolescents, *219*, 220, *221*
   concepts and definitions, 24
   diffusion weighted imaging, 28–29, *29*
   dynamic contrast-enhanced imaging, 30

magnetic resonance imaging (MRI) (Cont'd)
  first branchial cleft cyst, 56–57, *57*
  fluid attenuation inversion recovery, 28, *29*
  gadolinium contrast, 28, *28*
  gradient recalled echo imaging, 26, *27*
  hereditary and congenital conditions, 544, *546–547*, *551*
  HIV-associated lymphoepithelial lesions, 54
  innovations in salivary gland surgery, 609, 617–618
  Küttner tumor, 561, *562*
  malignancies, 60, *61*, 67
  mucous escape reaction, 54
  non-salivary tumors of the salivary glands, 471–473, *473–474*, 475–478, *478*, *496*, 498–501, *500–501*
  other techniques, 30–31
  parotid gland, 42–45, *43–44*
  proton density images, 25
  sarcoidosis, 56
  short tau inversion recovery, 26–27, *27*, *44*, *50*
  sialadenosis/sialosis, 54–55
  sialography, 35
  sialolithiasis, 55
  Sjögren syndrome, 55–56
  spin-echo T1, 25, *25*, **26**, *43–44*, *46–47*, *51*, *53*, *64*
  spin-echo T2, 25, **26**, *27*, *47*, *51*, *57*, *63–64*
  sublingual gland, 48–49, *48*
  submandibular gland, 45–48, *46–47*
  technique, 24–31
  traumatic injury to the salivary glands, *513*
  tumors of the minor salivary glands, *399*, *427–428*
  tumors of the parotid gland, 304, *306*, *316*, *322–323*, 325, *331*, *336*
  tumors of the submandibular and sublingual glands, *349*, *350*, *351*, *359*, *360*, *362*, *366–368*
  vascular lesions, 50–52, *50–51*
magnetic resonance spectroscopy (MRS), 30
malignancies
  children and adolescents, 201–202, 207–218, **208**, *210–213*, *215–218*
  classification systems for salivary gland tumors, 225–228, **227**, 234–253, *234–244*, *246–253*, 259–261, *260–262*
  complications of salivary gland surgery, 593–596, *594–596*
  cysts and cyst-like lesions, 130–138, *136–138*, **136**
  diagnostic imaging, 28–30, 42, 49, 60, *60–62*, 64–67, *65–66*
  grading of malignant salivary gland tumors, **228**, 253–256, **257–259**
  innovations in salivary gland surgery, 604–605, *605*
  molecular biology of salivary gland tumors, 269–299
  non-salivary tumors of the salivary glands, 478–503, *480–481*, *483–486*, *488–492*, *494–497*, *499–504*
  radiation therapy for malignant tumors, 435–454
  Sjögren syndrome, 177–180, *177–178*, 184–185
  systemic therapy for salivary gland cancer, 455–469
  tumors of the minor salivary glands, 373–379, **375**, **377–378**, 385, 387–424, *391–399*, *401–408*, *410–416*, *418–422*, 425, *426–430*
  tumors of the parotid gland, 301–315, *303*, 325–337, *328–332*, *336*
  tumors of the submandibular and sublingual glands, 345–372
  see also individual neoplasms
malignant melanoma (MM), 479, *482*, 490–493, *492*, *494–495*
MALT *see* mucosa-associated lymphoid tissue
mammary analogue secretory carcinoma (MASC) *see* secretory carcinoma
mandibular hypoplasia, 544
mandibular osteoma, 150, *153*
mandibulo-stylohyoid ligament, 4, *4*
marginal mandibular branch injury, 588
marginal mandibular resection, 359, *363*
marginal zone B-cell lymphoma, 483–484
marsupialization, 122–124, *123–124*
MASC *see* mammary analogue secretory carcinoma
masseteric hypertrophy, 304
masticator space (MS), 45
matrix metalloproteinases (MMP), 176, 280
maxillectomy
  complications of salivary gland surgery, 593, 596
  tumors of the minor salivary glands, 378, 392–394, *393–394*, *413*
measles–mumps–rubella (MMR) vaccine, 105
MEC *see* mucoepidermoid carcinoma
megaduct, 582–583, *582*, 620–621
Merkel cell carcinoma, 253
mesenchymal tumors

benign mesenchymal tumors, 471–478, *472–478*
children and adolescents, 201, 210–214, *210–213*
classification systems for salivary gland tumors, 252–253, *252–253*
malignant mesenchymal tumors, 478–479, *480–481*
non-salivary tumors of the salivary glands, 471–479
messenger RNA (mRNA), 275, 283, 288
metabolic syndrome, 302
metastatic disease
    classification systems for salivary gland tumors, 245
    complications of salivary gland surgery, 593
    diagnostic imaging, 49, 65–67, *66*
    molecular biology of salivary gland tumors, 280, 287–288
    non-salivary tumors of the salivary glands, 479, 486–503, *488–492*, *494–497*, *499–504*
    radiation therapy for malignant tumors, 436, 441
    systemic therapy for salivary gland cancer, 457–458, **458**, **460**, 465
    tumors of the minor salivary glands, 385, 389–390, 399–400, 404–406, 408
    tumors of the submandibular and sublingual glands, 355–359, *356–357*, *364–365*
methicillin-resistant *Staphylococcus aureus* (MRSA), 86, 88, 111–114, *112–113*
methylenetetrahydrofolate reductase (MTHFR), 16
microforceps, 613
microRNA, 283–284, 287
Mikulicz disease, 178–180, *179–182*
minimally invasive surgery
    parotid gland surgery, 602–606, *604–605*
    sublingual gland surgery, 606–608
    with sialendoscopy, 608–617
minor salivary glands
    amyloidosis, 560
    anatomy, embryology, and physiology, 13
    children and adolescents, 214–218
    complications of salivary gland surgery, 590–591, *590–592*
    diagnostic imaging, 49
    radiation therapy for malignant tumors, 439
    sarcoidosis, 187, 192
    sialolithiasis, 147, 162, *166*
    Sjögren syndrome, 180, *181–182*, 183, 185
    systemic therapy for salivary gland cancer, 456–457

tumors of the minor salivary glands, 373–433
    case presentation, 425, *426–430*
    chemotherapy for malignant tumors, 424
    diagnosis, 376, **377**
    epidemiology, 373–374, **375**
    etiology, 374–376
    general principles of surgery, 376–378
    radiation therapy for malignant tumors, 423–424
    surgical management of the neck for malignant tumors, 423
    surgical treatment of benign tumors, 378–386, *380–388*
    surgical treatment of malignant tumors, 387–423, *391–399*, *401–408*, *410–416*, *418–422*, 425, *426–430*
    treatment, 376–424
mixed ranula, 584
mixed tumor, 245
MM *see* malignant melanoma
MMP *see* matrix metalloproteinases
MMR *see* measles–mumps–rubella
molecular biology of salivary gland tumors, 269–299
    cell biology of salivary gland tumors, 271–274, *272–273*
    challenges and potential solutions, 269–271, *270*
    diagnostic applications, 284–288, *286*
    enhanced cellular proliferation, 276–277, *278*
    epigenetic alteration of gene expression, 283–284, 287
    evasion of apoptosis, 277–279
    fundamental paradigms of tumor biology, 274–275, *275–276*
    histogenetic versus morphogenetic classification, 271–274, *272–273*
    immortalization, 279
    invasion and metastasis, 280
    neovascularization, 279–280
    nucleic acid dysregulation, 281–284, *282*
    protein dysregulation and neoplasm phenotypes, 275–280, *278*
    systemic therapy for salivary gland cancer, 456
    therapeutic applications, 288–290, *289*
molecular systematics, 226, 253–255
monoclonal antibodies
    EFGR inhibition, 459–461
    molecular biology of salivary gland tumors, 288
    Sjögren syndrome, 178

monoclonal antibodies (*Cont'd*)
  tumors of the minor salivary glands, 424
  tumors of the parotid gland, 330
morphogenetic tumor classification, 271–274, *272–273*
MRA *see* magnetic resonance angiography
MRI *see* magnetic resonance imaging
mRNA *see* messenger RNA
MRS *see* magnetic resonance spectroscopy
MRSA *see* methicillin-resistant *Staphylococcus aureus*
MS *see* masticator space
MTHFR *see* methylenetetrahydrofolate reductase
mTOR inhibitors, 475
mucoceles
  complications of salivary gland surgery, 590–591, *590–592*
  esthetic defects following removal, 591, *592*
  incidence and diagnosis, 119, *119*
  innovations in salivary gland surgery, 606–607
  neurosensory change following removal, 591, *592*
  recurrence, 590–591
  submandibular gland mucocele, 125–126, *126*
mucoepidermoid carcinoma (MEC)
  children and adolescents, 201–202, 209–210, 214–223, *221–222*
  classification systems for salivary gland tumors, 234–236, *234–235*
  diagnostic imaging, 60, *60–61*
  grading and staging of salivary gland tumors, 254
  molecular biology of salivary gland tumors, 280, 282–283, 285–287
  radiation therapy for malignant tumors, 436, 438–441, 446–447
  systemic therapy for salivary gland cancer, 456–457, 460
  tumors of the minor salivary glands, 388, 389–399, *391–399*, 424, 425, *426–430*
  tumors of the parotid gland, 301–302, 314–315, 325, *329–330*, 333–337, *336*
  tumors of the submandibular and sublingual glands, 345–346, 349, *350*, 359, *361*, *363–365*
mucosa-associated lymphoid tissue (MALT) lymphoma
  amyloidosis, 560
  classification systems for salivary gland tumors, 252
  diagnostic imaging, 64–65, *65–66*
  non-salivary tumors of the salivary glands, 483–486, *486*

  Sjögren syndrome, 178, 180
mucosal primary cancer, 486–488
mucous escape reaction, 117–127
  children and adolescents, 203
  clinical features and treatment, 118–127
  cyst of Blandin and Nuhn's gland, 127, *127*
  diagnostic imaging, 54
  mucoceles, 119, *119*, 125–126, *126*
  nomenclature and classification, 117–118
  ranula and plunging ranula, 119–125, *119–121, 123–125*, 139–142, *139–142*
  submandibular gland mucocele, 125–126, *126*
mucous extravasation phenomenon *see* ranulas
mucous retention cyst, 127, *128–129*
multi kinase inhibition, 460
mumps
  children and adolescents, 202
  differential diagnosis, 85
  etiology and pathophysiology, 105
  treatment, 105, *107*
musculoskeletal system
  diagnostic imaging, 38, *39*
  parotid gland, 2–4, *2–4*
mycobacterial adenitis, 150, *151*
myeloma, 559–560
mylohyoid hiatus, 121–122
myoepithelial carcinoma
  classification systems for salivary gland tumors, 249–250
  molecular biology of salivary gland tumors, 271–274, 282
  tumors of the minor salivary glands, 389
myoepithelial cells, 14
myoepithelioma, 232, *232*

necrotic ulceration, 303, *303*
necrotizing sialometaplasia, 556–557, *557*
neoplasms *see* benign neoplasms; malignancies
neovascularization, 279–280
nephrolithiasis, 147, 166–168
neurilemmoma, 475–476
neurofibroma, 214, *215–216*, 475–476, *476*
neurofibromatosis, 214, *215–216*, 475
neurogenic tumors, 63–64, *63–64*
neutron therapy, 451
NHL *see* non-Hodgkin lymphoma
non-epithelial neoplasms, **227**, 251–252, *251–252*
non-Hodgkin lymphoma (NHL)

non-salivary tumors of the salivary glands, 479–486, *483*, *485*
    Sjögren syndrome, 178
non-salivary tumors of the salivary glands, 471–508
    case presentation, 498–503, *499–504*
    epithelial non-salivary tumors, 479, *482*
    mesenchymal tumors, 471–479, *472–478*, *480–481*
    miscellaneous, 497
    primary lymph node tumors, 479–486, *483–486*
    secondary lymph node tumors, 486–497, *488–492*, *494–497*
nontuberculous mycobacterial disease, 104–105, *106*
NOTCH gene, 456
NTRK inhibition, 461
nuclear protein of the testis (NUT) carcinoma, 302
nucleic acid dysregulation, 281–284, *282*
NUT *see* nuclear protein of the testis
nutritional disturbances, 192–194, *193*

OAVS *see* oculo-auriculo-vertebral spectrum
obesity, 302
oculo-auriculo-vertebral spectrum (OAVS), 544–545
oncocytes, 557
oncocytic carcinoma, *242*, 243
oncocytoma
    classification systems for salivary gland tumors, 231, *231*
    diagnostic imaging, 60
    ischemic/degenerative disease, 557
oncogenes, 275, 283, 287–288
oncoproteins, 456
OPC *see* oropharyngeal cancer
oral hemangioma, 150
oropharyngeal cancer (OPC), 552
osteoradionecrosis
    radiation therapy for malignant tumors, 446, 451
    tumors of the parotid gland, 330, 333
osteotomy, 314, *316–318*
oxalate, 145

p53, 279, 281, 287
PA *see* pleomorphic adenoma
paediatrics *see* children and adolescents
palatal tumors, 378–380, **378**, 390–394, *391–396*, *401–403*, *407–408*, *409*, *410–414*, *425*, *426–430*
papillary cystadenoma lymphomatosum *see* Warthin tumor

parapharyngeal space (PPS), 45
parasympathetic nervous system
    control of salivation, 14–16
    parotid gland, 8–9, *9*
    submandibular gland, 12, *12*
Parkinson disease and Parkinsonism, 554–555, 560
parotidectomy
    children and adolescents, *204–205*, 207, *212*
    chronic bacterial parotitis, 89–90, *95–96*, 97
    complications of salivary gland surgery, 570–573, *571–573*, **572**, *576*, *578*, *581–582*
    hereditary and congenital conditions, 545, *549*, *553*
    innovations in salivary gland surgery, 602–606, *604–605*
    non-salivary tumors of the salivary glands, 479, *482*, 490–493, *492*, 497, *501*, *503*
    sialolithiasis, 159, *162*
    systemic therapy for salivary gland cancer, 462
    traumatic injury to the salivary glands, 514–515, 519–521, 523–524
    tumors of the parotid gland, 306–308, *307*, *313–315*, 314–324, *319–320*, *322*, *327*, *328–329*, *332*
parotid gland, 2–9
    amyloidosis, 560
    anatomical structures, 2–4, *2–4*
    auriculotemporal nerve, 5–6
    children and adolescents, 203, *204–207*, 206–207, 214
    complications of salivary gland surgery, 570–583
    contents, 4–9
    cysts and cyst-like lesions, 127–138, *131–138*, **136**
    diagnostic imaging, *31–34*, 42–45, *43–44*
    embryology, 2
    external carotid artery, 8
    facial nerve, 4–5, *5–6*
    hereditary and congenital conditions, 543–548, *546–547*
    innovations in salivary gland surgery, 602–606, *604–605*, 616–617, *616*
    lymph nodes, 8
    malignancies, 49
    nerve supply, 8–9, *9*
    non-salivary tumors of the salivary glands, *472*, 473, 475–485, *476–477*, *482*, *484–486*, *487–503*, *499–504*

parotid gland (Cont'd)
  parotid duct, 8, *8*
  radiation therapy for malignant tumors, 437–438
  retromandibular vein, 6, *7*
  saliva, 555
  sarcoidosis, 186–187, *187–190*
  sialadenitis, 79, *80*
  sialolithiasis, 147–150, **147**, 159–162, *159–165*
  sialosis, 192–193, *193*
  Sjögren syndrome, 177–180, *179–185*, 183–185
  systemic therapy for salivary gland cancer, 456, 461–466, *463–465*
  traumatic injury to the salivary glands, 509–510, 512–515, *514–515*, 522–524, *531*
  tumors of the parotid gland, 301–343
    benign neoplasms, 301–304, *307*, 308, *309–313*, 315–325, *316*, *322–324*, *326–327*
    case presentation, 335–337, *336*
    diagnosis, 303–308, *303*, *305–307*
    etiology and epidemiology, 301–303
    malignancies, 301–315, *303*, 325–337, *328–332*, *336*
    surgical management, 308–335, *309–320*, *322–324*, *326–332*
  see also individual disorders
partial superficial parotidectomy, 602–603
PCR *see* polymerase chain reaction
PD *see* proton density
penetrating injuries, 509–529
  facial nerve injuries, 515–522, *516–522*
  Frey syndrome, 522–524, *524*
  hollowing, 524
  management algorithm, *534*
  salivary fistula, 509–512, *510–511*
  sialocele, 512–515, *512–515*
  stricture of the salivary duct, 529, *530*
  transection of the salivary duct, 524–529, *525–529*
perineural invasion
  non-salivary tumors of the salivary glands, 490
  radiation therapy for malignant tumors, 437, 438–439
  tumors of the minor salivary glands, 408
PET *see* positron emission tomography
phleboliths, 150, *152*
pilocarpine, 532–533
planning target volume (PTV), 442
platelet-rich plasma (PRP), 516
pleomorphic adenoma (PA)
  children and adolescents, 201–202, 208–209, 214, 218, *219*
  classification systems for salivary gland tumors, 228, *229*
  complications of salivary gland surgery, 593–596, *594–596*
  diagnostic imaging, 57–59, *58–59*
  grading and staging of salivary gland tumors, 254
  molecular biology of salivary gland tumors, *270*, 279, 282–283, 285
  radiation therapy for malignant tumors, 436
  tumors of the minor salivary glands, 378–385, *380–385*
  tumors of the parotid gland, 301–302, 304, *307*, 308, *309–313*, 315–324, *316*, *320–324*
  tumors of the submandibular and sublingual glands, 345–346, *349*, 351–353, *352–357*
plexiform neurofibroma, 475
plunging ranula *see* ranula and plunging ranula
PMAC *see* polymorphous adenocarcinoma
polycystic disease of the salivary glands, 545, *546–547*
polymerase chain reaction (PCR), 552–554
polymorphous adenocarcinoma (PMAC)
  classification systems for salivary gland tumors, 237–239, *238*
  complications of salivary gland surgery, 593–596, *594–596*
  grading and staging of salivary gland tumors, 255
  molecular biology of salivary gland tumors, 271
  non-salivary tumors of the salivary glands, 498–503, *499–504*
  tumors of the minor salivary glands, 389, 406–414, *408*, *410–416*
  tumors of the parotid gland, 302–303
  tumors of the submandibular and sublingual glands, 345, *351*, 359
poorly differentiated adenocarcinoma, 462
poorly differentiated carcinoma
  classification systems for salivary gland tumors, 247–248, *247*
  radiation therapy for malignant tumors, 436, 439–440
  tumors of the parotid gland, 302, *303*, 325
PORT *see* postoperative radiation therapy
positron emission tomography (PET)
  advanced techniques, 42
  benign neoplasms, 59, *59*

children and adolescents, 220, *221*
malignancies, 64–67, *65–66*
non-salivary tumors of the salivary glands, *489*
radionuclides, 38–39
standardized uptake values, 39–41, *41*, **42**
sublingual gland, 48–49, *49*
submandibular gland, 45–48, *47*
systemic therapy for salivary gland cancer, *463*
technique and clinical application, 36–41, *39–41*
tubarial salivary glands, 13
tumors of the parotid gland, 304, 325
postoperative radiation therapy (PORT)
   high-risk malignancies, 441
   low-risk malignancies, 437
   moderate-risk malignancies, 439
   traumatic injury to the salivary glands, 522, 532
   tumors of the minor salivary glands, 400
   tumors of the parotid gland, 324, 327–330, 333–335
   tumors of the submandibular and sublingual glands, 355–358, 360, 369
PPS *see* parapharyngeal space
pRb downregulation, 277, *278*
pregnancy, 108–110, *109*
propranolol, 473
prostate-specific membrane antigen (PSMA), 13, 534
proteasome inhibition, 460
protein dysregulation, 275–280, *278*
proteomics, 226, 285
proton density (PD) imaging, 25
proton therapy, 449–451, *450*
PRP *see* platelet-rich plasma
pseudocapsule, 379
pseudocyst, 123–125, *123–124*
Pseudomonas spp., 86
pseudopodia, 351
PSMA *see* prostate-specific membrane antigen
PTV *see* planning target volume

radiation exposure
   systemic therapy for salivary gland cancer, 455
   tumors of the minor salivary glands, 374–375
   tumors of the parotid gland, 301
radiation therapy
   advanced techniques, 449–451, *450*
   carbon ion therapy, 451
   complications of radiation therapy, 445–446, *445*
   complications of salivary gland surgery, 581
   concepts and definitions, 435–436
   diagnostic imaging, 39–41
   evolution of radiation techniques, 442–444, *442–444*
   high-risk malignancies, 436, *436–437*, 440–441, 447–449, *447*, *449*
   low-risk malignancies, 436–438, *436–437*, 446–447
   malignant tumors, 435–454
   moderate-risk malignancies, 436, *436–437*, 438–439, *440*, 446–447
   molecular biology of salivary gland tumors, 274
   neutron therapy, 451
   non-salivary tumors of the salivary glands, 479, 485, 488
   proton therapy, 449–451, *450*
   saliva, 552, 555
   technique for high-risk tumors, 447–449, *447*, *449*
   technique for low-/moderate-risk tumors, 446–447
   traumatic injury to the salivary glands, 522, 530–534, *531*
   tumors of the minor salivary glands, 374, 400, 409–414, 423–424
   tumors of the parotid gland, 301, 324, 327–330, 333–335
   tumors of the submandibular and sublingual glands, 355–358, 360, 369
radioactive iodine, 533–534
radiography
   children and adolescents, *211*
   complications of salivary gland surgery, *572*
   innovations in salivary gland surgery, 613
   sarcoidosis, *187*
   sialadenitis, *81*, *83*, *85*, 88–89, *100*
   sialolithiasis, *147–149*, 150, *151–153*, *156*, *160*, *163*, *169*
   traumatic injury to the salivary glands, *514–515*
   tumors of the minor salivary glands, *399*, *419–420*
radionuclide imaging (RNI), 36
ranula and plunging ranula
   complications of salivary gland surgery, 584–586, *584–586*
   hereditary and congenital conditions, 544
   innovations in salivary gland surgery, 606–608, 613
   lingual nerve injury, 585
   mucous escape reaction, 119–125, *119–121*, *123–125*, 139–142, *139–142*
   recurrence, 585

ranula and plunging ranula (*Cont'd*)
  submandibular duct injury, 585–586, 588
  tumors of the submandibular and sublingual glands, 347–348
RES *see* reticuloendothelial system
respiratory symptoms, 186, *187*
reticuloendothelial system (RES), 31
retromandibular incision, 571–572, *572*
retromandibular vein (RMV)
  anatomy, embryology, and physiology, 6, *7*
  diagnostic imaging of salivary gland pathology, 45
  tumors of the parotid gland, 304, *313*
rhabdomyosarcoma, 478–479, 493
rheumatoid arthritis, 186
rhinorrhea, 512
RMV *see* retromandibular vein
RNA interference (RNAi) targeting, 290
RNI *see* radionuclide imaging
robotic surgery, 355, 617

saliva, 548–556
  control of salivation, 14–16
  diagnostic applications, 548–554
  drooling, 554–556
  hypersalivation, 554–556
  hyposalivation, 590
  management of xerophthalmia, 556
  see also xerostomia
salivary carcinosarcoma, 245
salivary duct carcinoma (SDC)
  classification systems for salivary gland tumors, 243–244, *243*
  grading and staging of salivary gland tumors, 254
  molecular biology of salivary gland tumors, 271, 282
  radiation therapy for malignant tumors, 436, 440–441
  systemic therapy for salivary gland cancer, 460–461
salivary gland ducts
  anatomy, embryology, and physiology, 8, *8*, 11–12
  complications of salivary gland surgery, 570, *570*, 581–583, *581–583*, 585–587, *587*
  hereditary and congenital conditions, 544, *545*
  innovations in salivary gland surgery, 608, 617–621, *619–620*
  traumatic injury to the salivary glands, 524–529, *525–530*

  see also Stensen duct; Wharton duct
salivary gland tumors *see* benign neoplasms; malignancies
salivary leakage
  classification, 579
  management, 579–583
  parotid duct, 581–583, *581–583*
  parotid gland, 578–581, *579*
  postoperative infections, 581
sarcoidosis, 185–192
  children and adolescents, 203
  clinical manifestations, 186–187, *187–190*
  diagnosis with salivary gland biopsy, 187–192, *191–192*
  diagnostic imaging, 56
  extraglandular findings, 185, **185**
  minor salivary glands, 187, 192
  pathophysiology, 186
sarcoid-related sialadenitis, 110
sarcoma, 478–479, *480–481*
scanning electron microscopy (SEM), 146
SCC *see* squamous cell carcinoma
scintigraphy, 64–65
sclerosing agents
  children and adolescents, 211
  complications of salivary gland surgery, 580
  non-salivary tumors of the salivary glands, 475
sclerosing polycystic adenoma, 233–234, *233*
SCM *see* sternocleidomastoid muscle
SCNEC *see* small cell neuroendocrine carcinoma
scopolamine, 580
scrofula *see* mycobacterial adenitis
SDC *see* salivary duct carcinoma
sebaceous adenocarcinoma, 242, *242*
sebaceous adenoma, *231*, 232
sebaceous lymphadenocarcinoma, 242–243
sebaceous lymphadenoma, 232
secretory carcinoma
  case presentation, 259–261, *260–262*
  classification systems for salivary gland tumors, 250–251, *250*
  grading and staging of salivary gland tumors, 255
  molecular biology of salivary gland tumors, 285
  systemic therapy for salivary gland cancer, 456
  tumors of the minor salivary glands, 417, 423
  tumors of the parotid gland, 334
  tumors of the submandibular and sublingual glands, 345

SEM *see* scanning electron microscopy
sensory innervation, 12–13
serous cells, 14
shock wave lithotripsy, 154–158, 160–162, 206, 614–615, *614–615*
short tau inversion recovery (STIR), 26–27, *27*, *44*, *50*
shotgun wounds, 510, *511*, 522
sialadenectomy
  complications of salivary gland surgery, 586, *586*, 588–590
  innovations in salivary gland surgery, 608–609
sialadenitis, 79–115
  acute bacterial parotitis, 82, *83–84*, 85–89, *87–88*, *90–91*, 111–114, *112–113*
  acute bacterial submandibular sialadenitis, 98–99, *98–99*
  autoimmune sialadenitis and IgG4-related disease, 110–111
  bacterial sialadenitis in pregnancy, 108–110, *109*
  case presentation, 111–114, *112–113*
  cat-scratch disease, 99–102, *103–104*
  children and adolescents, 203–207, *204–207*
  chronic bacterial parotitis, 89–97, *91–96*
  chronic recurrent juvenile parotitis, 97–98
  chronic recurrent submandibular sialadenitis, 99, *100–102*
  classification, **81**
  complications of salivary gland surgery, *570*
  diagnostic imaging, 52, *52–53*
  HIV/AIDS, 82, 105–107, *108*
  influenza A, 107–108
  introduction and general considerations, 79–85
  Küttner tumor, 557–558
  mumps, 85, 105
  nontuberculous mycobacterial disease, 104–105, *106*
  risk factors, 79–85, **81–82**
  sialolithiasis, 145, 146, 148–149
  tuberculous mycobacterial disease, 102–104
  tumors of the submandibular and sublingual glands, 346
sialadenoma papilliferum (SP), 233, *233*
sialadenosis *see* sialosis
sialendoscopy and sialography
  basket retrieval of stones, 610–613, *611–613*
  children and adolescents, 206–207
  chronic bacterial parotitis, 89, *92–94*
  chronic recurrent juvenile parotitis, 97

chronic recurrent submandibular sialadenitis, 99
clinical indications, 32, *33*
combined open and endoscopic stone removal, 616–617, *616*
complications of salivary gland surgery, *570*, 581–583, *581–582*, 586–587, *587*
concepts and definitions, 32
fragmentation of stones, 613–615, *614–615*
imaging modalities for sialolithiasis, 609, *609–610*
intraoral stone release, 615–616, *615*
minimally invasive surgery, 608–617
salivary duct strictures, 617–621, *619–620*
sialolithiasis, 146, 149, 157–158, *158*
technique and equipment, 33–35, 609–610, *610–611*
traumatic injury to the salivary glands, 515, 529, *530*, 533–534
sialoblastoma, 245–246
sialoceles
  complications of salivary gland surgery, 578–579, *579*
  traumatic injury to the salivary glands, 512–515, *512–515*
sialodochoplasty
  complications of salivary gland surgery, *583*, 588, *589*
  hereditary and congenital conditions, *545*
  sialolithiasis, 152–153, *165*
  traumatic injury to the salivary glands, 529, *529*
sialolithiasis, 145–174
  case presentation, 168–172, *169–172*
  children and adolescents, 203–206
  clinical features, 147–149, *147–149*
  complications of salivary gland surgery, 578–579, *579*, 586, *588–589*
  composition of saliva, 146, **147**
  diagnosis and differential diagnosis, 150, *151–153*
  diagnostic imaging, 55, *55*
  etiology and epidemiology, 145
  innovations in salivary gland surgery, 608–609, *609*
  multiple and bilateral sialoliths, 149–150, 162, *164–165*
  nephrolithiasis, cholelithiasis, primary hyperparathyroidism, and gout, 147, 166–168
  parotid sialolithiasis, 147–150, **147**, 159–162, *159–165*
  pathophysiology, 145–146, **147**
  sialadenitis, 145, 146, 148–149

sialolithiasis (Cont'd)
    sublingual and minor salivary gland sialolithiasis, 147, 162, *166*
    submandibular sialolithiasis, 146–150, *147–149*, **147**, 152–158, *154–158*, *164–165*, 168–172, *169–172*
    treatment, 150–162
    tumors of the submandibular and sublingual glands, 346
sialolithotomy, 152, 160
sialosis, 192–194
    clinical manifestations, 193
    diagnosis with salivary gland biopsy, 193–194, *194*
    diagnostic imaging of salivary gland pathology, 54–55
    etiology and classification, 192–193, **192**
Sicca syndrome, 560
single photon emission computed tomography (SPECT), 46
sinuses, 545–548, *547*, *549–553*
Sjögren syndrome, 175–185
    amyloidosis, 560
    children and adolescents, 203
    clinical manifestations, 176–177, *177*
    complications of salivary gland surgery, 587
    diagnosis with salivary gland biopsy, 180–185, *183–185*
    diagnostic imaging, 34–35, *34*, 55–56, 64
    epidemiology, 175–176
    extraglandular findings, 175, **176**
    lymphoma, 177–180, *177–178*, 184–185
    Mikulicz disease, 178–180, *179–182*
    minor salivary glands, 180, *181–182*, 183, 185
    non-salivary tumors of the salivary glands, 483–485
    pathophysiology, 176
    sialadenitis, 110–111
skin cancers, 479, *482*, 486–493, *488–492*
SLE *see* systemic lupus erythematosus
small B-cell lymphoma, *252*
small cell neuroendocrine carcinoma (SCNEC), 248, 493–495, *496–497*
SMAS *see* superficial musculoaponeurotic system
smoking
    systemic therapy for salivary gland cancer, 456, 462
    tumors of the parotid gland, 302
SP *see* sialadenoma papilliferum
SPECT *see* single photon emission computed tomography

spindle cell tumor, *252–253*
spin-echo T1 MRI, 25, *25*, **26**, *43–44*, *46–47*, *51*, *53*, *64*
spin-echo T2 MRI, 25, **26**, *27*, *47*, *51*, *57*, *63–64*
squamous cell carcinoma (SCC)
    classification systems for salivary gland tumors, 246, *246*
    molecular biology of salivary gland tumors, 269
    non-salivary tumors of the salivary glands, 479, *482*, 486–493, *488–492*
    radiation therapy for malignant tumors, 436, 437, 440
    saliva, 550, 554
    tumors of the parotid gland, 302
standardized uptake values (SUV), 39–41, *41*, **42**, 63–64
Staphylococcus spp., 86, 206
stenosis
    innovations in salivary gland surgery, 619–621
    parotid duct orifice, 583
Stensen duct
    complications of salivary gland surgery, 583
    sialadenitis, 82, *84*, 85, 97, 111–114, *112–113*
    sialolithiasis, 147, *148*, 160, *160–161*
    traumatic injury to the salivary glands, 524–525, *526–527*, 530
sternocleidomastoid muscle (SCM)
    complications of salivary gland surgery, 577, 578
    diagnostic imaging, 44–45
    tumors of the parotid gland, 308–312
STIR *see* short tau inversion recovery
Streptococcus spp., 86, 97, 146, 206
stricture formation
    classification of salivary duct strictures, 618
    complications of salivary gland surgery, 586–587, *587*
    dilatation techniques, 618–619, *619–620*
    imaging modalities, 617–618
    innovations in salivary gland surgery, 617–621
    treatment and outcomes, 618–621, *619–620*
stroke, *518*
stylomandibular ligament, 4–5, *4*
sublingual gland
    anatomy, embryology, and physiology, 13
    complications of salivary gland surgery, 583–588
    cysts and cyst-like lesions, 121–125, *123–124*
    diagnostic imaging, 48–49, *48–49*
    innovations in salivary gland surgery, 606–608

non-salivary tumors of the salivary glands, *483*, 487–488
saliva, 555–556
sialolithiasis, 147, 162, *166*
Sjögren syndrome, 177
systemic therapy for salivary gland cancer, 456
tumors of the sublingual glands, 345–372
    case presentation, 365–370, *366–368*
    diagnosis, **347**, 350–351, *351*
    epidemiology and etiology, 345–346
    management, 359–363, *359–365*
submandibular gland, 9–13
  agenesis, 16–17, *17*
  amyloidosis, 560
  anatomical structures, 10–13, *10–12*
  blood supply and lymphatic drainage, 12
  children and adolescents, 203–206, *205*, 214
  complications of salivary gland surgery, 570, *570*, 583–590
  cysts and cyst-like lesions, 125–126, *126*
  deep lobe, 11, *12*
  diagnostic imaging, *31*, *33*, 45–48, *46–47*
  embryology, 9–10
  hereditary and congenital conditions, 544–545
  IgG4-related disease, 196–199, *197–198*
  innovations in salivary gland surgery, 608, 615–616, *615*
  nerve supply, 12–13, *12*
  non-salivary tumors of the salivary glands, 478–479, *478*, 483, 487
  radiation therapy for malignant tumors, 439
  saliva, 555–556
  sarcoidosis, 186–187, *191*
  sialadenitis, 79, *81*
  sialolithiasis, 146–150, *147–149*, **147**, 152–158, *154–158*, *164–165*, 168–172, *169–172*
  Sjögren syndrome, 177
  submandibular duct, 11–12
  superficial lobe, 11, *11*
  systemic therapy for salivary gland cancer, 456
  traumatic injury to the salivary glands, 510–512, 529, 531, *531*, 533
  tumors of the submandibular glands, 345–372
    case presentation, 365–370, *366–368*
    diagnosis, 346–349, *347–350*
    epidemiology and etiology, 345–346
    management, 351–359, *352–357*

see also individual disorders
superficial lobe
  anatomy, embryology, and physiology, 11, *11*
  tumor, *315*, *328–329*
superficial musculoaponeurotic system (SMAS), 2–3, 308, 523–524, 577, *577*, 578
suppurative parotitis, 111–114, *112–113*
  children and adolescents, 206, *206*
sural nerve graft, 517–519, *522*
SUV *see* standardized uptake values
sympathetic nervous system, 12, 14–16
synovial cell carcinoma, 480–481
syringoma, 488, *488*
systemic lupus erythematosus (SLE), 110
systemic therapy *see* chemotherapy

TB *see* tuberculosis
tear flow tests, 177
temporalis fascia, 581
temporoparietal flap (TPF), 523–524, 576, 578
three-dimensional conformal radiation therapy (3D-CRT), 442–443, *443*
tissue inhibitors of matrix metalloproteinases (TIMP), 176, 280
TNM staging, 255–256, **257–259**
tongue tumors, 379, *404–406*, 487–488
TPF *see* temporoparietal flap
traumatic injury to the salivary glands, 509–541
  barotrauma, 534–535
  blunt trauma, *535*
  penetrating injuries, 509–529
    facial nerve injuries, 515–522, *516–522*
    Frey syndrome, 522–524, *524*
    hollowing, 524
    management algorithm, *534*
    salivary fistula, 509–512, *510–511*
    sialocele, 512–515, *512–515*
    stricture of the salivary duct, 529, *530*
    transection of the salivary duct, 524–529, *525–529*
  radiation injury, 530–534, *531*
trumpet blower's syndrome, 82
tubarial salivary glands, 13–14
tuberculosis (TB), 102–104
tumorigenesis, 271, 275, 283, 288
tumor initiation cell theory, 274
tumors *see* benign neoplasms; malignancies
tumor suppressor genes, 271, 275, 283

tympanic neurectomy, 580–581
tyrosine kinase inhibitors, 285, 288–290

ulceration, 376
ultrasonography (US)
   concepts and definitions, 31–32, *31–32*
   hereditary and congenital conditions, 544
   image-guided biopsies, 35–36, *37*
   innovations in salivary gland surgery, 609, *609*, 617
   Küttner tumor, 561, *562*
   non-salivary tumors of the salivary glands, 471–473
   sarcoidosis, 56
   technique, 32
   tumors of the parotid gland, 304
   tumors of the submandibular and sublingual glands, 349, *350*
undifferentiated carcinoma
   classification systems for salivary gland tumors, 248–249, *248–249*
   molecular biology of salivary gland tumors, 274
   radiation therapy for malignant tumors, 436, 440
   tumors of the parotid gland, 325
uric acid, 147, 166–168
US *see* ultrasonography

vaccination, 105
vascular endothelial growth factor (VEGF), 279–280
vascular lesions
   diagnostic imaging, 50–52, *50–51*
   non-salivary tumors of the salivary glands, 473
vascular malformation
   non-salivary tumors of the salivary glands, 473
   tumors of the submandibular and sublingual glands, 347–348
vascular tumors, 210–211, *210–212*

VEGF *see* vascular endothelial growth factor
volumetric modulated arch therapy (VMAT), 442–447, *444*, 449–451
Warthin tumor
   children and adolescents, 209–210
   classification systems for salivary gland tumors, 230, *230*
   diagnostic imaging, 59, *59*, 68, *68–74*
   systemic therapy for salivary gland cancer, 456
   tumors of the parotid gland, 302, *305*, 324–325, *326–327*
Wharton duct
   complications of salivary gland surgery, *584*
   cysts and cyst-like lesions, 122, *123–124*
   hereditary and congenital conditions, 544, *545*
   innovations in salivary gland surgery, 620
   sialadenitis, 85, 98
   sialolithiasis, 146, 152, *155*, 164–166
   traumatic injury to the salivary glands, 529, *529*
   tumors of the submandibular and sublingual glands, 355
Wnt/β-catenin pathway, 277
World Health Organization (WHO), **227**

xerophthalmia, 556
xerostomia
   hereditary and congenital conditions, 543–544, 550–554, 556
   IgG4-related disease, 196
   radiation therapy for malignant tumors, 445–446, *445*
   sialolithiasis, 172
   Sjögren syndrome, 175–177
   traumatic injury to the salivary glands, 532–534
X-ray diffraction analysis (EDX), 146